FOUNDATIONS OF NORMAL AND THERAPEUTIC NUTRITION

SECOND EDITION

T. Randall Lankford, M.S.

Professor of Biology
Department of Math and Science
Galveston Community College
Galveston, Texas

Contributing Author:

Paula Verry Gribble, R.N., B.S.N., M.S.

Chair Nursing and Allied Health
Coastal Carolina Community College
Jacksonville, North Carolina

D1529801

Delmar Publishers Inc.™
I(T)P™

NOTICE TO THE READER

Publisher does not warrant or guarantee any of the products described herein or perform any independent analysis in connection with any of the product information contained herein. Publisher does not assume, and expressly disclaims, any obligation to obtain and include information other than that provided to it by the manufacturer.

The reader is expressly warned to consider and adopt all safety precautions that might be indicated by the activities described herein and to avoid all potential hazards. By following the instructions contained herein, the reader willingly assumes all risks in connection with such instructions.

The publisher makes no representations or warranties of any kind, including but not limited to, the warranties of fitness for particular purpose or merchantability, nor are any such representations implied with respect to the material set forth herein, and the publisher takes no responsibility with respect to such material. The publisher shall not be liable for any special, consequential or exemplary damages resulting, in whole or in part, from the readers' use of, or reliance upon, this material.

Cover design: Paul Koziarz, Precision Graphics

Delmar staff:
Publisher: David C. Gordon
Administrative Editor: Patricia Casey
Developmental Editor: Marjorie A. Bruce
Project Editor: Danya M. Plotsky
Production Coordinator: Jennifer Gaines
Art and Design Coordinator: Mary E. Siener

For information, address

Delmar Publishers, Inc.
3 Columbia Circle, Box 15015
Albany, NY 12212-5015

COPYRIGHT © 1994 BY DELMAR PUBLISHERS INC.™

The trademark ITP is used under license.

All rights reserved. Certain portions of this work © 1986. No part of this work covered by the copyright hereon may be reproduced or used in any form, or by any means—graphic, electronic, or mechanical, including photocopying, recording, taping, or information storage and retrieval systems—without written permission of the publisher.

Printed in the United States of America
Published simultaneously in Canada
by Nelson Canada,
a division of The Thomson Corporation

2 3 4 5 6 7 8 9 10 XXX 00 99 98 97 96 95 94

Library of Congress Cataloging-in-Publication Data

Lankford, T. Randall, 1942-
     Foundations of normal and therapeutic nutrition / T. Randall
Lankford ; contributing author, Paula Verry Gribble. — 2nd ed.
          p.   cm.
     Previously published: 1986.
     Includes bibliographical references and index.
     ISBN 0-8273-5268-9
     1. Diet therapy. 2. Nutrition. I. Gribble, Paula Verry.
II. Title
RM216.L26 1993
615.8'54—dc20   93-35725
                                                    CIP

To my parents for their encouragement

To my wife, Billie Jo, whose sacrifices and support made completion of this text possible

To my sons, Christopher and Nicholas, whose nutritional state, I hope, will always be optimal

T.R.L.

PREFACE

INTRODUCTION

Nutrition is a complex, dynamic field in which new information is disclosed daily. The application of nutritional principles by health professionals is essential in preventing disease, protecting the general health and well-being of the public, diagnosing diseases, and minimizing complications of illnesses. To accomplish these goals health professionals need a sound nutritional background. This includes a knowledge of the chemical principles of nutrients, the ability to integrate nutritional concepts to the functioning of the organ systems, and the application of this information to clinical situations.

PURPOSE OF TEXT

Foundations of Normal and Therapeutic Nutrition, second edition, is written for students in nursing, nutrition, and allied health programs. The primary goal is to present the study of normal and therapeutic nutrition in as clear and informative a manner as possible to encourage maximum retention of the material by students and help them to apply the concepts effectively to daily practice. With this purpose in mind, the text is organized to show the relationship of basic science principles (chemistry and anatomy and physiology) to nutrition and to give students the opportunity to measure their progress in learning the material. This goal is achieved in the following ways.

First, the text provides students with a thorough introduction to the chemical principles of nutrients. These principles are of primary importance to health professionals. The material is presented with the assumption that the student has *no* prior chemistry background. Many explanatory figures are provided to help students learn these concepts.

Second, the text helps students relate the chemical principles of nutrients to the normal and abnormal functions of the organ systems. The clinical applications in Part I are unique tools that integrate chemistry with nutritional therapy examples and are designed to attract and increase student interest.

Third, students learn how to apply nutritional concepts to clinical situations. The normal functioning of various body systems is discussed first. Then, diseases and disorders that can affect these systems are explained together •with the role therapeutic diets play in patient recovery. Thus, a logical cause-and-effect relationship is established so that students can see the association between illness and therapeutic nutrition. In particular, the case studies in each of the therapeutic chapters reinforce the concepts learned earlier in the text and help students apply the principles to actual clinical situations.

ORGANIZATION

The text is divided into three parts: Principles of Nutrition, Nutrition Throughout the Life Cycle, and Therapeutic Nutrition. Part I discusses dietary planning (including food guides and RDAs), the food exchange system, and the six basic nutrients (carbohydrates, lipids, proteins, vitamins, minerals, and water).

Part II discusses the measurement of and types of energy; causes and treatment of obesity, underweight, anorexia nervosa, bulimia, and bulimamexia; and presents nutritional requirements for the different phases of the life cycle from pregnancy through the elder years.

In Part III, Chapter 13 presents the steps in the clinical process (assessment, planning, implementation, and evaluation) and how they are applied to the nutritional care of the patient. A separate chapter (14) is presented on enteral-parenteral nutrition due to the importance of the topic. Chapters 15 through 20 discuss diseases and disorders of organ systems and the use of therapeutic nutrition in alleviating the symptoms of these illnesses. Chapters 21 and 22 contain material on diet and cancer prevention, diet therapy for cancer patients, and pre- and postoperative nutrition. Throughout these chapters, sample menus of therapeutic diets with analysis and comments are provided.

The organizational format of the text includes numerous, well-designed pedagogical aids. These aids include the following:

- *Objectives.* Objectives appear at the beginning of each chapter to identify important concepts for students and to assist instructors in planning and organizing lectures.
- *Definition of terms.* Important terms and definitions are placed in the margin next to the first usage of the term in the text.
- *Chapter summaries.* Bulleted reviews of each chapter are included to aid students in preparing for tests and for quick reference. They are also helpful to instructors as a source of lecture information. Detailed outlines of chapters are provided in the Instructor's Guide.

- *Chapter review questions.* True-false, multiple-choice (answers are given in the Appendix of the text for both types of questions), and discussion questions are given at the end of each chapter.
- *Critical thinking challenge questions.* Questions are given at the end of the chapter to challenge students to develop their problem-solving skills. Answers and explanations for these questions are provided in the Instructor's Guide.
- *NCLEX-RN style questions.* Questions simulating those on the NCLEX-RN examination are provided at the end of each chapter with answers in the Appendix of the text.
- *Clinical applications.* These applications in Part I help students apply nutritional concepts to the clinical setting.
- *Case studies.* Case studies are provided at the end of Chapters 15–22 to facilitate application of therapeutic nutrition in clinical setting. The case study format includes a general description of a clinical disorder, relevant data (laboratory, anthropometric and pharmacology with normal values given in parentheses), and objective questions. The questions help students analyze the data and integrate information from previous chapters. Answers to the case study questions are provided in the Instructor's Guide.
- *Explanatory figures.* Many of the figures in the text are designed to explain certain difficult concepts or a series of interrelated changes.
- *Glossary.* The end-of-book glossary presents a comprehensive summary of the important terms that appear in boldface type in the text and are defined in the margin.
- *Appendixes.* The Appendixes provide valuable reference material with easy access.

CHANGES FOR THE SECOND EDITION

- Addition of NCLEX-RN style questions to familiarize students with the format of examination questions
- Critical Thinking Challenge Questions to promote the development of problem-solving skills
- Bulleted chapter end summary to highlight important concepts; format is more conducive to ready reference than previous detailed summary
- All nutritional data updated as necessary using the latest references from the National Academy of Science, National Research Council, Food and Nutrition Board, and U. S. Department of Agriculture
- Nursing content enhanced through case studies, clinical applications, and NCLEX-RN style questions for each chapter
- Revised menus to include nutritional values reflecting current guidelines/data from regulatory agencies

- Updated chapter references
- Topics for which content was revised and/or added include the food pyramid, commercial food labeling for foods regulated by Food and Drug Administration, dietary fiber, digestion of carbohydrates, artificial fats, omega-3 and omega-6 fatty acids, digestion of proteins, selenium as a trace mineral, energy expenditure and REE (resting energy expenditure), calculating total energy requirements, suggested weights for adults in relation to body composition, nutritional requirements for the elderly, treatment and prevention of elevated cholesterol, and diet and cancer prevention

SUMMARY

The approach used in this text to present normal and therapeutic nutrition is an instructive and interactive one. By becoming familiar with the concepts and examples provided, students will gain the knowledge and confidence to plan and implement effective nutritional care for their clients.

T. Randall Lankford

ACKNOWLEDGMENTS

The author wishes to thank Paula Gribble for her contributions to the second edition of the text. Ms. Gribble critiqued and reworked content within the case studies, the critical thinking questions, and the review questions to ensure that they reflect current clinical nursing situations and evaluations. Ms. Gribble is the Chair of Nursing and Allied Health at Coastal Carolina Community College in Jacksonville, North Carolina.

Appreciation is also extended to the following nutrition instructors and nursing instructors who evaluated the manuscript for the revised text and supplied valuable feedback.

Ann Feins, MS, RD: St. Anselm College, Manchester, NH

Kenneth I. Burke, PhD, RD: Loma Linda University, Loma Linda, CA

Lois Bodinski: (Formerly Department Chair, Nursing, Community College of Rhode Island) North Attleboro, MA

Sheila F. Guidry: Wallace Community College, Selma, AL

Marilyn Robinson Neumann, RN, MS, MA: Central Texas College, Killeen, TX

Jean Hassell, RD: Youngstown State University, Warren, OH

Elaine Mohn: Chemeketa Community College, Salem, OR

Carol Beyer: Paducah Community College, Paducah, KY

The following figures were drawn by Masako Herman:
Figures 2-2, 3-3, 3-6, 3-8, 3-10, 3-14, 3-15, 4-8, 4-10, 4-11, 4-12, 5-5, 5-8, 5-9, 6-5, 6-6, 6-12, 6-16, 6-17, 6-18, 6-19, 7-1, 7-5, 7-6, 7-8, 7-9, 7-10, 7-11, 7-12, 7-13, 8-4, 9-1, 9-6, 9-7, 9-8, 14-1, 14-3, 14-4, 15-2, 15-5, 16-3, 16-6, 16-7, 16-8, 16-10, 16-13, 16-15, 17-1, 17-3, 17-4, and 20-3.

T. Randall Lankford

CONTENTS

LIST OF TABLES

PART

I

PRINCIPLES OF NUTRITION

1

INTRODUCTION TO NUTRITION

Upon completion of this chapter, you should be able to:

1. Define nutrition and describe the four main components of the study of nutrition.
2. List the energy nutrients.
3. Define an organic compound and list the four classes of organic nutrients.
4. List the two inorganic nutrients and two of their functions.
5. Define culture and describe four ways in which culture relates to food and eating habits.
6. Explain two ways in which cultural influence is important to health professionals.
7. List three ways in which food faddism may adversely affect a person.
8. Define food fad, natural food, organically grown food, and megadose.
9. State the Senate Select Committee's recommended dietary guidelines in terms of percentages of fat, protein, and carbohydrates.

INTRODUCTION

Nutrition is a human need and is recognized by consumers as essential to life itself. Food and eating are among the great pleasures of life. In the last few years, the public has become more concerned about the relationship of nutrition and general health. As a result, the public is being bombarded with nutritional information and claims in books, magazines, newspapers, and even grocery stores. As a result, many consumers are confused by conflicting food and health claims. Food manufacturers are providing more information about nutrients on labels, but many consumers do not understand how to read or analyze it.

To help consumers understand nutritional information they read and to explain the relationship of nutrition to normal health and disease are two reasons why health professionals need to study nutrition. In addition, health professionals must study nutrition in order to provide preventive health care on the **primary, secondary,** and **tertiary** levels. Knowledge of nutrition is important in primary prevention because it prevents the occurrence of disease and protects the general health and well-being of the public. To do this, health professionals must be knowledgeable about nutritious diets, foods, and exercise. In addition, they need to be aware of government primary prevention programs such as Head Start preschool programs, breakfast programs, and food stamp programs.

primary level   Health care that is aimed at averting the occurrence of disease and protecting the health of the general public.

secondary level   Health care that is utilized for early diagnosis of disease and prevention of further complications.

tertiary level   Health care that is designed to educate a patient for the maximum use of his or her remaining capacities.

Nutritional information is important in secondary preventive health care in that it can be utilized for early diagnosis of diseases and prevention of further complications. Specifically, the health professional frequently alerts the medical service or physician to abnormal laboratory values and is aware of the patient's tolerance of the prescribed therapeutic diet.

Tertiary preventive health care involves the health professional in retraining and educating patients for the maximum use of their remaining capacities. For example, this involves advising paraplegics and quadriplegics about the possible dietary side effects of their immobility, such as constipation, kidney stones, and dietary measures to help prevent or alleviate such problems.

In summary, nutritional information is increasing at a rapid rate. This challenges health professionals to be knowledgeable about nutrition so that they can provide competent health care on all three levels. Nutritional knowledge will enrich a health professional's personal life.

DEFINITION OF NUTRITION

Nutrition is the combination of processes by which the body receives and utilizes the materials necessary to maintain homeostasis. These pro-

nutrition The combination of processes by which the body receives and utilizes the materials necessary to maintain homeostasis.

cesses are also important in their relationship to health and disease. In addition, nutrition is concerned with the social, economic, cultural, and psychological implications of food and eating.

FOUR MAIN COMPONENTS OF THE STUDY OF NUTRITION

The study of nutrition involves four main components (see Fig. 1-1):

Nutrients. Substances that are necessary for the metabolic processes of the body.

Body processes. Physiological activities (e.g., digestion and absorption) that interact with nutrients to maintain homeostasis.

Nutrient requirements. Individual nutritional requirements to maintain homeostasis depend upon various factors (age, sex, and physical condition).

Homeostasis. The maintenance of organ systems, such as the respiratory and cardiovascular systems, in a dynamic state. The above three components are essential for homeostasis, as shown in Figure 1-1.[1]

Nutrients

There are six classes of nutrients:

Carbohydrate	Vitamins
Lipid (Fat)	Minerals
Protein	Water

These classes are subdivided into energy, organic, and inorganic nutrients.

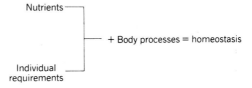

FIGURE 1-1 Interaction of four components of the study of nutrition.

oxidation A chemical reaction in which an atom or molecule either loses hydrogen atoms and electrons or accepts oxygen.

organic compounds Substances that contain carbon atoms.

inorganic nutrients Substances that do not contain carbon atoms.

Energy Nutrients

Carbohydrate, fat, and protein are designated as energy nutrients, since they release energy when **oxidized** (chemical reaction). The maintenance of homeostasis depends upon continual input of energy.

Organic Nutrients

Carbohydrate, fat, protein, and vitamins (see Table 1-1) are composed of **organic compounds.** Vitamins are the only type of organic nutrients that do not provide energy. Organic nutrients have many functions, such as building, maintaining body tissues and regulating body processes, which will be discussed in detail in later chapters.

Inorganic Nutrients

Minerals and water are **inorganic nutrients** (see Table 1-1). Minerals are required in minute amounts and are essential for many body functions such as bone formation, conduction of nerve impulses, and synthesis of red blood cells. Water is the most prevalent nutrient, as well as the most important. This is evidenced by the fact that a person can live for about 40 days in a fasting state, but can live for only about 3 days without taking in water. Examples of body functions for which water is important are as a medium for chemical reactions, in transporting materials, and in helping to maintain body temperature.[2]

TABLE 1-1 SUMMARY OF CLASSES OF NUTRIENTS

Description	Classes	Functions
Energy nutrients	Carbohydrate Fat Protein	Release energy for maintenance of homeostasis
Organic nutrients	Carbohydrate Fat Protein Vitamins	Build and maintain body tissues Regulate body processes
Inorganic nutrients	Water Minerals	Medium for chemical reactions Transport materials Maintain body temperature Bone formation Conduction of nerve impulses

IMPORTANT NUTRITIONAL TERMS

A meaningful discussion of nutrition must contain words and terms that are clearly defined. The following list of terms will appear in many places throughout the text; therefore, knowledge of them is essential.

Health. State of optimal physical, mental, and social well-being, not just the absence of illness.

Nutritional status. An individual's condition of health in relation to the digestion and absorption of nutrients.

Nutritional care. Application of the science of nutrition in nourishing the body regardless of health problems or potential problems.[1]

anemia A condition in which the total quantity of red blood cells and hemoglobin is less than normal. See iron deficiency anemia (Chapter 7) and pernicious anemia (Chapter 6).

Malnutrition. A condition of the body that arises from a prolonged lack or excessive intake or impaired utilization of food. This condition is often evidenced by the appearance of specific clinical conditions such as **anemia, goiter,** and **rickets.**[3]

Nutritious. Food in a diet that provides needed nutrients for maintenance of homeostasis. A food cannot be determined to be nutritious when considered by itself, but rather in relation to the total diet.

goiter Abnormal enlargement of the thyroid gland due to an imbalance in the amount of the mineral iodine (see Chapter 7).

Junk food. A term for which there is no acceptable scientific definition, but in popular usage refers to foods that are harmful, for example, foods high in salt, sugar, or fat content.[4]

Health food. Another term for which there is no scientifically accepted definition; however, it usually refers to foods that have been subjected to less processing than usual (for example, hydrogenated nut butter and whole grain flour).

rickets A condition caused by a deficiency of vitamin D that leads to decreased absorption of calcium by the bones.

CULTURAL INFLUENCE ON FOOD HABITS AND IMPORTANCE TO HEALTH PROFESSIONALS

Food habits are the result of many influences such as personal, cultural, social, and psychological factors. A full discussion of each is beyond the scope of this text. However, we will discuss the cultural influence on food habits and why it is important for health professionals to understand it.

culture The concepts, skills, and broad-based characteristics of a given population.

Culture relates to food and eating habits in a variety of ways.[5] Culture determines:

- Acceptable foods
- Appropriate methods of food handling, preparation, and storage
- Table manners

- Attitudes toward eating
- Attitudes toward obesity and other aspects of body size
- Attitudes about the relationship of food and health[6]

One might ask, of what importance is cultural influence on food habits to a health professional? The answer is related essentially to the roles of health team members in teaching nutrition concepts to patients and their families, as well as in assessment of patient responses to diets. In order to perform these roles effectively, a health professional needs to separate his or her own cultural background and apply the patient's cultural food patterns to the task at hand. Food patterns of two major U.S. cultures are given in Table 1-2.

FOOD FALLACIES, CONTROVERSIES, AND FACTS: A CHALLENGE FOR THE HEALTH PROFESSIONAL

food fallacies False, deceptive ideas about food and its effects in the body.

If a health professional is to teach nutrition concepts effectively to patients and their families, it is not enough to have only a good scientific foundation of nutritional knowledge. The professional needs to be informed about **food fallacies** and controversies in order to respond accurately and authoritatively to patients who have questions about food fallacies.

Health Dangers of Food Fallacies

There are three basic ways that food fallacies may adversely affect a person.

Increase the Risks of High-Risk People

People who are in high-risk health groups can be adversely affected by food fallacies. For example, people with a chronic illness (such as cancer, arthritis, or diabetes) may turn to food fads to alleviate their symptoms, since conventional treatments have not produced dramatic results. Teenagers can be harmed by food fallacies that promise to improve physique and figure development.[7]

Malnutrition

Some people may actually suffer from malnutrition as a result of a food fad. Vitamin A poisoning (see Chapter 6) can occur following consump-

TABLE 1-2 CULTURAL DIETARY PATTERNS CLASSIFIED ACCORDING TO THE DAILY FOOD GUIDE

	Chinese	Japanese	Filipino	American Indian	African-American
Milk Group	Intake of fluid milk usually limited; ice cream well accepted; flavored milk drinks preferred until taste is developed Limited intake of cheese; younger generations are consuming larger quantities of milk and cheeses	Milk and cheese consumed in larger quantities by the younger generations Ice cream and milk puddings are well accepted	Dairy foods are gaining acceptance and are tolerated Limited intake of milk and cheese Custards similar to Mexican flan Ice cream, flavored milk drinks, fresh white cheese	Most easily tolerate milk products in fermented form or in small quantities throughout the day Buttermilk, yogurt, cottage cheese, and Monterey Jack cheese Nonfat dry milk is used in cooking	Fresh homogenized milk, chocolate milk, buttermilk, evaporated and nonfat dry milk in cooking; ice cream, milk puddings, and custards Cheese (American, Cheddar, cottage, longhorn) Yogurt
Supplementary Source of Calcium	*Tofu* (soybean curd) has significant calcium content.* Canned fish with bones, sardines, small fried fish eaten whole (smelts), dried small fish, including bones Various leafy greens (amaranths, kale, Chinese cress, Chinese mustard greens, pickled mustard leaves)	*Tofu* (soybean curd) has significant calcium content* Whole dried fish, including bones	*Tofu* (soybean curd) has significant calcium content* *Alamang* and *bagoong* (fish sauce) *Dilis* (dried fish) *Malunggay* (dark green, leafy vegetables)		Dark green, leafy vegetables (collard greens, mustard greens, and kale) Sardines
Bread-Cereal Group	Large intake of rice, rice cakes, rice noodles, rice flour; wheat products (breads, noodles, spaghetti, macaroni); millet, oats *Won ton* (stuffed noodles) *Bow* (filled buns)	Large quantities of rice and rice products used; *Mochiko* (rice flour) often used; rice cakes, breads, and crackers *Sushi* (rice wrapped in seaweed) *Somen* and *soba* (noodles), millet and barley are commonly used	Rice is the staple food. Some noodles used also. *Won ton* used in soups as in Chinese diet Cooked cereals; various kinds of bread including *Pan de Sal* (white bread) *Mochiko* (rice flour)	Cornmeal and flours made from ground sweet acorn, wheat, or rye; white flour used for *fry bread* (fried biscuit dough); tortillas also popular Cornbread, rice, *bean bread* (shelled bean and cornmeal mixture), *ta fulla* (hominy and cake of bean ashes), *shinish-bay* and *buh-kway-shee* (fried bread), *bota-cuppa* (Cherokee poached corn and water with sugar), *walakshi* (fruit-flavored cornmeal dumplings)	Homemade bread, white and whole-wheat breads, biscuits, cornbread (also cornpone, hush puppies, spoon bread, cracklin' bread), pancakes, grits, rice, macaroni, spaghetti Whole-grain cereals and cooked cream of wheat, oatmeal, and rice cereals Dry cereals (corn flakes, rice, or wheat)

(continued)

TABLE 1-2 CULTURAL DIETARY PATTERNS (Continued)

	Chinese	Japanese	Filipino	American Indian	African-American
Sources of Vitamin A	*Napa* (Chinese celery cabbage), *gai choy* (Chinese mustard greens), watercress, *yin choy* (amaranth greens), leaf lettuce. *oong choy* (water convolvulus), *gou gay* (wolfberry leaves), *lo bok* (Chinese turnips) Green peppers, tomatoes, spinach, Chinese chard, carrots, sweet potatoes, pumpkin, coriander, squash, apricots, peaches	Spinach, carrots, tomatoes, yellow squash, sweet potatoes, parsley, Japanese persimmons, mustard greens *Laver, nori, wakame, kombu* (types of seaweed)	*Camotes* (sweet potatoes), tomatoes, squash, *saluyot* (leafy green, slimy vegetable), *malunggay* (dark green leafy vegetable)	Pumpkin and all squash very popular Carrots, onions, potatoes, celery, cabbage, peas Dandelion greens, milkweed Wild and cultivated berries, yellow corn, eaten very commonly	Leafy greens—fresh preferred (collards, mustard, turnip greens, kale, spinach, chard, beet tops); encourage use of the pot liquor (the liquid in which vegetables are cooked) Tomatoes, sweet potatoes, carrots, pumpkins, yellow squash, green peppers, okra, lettuce Melons, peaches
Vegetable-Fruit Group Sources of Vitamin C	*Gai lan* (Chinese broccoli), Chinese cabbage, green peppers, fresh tomatoes, watercress, broccoli, spinach, leafy greens, celery, turnips, cauliflower, *daikon* (white radish), *chow yuk* (stir-fried vegetables) Fruits not eaten frequently; more widely used in younger generations. Oranges, papayas, tangerines, melons, guavas, lemons	Fresh tomatoes, broccoli, *napa* (cabbage), *kimchee* (pickled cabbage), *daikon* (white radish), turnips, potatoes (eaten in limited amounts) Oranges	Cabbage, cauliflower, corn, pith of sago palm, potatoes, turnips, avocados *Achara* (papaya and peppers), melons, guavas, jackfruit, limes, mangoes, oranges, papayas, pomelos, strawberries, *naranghita* (tangelo)	Mustard greens, watercress, cabbage, turnips, potatoes (sweet and white) Lemons, oranges, melons, grapefruit, strawberries, dried fruit (wild cherries, berries, and grapes)	Broccoli, turnips, green peppers, cabbage, mustard greens, tomatoes, potatoes (sweet and white) Oranges, grapefruit, melons, lemons, strawberries
Other Vegetables and Fruits	Snow peas (Chinese pea pods), Chinese okra, bamboo shoots, soybean sprouts, mung bean sprouts, alfalfa sprouts, taro roots, lotus tubers, dried day lillies, *Black Juda's ear* (high-fiber dry fungus) Eggplant, cucumbers, green beans, mushrooms, onions, leeks Plums, prunes, persimmons, apples, bananas, pears, figs, grapes, pineapples, pomegranates	String beans, onions, eggplant, cucumbers, pickled vegetables (as dessert), mushrooms, celery, *gobo* (burdock), *takenoko* (bamboo shoots), *seri* (Japanese parsley), *renkon* (lotus root), *wasabi* (horseradish) *Mizutaki* (vegetable soup)	Mung beans, bean sprouts, okra, eggplant, celery, onions, radishes, bamboo shoots, *gabi* (root crop), mushrooms, onions *Tamarind* (pod fruit), *ampalaya* (bitter melon), bananas, pineapple	Eggplant, wild tullies (tuber used as vegetable), green peas, green beans, beets, onions, corn, cucumbers, cassava Grapes, apples, pears, bananas	Green peas, green beans, beets, onions, cucumbers, eggplant, corn, radishes Grapes, bananas, pears, fruit cocktail, apples, pineapple

(continued)

TABLE 1-2 *(Continued)*

	Chinese	Japanese	Filipino	American Indian	African-American
Meat Group (includes Meat, Poultry, Game, Fish, Eggs, Dried Peas and Beans, and Nuts)	Large intake of pork and pork products (sausage, BBQ pork, roast pork, pig knuckles), fish of various kinds (fresh, canned, salted); seafoods (shrimp, crabs, squid, oysters, clams, octopus, abalone) Poultry (chicken, duck); eggs (chicken, duck); organ meats (liver, heart, tongue, maws, kidney, spleen) Peanuts, almonds, walnuts; dried beans (soybeans, black beans, red beans, white beans); *tofu* (soybean curd)	Pork, beef, chicken; large intake of fish and shellfish dishes; *sashimi* (raw fish), *kamaboko* (fish cake) Soybeans, *miso* (fermented soybean), soya cake, *tofu* (soybean curd) Eggs; peanuts, chestnuts; *azuki beans* (red beans), lima beans *Hekka* (seasoned chicken dish)	Fresh and dried fish as well as shellfish are major sources of protein; *dilis* (dried fish) Chicken, duck, pork, beef, *adobo* (pieces of pork and chicken in soy sauce), *relleno* (chicken) *Tortilla* (an omelet) and *lumpia* (egg roll) also popular *Lechon* (barbequed pig) is considered a specialty Organ meats (liver, heart, intestines) Various sausages, ham and cured meats, canned meats Eggs, dried beans, soybeans, garbanzo beans, peanut butter, *tofu* (soybean curd)	When available in hunting areas, wild rabbit, venison, wild geese, duck, groundhog are popular Fresh fish, pork, chicken; eggs eaten in large quantities Dried peas and beans (kidney, pinto, and lentils very common in diet and usually eaten with rice and other grains) *Roe* (fish eggs) Pinenuts, acorns, peanuts, and other nut sources of protein	Large intake of pork (fresh and cured) and pork products such as sausage (mild or hot) Scrapple (pork and cornmeal), cold cuts, organ meats, including chitterlings (pork intestines), kidney, liver, tongue Beef, lamb, tripe, chicken, turkey, duck, goose Game such as rabbit and venison; fresh and canned fish (buffalo, catfish, trout, shellfish, tuna, salmon, mackerel, sardines) Eggs; walnuts, pecans, peanuts; dried peas and beans (black-eyed peas, chickpeas; kidney, pink and red beans, navy beans) Peanut butter Lower-protein, high-fat meat sources (cured bacon—thin slices or slab, pig's feet, pig ears, souse, pork neck bones)

*6 oz of tofu contains an amount of calcium comparable to 1 c of milk.
Reproduced with permission from *Extension of Guide to Good Eating*. Sacramento, Calif., Dairy Council of California.

rebound scurvy A condition that occurs when a pregnant woman takes megadoses of vitamin C, causing the fetus to adapt to the massive doses. After birth, without continued ingestion of vitamin C, the infant shows signs of scurvy.

tion of large doses of vitamin A for acne. Excessive intake of vitamin C has been found to cause kidney stones, impaired ability of white blood cells to kill bacteria, and **rebound scurvy** in infants born to mothers who take megadoses of vitamin C.[8]

Economics

Consumers are frequently confused by claims made for organic, natural, and health foods. As a result, they tend to buy these more expensive foods in the belief that if it costs more, it must be better. Often the consumer who spends excessively on food fads cannot afford to do so.

Definitions

Some terms and their definitions are necessary to discuss food fallacies and controversies.

Food fad. Any dietary concept that remains scientifically unproven.

Natural food. A term for which there is little agreement on meaning. It is marketed as a food that is produced with minimal processing and without the use of preservatives, additives, or other artificial ingredients.

Organically grown food. Food fertilized with manure rather than chemical fertilizers and processed without additives or chemicals.[9]

Megadose. A quantity that exceeds by 10 times or more the normal recommended amount of a vitamin.

Table 1-3 briefly presents examples of various fallacies; details are given in later chapters.

DIETARY GOALS FOR THE UNITED STATES

In the 1960s, the Senate Select Committee on Nutrition and Human Needs was formed to study the nutritional status of the public. The committee held hearings for several years before publishing a number of recommendations in its publication entitled *Dietary Goals for the U.S.* (1977). The seven goals stated in the revised edition are:

calorie A measure of the energy value of substances; defined as the amount of heat required to raise the temperature of 1 g of water 1° Celsius (C).

naturally occurring sugars Sugars found naturally in foods, such as glucose and fructose, as opposed to artificial sugars, such as sorbital and xylitol (see Chapter 16).

1. To avoid becoming overweight, consume only as much energy (**calories**) as is expended. If you are overweight, decrease energy intake and increase energy expenditure.
2. Increase the consumption of complex carbohydrates and **naturally occurring sugars** from about 28% to about 48% of energy intake.
3. Reduce the consumption of refined and processed sugars by about 45% to about 10% of total energy intake.
4. Reduce overall fat consumption from approximately 40% to about 30% of energy intake.
5. Reduce saturated fat consumption to about 10% of total energy intake and balance that consumption with polyunsaturated and monounsaturated fats, which should each account for about 10% of energy intake.
6. Reduce cholesterol consumption to about 300 mg a day.

TABLE 1-3 FOOD FALLACIES VERSUS FACTS

Fallacy	Facts
1. Vitamin C prevents common colds.	1. Extensive research shows that megadoses of vitamin C do not prevent common colds, but can be toxic when taken over a long period (see Chapter 6 for details).
2. Vitamin A can help reduce acne.	2. Megadoses of vitamin A for acne caused many toxic problems. A derivative of vitamin A (accutane) has shown success in reducing acne when given in megadose amounts. People are carefully monitored for toxic effects.[7]
3. Orange juice is too acid for infants.	3. Citrus fruits are not acid formers in the body of an adult or an infant, but rather are base formers.
4. Adolescent acne is caused by eating too much chocolate and junk foods.	4. Acne in adolescents is a result of an increase in sex hormones and their interaction with oil-producing (sebaceous) glands.
5. Food grown with natural organic fertilizers is superior to that grown with chemical fertilizers.	5. Natural organic and chemical fertilizers essentially contain the same nutrients necessary for plant growth.
6. Fad weight loss diets (for example, the Beverly Hills Diet, Cambridge Diet, Dr. Atkins Diet) are equal to or better than medically prescribed and supervised diets.	6. Best-seller fad diets will help some people lose weight, but 80–90% of them regain the weight. These diets do not attack the psychological problems that cause overeating. A medical diet is designed to help a person lose weight permanently by changing the person's eating habits.[7]

7. Limit the intake of sodium by reducing the intake of salt to about 5 g a day.

The Senate Select Committee compared the current American diet with its recommended diet as set forth in its dietary goals:

Current Diet	*Dietary Goals*
Fat: 42%	Fat: 30%
Protein: 12%	Protein: 12%
Carbohydrates: 46%	Carbohydrates: 58%
Complex carbohydrate: 22%	Complex carbohydrate: 48%
Sugar: 24%	Sugar: 10%

It should be emphasized that the committee's dietary goals were criticized by many groups. Other dietary reports have been published by other committees, such as the joint committee of the U.S. Department of

Agriculture and the former Department of Health, Education and Welfare. They published a set of dietary guidelines for Americans called "Nutrition and Your Health" (1980), which recommended the following:

1. Eat a variety of foods.
2. Maintain ideal weight.
3. Avoid too much fat, saturated fat, and cholesterol.
4. Eat foods with adequate starch and fiber.
5. Avoid too much sugar.
6. Avoid too much sodium.
7. If you drink alcohol, do so in moderation.

SUMMARY

- Nutrition is the combination of processes by which the body receives and utilizes the materials necessary to maintain homeostasis.
- Carbohydrates, proteins, and fats are energy nutrients.
- Organic nutrients contain carbon atoms; four classes of organic nutrients include carbohydrates, proteins, fats, and vitamins.
- Culture is the concepts, skills, and broad-based characteristics of a given population; four ways in which culture relates to food and eating are: acceptable foods, appropriate methods of food handling, and table manners.
- Two ways cultural influence is important to health professionals are as aids in teaching nutrition concepts to patients and families, and in assessment of patients' responses to diets.
- Three ways in which food fallacies may adversely affect a person are: increasing the risks of high-risk people, promoting malnutrition, and causing one to overspend.
- Food fad: any dietary concept that remains scientifically unproven; natural food: food that is produced with minimal processing and without the use of preservatives; organically grown food: food fertilized with manure rather than chemical fertilizers and processed without additives or chemicals; megadose: a quantity that exceeds 10 times or more the normal recommended amount of a vitamin.
- Senate Select Committee recommended dietary guidelines are: fat: 30% of daily kcal; protein: 12% of daily kcal; carbohydrates: 58%—complex carbohydrates 48% and sugar 10%.

REVIEW QUESTIONS

True (A) or False (B)

1. Nutrition is defined as the maintenance of organ systems (respiratory and cardiovascular) in a dynamic state. (F)
2. The four main components of the study of nutrition include nutrients, body processes, nutrient requirements, and homeostasis. (T)
3. Energy nutrients include carbohydrate, fat, and vitamins. (F)
4. Organic nutrients do not contain carbon atoms and function only to release energy. (F)
5. Inorganic nutrients contain carbon atoms and include water and minerals. (F)
6. Cultural influence is important to health team members in teaching nutrition concepts and assessment of patient responses to diets. (T)
7. Food fallacies may adversely affect a person by increasing the risks of high-risk people, causing malnutrition, and causing people to spend excessive amounts of money. (T)

Matching

8. D Homeostasis
9. B Minerals
10. E Energy nutrients
11. C Culture
12. A Food fad

A. dietary concept that remains scientifically unproven.
B. conduction of nerve impulses
C. concepts, skills, and broad-based characteristics of a given population.
D. maintenance of organ systems in a dynamic state.
E. carbohydrate, fat, and protein.

Multiple Choice

13. The components of the study of nutrition are
    1. nutrients
    2. organic compounds
    3. body processes
    4. inorganic compounds
    A. 1, 2, 3 B. 1, 3 C. 2, 4 D. 4
    E. All of these
14. Inorganic nutrients include:
    A. minerals
    B. vitamins
    C. water
    D. A, C
    E. B, C
15. Which of the following is (are) *incorrectly* paired?
    A. food fad—dietary concept that remains scientifically unproven.

15

B. natural food—foods fertilized with manure rather than chemical fertilizers.

C. fallacy—a false, deceptive idea.

D. none of these.

Completion

16. Describe the four main components of nutrition that you will be studying in this course.
17. Define the terms *food fad*, *nature food*, *health food*, and *megadose*.
18. Give the Senate Select Committee's recommended dietary goals in terms of percentages of fat, protein, and carbohydrates in the diet.

CRITICAL THINKING CHALLENGE

1. Analyze the diet below and calculate the following:
   a. Percentage of the total calories from fat.
   b. Percentage of the total calories from carbohydrates.
   c. Percentage of the total calories from protein.
   d. How do the above percentages compare to the Dietary Goals?
   Total calories = 2,000
   Calories from fat = 840
   Calories from protein = 240
   Calories from carbohydrate = 920
2. Suppose that you know someone who has colon cancer and he tells you he is buying a bottle of "Colocancer Tablets," 100 tablets for $99.95. He tells you that these tablets contain a newly discovered natural food that is guaranteed to eliminate the cancer condition or money back.
   Which term or definition (studied in this chapter) correctly describes the claim made for the natural food in these Colocancer Tablets? Give three ways (studied in this chapter) that buying and consuming these tablets could adversely affect the person.

REVIEW QUESTIONS FOR NCLEX

Situation. A nutrition student, studying with other students in a study group for an exam, was asking other members of the group the following questions.

1. The energy nutrients include
   A. carbohydrate
   B. minerals
   C. water
   D. vitamins
2. Inorganic nutrients include
   A. carbohydrates
   B. water
   C. protein
   D. vitamins
3. Which of the following correctly states what culture determines in relation to food and eating habits?
   Culture determines:
   A. acceptable foods.
   B. knowledge of foods.
   C. interest in nutrition.
   D. level of exercise.
4. The Senate Select Committee's recommended dietary goals as to percentages of fat, protein, and carbohydrates are:
   A. fat: 42%
      protein: 20%
      carbohydrate: 38%
   B. fat: 20%
      protein: 50%
      carbohydrate: 30%
   C. fat: 30%
      protein: 12%
      carbohydrate: 58%
   D. fat: 10%
      protein: 60%
      carbohydrate: 30%
5. Which of the following are components in the study of nutrition?
   A. nutrients
   B. organic compounds
   C. diseases
   D. inorganic compounds

REFERENCES

1. Brown, J. E. (1990). *The science of human nutrition* (pp. 46–47). San Diego: Harcourt Brace Jovanovich.
2. Christian, J. L., & Greger, J. L. (1991). *Nutrition for living* (3rd ed.) (pp. 6–9). Redwood City, CA: Benjamin Cummings.

3. Nieman, D. C., Butterworth, D. E., & Nieman, C. N. (1990). *Nutrition.* Dubuque: W. C. Brown.
4. Food and Nutrition Board. (1986). *What is America eating?* Washington, DC: National Academy Press.
5. Food Technology. International foods—A growing market in the U.S. (1987). *Food Technology, 41,* 120–134.
6. Harper, A. E. (1988). Nutrition: From myth and magic to science. *Nutrition Today, 23,* 8–17.
7. Hornig, D. H., Moser, U., & Glatthaar, B. E. (1988). Ascorbic acid. In M. E. Shils & V. R. Young (Eds.), *Modern nutrition in health and disease.* Philadelphia: Lea and Febiger.
8. The American Medical Association Council on Scientific Affairs. (1987). Vitamin preparations as supplements and therapeutic agents. *Journal of the American Medical Association, 257,* 1927–1936.
9. Salunkke, D. K., & Desai, B. B. (1988). Effects of agricultural practices, handling, processing, and storage on vegetables. In E. Karmas & R. S. Harris (Eds.), *Nutritional evaluation of food processing.* New York: Van Nostrand Reinhold.

2 DIETARY PLANNING

Upon completion of this chapter, you should be able to:

1. Define the four components of a nutritious diet.
2. List the five food groups in the food pyramid and range of servings for each food group.
3. Describe the difference between a vegan and a lacto-ovo vegetarian diet.
4. Discuss three possible deficiencies of a vegetarian diet.
5. Discuss four advantages of a vegetarian diet.
6. Name the six exchange lists.
7. Give the grams of carbohydrate, protein, and fat and the kilocalories for one exchange on each list.
8. Take a meal and calculate the grams of carbohydrate, fat, protein, and kilocalories for each food, as well as the total kilocalories.
9. Utilize information from objective 8 to calculate the percentage of the total kilocalories in the meal due to carbohydrate, fat, and protein.
10. Utilize information from objective 9 to determine whether the meal is balanced in regard to the distribution of carbohydrate, fat, and protein.
11. Distinguish between RDAs and U.S. RDAs.
12. Name the nutrients that have established RDA values.

INTRODUCTION

The maintenance and restoration of good health are objectives with which consumers and health professionals are concerned. One way to achieve these objectives is by eating a nutritious diet. Four components of a nutritious diet are:

essential nutrients Compounds that the body cannot synthesize.

Adequacy. Foods that provide all of the **essential nutrients** and calories in the proper amounts.

Nutrient density (calories control). Refers to the content of specific nutrients in relation to kcal. High nutrient density foods are those that have a high level of nutrients with a low level of kcal. An example is skim milk compared to whole milk (see Table 2-5 for details).

Balance. Distribution of daily calories among fat, protein, and carbohydrate in a certain ratio. The normal ratio is: fat 30%, carbohydrate 55–60%, and protein 10–15% of calories.

Variety. Inclusion of a variety of foods in the daily diet.[1]

FOOD GUIDES FOR PLANNING NUTRITIOUS DIETS

Two commonly used guides in planning nutritious diets are the Food Guide Pyramid and the Food Exchange System. These two guides allow one to plan a diet and achieve the four dietary components.

Food Guide Pyramid

The Food Guide Pyramid (Figure 2-1) developed by the United States Department of Agriculture (USDA) is designed to help people both choose what food groups to consume and determine how many servings of each to eat. The main focus of the pyramid is to educate people about the high amount of fat, sugar, and salt in the foods that most Americans eat. In addition, the pyramid provides a recommended range of servings for each food group necessary to achieve a nutritious diet.

Figure 2-1 shows the bread group at the base of the pyramid. This group includes breads, cereals, rice, and pasta (all of which come from grains). A person needs more servings from the bread group than any other because of the high levels of complex carbohydrates and low levels of fat, salt, and sugar. The next level of the pyramid, fruits and vegetables, is important because these foods provide vitamins, minerals, and fiber. The third level of the pyramid includes the meat and milk groups, which are rich in protein, calcium, iron, and zinc. The tip of the pyramid is fats, oils, and sweets, which come from foods such as salad dressings

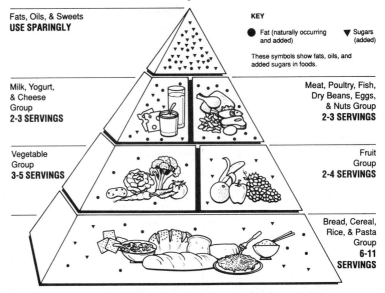

Food Guide Pyramid
A Guide to Daily Food Choices

Fats, Oils, & Sweets
USE SPARINGLY

KEY
● Fat (naturally occurring and added)   ▼ Sugars (added)

These symbols show fats, oils, and added sugars in foods.

Milk, Yogurt, & Cheese Group
2-3 SERVINGS

Meat, Poultry, Fish, Dry Beans, Eggs, & Nuts Group
2-3 SERVINGS

Vegetable Group
3-5 SERVINGS

Fruit Group
2-4 SERVINGS

Bread, Cereal, Rice, & Pasta Group
6-11 SERVINGS

FIGURE 2-1   Food guide pyramid. The food group for each level and the number of servings are given. (Courtesy of USDA April 1992. Home and Garden Bulletin (249), 5).

and oils, cream, butter, margarine, sugars, soft drinks, candies, and sweet desserts. These foods provide almost no nutrients but are high in calories, which is why there is no recommended number of servings.

Number of Servings and Kilocalories (kcal)

In order to plan a nutritious diet, a person must know how many servings of each food group and how many kcal should be consumed. Figure 2-1 shows a range of servings for each food group. In addition to the number of servings, Table 2-1 shows how many kcal a person should consume depending on age, sex, and activity level.

Notice in Figure 2-1 that the meat group shows 2–3 servings, but in Table 2-1 the meat group servings are in total ounces. The following equivalents must be used to understand servings of meat and then convert them to ounces of meat:

> 2–3 oz of meat, fish, poultry = 1 serving
> 3 oz piece of meat = 1 average hamburger patty

TABLE 2-1 SUMMARY OF FOOD GUIDE PYRAMID

Food Group	1,600 kcal (many sedentary women and some older adults)	2,200 kcal (most children; teenage girls; active women; many sedentary men)	2,800 kcal (teenage boys; many active men; some very active women)
Bread (1 serving = 1 slice of bread; 1 oz. ready-to-eat cereal; 1/2 cup of cooked cereal, rice, or pasta)	6	9	11
Vegetable (1 serving = 1 cup raw leafy vegetables; 1/2 cup cooked or chopped raw)	3	4	5
Fruit (1 serving = 1 medium apple, banana, orange; 1/2 cup chopped, cooked, canned fruit; 3/4 cup fruit juice)	2	3	4
Milk (1 serving = 1 cup of milk or yogurt; 1 1/2 oz of natural cheese; 2 oz processed cheese)	2–3[a]	2–3[a]	2–3[a]
Meat (1 serving = 2–3 oz of cooked lean meat, poultry, or fish; 1/2 cup cooked dry beans; 1 egg or 2 tablespoons of peanut butter)	5[b]	6[b]	7[b]
Total fat (g)	53[c]	73[c]	93[c]
Total Added Sugars (tsp)	6[d]	12[d]	18[d]

[a]Women who are pregnant or breastfeeding, teenagers, and young adults to age 24 need 3 servings.
[b]Meat group amounts are in total ounces. See text for details as to how to count amounts of meat and other foods in this group.
[c]See text as to how to calculate total fat and Table 2-2 for the amount of fat for common foods in each food group.
[d]See Table 2-3 for the amount of added sugars in common foods for each food group.
Source: Adapted from USDA Food Guide Pyramid. April 1992. *Home and Garden Bulletin* (249), 9.

3 oz piece of meat = 1/2 chicken breast
1 oz meat = 1/2 cup of cooked dry beans
or
1 egg
or
2 tablespoons of peanut butter

Fat in the Food Groups

In order to help a person calculate total fat (grams), the following equivalent should be used:

1 pat of butter or regular margarine = 4 g of fat
4 g of fat = 1 tsp

It should be pointed out that some margarines are lower in fat and cholesterol than others; therefore, a person should compare food labels on margarines. See Table 2-2 for grams of fat in the most commonly used foods in each food group. This table, along with the recommended number of grams of fat for each kcal (Table 2-1) category, allows a person to plan a diet that will have 30% or less of the total kcal from fat and achieve a balanced, nutritious diet.

TABLE 2-2 FAT CONTENT OF COMMON FOODS IN EACH FOOD GROUP

For this amount of food ...	count this many ...	
Bread, Cereal, Rice, and Pasta Group		
Eat 6 to 11 servings daily	Servings	Grams of Fat
▲ Bread, 1 slice	1	1
▲ Hamburger roll, bagel, english muffin, 1	2	2
Tortilla, 1	1	3
▲ Rice, pasta, cooked, 1/2 cup	1	Trace
Plain crackers, small, 3-4	1	3
Breakfast cereal, 1 oz.	1	*
Pancakes, 4" diameter, 2	2	3
Croissant, 1 large (2 oz.)	2	12
Doughnut, 1 medium (2 oz.)	2	11
Danish, 1 medium (2 oz.)	2	13
Cake, frosted, 1/16 average	1	13
Cookies, 2 medium	1	4
Pie, fruit, 2-crust, 1/6 8" pie	2	19
Vegetable Group		
Eat 3 to 5 servings daily	Servings	Grams of Fat
▲ Vegetables, cooked, 1/2 cup	1	Trace
▲ Vegetables, leafy, raw, 1 cup	1	Trace
▲ Vegetables, nonleafy, raw, chopped, 1/2 cup	1	Trace
Potatoes, scalloped, 1/2 cup	1	4
Potato salad, 1/2 cup	1	8
French fries, 10	1	8

TABLE 2-2 *(Continued)*

For this amount of food ...		count this many ...
Fruit Group		
Eat 2 to 4 servings daily		
▲ Whole fruit: medium apple, orange, banana	1	Trace
▲ Fruit, raw or canned, 1/2 cup	1	Trace
▲ Fruit juice, unsweetened, 3/4 cup	1	Trace
Avocado, 1/4 whole	1	9

Meat, Poultry, Fish, Dry Beans, Eggs, and Nuts Group		
Eat 5 to 7 oz. daily	*Servings*	*Grams of Fat*
▲ Lean meat, poultry, fish, cooked	3 oz	6
Ground beef, lean, cooked	3 oz	16
Chicken, with skin, fried	3 oz	13
Bologna, 2 slices	1 oz	16
Egg, 1	1 oz	5
▲ Dry beans and peas, cooked, 1/2 cup	1 oz	Trace
Peanut butter, 2 tbsp.	1 oz	16
Nuts, 1/3 cup	1 oz	22

Milk, Yogurt, and Cheese Group		
Eat 2 to 3 servings daily	*Servings*	*Grams of Fat*
▲ Skim milk, 1 cup	1	Trace
▲ Nonfat yogurt, plain, 8 oz.	1	Trace
Lowfat milk, 2 percent, 1 cup	1	5
Whole milk, 1 cup	1	8
Chocolate milk, 2 percent, 1 cup	1	5
Lowfat yogurt, plain, 8 oz.	1	4
Lowfat yogurt, fruit, 8 oz.	1	3
Natural cheddar cheese, 1-1/2 oz.	1	14
Process cheese, 2 oz.	1	18
Mozzarella, part skim, 1-1/2 oz.	1	7
Ricotta, part skim, 1/2 cup	1	10
Cottage cheese, 4 percent fat, 1/2 cup	1/4	5
Ice cream, 1/2 cup	1/3	7
Ice milk, 1/2 cup	1/3	3
Frozen yogurt, 1/2 cup	1/2	2

*Check product label.
▲Food is one of the lowest fat choices you can make in that food group.
Source: USDA Food Guide Pyramid. April 1992. *Home and Garden Bulletin* (249), 25–27.

Added Sugars in the Food Groups

As discussed in Chapter 1, the amount of sugar in American diets is too high. Table 2-1 gives the recommended number of added teaspoons of sugar for each food group according to a person's kcal category. Table 2-3 gives the actual number of teaspoons of added sugars for common foods in each food group.

Salt and Sodium in Food Groups

Most Americans consume too much salt in their daily diets. Some health authorities say that sodium intake should not be more than 2,400–3,000 milligrams (mg) per day. Table 2-4 gives the mg of sodium in the common foods for each food group. One teaspoon of salt provides about 2,000 mg of sodium.

Food Labels—New Guidelines

As of spring 1993, new food labels have begun appearing on processed foods, and by May 1994 all foods regulated by the Food and Drug Administration will have the new labels.

The new food labels were created to end confusion caused by the old labels and to help consumers choose a healthier diet. These labels are the product of regulations from the Food and Drug Administration (FDA), an agency of Health and Human Services (HHS), to implement the provisions set forth in the Nutrition Labeling and Education Act (NLEA) passed by Congress in 1990. Four broad categories are covered in the NLEA: nutrition labeling, serving sizes, descriptors, and health claims.

The new labels will differ from the old labels in two basic ways: the amount and type of nutrients that will be required to be listed and health claims that will be allowed. FDA will permit health claims for seven correlations between a food or a nutrient and the risk of a disease or health-related condition. Health claims will be allowed for the following: calcium and osteoporosis; fat and cancer; saturated fat and cholesterol and the risk of coronary heart disease (CHD); sodium and hypertension; fiber-containing grain products, fruits and vegetables and cancer; fruits, vegetables, and grain products that contain fiber, particularly soluble fiber, and the risk of CHD; and fruits and vegetables and cancer.

The items (and a description of each) that will appear on food labels (see Fig. 2-2) are as follows:

TABLE 2-3 ADDED SUGAR IN COMMON FOODS OF THE FOOD GROUPS

WHERE ARE THE ADDED SUGARS?

Food Groups	Added Sugars (teaspoons)
Bread, Cereal, Rice, and Pasta	
Bread, 1 slice	0
Muffin, 1 medium	★ 1
Cookies, 2 medium	★ 1
Danish pastry, 1 medium	★ 1
Doughnut, 1 medium	★ ★ 2
Ready-to-eat cereal, sweetened, 1 oz.	*
Pound cake, no-fat, 1 oz.	★ ★ 2
Angelfood cake, 1/12 tube cake	★ ★ ★ ★ ★ 5
Cake, frosted, 1/16 average	★ ★ ★ ★ ★ ★ 6
Pie, fruit, 2 crust, 1/6 8" pie	★ ★ ★ ★ ★ ★ 6
Fruit	
Fruit, canned in juice, 1/2 cup	0
Fruit, canned in light syrup, 1/2 cup	★ ★ 2
Fruit, canned in heavy syrup, 1/2 cup	★ ★ ★ ★ 4
Milk, Yogurt, and Cheese	
Milk, plain, 1 cup	0
Chocolate milk, 2 percent, 1 cup	★ ★ ★ 3
Lowfat yogurt, plain, 8 oz.	0
Lowfat yogurt, flavored, 8 oz.	★ ★ ★ ★ ★ 5
Lowfat yogurt, fruit, 8 oz.	★ ★ ★ ★ ★ ★ ★ 7
Ice cream, ice milk, or frozen yogurt, 1/2 cup	★ ★ ★ 3
Chocolate shake, 10 fl. oz.	★ ★ ★ ★ ★ ★ ★ ★ ★ 9
Other	
Sugar, jam, or jelly, 1 tsp.	★ 1
Syrup or honey, 1 tbsp.	★ ★ ★ 3
Chocolate bar, 1 oz.	★ ★ ★ 3
Fruit sorbet, 1/2 cup	★ ★ ★ 3
Gelatin dessert, 1/2 cup	★ ★ ★ ★ 4
Sherbet, 1/2 cup	★ ★ ★ ★ ★ 5
Cola, 12 fl.oz.	★ ★ ★ ★ ★ ★ ★ ★ ★ 9
Fruit drink, ade, 12 fl.oz.	★ ★ ★ ★ ★ ★ ★ ★ ★ ★ ★ ★ 12

*Check product label. ★ = 1 teaspoon sugar.
Note: 4 grams of sugar = 1 teaspoon.
Source: USDA Food Guide Pyramid. April 1992. Home and Garden Bulletin (249), 16.

TABLE 2-4 AMOUNT OF SODIUM IN COMMON FOODS OF THE FOOD GROUPS

WHERE'S THE SALT?	
Food Groups	*Sodium, mg*
Bread, Cereal, Rice, and Pasta	
Cooked cereal, rice, pasta, unsalted, 1/2 cup	Trace
Ready-to-eat cereal, 1 oz.	100–360
Bread, 1 slice	110–175
Vegetable	
Vegetables, fresh or frozen, cooked without salt, 1/2 cup	Less than 70
Vegetables, canned or frozen with sauce, 1/2 cup	140–460
Tomato juice, canned, 3/4 cup	660
Vegetable soup, canned, 1 cup	820
Fruit	
Fruit, fresh, frozen, canned, 1/2 cup	Trace
Milk, Yogurt, and Cheese	
Milk, 1 cup	120
Yogurt, 8 oz.	160
Natural cheeses, 1-1/2 oz.	110–450
Process cheeses, 2 oz.	800
Meat, Poultry, Fish, Dry Beans, Eggs, and Nuts	
Fresh meat, poultry, fish, 3 oz.	Less than 90
Tuna, canned, water pack, 3 oz.	300
Bologna, 2 oz.	580
Ham, lean, roasted, 3 oz.	1,020
Other	
Salad dressing, 1 tbsp.	75–220
Ketchup, mustard, steak sauce, 1 tbsp.	130–230
Soy sauce, 1 tbsp.	1,030
Salt, 1 tsp.	2,000
Dill pickle, 1 medium	930
Potato chips, salted, 1 oz.	130
Corn chips, salted, 1 oz.	235
Peanuts, roasted in oil, salted, 1 oz.	120

Source: USDA Food Guide Pyramid. April 1992. *Home and Garden Bulletin* (249), 18.

FIGURE 2-2. Sample of a Nutritional Label

NUTRITION FACTS

Serving Size 1/2 cup (114 g)	Servings per container 4

Amount Per Serving	
Calories 250	Calories from Fat 135
	% Daily Value*
Total Fat 15g	23%
Saturated fat 7g	35%
Cholesterol 20mg	7%
Sodium 565	24%
Total Carbohydrate 30g	10%
Dietary Fiber 5g	20%
Sugars 0g	
Protein 5g	

Vitamin A	6%	Vitamin C	2%
Calcium	10%	Iron	5%

*Percent Daily Values are based on a 2,000 calorie diet. Your daily values may be higher or lower depending on your calorie needs:

	Calories	2,000	2,500
Total fat	less than	65g	80g
Sat Fat	less than	20g	25g
Cholesterol	less than	300mg	300mg
Sodium	less than	2,400mg	2,400mg
Total Carbohydrate		300g	375g
Fiber		25g	30g

Calories per gram:		
Fat 9	Carbohydrates 4	Protein 4

Standardized serving sizes. Sizes will be standardized based on food consumption surveys. Formerly, a company could reduce the quantity of fat in a food by reducing a serving size.

Saturated fat. While the total amount of fat from calories should be no more than 30%, saturated fat should be no more than 10%, or only one-third of the total fat intake.

Dietary fiber. Americans are advised to increase their daily intake of fiber from a current average of 10–12 grams to about 20 grams. This component on the label will allow a person to choose more fiber-rich foods.

Percent daily values. Based on what experts determine to be 100% of fat, saturated fat, cholesterol, sodium, carbohydrate, and fiber that should be consumed per day, the numbers indicate the percentage contributed by a single serving of a food. Using 2,000 calories per day as a standard, the 100% figure for each nutrient is:

- Sodium—no more than 2,400 mg/day
- Cholesterol—no more than 300 mg/day
- Vitamins and minerals—not based on kcal intake and vary for each vitamin or mineral
- Total fat—no more than 30% of kcal consumed
- Total carbohydrate—60% of total kcal
- Fiber—11.5 g/1,000 kcal
- Protein—10% of total kcal

Nutrition Information Not Included on the New Labels

The following are examples of nutritional information that does not have to be included on the new food labels.

Quantities of the B vitamins—thiamin, riboflavin, and niacin. Unless the manufacturer makes a claim about the above-mentioned nutrients, no information will be provided.

Nutrition information on small packages. Packages smaller than 12 square inches (a small candy bar) do not have to provide nutrition information.

Fat levels in children's foods. Since fat is important during the first few years of life to ensure adequate growth and development, food labels for children under age 2 may not carry information related to calories from fat and saturated fat, in order to prevent parents from thinking that infants and toddlers should restrict fat intake.

Nutrition information about food served in restaurants. Nutrition labeling is exempt for food served in restaurants, cafeterias, and airplanes.

Information on how to eat a balanced diet. The labels can only give so much information; therefore, guidelines for a balanced nutritious diet will have to be acquired elsewhere. For examples, see the Food Guide Pyramid (pp. 19–29) or the Exchange System (pp. 31-34).

Standardized Definitions of Label Terms

Under the new labeling laws, terms such as *light* or *low fat* will have standardized definitions. Examples are:

Free. Indicates that a product contains none or only neglible amounts of fat, saturated fat, cholesterol, sodium, sugar, and/or calories.

Low. The term *low* along with *fat, saturated fat, cholesterol, sodium, sugar,* and/or *kcal.*

- Low fat—3 g or less per serving
- Low saturated fat—no more than 1 g per serving
- Low sodium—fewer than 140 mg per serving
- Very low sodium—fewer than 35 mg per serving
- Low cholesterol—fewer than 20 mg per serving
- Low calorie—40 calories or fewer per serving; for meals and main dishes the product contains 120 calories or fewer per 100 g.

Lean and extra lean. These terms describe the fat content of meats, poultry, seafood, and game meats.

- Lean—fewer than 10 g of fat, fewer than 4 g of saturated fat, and fewer than 95 mg of cholesterol per serving.
- Extra lean—fewer than 5 g of fat, fewer than 2 g of saturated fat, and fewer than 95 mg of cholesterol per serving.

High. A serving of food contains 20% or more of the Daily Value for a particular nutrient.

Good source. A serving supplies 10–19% of the Daily Value for a particular nutrient.

Reduced. A product has been nutritionally altered and contains 25% less of a nutrient (such as fat) than the regular product.

Less or fewer. A food contains 25% less of a nutrient than a comparable food.

Light in sodium. Sodium is reduced 50% in a food.

Light (when used in reference to a meal or main dish). The meal is 50% lower in calories or sodium than the regular meal.

More. A serving of food contains at least 10% or more of the Daily Value.

REFERENCES

1. FDA Backgrounder: The new food label. (Dec. 10, 1992.) Food and Drug Administration, BG92-4.
2. Couig, M. P. 1993. The new food label. *American Journal of Nursing, 93*(2), 68–71.

Vegetarian Diets

Some people choose to follow a vegetarian diet for religious reasons, health concerns, environmental considerations, humanitarian issues, or economic or political reasons. There are two major classes of vegetarians (approximately four other variations exist):

vegan Pure vegetarian diet that uses no animal or dairy products.

lacto-ovo vegetarian A vegan diet that includes milk, eggs, and other dairy products.

Vegan (*pure vegetarian*). A strict vegetarian diet, using no animal or dairy products. This diet may be inadequate in vitamins B_{12} and D, riboflavin, calcium, iron, and zinc. Supplements of each are recommended.

Lacto-ovo vegetarian (*lacto-milk, ovo-egg*). This diet is a vegan diet, except that milk, eggs, and other dairy products are included. This diet may be inadequate in iron, since meats are a good source of iron.

Disadvantages of Vegetarian Diets

As indicated above, vegetarian diets can be deficient in certain nutrients. A large quantity of food must be consumed in vegetarian diets in order to meet calorie needs and can be difficult for some people to do, especially children. A person needs to know how to combine protein foods in order to obtain all of the essential amino acids, a process known as **complementary protein supplementation** (discussed in Chapter 5).

complementary protein supplementation A strategy that involves eating two or more foods that are complementary to each other in amino acids.

Advantages of Vegetarian Diets

While there are several disadvantages to a vegetarian diet, there also are some advantages, such as these:

It increases fiber. Vegetables are high in fiber compared to meat, which is eliminated in this diet. Increased fiber aids in bowel movements and possibly helps to prevent problems like **diverticulitis** and colon cancer.

diverticulitis Inflammation of diverticuli (outpouching of the colon lining) (see Chapter 16).

It decreases daily caloric intake. Vegetables tend to be low in calories; therefore, a vegetarian diet should be beneficial to people on a low-kilocalories weight-loss diet.

It decreases total fat, saturated fat, and cholesterol. Vegetables are low in fat and cholesterol compared to meat. This diet can be beneficial to people who have **hyperlipidemia** (elevated level of lipids in blood) and decreases the chances of developing **atherosclerosis.**

hyperlipidemia Elevated level of lipids in the blood (see Chapter 18).

atherosclerosis Accumulation of fatty plaques within medium-sized and large arteries (see Chapter 18).

It provides a more economical source of protein than meat. For some societies, especially those of developing countries, meat is not readily available and can be very expensive. A vegetarian diet provides an affordable source of protein; however, it lacks some essential nutrients, and protein supplementation has to be practiced to overcome this deficiency.[2]

The Food Exchange System

The Food Exchange System is important in planning a nutritious diet, since two components, nutrient density and balance, are achieved when the guide is utilized. Essentially, the Food Exchange System can be used to select foods that are high in nutrient content but low in **kilocalories.** In order to make these calculations, one needs to know that:

kilocalorie (kcal) A unit of energy measurement that is calculated and expressed in relation to nutrition. A *calorie* is often called a *small calorie*, since 1,000 small calories equal 1 kilocalorie. Although it is not technically correct, some nutritional books and consumer literature refer to energy units in food as calories. To avoid confusion between the small physical calorie and the nutritional calorie, the unit *kcal* will be used throughout this book.

$$1 \text{ g of carbohydrate} = 4 \text{ kcal}$$
$$1 \text{ g of lipid (fat)} = 9 \text{ kcal}$$
$$1 \text{ g of protein} = 4 \text{ kcal}$$

As an example, compare whole milk with skim or nonfat milk:

	Carbohydrate (g)	Protein (g)	Fat (g)	Total kcal
Whole milk	12	8	8	150
Skim milk	12	8	Trace	90

As we can see, whole milk and skim milk contain the same amounts of carbohydrate and proteins; however, whole milk also contains 8 g of fat, which contributes 60 kcal more than skim milk. Therefore, skim milk is a better nutrient density choice than whole milk.

In order to understand how the Food Exchange System allows one to choose foods high in nutrient density, a person must know the following important points about the system:

- Foods in the food guide pyramid are separated into six exchange lists (see Table 2-5).
- Each list consists of foods of specific serving sizes that are equal in kilocalories, protein, fat, and carbohydrate (see Appendix A).

Some important points about each exchange list are as follows:

1. Starch/bread List. This list includes cereals/grains/pasta, dried beans/peas/lentils, starchy vegetables, and bread. Whole-grain products average about 2 grams of fiber per serving. Some foods are higher in fiber and those in Appendix A that contain 3 or more grams of fiber per serving are identified with the fiber symbol. (See Appendix A for specific details of this list.)
2. Meat List. Each serving of meat and substitutes on this list contains about 7 grams of protein. The amount of fat and number of calories varies, depending on what kind of meat or substitute you choose. The list is divided into three parts based on the amount of fat and calories. (See Appendix A for details.)

TABLE 2-5 THE SIX EXCHANGE LISTS

Exchange List	Carbohydrate (grams)	Protein (grams)	Fat (grams)	Calories
Starch/bread	15	3	Trace	80
Meat				
Lean	—	7	3	55
Medium-fat	—	7	5	75
High-fat	—	7	8	100
Vegetable	5	2	—	25
Fruit	15	—	—	60
Milk				
Skim	12	8	Trace	90
Lowfat	12	8	5	120
Whole	12	8	8	150
Fat	—	—	5	45

3. Vegetable List. Vegetables on this list include only low-calorie vegetables; therefore, higher calorie vegetables (corn, potatoes, and lima beans) are not included on this list but rather on the bread list. Vegetables contain 2–3 grams of dietary fiber. Vegetables that contain 400 mg of sodium per serving are identified with a special symbol. (See Appendix A for details.)

4. Fruit List. Each item on this list contains about 15 grams of carbohydrates and 60 calories. Fresh, frozen, and dry fruits have about 2 grams of fiber per serving. Fruits that have 3 or more grams of fiber per serving have a special symbol. Fruit juices have little dietary fiber. (See Appendix A for details.)

5. Milk List. Each serving of milk or milk product contains about 12 grams of carbohydrate and 8 grams of protein. The amount of fat in milk varies and is the basis for the three categories: skim/very low fat milk, lowfat milk, and whole milk. (See Appendix A for details.)

6. Fat List. Each serving on the fat list contains about 5 grams of fat and 45 calories. The foods on the fat list contain mostly fat, although some items may also contain a small amount of protein. (See Appendix A for details.)

Use of the Food Exchange System to Achieve Balance

The Food Exchange System can be used to achieve the balance component of a nutritious diet. Previously, it was stated that a balanced diet is one that distributes kilocalories among fat, protein, and carbohydrate in the following proportions:

fat: 30% of total kilocalories
carbohydrate: 55–60% of total kilocalories
protein: 10–15% of total kilocalories

Since the number of grams of carbohydrate, fat, and protein within each food exchange is known, it can then be calculated how many grams and kilocalories are present in a meal. Also, meals can be planned to achieve these or modified percentages of fat, carbohydrate, and protein.

An example of a meal in which these calculations can be made is shown in Table 2-6. The calculations for the foods in Table 2-6 are explained below.

1. Total kilocalories = 460
2. Calculations of carbohydrate
   a. Total grams of carbohydrate = 32
   b. Total kilocalories due to carbohydrate = $\dfrac{32\,g}{1} \times \dfrac{4 \text{ kcal}}{g} = 128 \text{ kcal}$

      (1g = 4 kcal)
   c. Percentage of total kilocalories due to carbohydrate = $\dfrac{128 \text{ kcal}}{460 \text{ kcal}} \times$

      100 = 28%
3. Calculation of fat
   a. Total grams of fat = 17
   b. Total kilocalories due to fat = $\dfrac{17\,g}{1} \times \dfrac{9 \text{ kcal}}{g} = 153 \text{ kcal}$

      (1g = 9 kcal)
   c. Percentage of total kilocalories due to fat = $\dfrac{153 \text{ kcal}}{460 \text{ kcal}} \times 100 =$

      33%

TABLE 2-6

	Exchange(s)	Carbohydrate (g)	Fat (g)	Protein (g)	Kcal
1 cup skim milk	milk	12	Trace	8	90
½ cup green beans	vegetable	5	0	2	25
1 small potato	bread	15	Trace	3	80
1 pat margarine	fat	0	5	0	45
4 oz fish	4 meat (lean)	0	12	28	220 (4 × 55)
		32	17	41	460

Calculating the total Kcal value for a meal or a diet will be done by adding up the kcal for each exchange or multiples of exchanges, as shown above. This method will be used throughout the text.

4. Calculations of protein
   a. Total grams of protein = 41
   b. Total kilocalories due to protein = $\dfrac{41\cancel{g}}{1} \times \dfrac{4 \text{ kcal}}{\cancel{g}} = 164 \text{ kcal}$

   (1g = 4 kcal)

   c. Percentage of total kilocalories due to protein = $\dfrac{164 \text{ kcal}}{460 \text{ kcal}} \times$ 100 = 36%

5. Summary of calculations

   The meal in Table 2-6 is low in carbohydrates, since 28% of the total kilocalories are due to carbohydrates compared to 55–60%. The meal is slightly high in fat, since 33% of the total kilocalories are due to fat compared to 30%. The meal is quite high in protein, since 36% of the total kilocalories are due to protein compared to 10–15%.

This meal is not exactly balanced, but the next two meals can be planned so that carbohydrates are increased (possibly by including fruits) and proteins are decreased (possibly by decreasing the serving sizes of high-protein foods) to achieve the recommended percentages.

Health professionals use the Food Exchange System in planning diets for hospitalized patients (see the Clinical Application "Planning a Hospital Diet Using the Food Exchange System", page 35).

The fourth component of a nutritious diet is variety. People should eat a variety of foods rather than the same ones each day. A variety of foods enables a person to achieve adequacy more easily than by consuming only a few foods. The adherence of hospital patients to their diets is increased if a variety of foods are served. Most foods contain some additives, some of which can be toxic at high levels; by eating a variety of foods, the possibility of developing a toxic condition is reduced.

RECOMMENDED DIETARY ALLOWANCES (RDAs)

Recommended Dietary Allowances (RDAs)
Recommended allowances of certain nutrients that are established by the Food and Nutrition Board of the National Academy of Sciences–National Research Council (NAS–NRC).

Nutritionists and health professionals frequently refer to **Recommended Dietary Allowance (RDA)** values when planning an adequate diet. The recommendations are established by the Food and Nutrition Board of the National Academy of Sciences–National Research Council (NAS–NRC) and published by the U.S. government.[3] Approximately every 5 years, the Committee on RDA meets to reexamine and revise these recommendations on the basis of new evidence regarding people's nutrient needs. The most recent recommendations were published in 1989 (see inside front cover).

Clinical Application: Planning a Hospital Diet Using the Food Exchange System

In planning a diet for a hospitalized patient, health professionals utilize the Food Exchange System. First, the total kilocalories for a day is established; then the percentage of protein, carbohydrate, and fat that is to make up the total kilocalories is calculated. The amount of carbohydrate, fat, and protein in grams can then be determined. A calculation of the total number of exchanges for each list necessary to meet the above requirements has to be made. Then the distribution of these exchanges into actual recommended foods for breakfast, noon, evening, and bedtime meals is planned.

The following example illustrates these points. The patient has been prescribed a 1,500 kcal/day diet.

15% protein	225 kcal	56 g	$4 \frac{kcal}{g}$
55% carbohydrate	825 kcal	206 g	$4 \frac{kcal}{g}$
30% fat	450 kcal	50 g	$9 \frac{kcal}{g}$

Exchange List	Number of Exchanges
1. Milk, skim	2
2. Vegetable	4
3. Fruit	7
4. Bread (starch)	4
5. Meat	3
6. Fat	7

Exchange	Foods
Breakfast	
1 Milk (skim) exchange	1 cup skim milk
2 fruit exchange	1 banana
1 Bread (starch) exchange	1 slice whole wheat bread
1 Meat exchange (med.-fat)	1 poached egg
2 Fat exchange	2 tsp margarine

Noon

<u>0</u> Milk (skim) exchange	
<u>2</u> Vegetable exchange	1 whole tomato
	2 medium carrots
<u>2</u> Fruit exchange	½ cantaloupe
<u>1</u> Bread exchange	1 slice whole wheat bread
<u>1</u> Meat exchange (lean)	1 oz white tuna
<u>3</u> Fat exchange	3 tsp. mayonnaise

Evening

<u>0</u> Milk exchange	
<u>2</u> Vegetable exchange	2 cups broccoli
<u>1</u> Fruit exchange	1 small apple
<u>1</u> Bread exchange	1 small baked potato
<u>1</u> Meat exchange (lean)	1 oz lean roast beef
<u>2</u> Fat exchange	2 tsp margarine

Bedtime Snack

<u>1</u> Milk exchange	1 cup skim milk
<u>2</u> Fruit exchange	1 banana
<u>1</u> Bread exchange	1 serving all-bran cereal

Nutrients Recommended and Division of RDA into Age and Sex Groups

The main RDA table contains recommendations for protein, 11 vitamins, and 7 minerals. In addition to the main table, there is the Estimated Safe and Adequate Daily Dietary Intake (ESADDI) table (see inside back cover) of recommended values for more vitamins and minerals. These nutrients are listed in a separate table, since there is less information on which to base the allowances, and the figures are in the form of ranges of recommended intakes.

The recommendations are made for different groups—infants, children, men, women, and pregnant and lactating women. Each grouping is further subdivided into age groups.

Important points about the RDAs are as follows:

- They are recommendations, not requirements.
- They include a substantial margin of safety; therefore, two-thirds of the RDA is often deemed adequate, except for energy.
- The recommendations are for healthy people only; therefore, for ill people, the values could be higher or lower.
- There is a recommendation for protein but not for carbohydrate and fat.

U.S. RDAs

U.S. RDAs Nutrient recommendations established by the U.S. Food and Drug Administration (FDA) that are used as a standard for nutritional labeling.

The **U.S. RDAs** are used as a standard for nutritional labeling. For example, a food label on a cereal box might state that one serving provides about 25% of the U.S. RDA for iron.

There are four different sets of U.S. RDAs:

- Baby food set. These recommendations are for infants 12 months of age or under and are used with baby foods.
- Junior food set. These recommendations are for children between the ages of 1 and 4 years and are used with junior foods.
- Pregnant and lactating women. These recommendations are for increases in certain nutrients for women in these special situations.
- Adults and children over the age of 4. This is the set that is used on the majority of food labels that a person reads.

Although the 1980 revised RDA tables included a few changes for certain nutrients, the rest of the recommendations are based on 1968 RDAs. The U.S. RDA values were chosen from among the highest amounts recommended for each nutrient in the 1968 RDA table. Therefore, most of the U.S. RDA values are the same as the RDAs for a man, since they have the greatest nutrient requirements of any group. The exceptions to this statement are iron, thiamin, niacin, iodine, and magnesium. Women have a greater need for iron than men and, as a result, the woman's RDA for iron is used for the U.S. RDA. The RDAs for thiamin, niacin, iodine, and magnesium are based on the needs of an adolescent boy, since they are even higher than adult RDAs.

The highest RDA values are used for each nutrient to ensure that the nutrient needs of all persons are met. Therefore, when a person reads that a label provides 100% of the U.S. RDA for iron, whether the person is a 7-year-old boy or a 60-year-old woman, he or she can be assured that the need for iron is being met for that age group.

SUMMARY

- Four components of a nutritious diet: adequacy, nutrient density, balance, and variety.
- The five food groups in the Food Guide Pyramid are as follows: bread, 6–11 servings; vegetable, 3–5 servings; fruit, 2–4 servings; milk, 2–3 servings; meat, 2–3 servings.
- The differences between a vegan and lacto-ovo vegetarian diet are that a vegan diet is strictly vegetables whereas lacto-ovo diet includes eggs and milk.
- Three possible deficiencies in a vegetarian diet are vitamins B_{12} and D, and riboflavin.
- Four advantages of a vegetarian diet are an increase in fiber, a decrease in daily kcal intake, a decrease in total fat, and utilization of a more economical source of protein.
- The six exchange lists and the g of carbohydrate, protein, and fat for each are as follows: starch—15, 3, 0; meat—0, 7, 3; vegetable—5, 2, 0; fruit—15, 0, 0; milk—12, 8, 0; fat—0, 0, 5.
- RDAs are distinguished from U.S. RDAs by the fact that RDAs are recommendations for nutrients utilized by health professionals in planning nutritional diets; U.S. RDAs are used as standards for nutritional labeling and the values are chosen from the highest amount recommended for each nutrient in the RDA table.
- The nutrients that have established RDA values are protein, vitamin A, vitamin D, vitamin E, ascorbic acid, folacin, niacin, riboflavin, thiamin, vitamin B_{12}, vitamin B_6, calcium, phosphorus, iodine, magnesium, and zinc.

REVIEW QUESTIONS

True (A) or False (B)

1. The four components of a nutritious diet are adequacy, nutrient density, balance, and high fiber. (F)
2. An adequate diet is defined as a diet that is composed of foods that provide all of the essential nutrients and calories in the proper amounts. (T)
3. A balanced diet is one that distributes daily kilocalories in the following proportions: fat 55–60%, carbohydrate 30%, and protein 10–15%. (F)
4. Two diet planning guides that help people achieve a nutritious diet are the Food Guide Pyramid and the Cambridge Diet. (F)

5. The Food Guide Pyramid includes milk, meat, fruits and vegetable, and bread/cereal. (A)(T)
6. The two most common vegetarian diets are vegan and lacto-ovo vegetarian. (A)(T)
7. The only disadvantage of vegetarian diets is that a person does not receive an adequate amount of kilocalories without consuming a large amount of food. (F)
8. The Food Exchange System is most valuable in achieving adequacy. (F)
9. Any food on any exchange list can be exchanged for any food on any other list. (F)
10. A user of the Food Exchange System should think of skim milk as milk and whole milk as milk plus 8 g fat. (T)
11. Based upon the Food Exchange System, all meats are in the same group. (F)
12. If a person consumes 2,000 kcal/day, approximately 55–60%, or 1,100–1,200 kcal, should come from carbohydrate. (T)
13. RDA values are established for energy (kcal), protein, (g), vitamins (10), and minerals (6). (F)
14. RDAs are very valuable for planning therapeutic diets. (F)
15. RDAs are not expressed in group by age, sex, and weight. (F)
16. U.S. RDAs differ from RDAs in that they appear on food labels. (T)
17. Each U.S. RDA for persons aged 4 years or older was chosen from the highest amount for each RDA. (T)

Matching

These questions and answers are based on information in Table 2-5. Match each exchange on the left with nutritional information on the right.

Exchange List		Carbohydrate (g)	Protein (g)	Fat (g)	Energy (kcal)
18. Milk	A.	15	0	0	60
19. Vegetable	B.	0	7	3	55
20. Fruit	C.	15	3	Trace	80
21. Bread	D.	12	8	Trace	90
22. Meat	E.	5	2	0	25

Multiple Choice

Questions 23–28 are based on the following meal. An example of how to make the calculations necessary to answer these questions is given in Table 2-6. The values for the foods below are found in Appendix A.

½ cup spinach
1 cup whole milk
1 small potato
1 pat margarine
6 oz fish

23. The total kilocalories for the meal are _____.
    (See Table 2-6, p. 33 on how to calculate kcal for a meal.)
    A. 550
    B. 1,040
    C. 630
    D. 440
24. The total grams of carbohydrate in the above meal are _____.
    A. 32
    B. 17
    C. 25
    D. 62
25. The total grams of fat in the above meal are _____.
    A. 17
    B. 22
    C. 35
    D. 31
26. The total grams of protein in the above meal are _____.
    A. 40
    B. 55
    C. 45
    D. 65
27. The percentages of kilocalories due to carbohydrate (C), fat (F), and protein (P) in the above meal are:
    A. C—20%
       F—44%
       P—34%
    B. C—46%
       F—20%
       P—34%
28. In evaluating the balance of the meal, one could say that it is:
    A. about normal in carbohydrate, normal in fat, and high in protein.
    B. low in carbohydrate, high in fat, and high in protein.

Completion

29. Name and define the four components of a nutritious diet.
30. Give the grams of carbohydrate, protein, fat, and kilocalories for one exchange on each of the six lists.
31. Distinguish between RDAs and U.S. RDAs.

CRITICAL THINKING CHALLENGE

1. Use the information on the Food Guide Pyramid and analyze the meals below to determine how many servings of each food group are present.

   Breakfast
   3/4 cup citrus juice
   1 egg
   1 slice toast
   1 tsp butter
   1 tbsp jelly

   Lunch
   tuna fish sandwich (2 slices bread + 1 meat serving)
   1 apple
   2 pickles
   1 glass skim milk

   Dinner
   2 oz. roast beef
   1/4 cup gravy
   1 cup mashed potatoes
   1/2 cup carrots
   1 glass skim milk
   1 dinner roll

   a. Do these three meals provide the recommended range of servings from each of the food groups? Make recommendations to correct any deficiencies.
2. Use the number of exchanges below to calculate the following:

Exchange	# of Exchanges
Starch/bread	9
Meat (lean)	11

Exchange	# of Exchanges
Vegetable	5
Fruit	7
Milk (skim)	2
Fat	2

   a. total calories for all exchanges (See Table 2-6, p. 33, as to how to calculate kcal for all the exchanges.)
   b. total grams of carbohydrates
   c. total grams of lipids
   d. total grams of proteins
   e. percent of total calories supplied by carbohydrates
   f. percent of total calories supplied by lipids
   g. percent of total calories supplied by proteins
3. Your client has stated that he is aware of the four components of a nutritious diet. Which of the following statements indicates a need for additional teaching?
   a. "I know that I must include all the essential nutrients to meet my energy needs."
   b. "I always try to keep my meals colorful."
   c. "Sometimes I have trouble getting the right distribution of fat, protein, and carbohydrates during the day's meals."
   d. "Since I started using the exchange list I don't find it difficult to select foods of similar nutrient value."

REVIEW QUESTIONS FOR NCLEX

Situation. A health professional was describing and defining to a client the four components of a nutritious diet—adequacy, nutrient density, balance, and variety.

1. In a nutritious diet, adequacy is the component that provides _____.
   A. foods from all five food groups in the recommended amounts
   B. two servings from each of the exchange groups
   C. foods low in fat and cholesterol but also high in protein

   D. all of the essential nutrients and calories in the proper amounts
2. In a nutritious diet, nutrient density is one that provides _____.
   A. foods that have a high level of nutrients with a low level of kcal
   B. the number of kcal a person needs to grow and gain weight
   C. kcal according to a person's needs to lose weight
   D. kcal from carbohydrates, and proteins but none from fat
3. Balance, in a nutritious diet, is the component that provides _____.
   A. foods in proper amounts from each of the five food groups
   B. foods in proper amounts from the five food groups and exchange groups
   C. distribution of daily kcal among fat, protein, and carbohydrate in a certain ratio
   D. low kcal diet from low cholesterol and fat foods
4. Variety, in a nutritious diet, is the component that provides _____.
   A. a variety of foods in the daily diet
   B. foods from each of the five foods groups
   C. foods from each of the five exchange groups
   D. foods low in fat and cholesterol from each exchange group

REFERENCES

1. Cronin, F. J., Shaw, A. M., Krebs-Smith, S. M. (1987). Developing a food guidance system to implement the dietary guidelines. *Journal of Nutrition Education, 19,* 281–302.
2. ADA Reports. (1988). Position of the American Dietetic Association: Vegetarian diets. *Journal of the American Dietetic Association, 88,* 351–355.
3. Food and Nutrition Board, Committee on Recommended Allowances. (1989). *Recommended dietary allowances* (10th ed.). Washington, DC: National Academy of Sciences.

3

CARBOHYDRATES

Upon completion of this chapter, you should be able to:

1. List the names of the monosaccharides commonly found in food.
2. Describe a clinical application of glucose.
3. List the disaccharides found in foods and their monosaccharide components.
4. State where glycogen is stored and its function.
5. Identify the polysaccharide composing fiber and distinguish between insoluble and soluble fiber.
6. Describe two functions of fiber.
7. List the food groups rich in fiber together with the amount in a serving.
8. Describe two functions of carbohydrates.
9. Describe the digestion of starch in terms of location, enzymes, and products.
10. List the two phases of metabolism.
11. Describe glycolysis.
12. Describe a citric acid cycle.
13. Describe electron transport system.
14. Differentiate between glycogenesis and glycogenolysis, and give the functions of each process.
15. Compare the current U.S. diet with the recommended diet in regard to percentages of polysaccharides and disaccharides (sugar).
16. Give the type(s) and grams of carbohydrates in each of the six exchange lists.

INTRODUCTION

diabetes mellitus Disease of the pancreas that causes inadequate secretion of insulin, thereby resulting in an inability to regulate blood glucose level normally (see Chapter 15).

galactosemia A genetic disease in which galactose is not properly metabolized due to the lack of an enzyme.

Carbohydrates are important for both the normal functioning of the body and their possible cause–effect relationship with certain disorders. Health professionals need a knowledge of carbohydrates, their functions, metabolism, and food sources to help prevent diseases, as well as to treat **diabetes mellitus** and inborn errors of carbohydrate metabolism such as **galactosemia.** A knowledge of carbohydrates is also essential in order for a health professional to educate a patient effectively about quick-weight-loss fad diets.

CHEMISTRY OF CARBOHYDRATES

carbohydrate Organic compound composed of carbon, hydrogen, and oxygen, with a 2:1 ratio of hydrogen to oxygen atoms.

Each **carbohydrate** molecule is composed of three basic atoms: carbon (C), hydrogen (H), and oxygen (O). The hydrogen and oxygen atoms occur in the same 2:1 ratio as water.

For example:

$$C_6H_{12}O_6\text{—glucose}$$
$$C_{12}H_{22}O_{11}\text{—sucrose}$$

Health professionals frequently write the word *carbohydrate* in a shorthand way as CHO; however, it is more accurate to write it as CH_2O due to the 2:1 ratio of hydrogen to oxygen.

CARBOHYDRATES FOUND IN FOODS

saccharide Sugar unit.

The carbohydrates found in foods are divided into three classes according to the number of **saccharides** composing the molecule:

monosaccharide Simple sugar.

Monosaccharide. Each molecule in this class is composed of a simple sugar.

disaccharide Double sugar.

Disaccharides. Two monosaccharides bonded together compose each disaccharide molecule.

polysaccharide Complex sugar.

Polysaccharides. These complex molecules are composed of many monosaccharides bonded together.

Monosaccharides (Simple Sugars, $C_6H_{12}O_6$)

Three monosaccharides are commonly found in food: glucose, galactose, and fructose (see Fig. 3-1). Notice that they all have the same chemical formula, $C_6H_{12}O_6$, but differ slightly in the geometrical arrangement of their atoms. This class of carbohydrate is absorbed into the blood from the intestines as a result of their small size. Table 3-1 summarizes information about carbohydrates.

Glucose

Glucose is found free in foods such as honey and fruits. It is the major chemical building block of disaccharides and polysaccharides and is transported by the blood to the cells, where it is oxidized for energy. Glucose is present in the blood in a concentration of 70–120 mg/dl.* (See the Clinical Application "Clinical Importance of Glucose.")

Galactose

Galactose (Fig. 3-1) is not found in nature as a monosaccharide, but rather as a part of the disaccharide, *lactose* (Fig. 3-2). Lactose is broken down into glucose and galactose; the latter is then converted to glucose by the liver (see Fig. 3-3).

Milk is the primary food source of galactose. Mammary tissue in human breasts converts glucose to galactose and then synthesizes lactose. The presence of galactose in milk is a dietary planning problem for children who have galactosemia (see the Clinical Application "Clinical Importance of Disaccharides").

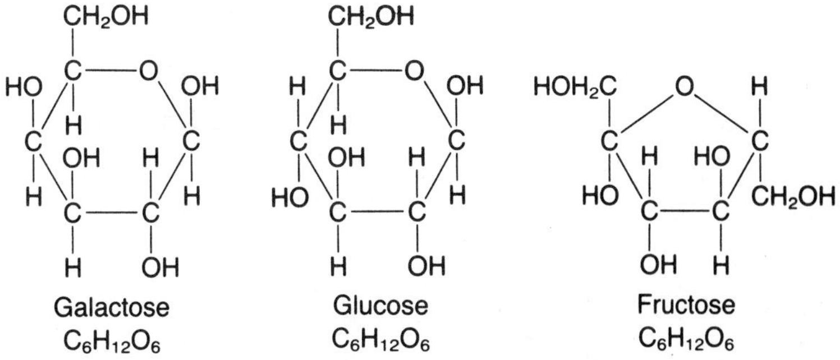

FIGURE 3-1 The three monosaccharides commonly found in food.

*Note: dl (deciliter) (*deci:* one-tenth); a deciliter is one-tenth of a liter, or 100 ml.

TABLE 3-1 SUMMARY OF INFORMATION ABOUT CARBOHYDRATES

Class	Composition	Food Sources	Comments
Monosaccharide ($C_6H_{12}O_6$)			
Glucose (Dextrose)		Found free in honey and fruits	Important as a primary source of energy; used as carbohydrate source in IVs
Galactose		Not found free in nature; found in human breast milk	Galactosemia, the inability to digest galactose, is an inherited trait
Fructose		Fruits and honey	Sweetest-tasting of the monosaccharides
Disaccharide ($C_{12}H_{22}O_{11}$)			
Sucrose	Glucose and fructose	Found naturally in sugar cane, maple syrup, bananas, green peas, and sweet potatoes	Commonly called *table sugar;* found in many convenience and fast foods
Lactose	Glucose and galactose	Milk is the main food source	Main source of carbohydrate for infants; some infants and adults develop the inability to digest lactose
Maltose	Glucose and glucose	Not found free in nature	Used in candy flavor and brewing beer
Polysaccharide ($(C_6H_{10}O_5)_n$)			
Glycogen	Many glucose molecules	Not found in foods	Synthesized in liver and muscles; important as a reserve source of blood glucose
Cellulose	Many glucose molecules	Found in many vegetables	Human body cannot digest it due to inability to synthesize enzymes needed for its digestion; important to the body in increasing motility, attracting water into intestines, and possibly preventing certain health conditions
Starch	Many glucose molecules	Plant seeds, cereal grains, and some vegetables	Major source of carbohydrate in many countries; for example, corn and rice

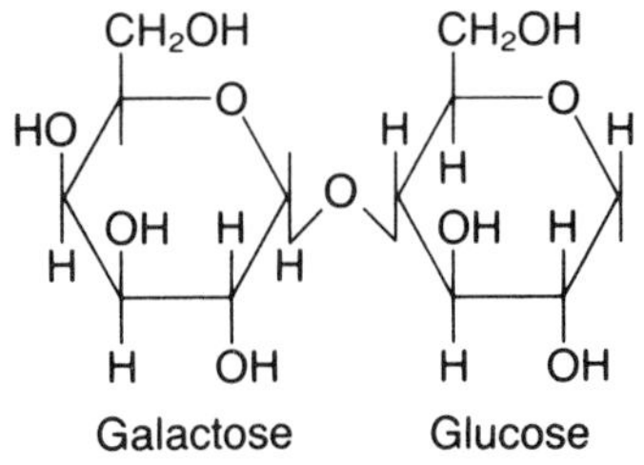

Galactose   Glucose

LACTOSE

FIGURE 3-2   Lactose is composed of galactose and glucose.

Clinical Application: Clinical Importance of Glucose

Some clinical conditions can be helped by the use of certain monosaccharides; other conditions require regulation and monitoring of the kinds and amounts of simple sugars. An example will be presented here, with more details presented in Part 3.

Use of Glucose (Dextrose) in Intravenous Therapy

Many clinical conditions (for example, inability to ingest fluids orally or severe burns, in which patients lose large amounts of fluids) require that a patient be given fluids directly into the veins or *intravenous (IV) therapy.* The most common type of IV contains dextrose (glucose used by hospitals) in a 5% concentration. It is commonly referred to as *D-5-W.* Each liter (1,000 ml) of 5% IV fluid provides only about 170 kcal. (See Chapter 14 for the kilocalorie values of dextrose infused parenterally.)

The reason why dextrose (a monosaccharide) is used in IVs instead of sucrose (a disaccharide) is that glucose is in a form that can be readily absorbed into the body's cells. Sucrose (a disaccharide) must undergo digestion before glucose and fructose can be absorbed.

Fructose

fructose   Fruit sugar.

Fructose (Fig. 3-1) is found in many fruits as well as in honey. It is also a component of sucrose (see Fig. 3-4). Fructose can be absorbed into the blood from food, but the majority of it is converted to glucose in the liver (see Fig. 3-3), most of which is stored in glycogen.[1] Fructose is the sweetest-tasting of the monosaccharides.

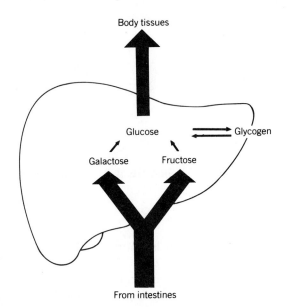

FIGURE 3-3   Conversion of galactose and fructose to glucose in the liver.

Disaccharides (Double Sugar, $C_{12}H_{22}O_{11}$)

A disaccharide is composed of two monosaccharides. Three disaccharides commonly found in foods are sucrose, lactose, and maltose.

Sucrose

sucrose   Table sugar.

Sucrose is composed of glucose and fructose (see Fig. 3-4). This disaccharide occurs naturally in foods such as sugar cane, maple syrup, ba-

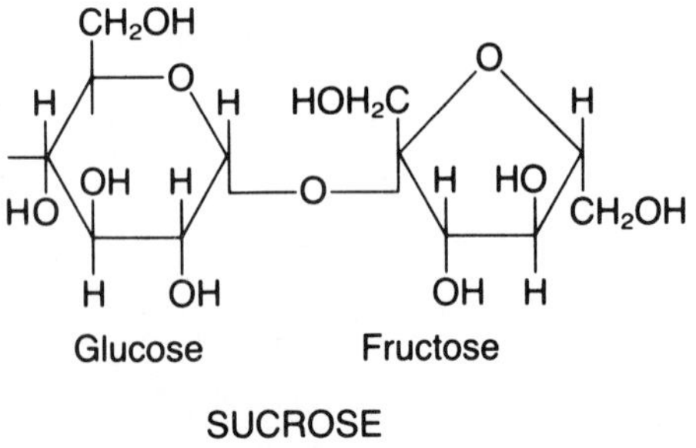

CH₂OH
H   O   H   HOH₂C   O
H   H
OH H   H   HO
HO   O   CH₂OH
H   OH   OH H
Glucose   Fructose

SUCROSE

FIGURE 3-4   Sucrose is a disaccharide composed of glucose and fructose.

Clinical Application: Clinical Importance of Disaccharides

Some human disorders and diets used in tube feedings are important in relation to certain disaccharides.

Lactose Intolerance

Some people lack the ability to produce the enzyme lactase, which is necessary to digest lactose into glucose and galactose. There are three types of lactose intolerances: congenital, primary, and secondary. Each of these types is discussed further in Chapter 16. This condition results in lactose not being digested, thereby passing intact into the intestines. The intestines then absorb large amounts of water, which causes bloating, abdominal discomfort, nausea, and vomiting.

Tube Feedings

Some hospitalized patients cannot ingest food through the mouth (for example, comatose patients or those with neck or facial surgery); therefore, they may require tube feeding. Usually the tube is inserted through the nasal openings down to the stomach. Liquid commercial formulas containing different carbohydrate sources are delivered through the tube.

---

nanas, green peas, and sweet potatoes. The sugar that is bought in supermarkets is sucrose that has been produced by purifying and granulating sugar cane and sugar beets. Many convenience and fast foods are prepared with sucrose, so that it comprises about 15–20% of the total calories in our daily food intake.

Lactose

lactose Milk sugar.

Lactose contains glucose and galactose bonded together (see Fig. 3-3). It is found in cow's milk and can be synthesized by women during lactation. Lactose in cow's milk is the energy source for bacteria that converts it to lactic acid which is the source of the taste in spoiled milk.

Newborn infants obtain the majority of their carbohydrates from lactose, since milk is their main food source. However, some children become unable to digest lactose at about 4 years of age and experience a variety of difficulties when they drink milk (see the Clinical Application "Clinical Importance of Disaccharides").

Maltose

maltose   Malt sugar.

Maltose is composed of two glucose molecules (see Fig. 3-5) and is not found naturally in foods. The maltose in beer is produced by the partial digestion of starch.

Maltose itself has no dietary significance in humans. After it is ingested, it undergoes digestion to release its two glucose molecules.

Polysaccharides (Complex Sugar $C_6H_{10}O_5)_n$

A polysaccharide is composed of many monosaccharides. The n in the above formula refers to the number of saccharide units composing the molecule; it varies from several hundred to over one-half million. Three polysaccharides will be discussed: glycogen, cellulose (fiber), and starch.

Glycogen

glycogen   Branched-chain polysaccharide composed of glucose molecules.

Glycogen (see Fig. 3-6) is synthesized and stored in the liver and skeletal muscles. Approximately 100 g of glycogen are stored in the liver and 200 g in skeletal muscle tissue.[2]

Glycogen is important as a source of glucose for the blood whenever the level drops too low. It can be quickly decomposed to glucose in time of need (details of this process are presented later in this chapter).

Cellulose

cellulose   Fiber

Cellulose is composed of many glucose molecules but is different from glycogen in that it is a straight-chain polysaccharide (see Fig. 3-7). It is found in plants, where it provides strength and support to cell walls.

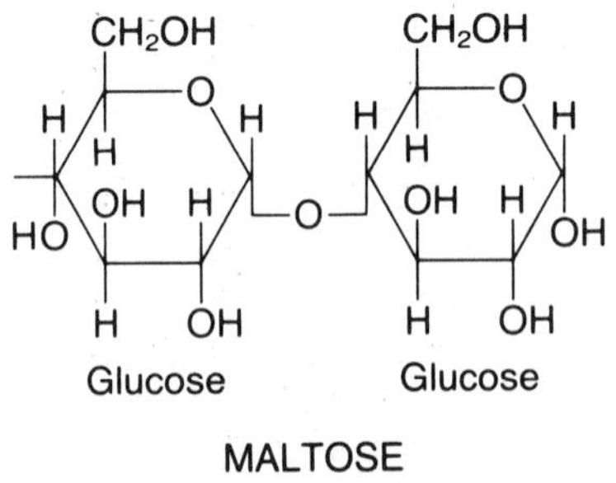

FIGURE 3-5 Two glucose molecules bonded together compose maltose.

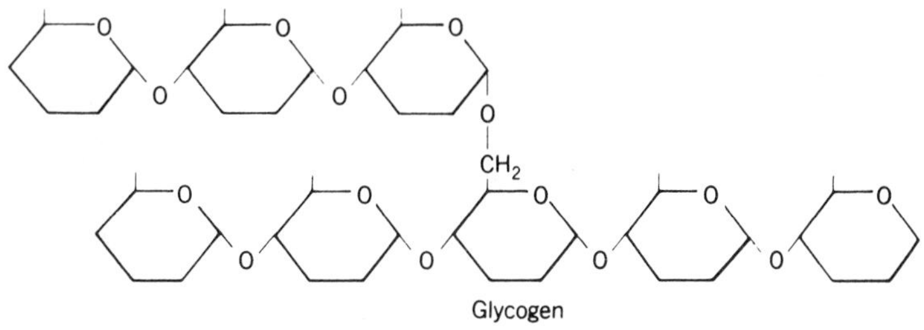

FIGURE 3-6 Glycogen is a branched chain polysaccharide composed of glucose molecules.

The human body does not synthesize any enzymes that will break down cellulose; therefore, it passes through the small intestine undigested. However, when fiber from fruits and vegetables reaches the large intestine, bacteria digest (see Fig. 3-8) or ferment these molecules. The end result is an increase in the bacterial mass, fatty acids, methane gas (or flatulence), and fiber residue.

dietary fiber Fiber resistant to the human digestive enzymes.

Dietary Fiber

Two types of fiber are commonly found in foods—insoluble fiber and soluble fiber.

Insoluble Fiber. This type of fiber holds water and is found in most whole grains and seeds. While the body cannot break down this type of carbohydrate, due to lack of enzymes, insoluble fiber does contribute to bulk and reduces constipation. However, this fiber does not have as many health benefits as soluble fiber.

Soluble Fiber. This type of fiber dissolves in water and results in the production of a gel. Food sources of this fiber are the pulp of fruits, vegetables, oat bran, and dried beans. Oat bran and oats are especially good

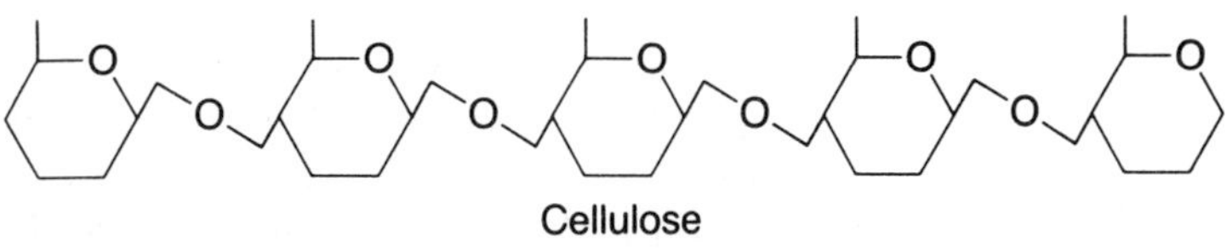

Cellulose

FIGURE 3-7 Cellulose is a straight chain polysaccharide.

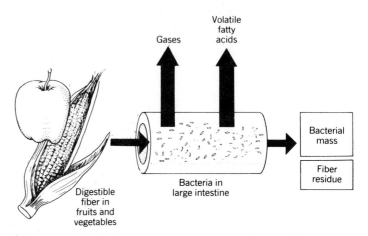

FIGURE 3-8   Breakdown of fiber by bacteria in the large intestine.

sources. Soluble fiber is more important healthwise than insoluble fiber because it has been found to reduce the level of LDL (low-density lipoproteins; see chapter 4) or the more undesirable form of blood cholesterol. Studies also show that soluble fiber can possibly benefit diabetics by decreasing absorption of glucose.

Functions of Fiber. The functions (see Fig. 3-9) of dietary fiber in the body are:

- To increase intestinal motility. Undigested fiber increases the peristaltic contractions of the intestines and thereby decreases the transit time of feces.
- To attract more water into the intestines. Increased attraction of water tends to soften stools and thereby helps prevent constipation.
- Possibly to prevent and treat certain health conditions (see the Clinical Application "Clinical Importance of Dietary Fiber").

Since the turn of the century, Americans have decreased their fiber consumption. This is the result of consuming more low-fiber foods such as meat, dairy products, and highly refined carbohydrate processed foods. Some scientists have attributed the increases in colon and rectum cancer, hemorrhoids, and **diverticulosis** to the low-fiber diet. Information on high-fiber diets and possible prevention of diseases is presented in the Clinical Application "Clinical Importance of Dietary Fiber."

diverticulosis Presence of diverticula (outpouching of the colon wall) (see Chapter 16).

Clinical Application: Clinical Importance of Dietary Fiber

hypoglycemia Abnormally low level of blood glucose (see Chapter 15).

hypercholesterolemia High level of cholesterol in the blood.

Much research has been done on the beneficial effects of high-fiber diets in preventing certain disorders: constipation, diverticulosis, colon cancer, obesity, **hypoglycemia,** and **hypercholesterolemia** (high level of cholesterol in the blood). Insulin-dependent diabetics can control their blood glucose levels more effectively and lower their insulin needs with an increased intake of fiber. Details concerning the relationship of fiber to these disorders will be presented in later chapters.

What is a high-fiber diet? Are there any disadvantages of increasing the fiber content of a person's diet? Most nutritional authorities define a high-fiber diet as one in which dietary fiber exceeds 40 g/day.[3] The average American now eats about 10–20 g of dietary fiber per day. This does not mean that the average person needs to double or quadruple the dietary fiber intake to help prevent the disorders discussed above. A desirable amount of fiber per day ranges from 25 to 35 g/day.[3] One does not have to sprinkle bran on all foods to achieve this intake. The average amounts of fiber in the fruit, bread and cereal, and vegetable groups are presented in this chapter. An example of three meals that contain a total of more than 35 g of dietary fiber is presented below.

Some of the disadvantages of increasing fiber in the diet are abdominal fullness and increased flatulence. These problems can be reduced or will disappear (except flatulence) by gradually decreasing the fiber content.

THREE TYPICAL MEALS THAT CONTAIN A TOTAL OF 37 G OF DIETARY FIBER

		Dietary fiber (g)
Breakfast	¾ cup All-Bran	11.2
	½ cup milk	0
	2 slices whole wheat toast with margarine	4.3
Lunch	2 slices whole wheat bread	4.3
	2 tbsp peanut butter	2.2
Dinner	3 oz beef	0
	1 baked potato with skin	7.0
	1 stalk broccoli	8.2
Total fiber content		37.0

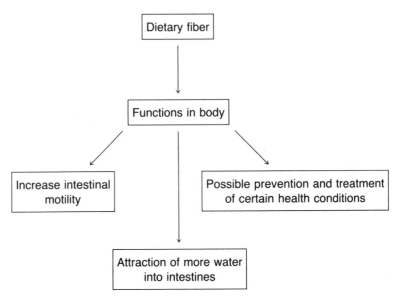

FIGURE 3-9 Functions of dietary fiber.

Starch

Starch is similar in structure to glycogen in that it is a branched polysaccharide molecule composed of glucose units. It is a storage form of glucose but is found only in plants. Starch is found in plant seeds, cereal grains, fruits, and roots.

Starch is a major source of carbohydrate and total energy intake in many countries. In the United States, wheat, oats, rye, barley, corn, potatoes, and rice are the primary food sources of starch. People in South American countries obtain most of their starch from corn, whereas Orientals use rice.

The digestion of starch begins in the mouth and is described later in this chapter.

Artificial Sweeteners

Sweeteners can be divided into two varieties: nutritive and nonnutritive.

Nutritive

Nutritive sweeteners contain 4 kcal/g as does sucrose. Fructose, sorbitol, and xylitol are examples.

Fructose. One advantage of using fructose is that it does not require insulin for absorption and metabolism. In addition, fructose is 15–80% sweeter than sucrose; therefore, it can provide the same degree of sweetness with fewer kilocalories.

Sorbitol. This nutritive sweetener is only half as sweet as sucrose. It is commonly found in sugar-free gums and candies. Like fructose, it does not require insulin to be absorbed.

Xylitol. The advantages of xylitol are the same as those of sorbitol. However, several animal species have developed tumors as a result of xylitol consumption.

Aspartame (Nutra Sweet). Aspartame is 180–220 times as sweet as sucrose. Therefore, only a small amount is needed to sweeten products. Nutra Sweet is used extensively in soft drinks, presweetened cold cereals, instant puddings, gelatins, dessert toppings, and chewing gum. In addition, Nutra Sweet is present in Equal, a low kilocalorie tabletop sweetener.

This product is not recommended for people with phenylketonuria and may be toxic to those with liver disease.

Nonnutritive

Nonnutritive sweeteners are often known as artificial and low-calorie sweeteners, since they contain very few kilocalories. The term *nonnutritive* also stems from the fact that they contribute almost no energy.

Saccharin. Saccharin is 300 times sweeter than sucrose and contains no kilocalories. It is controversial in that it has been determined to cause bladder cancer in laboratory rats. This relationship in humans has not been definitely established; however, saccharin is banned in Canada.

Saccharin is added to baked goods and is sold as a tabletop sweetener.

FUNCTIONS OF CARBOHYDRATES

Source of Energy

Glucose is the prime source of energy (see Fig. 3-10) for physiological activities (for example, muscle contractions and nerve impulse transmission). Each gram of glucose yields 4 kcal of energy when metabolized.

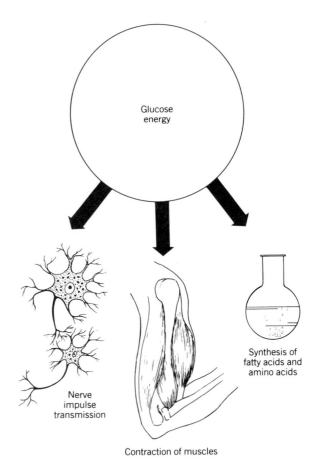

FIGURE 3-10 Glucose as a source of energy for physiological activities such as nerve impulse transmission and contraction of muscles, plus starting material for synthesis of other compounds.

triglyceride A lipid compound composed of three fatty acids attached to a glycerol molecule.

ketones Products of incomplete metabolism of fats (acetone is an example of a ketone).

blood acidosis A condition in which blood pH is below 7.35. This condition can result from an excess amount of ketones.

The brain tissue normally uses glucose as a source of energy. However, glycogen is not stored in nerve tissue; thus, the blood must continually bring glucose to the brain cells. Therefore, a low-calorie, low-carbohydrate diet can impair the normal functions of the brain.

If a person does not ingest an adequate amount of carbohydrates, **triglycerides** and proteins will be used as sources of energy. A danger in using triglycerides for energy is the release of **ketones,** which are acids. A high level of ketones can result in **blood acidosis,** which, if prolonged, can result in brain failure. Body proteins have many important functions (discussed in Chapter 5). If an adequate amount of carbohydrate is ingested, proteins are spared; therefore, carbohydrates are described as having "protein-sparing" action. A person must ingest a minimum of 50–100 g (200–400 kcal) of carbohydrate per day in order to spare proteins as a source of energy.

Starting Material for the Synthesis of Other Compounds

Glucose can be converted into other molecules, such as nonessential fatty acids and some amino acids, whenever their levels are inadequate.[3]

DIGESTION AND ABSORPTION OF CARBOHYDRATES

The carbohydrates in the foods we eat are usually disaccharides (sucrose is the most common) and polysaccharides (starch). These carbohydrates are too large to move from the intestines into the blood. Only monosaccharides can be absorbed into the blood; therefore, disaccharides and polysaccharides are broken down into their monosaccharide components by the digestive system.

Mouth

salivary amylase An enzyme secreted in the mouth that splits starch into smaller fragments.

Starch digestion begins in the mouth with the enzyme **salivary amylase** splitting starch into smaller fragments, disaccharide, and **dextrins** (see Fig. 3-11). Swallowing movements and **peristalsis** function to pass these fragments through the esophagus into the stomach.

There is no digestion of disaccharides in the mouth due to a lack of necessary enzymes.

dextrins Products of starch digestion in the mouth.

peristalsis Wavelike, muscular contractions that propel food and wastes through the gastrointestinal tract.

Stomach

Starch digestion continues for a short time before the **hydrochloric acid (HCl)** in gastric juice denatures (changes salivary amylase) into a nonfunctional state. No additional carbohydrate digestion occurs in the stomach due to its acidity and lack of enzymes.

hydrochloric acid Acid secreted by cells in the stomach that changes pepsinogen to pepsin.

duodenum First region of the small intestine.

Small Intestine

pancreatic amylase An enzyme secreted by the pancreas that breaks down dextrins into maltose.

Rhythmic contractions (*peristalsis*) of the stomach move maltose, dextrins, and other disaccharides that a person may have ingested into the **duodenum.** The pancreas secretes the enzyme **pancreatic amylase** into the duodenum, breaking down dextrins into maltose (see Fig. 3-11).

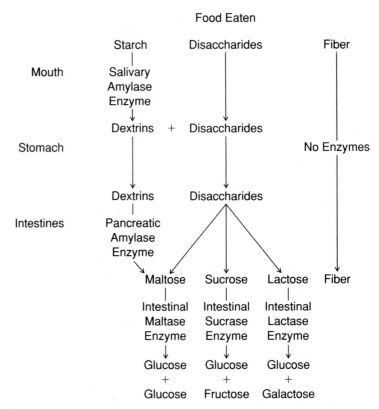

FIGURE 3-11 Digestion of carbohydrates in the mouth, stomach, and small intestine.

jejunum The region of the small intestine that extends from the duodenum to the ileum.

intestinal villi Small mucous projections lining the small intestine.

lumen The opening of the intestine.

blood capillary Microscopic blood vessels through which nutrients and wastes are exchanged.

diffusion Movement of molecules from high concentration in the intestines to low concentration in the blood capillary.

active transport Movement of molecules from a low concentration in the intestine to a high concentration in the blood. Energy is required and involves carrier molecules.

Disaccharide digestion begins at this point. Intestinal glands secrete maltase, lactase, and sucrase enzymes, which digest their respective disaccharides into their monosaccharides (see Fig. 3-11). Some people cannot synthesize the enzyme lactase and therefore have lactose intolerance (described earlier in the chapter).[4]

Absorption

Peristaltic contractions move monosaccharides into the **jejunum** where digestion is completed and absorption begins. Absorption is increased as a result of **intestinal villi** (see Fig. 3-12) projecting into the **lumen**. Each villus contains a **blood capillary** (see Fig. 3-13) into which the monosaccharides pass via **diffusion** and **active transport.**

Monosaccharides are absorbed at different rates; galactose, glucose, and fructose have decreasing rates of absorption.

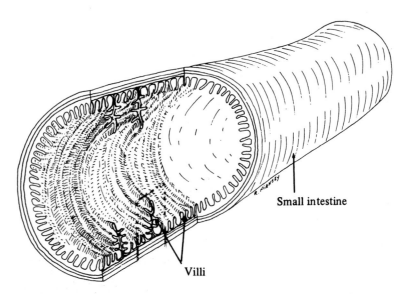

Small intestine

Villi

FIGURE 3-12 Intestinal villi, which increase absorption surface area, are shown.

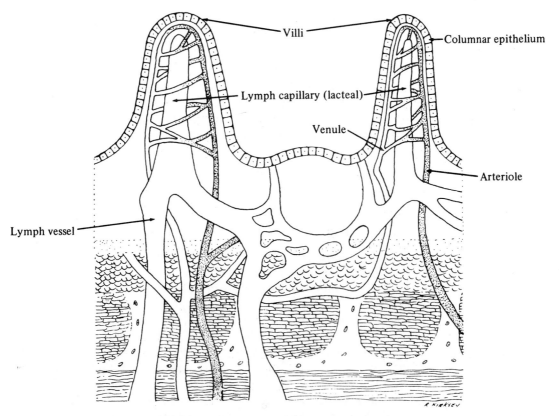

Villi

Columnar epithelium

Lymph capillary (lacteal)

Venule

Arteriole

Lymph vessel

FIGURE 3-13 Blood and lymph capillaries, which transport absorbed nutrients in villi, are shown.

METABOLISM OF CARBOHYDRATES

metabolism All chemical reactions that absorbed molecules undergo inside cells.

Metabolism is divided into two phases, **catabolism** and **anabolism.**

Catabolism

ATP Adenosine triphosphate. A high-energy compound that supplies energy for body processes.

Catabolism of glucose is important, since it results in the synthesis of the high-energy compound **ATP.**

Oxidation of Glucose and Synthesis of ATP

Three main processes are involved in the oxidation of glucose to synthesize ATP—glycolysis, citric acid cycle, and electron transport system.

Glycolysis. This process oxidizes glucose and removes hydrogen atoms. The hydrogen atoms along with energy from glucose are transported to the electron transport system by $NADH_2$ molecules. Two ATP molecules are formed.

Citric acid cycle (Krebs Cycle) A series of aerobic respiration reactions that result in the release of hydrogen atoms and CO_2 molecules and the synthesis of one ATP molecule.

Citric Acid Cycle. This process completes the removal of hydrogen atoms and energy that were originally a part of glucose. Carbon atoms also are removed in the form of CO_2.

electron transport system Composed of cytochrome molecules by which the pairs of hydrogen electrons released from glycolysis and citric acid cycles are carried.

Electron Transport System. This process takes the hydrogens that were removed by glycolysis and citric acid cycle and extracts energy from them to form ATP. Oxygen, as shown in Figure 3-14, acts as the final recipient of hydrogen atoms and electrons to form H_2O. If oxygen is absent, then hydrogens are not transported through this system and ATPs are not made.

insulin A hormone secreted by the pancreas that aids in both the diffusion of glucose into the liver and muscle cells and the synthesis of glycogen.

Anabolism and Interaction of Glycogenesis and Glycogenolysis

glycogenesis Synthesis of glycogen.

hyperglycemia A condition that pertains to high blood glucose.

A carbohydrate example of anabolism is the synthesis of glycogen (see Fig. 3-15) by liver and muscle cells. Figure 3-15 shows that **insulin** aids in both the diffusion of glucose into the liver and muscle cells and the synthesis of glycogen, which is called **glycogenesis.** It occurs whenever the blood glucose level becomes high. The normal blood glucose range is 70–120 mg per deciliter of blood. Whenever this upper limit is exceeded, a **hyperglycemia** condition exists. Persistent hyperglycemia can result in *diabetes mellitus* and other serious problems (see Chapter 15). The body normally corrects a hyperglycemic condition by glycogenesis.

glycogenolysis The catabolism of glycogen.

Whenever the blood glucose level drops below 70 mg/dl, a **hypoglycemic** condition exists. The liver cells correct this condition by **glycogenolysis** (see Fig. 3-15). This breakdown process releases glucose and,

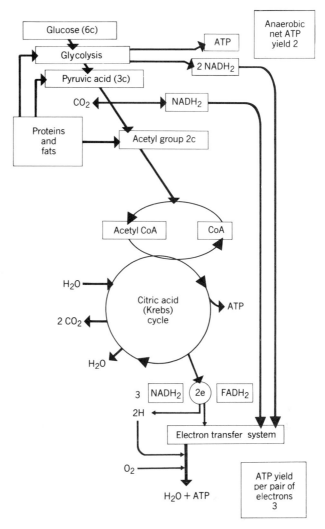

FIGURE 3-14 Metabolism of glucose resulting in the synthesis of ATP molecules.

glucagon A hormone secreted by the pancreas.

epinephrine A hormone secreted by the adrenal gland in times of stress.

therefore, blood glucose increases into the normal range. **Glucagon** and **epinephrine** (Fig. 3-15) stimulate the liver cells to undergo glycogenolysis. A continuous hypoglycemic condition is abnormal; its cause, symptoms, and diet are discussed in Chapter 15.

Glycogenesis (anabolism) and glycogenolysis (catabolism) interact to maintain a normal blood glucose range. In other words, the liver tissue alternates between anabolic and catabolic reactions with carbohydrates to regulate the blood glucose level.

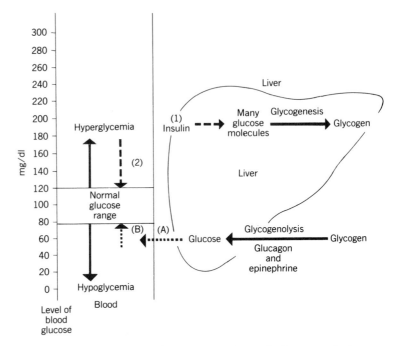

FIGURE 3-15 Interaction of glycogenesis and glycogenolysis to maintain the normal blood glucose range. Hyperglycemia results in excess glucose moving into liver, shown as (1). This action results in a lowering of blood glucose, shown as (2). The glucose is synthesized into glycogen by glycogenesis. Hypoglycemia results in release of glucose, supplied by glycogenolysis, into blood, shown as (A). This results in blood glucose rising to normal range, shown as (B).

AMOUNTS AND FOOD SOURCES OF CARBOHYDRATES IN DIETS OF DIFFERENT CULTURES

In the United States, a person currently obtains about 46% of the daily kilocalories from carbohydrates, with the amount of polysaccharides (complex carbohydrates) and disaccharides (sucrose) shown below. The Select Committee on Nutrition and Human Needs of the U.S. Senate has recommended that we increase from 46 to 58% the number of kilocalories derived from carbohydrates in the daily diet. The recommended amount of polysaccharide and disaccharide in the diet are compared to the current diet:

	Current U.S. Diet (%)	Recommended U.S. Diet (%)
Polysaccharide (complex carbohydrate)	22	48
Disaccharide (sucrose)	<u>24</u>	<u>10</u>
	46	58

These figures show that the recommended diet suggests an approximate doubling of the amount of complex carbohydrates consumed compared to the current diet. It is also recommended that the amount of disaccharides be cut approximately in half.[5]

It was mentioned in Chapter 2 that the bread and cereal food group contributes the bulk of carbohydrates. The specific foods in this group consumed to obtain carbohydrates vary from culture to culture.

As discussed in Chapter 1, it is important for health professionals to be knowledgeable about the food habits of different cultures. This knowledge of carbohydrates is important in order to counsel patients about achieving greater consumption of complex carbohydrates and reducing their intake of disaccharides (sugar).

CARBOHYDRATES AND THE EXCHANGE GROUPS

In Chapter 2, the exchange groups and the six exchange lists were discussed. These six lists are presented in this chapter for the purpose of discussing carbohydrate information for each list and for use in dietary planning to achieve recommended percentages of the nutrients.

Milk Group

One milk exchange is a serving of food equivalent to one cup of skim milk and 90 kcal. Table 3-2 shows that each milk exchange contains 12 g of carbohydrate and that disaccharide (lactose) is the primary type of carbohydrate.

As discussed in Chapter 2, one cup of whole milk is milk plus two fat exchanges, for a total of 150 kcal. However, whole milk does not contain more carbohydrate or protein than skim milk.

TABLE 3-2 CARBOHYDRATE CONTENT IN EXCHANGE GROUPS

Exchange Group	Grams of Carbohydrate	Type(s) of Carbohydrate(s)	Total kcal
Milk (1 cup)	12	Disaccharide (lactose)	90
Vegetable (½ cup)	5	Complex (starch); 2–3 g of fiber	25
Fruit (serving varies)	15	Monosaccharide (fructose); 2 g of fiber in dry fruits; 3 g of fiber in some fruits	60
Bread and starchy vegetables	15	Complex (starch); 2 g of fiber in whole-grain products and 3 g of fiber in some products	80

Vegetable Group

A vegetable exchange is one-half cup of a low-calorie vegetable and provides 25 kcal. One-half cup of vegetables contain 2–3 g of fiber.

This group is important, since it contains complex carbohydrates (starch) and fiber (Table 3-2). Increasing daily servings of vegetables will help one achieve the recommended 48% of the total kilocalories from complex carbohydrates.

Fruit Group

A fruit exchange varies from fruit to fruit in order that the exchange provides 15 g of carbohydrate and 60 kcal. Dry fruits contain 2 g of fiber and some fruits contain 3 g of fiber.

This exchange group is a good source of monosaccharides, especially fructose (Table 3-2), but it is a poor source of dietary complex carbohydrates (starch). However, some fruits are good sources of fiber.

Bread and Starchy Vegetable Group

A bread and starchy vegetable exchange varies, so that a serving provides 15 g of carbohydrate (Table 3-2). Whole-grain products contain 2 g of fiber and some products contain 3 g of fiber.

More complex carbohydrate, starch, and fiber are contributed by this group that any of the others. It is important to point out that some vegetables, such as corn and potatoes, are on this list rather than the vegetable list, since starchy vegetables contain 15 g of carbohydrate per serving compared to 5 g for those on the vegetable list.

Fat and Meat Groups

The fat and meat groups contain no dietary carbohydrates or fiber per exchange serving.

Sugar

The exchange lists do not include one that gives the amount of concentrated sugar found in various foods. Dietary planning cannot be realistically done unless this information is available. Each food presented below contains the equivalent of 4 g of pure white sugar.

Serving Size (1 tsp; 16 Kcal; 4 g)	Food
Brown sugar	Jam
Molasses	Jelly
Corn syrup	Candy
Honey	Maple syrup

Catsup lovers should be aware that each tablespoon contains 1 tsp of sugar. Also, people who drink regular 12-oz cans of soft drink beverages, as opposed to the diet drinks, ingest about 9 tsp of sugar per can.

SUMMARY

- Monosaccharides commonly found in food are glucose, galactose, and fructose.
- Glucose is used clinically as the energy source for cells in intravenous therapy.
- The disaccharides found in food and their monosaccharide components are as follows: sucrose—glucose and fructose; lactose—glucose and galactose; maltose—glucose and glucose.
- Glycogen is stored in skeletal muscles and liver as a source of glucose for the blood.
- Fiber is composed of polysaccharide celluose; insoluble fiber holds water and is found in most grains and seeds; soluble fiber results in the formation of gel and is able to lower low-density lipoproteins (LDL).
- Fiber functions to prevent constipation and diverticulosis.
- Carbohydrates are a source of energy for the body and starting material for synthesis of other compounds.
- Digestion of starch begins in the mouth with salivary amylase breaking down starch to disaccharides and dextrins; digestion ceases in the stomach when HCl breaks down amylase. Intestinal enzymes break down disaccharides to monosaccharides.
- The two phases of metabolism are as follows: anabolism, or the synthesis of new molecules from smaller ones, and catabolism, or the breakdown of large molecules to smaller ones.
- Glycolysis involves oxidation of glucose and removal of hydrogen atoms, with a net formation of two ATPs.
- The citric acid cycle completes the removal of hydrogen atoms and energy from glucose; carbon atoms are removed from glucose in the form of CO_2; one ATP is also made.
- The electron transport system combines the hydrogens from glycolysis and the citric acid cycle with oxygen to ultimately form ATPs and H_2O.
- Glycogenesis forms glycogen whenever blood glucose is above the normal range; glycogenolysis breaks down glycogen to glucose whenver blood glucose is below the normal range.
- The current carbohydrate intake of Americans is too low in terms of total carbohydrates (46% vs. 58%) and too low in terms of polysaccharides (22% vs. 48%).

- The types of carbohydrate and grams of each in the six exchange lists are: milk—12 g, lactose; vegetable—5 g, complex plus 2–3 g of fiber; fruit—15 g, fructose, and 2–3 g of fiber; bread—15 g, complex, and 2–3 g of fiber; fat—no grams of carbohydrate.

REVIEW QUESTIONS

True (A) or False (B)

1. Glucose, galactose, and sucrose are monosaccharides.
2. The body uses all of the monosaccharides as a source of energy.
3. Conversion of galactose and fructose to glucose occurs in the liver.
4. Glucose is the type of carbohydrate used in intravenous (IV) solutions.
5. Disaccharides include sucrose, lactose, and maltose.
6. Sucrose is composed of glucose and galactose.
7. Lactose is found only in cow's milk.
8. Lactose intolerance occurs only in people in their thirties.
9. Sucrose is also known as table sugar.
10. Honey is a better source of carbohydrate than refined sugar.
11. Polysaccharides important in the body are glycogen, cellulose, and starch.
12. Glycogen is important as a reserve source of blood glucose.
13. Most glycogen is stored in the liver.
14. Cellulose is second only to glycogen as a reserve source of blood glucose.
15. Glucose is a source of energy and a starting material for the synthesis of other compounds.
16. In order for carbohydrates to have a "protein-sparing" action, one must ingest 400–500 g/day.
17. Carbohydrate digestion begins in the mouth, with all types initially being broken down.
18. Disaccharide digestion begins in the small intestine with enzymes secreted by the pancreas.
19. Absorption of monosaccharides is increased by the intestinal villi.
20. Catabolism of glucose is important because it results in the synthesis of ATP molecules.
21. Glycogenesis or synthesis of glycogen occurs when a hyperglycemic condition exists.

22. Whenever the blood glucose level is above 120 mg/dl, glycogenolysis occurs to reduce it to normal.
23. A milk exchange contains more grams of carbohydrate than any other exchange.
24. The U.S. Senate Select Committee recommended that Americans reduce their intake of carbohydrates to 10–15% of their daily kilocalorie intake.
25. Each gram of carbohydrate yields 4 kcal of energy.
26. A meal that contains one exchange of milk, bread, and fruit has a total of 42 g of carbohydrate and 230 kcal from the three exchanges.

Multiple Choice

27. The shorthand way that health professionals write *carbohydrate* is:
    A. CHON.
    B. CARBO.
    C. CHO.
    D. none of these.
28. Two clinical applications of monosaccharides are the following:
    A. Glucose is a source of carbohydrate in intravenous (IV) therapy.
    B. Monosaccharides help reduce the chance of developing diverticulosis.
    C. Short-term studies have shown that fructose can reduce the need for insulin for diabetics.
    D. A, B.
    E. A, C.
29. The polysaccharide composing fiber is _____ _____ and dietary fiber is _____.
    A. glycogen—the residue left after the laboratory treatment of food with acid and alkali.
    B. starch—fiber resistant to human digestive enzymes.
    C. cellulose—the residue left after digestion.
    D. none of these.
30. Two functions of carbohydrates are _____ _____ and _____.
    A. a source of energy—amino acids.
    B. the starting material for the synthesis of other compounds—source of vitamins.
    C. a source of energy—starting material for the synthesis of other compounds.
    D. none of these.

Questions 31–36 apply to the meals below. The information necessary to answer them is found in Table 3-2.

	Exchanges	Grams of Carbohydrate	kcal
Breakfast			
1 egg	1 meat and ½ fat		75
1 slice toast	1 bread		70
1 tsp margarine	1 fat		45
Lunch			
1 cup skim milk	1 milk		90
2 slices bread	2 bread		160
1 oz cottage cheese	1 lean meat		55
1 banana	2 fruit		120
Dinner			
6 oz fish	6 oz lean meat		330
½ cup green beans	1 vegetable		25
½ cup carrots	1 vegetable		25
1 plain roll	1 bread		80
1 tsp margarine	1 fat		45
1 cup skim milk	1 milk		90

31. The breakfast meal contains _____ g carbohydrate and _____ kcal.
    A. 25—190
    B. 0—250
    C. 15—190
    D. none of these
32. Lunch contains _____ g of carbohydrate and _____ kcal.
    A. 82—215
    B. 72—425
    C. 37—215
    D. none of these
33. The dinner meal contains _____ g of carbohydrate and _____ kcal.
    A. 37—595
    B. 25—425
    C. 45—635
    D. none of these

34. The three meals contains a total of _____ g of carbohydrate and _____ kcal.
    A. 134—1210
    B. 114—1,120
    C. 105—955
    D. none of these
35. For all three meals, the number of kilocalories contributed by carbohydrates is _____ kcal, which is _____% of the total kilocalories.
    A. 536—44
    B. 420—49
    C. 456—41
    D. none of these
36. In reference to adequacy, the total kilocalories contributed by the carbohydrates is _____.
    A. higher than the recommended 55–60% of total kilocalories per day.
    B. within the recommended 55–60% of total kilocalories per day.
    C. lower than the recommended 55–60% of total kilocalories per day.

Completion

37. Distinguish between insoluble and soluble fiber.
38. List the disaccharides found in foods and their monosaccharide components.
39. Compare the current U.S. diet with the recommended diet with regard to percentages of polysaccharides and disaccharides (sugar).

CRITICAL THINKING CHALLENGE

1. Carbohydrate information

	1 oz cereal	With ½ cup skim milk
Dietary fiber	3 g	3 g
Complex carbohydrate	17 g	17 g
Maltose and other sugars	3 g	9 g
Total carbohydrate	23 g	29 g

Use the food label information above to answer the following questions.

a. Assuming there are no other nutrients in this food, what is the total number of calories for the cereal with skim milk?
b. What percent of the total carbohydrate is due to complex carbohydrate? How does this compare with the dietary goals in Chapter 1?
c. What percent of the total carbohydrate is due to "maltose and other sugars"? How does this compare with the dietary goals in Chapter 1?
d. Your client has a lactose intolerance and has asked if he can eat the above cereal and skim milk for breakfast. Which of the following statements is correct and must be considered before you respond?
   1. Lactose is not listed; therefore, the foods can be eaten.
   2. Milk is a food source of lactose.
   3. Skim milk does not contain lactose.
   4. Many people think they have lactose intolerance when they actually do not.
2. Your client asks why he is receiving glucose (dextrose) in his intravenous fluids. Which of the following facts will be the basis for your response?
   A. Glucose is a source of energy.
   B. Glucose is a building block for other sugars.
   C. Glucose is readily absorbed into the body's cells.
   D. Glucose is present in the blood in a concentration of 70–120 mg/dl.
3. Which of the following statements supports the need for school children to eat a nourishing breakfast that provides some glucose?
   A. The blood must continually provide glucose to the brain cells.
   B. Glucose is the primary source of energy.
   C. Approximately 100 g of glycogen is stored in the liver.
   D. Each gram of glucose yields 4 kcal of energy when metabolized.
   E. Both A and B.

REVIEW QUESTIONS FOR NCLEX

Situation. A client asked a health professional to explain to her what the advantages are of increasing fiber in her diet, which foods are good sources of fiber and the differences between soluble and insoluble fiber.

1. The advantages of increasing fiber in a person's diet are _____ .
   A. to decrease the kcal intake, decrease fat intake, increase weight loss, and increase satiety
   B. to possibly prevent or reduce certain disorders—constipation, diverticulosis, and colon cancer
   C. to decrease consumption of fats, cholesterol, and kcal
   D. to increase nutrient density, lower kcal intake, and decrease consumption of fatty foods
2. Exchange or food groups that are good sources of fiber are _____ .
   A. fruit, bread and cereal, vegetable
   B. meat, milk, fat, bread and cereal
   C. fruit, milk, meat, fat
   D. vegetable, meat, milk, fat
3. Soluble fiber differs from insoluble fiber and the advantages of it are _____ .
   A. it can be digested by intestinal enzymes and it can provide kcal
   B. it is a better source of glucose that insoluble fiber and it can prevent breast cancer
   C. it can dissolve in water to form a gel and can reduce the level of undesirable form of blood cholesterol
   D. it is more readily available from foods and helps in weight loss by reducing the amount of nutrients that are absorbed from the intestines
4. Insoluble fiber differs from soluble fiber and the advantages of it are _____ .
   A. it can hold water and reduces constipation
   B. it can be broken down to provide glucose and provides a good source of energy
   C. it can provide monosaccharides to the blood and that it helps to maintain constant blood glucose
   D. it forms a gel
5. Food sources of insoluble fiber are _____ .
   A. fruits and vegetables
   B. breads and meats
   C. whole grains and seeds
   D. milk and vegetables
6. Food sources of soluble fiber are _____ .
   A. breads and meats
   B. fruits, vegetables, oat bran, and dried beans
   C. milk, fats, meat, and bread
   D. sweets, meats, vegetables, and milk

Situation. A hospitalized patient's chart showed he was lactose intolerant and had received 1 unit (1 liter) 5% DSW (5% dextrose or glucose in water) intravenously (solution is injected into veins).

7. Glucose is used intravenously, as an energy source, as opposed to sucrose because _____ .
   A. it supplies more kcal (energy) per gram than does sucrose
   B. it does not have to be digested since it is already in the monosaccharide form
   C. the person does not have the enzyme to break down sucrose, therefore, it cannot be digested and absorbed into the blood
   D. the blood has more enzymes to break down glucose, for absorption into cells, than enzymes for sucrose
8. The diet this patient receives has to contain no foods that contain the carbohydrate _____ .
   A. sucrose
   B. glycogen
   C. maltose
   D. lactose
9. A food source of the carbohydrate given in the previous question is _____ .
   A. milk
   B. bread
   C. vegetables
   D. fruit

REFERENCES

1. Bailey, L. L., Duewer, F., Gray, R., Hoskin, J. et al. (1988). Food consumption. *National Food Review*, *11*, 1–11.
2. Hole, J. W. (1991). *Human anatomy and physiology* (5th ed.). Dubuque: W. C. Brown.
3. Greenwald, P. E., Lanza, E., & Eddy, G. A. (1987). Dietary fiber in the reduction of colon cancer risk. *Journal of the American Dietetic Association, 87*, 1172–1177.
4. Nieman, D. C., Butterworth, D. E., & Nieman, C. N. (1992). *Nutrition* (rev. 1st ed., p. 113). Dubuque: W. C. Brown.
5. National Research Council. (1989). *Recommended Dietary Allowances* (10th ed., pp. 92–93) Washington.

4

LIPIDS

Upon completion of this chapter, you should be able to:

1. Describe the structure of a triglyceride molecule.
2. Distinguish between saturated and unsaturated fatty acids and name three polyunsaturated fatty acids.
3. List two functions of saturated and unsaturated fats.
4. Distinguish between essential and nonessential fatty acids and give an example of a polyunsaturated essential fatty acid.
5. Describe the structure of phospholipids and name two phospholipids that are important in the body.
6. Describe three functions of phospholipids and two food sources.
7. Recognize the structure of a cholesterol molecule and name the origin of the majority of cholesterol in the body.
8. Give the functions of cholesterol and three food sources.
9. Differentiate between low-density lipoproteins (LDL) and high-density lipoproteins (HDL) in terms of their

functions and correlation with increased heart attack.
10. Give six functions of lipids.
11. Describe what emulsification and digestion to globules accomplish.
12. Discuss what happens to glycerol and fatty acids when they pass into intestinal wall cells.
13. Discuss what transports short chain and long chain fatty acids.
14. Describe the basic symptom that indicates the inability to digest and absorb fats and give three conditions that can cause this symptom.
15. List three reasons why medium chain triglycerides (MCTs) can compensate for fat malabsorption problems.
16. Differentiate between low-, medium-, and high-fat meats in terms of their fat content.
17. Analyze different diets in terms of which ones are higher in fat and be able to calculate the total kilocalories and percentage due to fat.

INTRODUCTION

lipid A biological substance that has an oily or greasy touch and is insoluble in water. Lipids are soluble in organic solvents such as ether and alcohol.

Lipids are a very diverse group of organic compounds that includes oils, fats, resins, and waxes that originate in plants and animals. Subclasses of lipids that are important in the body are **glycerides, phospholipids, sterols,** and **lipoproteins.** Despite their diversity all classes of lipids have one thing in common, they are insoluble in water.

CHEMISTRY OF LIPIDS

Glycerides

triglyceride A molecule that is composed of a glycerol molecule to which is attached three fatty acids.

Glycerides compose about 95–98% of the fats in food and in the body. **Triglyceride** is the most common example in this subclass (see Fig. 4-1). A triglyceride molecule is composed of a glycerol to which is attached three fatty acids. A fatty acid is a straight, even-numbered carbon chain.

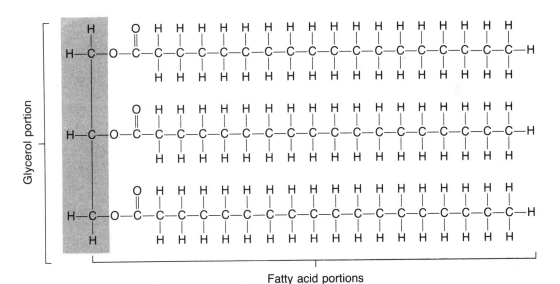

FIGURE 4-1 A triglyceride molecule is composed of a glycerol molecule that is attached to three fatty acids (FA). (From Hole, John W., Jr., *Human Anatomy and Physiology,* 3d ed. (c) 1978, 1981, 1984 Wm. C. Brown Publishers, Dubuque, Iowa. All rights reserved. Reprinted by permission.)

fatty acid Chain of carbon and hydrogen atoms that functions as a building block of fat molecules.

long chain fatty acids Fatty acids that are 18 to 20 carbon atoms in length.

medium chain fatty acids Fatty acids that contain 14 to 16 carbon atoms.

short chain fatty acids Fatty acids that contain 8 to 12 carbon atoms.

saturated fatty acid A fatty acid whose carbon atoms are linked by single bonds, and are bonded to as many hydrogen atoms as possible.

unsaturated fatty acid A fatty acid whose carbon atoms are linked by double or triple bonds, and therefore are not bonded to as many hydrogen atoms as possible.

monounsaturated fatty acid A fatty acid that contains one double bond.

polyunsaturated fatty acid A fatty acid that contains two or more double bonds.

hydrogenation A process by which an unsaturated fat is changed to a solid saturated fat by forcing hydrogens into the substance.

PUFA Polyunsaturated fatty acids.

cholesterol A lipid that is produced by the body and used in the synthesis of steroid hormones and excreted in bile.

One end of the chain is a carboxyl acid radical $\left(-C{\overset{\displaystyle O}{\underset{\displaystyle OH}{}}}\right)$, which gives off hydrogen ions (H^+) and therefore is the source of the acid part of the **fatty acid**.

Fatty acids vary in length from 4 to 24 carbon atoms. The more common fatty acids in dietary fat are called **long chain fatty acids. Medium chain fatty acids** contain 14 to 16 carbon atoms, whereas **short chain fatty acids** contain 8 to 12. Triglycerides are named long, medium, or short chain triglycerides, depending on the number of fatty acids present in the three chains.

Saturated and Unsaturated Fatty Acids

Double bonds may or may not be present between carbon atoms in fatty acids. There are two types of fatty acids: **saturated** and **unsaturated.** The term *saturated* comes from the fact that the fatty acid contains as many hydrogen atoms as possible (Fig. 4-2). Unsaturated fatty acids contain fewer hydrogen atoms due to the double bonds. For every double bond in a fatty acid, there are two fewer hydrogen atoms (Fig. 4-2). A **monounsaturated fatty acid** has one double bond, whereas a **polyunsaturated fatty acid** has two or more.

The dietary sources of saturated fatty acids are animal fat, beef, butter, chicken eggs, and whole milk. Unsaturated fatty acids are obtained from vegetable oils: corn, olive, soybean, peanut, and safflower.

The more saturated a fat is, the harder it is at room temperature. Likewise, unsaturated fats are more liquid at room temperature. As a rule of thumb, a person who wanted to buy unsaturated fatty acids would buy the more liquefied ones, which are generally the vegetable and fish oils.

Margarine is an example of a fat that must be somewhat hard in order to be spread. To make a margarine from a polyunsaturated oil such as corn oil, the producer will put it through **hydrogenation.**[1]

Polyunsaturated Fatty Acids (PUFA)

The ratio of **PUFA** to saturated fatty acids (i.e., the P/S ratio) in the total diet concerns nutritionists because of the potential health benefits of the unsaturated plant–derived PUFA. Research shows that polyunsaturated fat can reduce the **serum cholesterol** level.

Three PUFA that are important in the body are **linoleic, arachidonic,** and **linolenic** acids (see Fig. 4-3). Table 4-1 presents the number of carbon atoms, double bonds, and food sources of these PUFA.

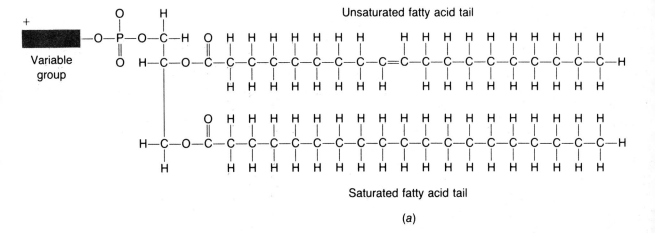

Variable group

Unsaturated fatty acid tail

Saturated fatty acid tail

(a)

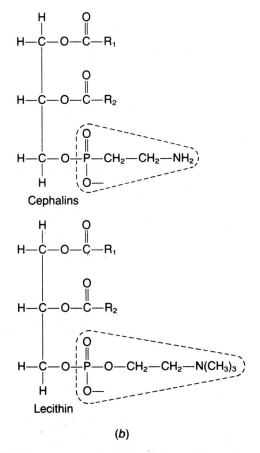

Cephalins

Lecithin

(b)

FIGURE 4-2 (a) A phospholipid is composed of two fatty acids and a phosphate group, with an attached nitrogen group in place of the third fatty acid. (b) Lecithin and cephalin are two important phospholipids in the body.

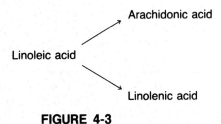

FIGURE 4-3

Polyunsaturated versus Saturated Fats

Research shows that an increase in polyunsaturated fats can reduce the serum cholesterol level. The desirable ratio of polyunsaturated to saturated fats (P:S) is 1:1 and may be achieved in three ways. One way is to add polyunsaturated fat to the diet. The second way is to consume less saturated fat. Table 4-2 presents some suggestions on how to decrease the amount of saturated fat in the diet. The third way is to decrease saturated fat and increase unsaturated fat until a ratio of 1:1 is achieved. Table 4-3 ranks fats and oils from most polyunsaturated to most saturated.

Functions of Saturated and Unsaturated Fats

Saturated Fats	Unsaturated Fats
Source of energy (9 kcal/g)	Source of energy (9 kcal/g)
Raise the serum cholesterol level and increase the risk of developing atherosclerosis	Aid the liver in converting cholesterol to bile acids
	Enhance the liver's ability to decrease excess fatty acids (see Fig. 4-4)

TABLE 4-1 COMMON FATTY ACIDS IN THE BODY

Common Name of Fatty Acid	Number of Carbons: Number of Double Bonds	Food Sources
Linoleic acid	18 : 2	Safflower oil, sunflower oil, and corn oil
Linolenic acid	18 : 3	Soybean oil
Arachidonic acid	20 : 4	Animal fat

Coconut oil is a vegetable oil that is actually more saturated than some animal fats. Coconut oil is often used in nondairy creamers and nondairy whipped toppings.

Essential and Nonessential Fatty Acids

essential fatty acid A fatty acid (e.g., linoleic acid) that cannot be manufactured by the body in adequate quantities and therefore must be obtained from the diet. Its absence results in a specific deficiency disease.

A fatty acid may be described as being either **essential** or nonessential. Linoleic acid, a polyunsaturated fatty acid, is the essential fatty acid required by the body for healthy cell membranes.

TABLE 4-2 HOW TO DECREASE FAT, ESPECIALLY SATURATED FAT

1. Limit beef, pork, lamb, and whole milk cheese consumption to a combined total of 20 ounces per week. (Each ounce contains approximately 1 teaspoon of saturated fat.)
2. When you do eat meat, select the leanest cuts and remove all visible fat before eating.
3. Use poultry, fish, and legumes to replace red meat several times a week.
4. Avoid luncheon meats, frankfurters, and sausage because they are so high in fat.
5. Skim the fat off broths, soups, and gravies.
6. Bake, broil, and boil meats. Avoid frying whenever possible.
7. Switch to nonfat or lowfat milk.
   a. Whole milk contains the equivalent of 2 teaspoons of butter per cup.
   b. Lowfat milk contains only about 1 teaspoon of butter per cup.
   c. Nonfat or skim milk contains no butter.
   d. If you prefer whole milk, you can reduce your intake of fats from other sources.
8. Use cheeses made with part skim milk rather than those made with whole milk. Recommended cheeses include:
   a. Cottage, Farmer, Sapsago, Edam, Gouda.
   b. Ricotta, Parmesan, Mozzarella, Gruyère, Jarlesberg Swiss.
9. Decrease your intake of rich dishes made with butter, cream, palm oil, coconut oil, and/or cocoa butter.
10. Avoid food products bearing the terms *hardened* or *hydrogenated* vegetable oil.
11. Use only small portions of fresh butter, margarine (listing liquid oil as the first ingredient), and mayonnaise as spreads.
12. Use salad dressings sparingly. (One ladleful can contain as much as 200 calories of fat!)

Source: High Level Health: A Proven Health Promotion Program. Green Bay, WI: Sun Valley Health Institute, 1982. Reprinted with permission.

TABLE 4-3 POLYUNSATURATED OILS

Safflower	Most
Sunflower	polyunsaturated
Corn	
Walnut	
Soybean	
Wesson	
Crisco	
Sesame	Least
Cottonseed	polyunsaturated

Source: High Level Health: A Proven Health Promotion Program. Green Bay, Wisc.: Sun Valley Health Institute, 1982. Reprinted with permission.

Deficiency of Essential Fatty Acids

dermatitis Inflammation of the skin, evidenced by itching and redness.

Diets that are deficient in linoleic acid are rare, but when they occur the skin may become irritated and reddened (**dermatitis**). Deficiencies are usually seen in hospital patients receiving liquid diets intravenously and infants fed formulas that are lacking in linoleic acid. Foods that are rich in linoleic acid are presented in Table 4-4.

The prevention or relief of dermatitis is actually not the result of linoleic acid; rather, it is due to the presence of arachidonic and linolenic acids. Since linoleic acid is widely available in foods compared to arachidonic and linolenic acids, linoleic acid is important as a precursor for the synthesis of the other two.[1]

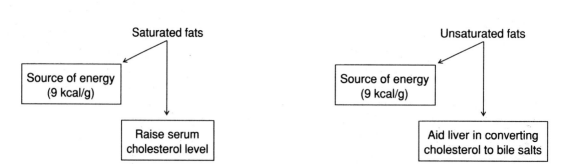

FIGURE 4-4 Functions of saturated and unsaturated fats.

TABLE 4-4 FOODS RICH IN LINOLEIC ACID

Plant Foods	% Linoleic Acid	Animal Foods	% Linoleic Acid
Safflower oil	74.1	Poultry	19.5
Sunflower oil	65.7	Fish, salmon	4.0
Corn oil	58.0	Pork	10.2
Wheat germ oil	54.8	Shortening	6.0
Cottonseed oil	51.5		

Fish Oils: Good or Bad?

Omega Fatty Acids

Omega-3 fatty acids and benefits of fish and fish oils are very popular topics. The terms *omega-3* or *omega-6 fatty acids* refer to the distance of the first double bond from the omega end (the -CH_3 end) of the fatty acid. As an example, linoleic acid is classified as an omega-6 fatty acid since the first double bond is six carbons from the omega end. (see Fig. 4-2 for -CH_3 end of fatty acids.) However, omega-3 fatty acids found in fish oils are what have made the omega term popular.

Importance of Omega-3 Fatty Acids

Several population surveys and clinical reports suggest that omega-3 fatty acids can help combat heart disease. Recent studies in the United States have shown that two to three servings of fish (which is a good source of omega-3 fatty acids) may reduce mortality by about 30% among patients who have survived their first myocardial infarction.[1]

It is important to point out that studies that have used fish oil concentrates to prevent and treat coronary artery disease, cardiovascular complications of diabetes, and rheumatoid arthritis have achieved mixed results. While many studies show that taking large doses (pharmacological doses in several studies) of these omega-3 fish oil supplements can help these conditions, they also produced some undesirable effects. Examples are raised low-density lipoproteins, raised blood glucose levels in diabetics, decreased blood clotting, and toxicities of vitamins A and D.[2,3]

Food Sources of Omega-3 Fatty Acids

The best sources are seafoods with sardines, salmon, tuna, mackerel, and trout being the best. Capsules containing these fatty acids are available but should be used with caution since, as pointed out above, they can produce some very undesirable effects.[4]

REFERENCES

1. Burr, M. L., Gilbert, J. F. et. al. (1989). Effects of changes in fat, fish and fibre intakes on death and myocardial reinfarction: Diet and reinfarction trial (DART). *Lancet, 2,* 757.
2. Simopoulos, A. P. (1991). Omega-3 fatty acids in health and disease and in growth and development. *American Journal of Clinical Nutrition, 54,* 438.
3. Sorisky, A., & Robbins, D. C. (1989). Fish oils and diabetes: The net effect. *Diabetes Care, 12,* 302.
4. Hepburn, F. N., Exler, J., & Weihrauch, J. L. (1986). Provisional tables on the content of omega-3 fatty acids and other fat components of selected foods. *Journal of the American Dietetic Association, 86,* 788–793.

PHOSPHOLIPIDS

A phospholipid molecule is very similar to a triglyceride. It is composed of glycerol and two fatty acids, but in place of the third fatty acid there is a phosphate and nitrogenous compound (see Fig. 4-5). Two important phospholipids in the body are **lecithin** and **cephalin.** Phospholipids differ from each other according to the nitrogenous compound they contain.

lecithin A phospholipid found in the body.

cephalin A phospholipid found in the body.

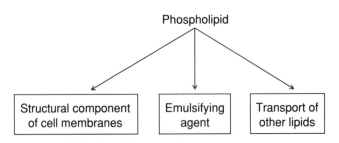

FIGURE 4-5 Functions of phospholipids.

Location and Functions

All cell membranes are composed of proteins and phospholipids. The cells in the brain, nervous tissue, and liver are especially rich in phospholipids. The functions of phospholipids are (see Fig. 4-5):

emulsifying agents
Substances that increase the surface area of fats for ease of absorption.

- Structural components of cell membranes
- Powerful **emulsifying agents**
- Transport agents of other lipids in the body

Phospholipids are nonessential nutrients. Liver, brains, heart, and egg yolk are good food sources.

STEROLS

Sterols, a subclass of lipids, have a completely different chemical structure from the triglycerides and phospholipids. Their chemical structure consists of four fused rings (see Fig. 4-6). Cholesterol is the most important nutritional sterol.

Location and Function

steroid hormones Hormones secreted by the adrenal cortex and other endocrine glands that have a typical steroid shape.

Cholesterol is located in cell membranes. It is a precursor of both **steroid hormones** such as estrogen, testosterone, aldosterone, and cortisone and of bile acids. Cholesterol can be synthesized by the body, and about 60% of it in the body is synthesized by the liver and intestine.

The functions of cholesterol are (see Fig. 4-7):

- A component of cell membranes
- A precursor of steroid hormones
- Formation of vitamin D

Cholesterol has many beneficial functions in the body; however, high levels in the blood have been associated with the development of fatty

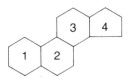

FIGURE 4-6 A cholesterol molecule as well as other steroids are composed of four fused rings.

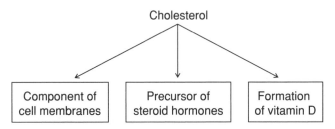

FIGURE 4-7 Functions of cholesterol.

plaques Mounds of lipid material, smooth muscle cells, and calcium.

Cardiovascular disease Disease of the blood vessels and the heart.

plaques in arteries and ultimately with atherosclerosis. The normal concentration of cholesterol in the blood ranges from 150 to 200 mg/100 ml (150 to 200 mg%) of blood. When the concentration is persistently well above 200 mg%, the chances of developing **cardiovascular disease** are higher than if the cholesterol level is within the normal range.

Food Sources of Cholesterol

Since approximately 40% of cholesterol comes from food, we need to be aware of which foods are rich in it. They include egg yolks, butter, cream, cheese, sweetbreads, liver, and other organ meats, and shellfish (lobster, shrimp, and oysters).[2]

ARTIFICIAL FATS

Companies are developing artificial fats to meet the demands for low-calorie foods. Two products that have been developed in this category are Olestra and Simplesse.

Olestra

"Artificial" correctly describes this product since it is not composed of fat at all but rather sucrose and long chain fatty acids. It has the taste and texture of fat but is not digested or absorbed, therefore, contributing no kcal. It is heat-stable and can be used in cooking oils, shortenings, bakery products, and snack foods.

Simplesse

This product, like Olestra, is not composed of fat at all but rather is made from egg-white protein or cow's milk protein. It is partially digested by the body and provides 1.3 calories per gram. Unlike Olestra, it is not heat-stable and can only be used in ice cream, yogurt, margarine, salad dressings, mayonnaise, and cheese.

It is important to be aware of some of the side effects of artificial fat usage in humans. Some studies have shown that it can decrease the absorption of vitamins A and E, and cause diarrhea and flatulence.

LIPOPROTEINS

lipoprotein Lipid with a protein coat around it.

A **lipoprotein** is a lipid with a protein coat around it. The body combines the two together so that the lipids are soluble in blood and **lymph** (remember, lipids are insoluble in water and blood is primarily water). Lipoproteins are synthesized in intestinal cells and the liver. The lipids transported are primarily triglyceride, cholesterol, and phospholipids.

blood lipid profile A measurement of the amounts of different classes of lipoproteins.

The level of lipoproteins in the blood can be determined by a **blood lipid profile,** and if low-density lipoproteins (LDL) are abnormally high, a person has a greater risk of developing cardiovascular disease. The classes of lipoproteins and their composition are discussed next.

Classification and Composition of Lipoproteins

Lipoproteins are classified into five types on the basis of their lipid composition and density of the protein coat:

Chylomicrons. Made in the intestinal cells and transport just-eaten triglycerides to the liver, where they are dismantled and new lipids synthesized. Chylomicrons have a thin protein coat and therefore a low density. They can be seen floating at the top of a blood sample, where they form a creamy layer.

VLDL (very low density lipoproteins). Made primarily by liver cells and transport triglycerides and some cholesterol to the tissues. They circulate in the blood for a few hours and are then converted to IDL.

IDL (intermediate-density lipoproteins). Formed in the liver after triglycerides are removed from VLDL and then converted to LDL.

LDL (low-density lipoproteins). Made in the liver, they are composed of about 50% cholesterol, which they transport to the tissues (see Fig. 4-8). LDL can combine with blood calcium to form **plaques** in arteries.

HDL (high-density lipoproteins). Very dense due to the amount of protein coat they contain. HDL contain about 20% cholesterol, which they transport from tissues and plaques to the liver (see Fig. 4-8), where the cholesterol is degraded and secreted in bile.

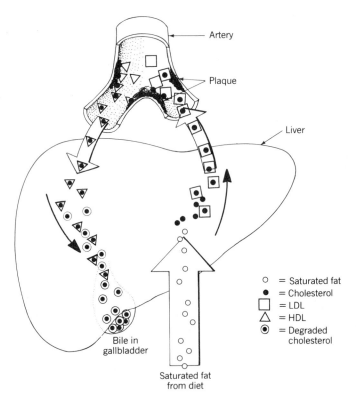

FIGURE 4-8 Formation and function of LDL and HDL are shown. Saturated fat in the diet is converted to cholesterol by the liver. LDL carries cholesterol from the liver through the blood, possibly resulting in the formation of plaques. HDL transports cholesterol from plaques to the liver, where it is degraded and secreted in bile. Plaques tend to form at points where arteries branch, since mechanical stresses are greater at these points.

Cardiovascular Disease and Lipoproteins

Research has shown that there is a correlation between the levels of LDL and HDL and the risk of developing cardiovascular disease. The risk of plaque formation and cardiovascular disease increases with a high level of blood cholesterol. Cholesterol is transported through the blood by lipoproteins, especially LDL; therefore, a high level of LDL correlates closely with an increased risk of cardiovascular disease. LDL have a tendency to accumulate in the inner lining of arteries, possibly as a result of their protein coat.

Since HDL transport cholesterol as well as LDL, why is there a reduced risk of cardiovascular disease with an increase in the level of HDL? The reason is that as described above, HDL transport cholesterol from the tissues and plaques to the liver, where it is decomposed. Since HDL tend to reduce the risk of cardiovascular disease, they are sometimes called "good cholesterol." Research on raising HDL shows that consumption of fish rather than meat is helpful. However, the best way to raise HDL is by exercise—prolonged, intense, and frequent.

$$\uparrow \text{ LDL level} = \uparrow \text{ cholesterol level} = \uparrow \text{ risk of heart attack}$$

$$\uparrow \text{ HDL level} = \downarrow \text{ cholestrol level} = \downarrow \text{ risk of heart attack}$$

FUNCTIONS OF LIPIDS

Much information has been published in recent years on the harmful effects of cholesterol and saturated fats in the body. Logically, then, many people may conclude that fats should be eliminated from the diet as much as possible. This belief is incorrect. Lipids have some very important functions in the body, such as (see Fig. 4-9):

Concentrated source of energy. Fat provides more than twice as much as energy as carbohydrates and proteins: 9 kcal/g for fat as opposed to 4 kcal/g for carbohydrates and proteins.

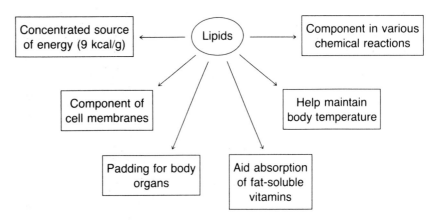

FIGURE 4-9 Functions of lipids.

Important component of cell membranes. Phospholipids and cholesterol are important structural components of cell membranes. One reason why swallowing kerosene, gasoline, or paint thinner is often fatal is that these compounds dissolve the phospholipids and cholesterol in the cells composing the digestive tract.

Aid absorption of fat-soluble vitamins. Fat-soluble vitamins cannot be absorbed into the blood and lymph unless fat is present.

Padding for the body's organs. All of the vital organs that maintain homeostasis are surrounded by a layer of fat. The kidneys, eyeballs, and heart are three examples.

Help maintain body temperature. Fat located below the skin helps to insulate the body against rapid loss of heat during the winter. This function results from the fact that fat does not conduct heat.

Component of various important chemical reactions. Bile salts help emulsify fats for fat digestion. All of the steroid hormones and vitamin D are synthesized from cholesterol.

DIGESTION AND ABSORPTION OF LIPIDS

Triglycerides, phospholipids, cholesterol, and sterols all are composed of large molecules. They cannot be absorbed into the blood and lymph from the digestive tract until they have been digested to smaller molecules. In this section, we will discuss how triglycerides are prepared by digestion for absorption and then used by the body.

Emulsification and Digestion

globules Small masses of material. Fat globules are small masses of fat.

bile salts Clear yellow or orange fluid secreted by the liver.

No chemical digestion of triglycerides occurs until they reach the duodenum of the small intestine. When fats reach the duodenum, they are in the form of **globules,** which cannot be effectively broken down. The entrance of fats into the duodenum stimulates the release of **bile salts** from the gallbladder into this organ. Bile acts as an emulsifier and breaks up globules into small droplets (see Fig. 4-10). Emulsification increases the surface area of fat molecules, enabling pancreatic lipase enzymes to break down the triglyceride molecules more rapidly. The pancreatic enzymes are emptied into the duodenum by the pancreatic duct at the same point at which bile enters through the common bile duct.

monoglycerides Glycerides that contain one fatty acid chain.

Lipase enzymes break down about 25% of the triglycerides into fatty acids and glycerol. The other 75% are broken down into **monoglycerides.** Enzymes split off two of the fatty acids (usually the ones on the ends) in a triglyceride molecule, resulting in the formation of a monoglyceride.

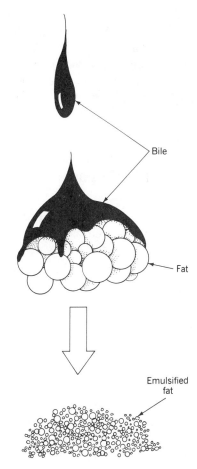

FIGURE 4-10 Emulsification of fat by bile.

Absorption

water soluble Refers to substances that dissolve in water. Fats become water soluble when a protein coat is secreted around them (see the discussion of water-soluble vitamins in Chapter 6).

chylomicrons Lipoproteins synthesized in the intestines that transport triglycerides through the lymph and blood to the liver.

After triglyceride molecules have been digested, they are absorbed through the intestinal lining into either blood vessels or lymph vessels.

In order for these digested materials (three triglycerides and one glycerol) to be absorbed, they must become **water soluble** (remember, lipids are insoluble in water), since blood and lymph are composed primarily of water. This process is accomplished by two methods—by combining with bile salts and by forming lipoproteins (**chylomicrons**). Bile salts combine with fatty acids and monoglycerides, which then pass into intestinal wall cells. The intestinal cells synthesize new triglyceride molecules, which are then wrapped in a thin membrane of phospholipid and lipoprotein. This water-soluble package is a chylomicron, and the larger

lacteals Lymph vessels.

left subclavian vein Vein that receives the majority of lymph and chylomicrons.

portal vein Vein that brings blood rich in nutrients into the liver. Blood from the intestines, stomach, and spleen drain into the portal vein.

ones are absorbed into the **lacteals** (see Figs. 4-11 and 4-12), whereas the smaller ones and short chain fatty acids are absorbed into the blood. The lymph vessels transport the larger chylomicrons into the blood (**left subclavian vein**) near the heart (see Fig. 4-12). Blood carries the smaller chylomicrons and short chain fatty acids initially into the liver through the **portal vein** (see Fig. 4-12).

Metabolism

The liver, cardiac, and skeletal muscle cells metabolize triglycerides for energy. The majority of triglycerides, however, are removed by fat depots and stored as energy.

In addition to metabolizing triglycerides for energy, the liver cells carry out the following fat metabolism functions:

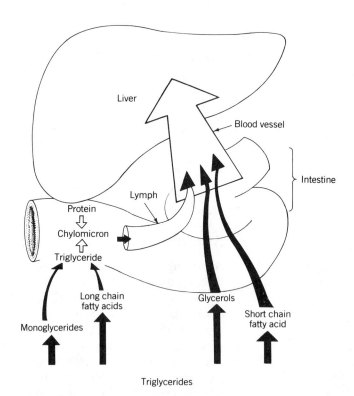

FIGURE 4-11 Absorption, synthesis, and transport of lipids.

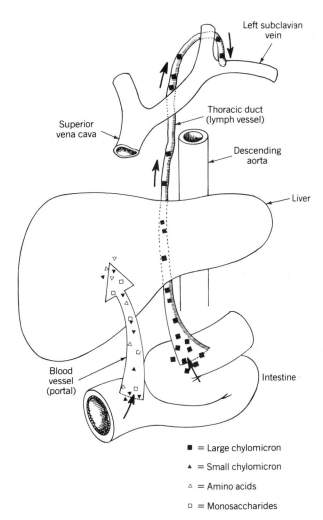

FIGURE 4-12 Large chylomicrons are absorbed into lacteals and transported by lymph into the left subclavian veins. Small chylomicrons, together with amino acids and monosaccharides, are transported by blood from the intestines to the liver.

- Synthesis of triglycerides from carbohydrates
- Synthesis of phospholipids and lipoproteins from proteins
- Synthesis of cholesterol from triglycerides
- Clearance or degradation of phospholipids, cholesterol, and lipoproteins from the blood

STORAGE OF FAT

adipose tissue Fat tissue.

The majority of triglycerides in the body are stored in fat cells composing **adipose tissue.** The number of fat cells probably reaches its maximum at adulthood or during pregnancy. Therefore, increased deposition of fat in an adult occurs primarily by increasing the amount of fat in each cell. Research shows that fat cells in an obese person may be 100 times larger than in a thin person. The size of fat cells also depends on their location in the body. In children, the cells of **subcutaneous** adipose tissue are larger than those in deeper tissues. In an adult, regions where fat is stored and percentages for each are:

subcutaneous Under the skin.

Subcutaneous tissue—50%

Around kidneys—12%

omenta A serous membrane attached to the visceral organs.

Omenta—10–15%

Genital areas—20%

Between muscles—5–8%[3]

PROBLEMS ASSOCIATED WITH DIGESTION AND ABSORPTION OF FATS

steatorrhea Abnormally large amounts of fats in the feces.

dehydration Excessive water loss from the tissues (see Chapter 8).

pancreatic enzyme deficiency A deficiency in the amount of enzymes secreted by the pancreas. This deficiency is especially a problem with pancreatic lipase, which breaks down triglycerides.

Cystic fibrosis A hereditary disease characterized by secretion and accumulation of excessively thick mucus that blocks the secretion of pancreatic enzymes (see Chapters 17 and 19).

There are several conditions that can result in an inability to digest and absorb fats normally. The basic symptom that indicates the existence of this malabsorption problem is **steatorrhea.** The stools are light, mushy, greasy, and foul-smelling. This malabsorption problem may also result in severe diarrhea, **dehydration,** and electrolyte depletion.

Some conditions that can result in steatorrhea and other previously described problems are:

Pancreatic enzyme deficiency

Cystic fibrosis

Bile salts deficiency

Lymphatic obstruction

Liver disease

Short bowel

Gluten intolerance

In each of the above conditions, *long chain triglycerides (LCT)* are not absorbed and are lost in feces. The reason is that they must go through the complex digestive processes in order to be absorbed, and due to the

short bowel Surgical shortening of the length of the small intestine. Normally done as a therapeutic procedure to aid person in losing weight.

gluten intolerance A disorder in which gluten (protein) causes the destruction of intestinal villi, thereby preventing the absorption of fats and other nutrients (see Chapter 16).

above problems, this does not effectively occur. In order to compensate for these problems, *medium chain triglycerides (MCT)* were developed synthetically several years ago. These MCT can provide compensation for the following reasons:

- They do not require bile salts for digestion or absorption.
- They are rapidly absorbed, even with a short bowel.
- They are digested to yield fatty acids that are absorbed into the portal vein rather than the lymphatic vessels.
- They can be mixed with LCT, which improves LCT digestion and absorption.[4]

FAT AND THE EXCHANGE GROUPS

Two food exchange groups that contain considerable amounts of fat are meat and fat. Some foods on the bread and milk exchange lists also contain fat (see below). The meat and fat exchange lists whose foods contain considerable amounts of fat will be discussed below.

Meat

This group is subdivided into three categories according to fat content:

Low-fat meats (lean). These meats contain 3 g of fat per exchange and a total of 55 kcal. Examples of low-fat meats are given in the meat exchange list in Appendix A.

Medium-fat meats. This category contains 5.0 g of fat per exchange and a total of 75 kcal or add one-half of a fat exchange (see the meat list in Appendix A).

High-fat meats. Meats in this category contain 8 g of fat per exchange and 100 kcal or add one fat exchange (see the meat list in Appendix A).

Many people believe that meats in the high-fat category are better quality than meats in the medium- and low-fat categories. There are 7 g of protein per exchange in each of the three meat categories. The quantity of fat does increase from 3 to 8 g per exchange in moving from the low- to high-fat meats categories. Therefore, high-fat meats are certainly not better in terms of protein but, rather, contain more fat and are more tender than the low- and medium-fat meats.

One should be aware that a meat exchange is 1 oz of meat, which is not a normal serving size. For meal planning, 4 oz of meat or four meat exchanges is considered normal (2–3 oz for hospitalized patients). A small fast-food hamburger is about 2 oz when cooked.

Fat

A fat exchange is a serving of food that contains about 5 g of fat and about 45 kcal. The protein and carbohydrate contents are negligible.

Some examples of foods that contain 1 fat exchange are:

1 tsp of butter or margarine

⅛ of an avocado

5 small olives

2 large pecans

1 tsp french dressing

2 tbsp sour cream

1 tbsp heavy cream

1 strip of bacon

The milk exchange group list is based on 1 cup of skim milk. Therefore, if a person drinks 1 cup of whole milk, he or she is actually getting 8 g of invisible fat. In other words, "invisible" fat is not obvious when one looks at foods. Visible fat is that which can be seen, such as the strip of fat around beef cuts.

Some bread exchanges contain fat. Examples are:

1 biscuit—2-in. diameter (add 1 fat exchange)

1 piece of cornbread—2 × 2 × 1 in. (add 1 fat exchange)

8 french fried potatoes—(add 1 fat exchange)

15 potato chips—(add 2 fat exchanges)

1 pancake—5 × ½ in. (add 1 fat exchange)

1 waffle—5 × ½ in. (add 1 fat exchange)

SUMMARY

- A triglyceride molecule is composed of three fatty acids and glycerol.
- Saturated fatty acids contain no double bonds whereas unsaturated fatty acids do.
- Saturated fatty acids provide energy and raise the blood cholesterol level; unsaturated fatty acids provide energy and aid the liver in converting cholesterol to bile acids.
- Essential fatty acids cannot be synthesized by the body whereas nonessential fatty acids can be. An example of a polyunsaturated fatty acid is linoleic acid.
- A phospholipid contains two fatty acids and a phosphate group in place of the third fatty acid. Two fatty acids important in the body are lecithin and cephalin.
- A cholesterol molecule is composed of four fused rings of carbon and hydrogen atoms. 40% of cholesterol comes from food and 60% is synthesized by the body.
- Cholesterol functions in the body as a component of the cell membrane and as a precursor of steroid hormones; three food sources of cholesterol are egg yolks, butter, and cream.
- LDL function to transport triglycerides and cholesterol through the blood from the liver to the tissues; HDL function to transport triglycerides and cholesterol from the tissues to the liver where they are degraded to bile. An increase in LDL increases risk of heart attack or cardiovascular disease whereas an increase in HDL decreases the risk.
- Six functions of lipids are as follows: a concentrated source of energy; a component of cell membranes; a padding for body organs; an aid to absorption of fat-soluble vitamins; an aid in maintaining body temperature; and a component in various chemical reactions.
- Emulsification breaks large globules of fats into smaller globules without chemically breaking bonds; digestion chemically breaks the bonds in triglycerides and fatty acids plus monoglycerides are produced.
- Glycerol and monoglycerides plus fatty acids are recombined together to form triglycerides as they are absorbed through the small intestine.
- Short chain fatty acids are transported through the blood whereas long chain fatty acids are transported through lymph to body tissues.
- Steatorrhea is the basic symptom indicating that a person has an inability to digest and absorb fat. Three conditions that can cause steatorrhea are pancreatic enzyme deficiency, cystic fibrosis, and bile salts deficiency.
- Three reasons why MCTs can compensate for fat malabsorption are 1) they do not require bile salts for digestion or absorption, 2) they are rapidly absorbed, and 3) they are absorbed into the portal vein rather than lymphatic vessels.
- Low-, medium-, and high-fat meats differ only in their fat content: low—3g, medium—5g, high—8g.

REVIEW QUESTIONS

True (A) or False (B)

1. A triglyceride molecule is composed of a glycerol atom and three fatty acid atoms.
2. A saturated fat differs from an unsaturated fat in that saturated fats contain hydrogen atoms at every possible carbon bond.
3. Polyunsaturated fatty acids (PUFA) are valuable nutritionally because they are low in kilocalories compared to saturated fatty acids.
4. Three essential PUFA are glycerol, cholesterol, and arachidonic acid.
5. An essential fatty acid is one that the body has to make for physiological activities.
6. Three functions of phospholipids are: precursor of steroid hormones, component of fatty plaques, and powerful emulsifying agents.
7. The majority of cholesterol in the body is synthesized by liver and intestine cells.
8. Foods rich in cholesterol are egg yolks, butter, cream, cheese, sweetbreads, and shellfish.
9. Emulsification of globules increases their surface area, which enables lipase enzymes to break down the molecules.
10. Most glycerol and fatty acids are not changed as they pass through intestinal cells into the blood or lymph.
11. High-density lipoproteins (HDL) tend to lower blood cholesterol levels by transporting cholesterol from tissues to the liver, where it is broken down.
12. Steatorrhea is a basic symptom of abnormal fat digestion and absorption.

13. Some examples of fat digestion and absorption disorders are atherosclerosis, eczema dermatitis, and steatorrhea.
14. High-fat meats not only contain more fat but also more protein than low-fat meats.
15. People should be aware that some foods, such as biscuits, cornbread, and waffles, contain invisible fat.
16. A balanced diet should derive no more than about 30% of the total kilocalories from fat.

Multiple Choice

17. Functions of unsaturated fats are:
    A. a source of energy (9 kcal/g).
    B. to raise the serum cholesterol level.
    C. to aid the liver in converting cholesterol to bile acids.
    D. A, C
    E. B, C
18. A phospholipid is composed of:
    1. glycerol
    2. three fatty acids
    3. phosphate and nitrogenous compound
    4. fused rings
    A. 1, 2, 3.   B. 2, 4.   C. 1, 3.   D. 4.
    E. all of these.
19. The formation of lipoproteins is important because they:
    A. contain essential fatty acids.
    B. enable insoluble fats to be transported in blood and lymph.
    C. are precursors of steroid hormones.
    D. are stored in fat cells.
    E. none of these.
20. Lipase enzymes break down triglycerides to:
    A. fatty acids.
    B. glycerol.
    C. monoglycerides.
    D. A, C.
    E. A, B, C.
21. Short chain fatty acids are absorbed and transported by:
    A. lymph.
    B. blood.
    C. protoplasm.
    D. cellular fluid.
    E. none of these.

22. Medium chain triglycerides (MCT) can compensate for fat malabsorption problems by:
    A. not requiring bile salts to be absorbed.
    B. being absorbed slowly.
    C. being absorbed into blood.
    D. A, B.
    E. A, C.
23. Which of the following in regard to meat categories and fat plus kilocalories is (are) incorrect?
    A. low fat—3 g and 55 kcal.
    B. medium fat—5.5 g and 80 kcal.
    C. high fat—8 g and 100 kcal.
    D. all of these.
    E. none of these.

Questions 24–29 apply to the meals below. The information necessary to answer these questions is found in Table 2-5.

	Exchanges	Fat (g)	Saturated (S), Unsaturated (U)	kcal
Breakfast				
1 egg	1 meat + ½ fat	—	S	—
1 slice toast	—	0		80
1 tsp margarine	1 fat	—	U	45
Lunch				
1 cup skim milk	1 milk	0		—
2 slices bread	2 bread	0		160
1 oz cottage cheese	—	—	S	55
1 banana	2 fruit	0		—
Dinner				
6 oz fish	6 oz low-fat or lean meat	—	S	330
½ cup green beans	1 vegetable	0		25
½ cup carrots	—	0		25
1 plain roll	1 bread	0		80
1 tsp margarine	—	—	U	45
1 cup skim milk	1 milk	0		90

24. The breakfast meal contains _____ g fat and _____ kcal.
    A. 10–225
    B. 5–190
    C. 0–115
    D. 10–200

25. The lunch meal contains _____ g of fat and _____ kcal.
    A. 3–425
    B. 10–215
    C. 6–160
    D. 0–245
26. The dinner meal contains _____ g of fat and _____ kcal.
    A. 3–675
    B. 9–525
    C. 23–595
    D. 14–425
27. The three meals contain a total of _____ g of fat and _____ kcal.
    A. 13–1365
    B. 36–1220
    C. 25–1575
    D. 23–925
28. For all three meals, the number of kilocalories contributed by fats is _____ kcal, which is _____ % of the total kilocalories for all three meals.
    A. 324–27
    B. 258–39
    C. 456–47
    D. 189–25
29. In reference to adequacy, the total kilocalories contributed by fats is _____.
    A. higher than the 30% of total kilocalories/day.
    B. within the recommended 30% or less of total kilocalories/day.

Completion

30. Differentiate between low-density lipoproteins (LDL) and high-density lipoproteins (HDL) in terms of functions and correlation with increased heart attack.
31. Give six functions of lipids.
32. Describe the basic symptom that indicates the inability to digest and absorb fats and give three conditions that can cause this symptom.

CRITICAL THINKING CHALLENGE

1. Use the information below about a fast food meal to answer the questions that follow:

	calories	unsat. fat (g)	total fat (g)
Hamburger	562	10	32
French fries	220	5	12
Diet drink	0	0	0

   a. What percent of the total calories are the result of calories from fat?
   b. What is the ratio of unsaturated fat versus saturated fat? [Assume the amount of saturated fat is the difference between the total fat (g) and unsaturated fat (g).]
2. Use the following label from a tub margarine container to answer the following questions:
   Calories 90
   Fat (99% of calories) 10 g
   Polyunsatureted 5 g
   Saturated 2 g
   Ingredients: liquid soybean oil and partially hydrogenated soybean oil, sweet cream buttermilk, water, salt, and artifically colored with beta carotene.
   a. What is the ratio of polyunsaturated to saturated fat?
   b. What ingredients are the source of polyunsaturated fat?
   c. What ingredients are the source of saturated fat?
3. Your neighbor has a family history of heart disease and asks you for suggestions to decrease the risk of heart attack. Which of the following suggestions will be *most* beneficial to increase high-density lipoproteins (HDL)?
   a. Increase consumption of saturated fats.
   b. Increase consumption of polyunsaturated fats.
   c. Consume more fish than meat.
   d. Participate in an intense, prolonged exercise program.

REVIEW QUESTIONS FOR NCLEX

Situation. A 2-year-old child has cystic fibrosis (see p. 83). This condition is characterized by excessive secretion of thick mucus which blocks the entrance of pancreatic enzymes (ex. lipase). The child has steatorrhea (fatty stools) and is very much underweight for her age.

1. The blockage of pancreatic lipase and bile from entering the duodenum results in _____.
   A. triglycerides being absorbed into the blood without being digested
   B. triglycerides not being digested to monoglycerides + glycerol
   C. cholesterol and phospholipids not being digested to fatty acids + glycerol
   D. saturated fats being digested and absorbed but not polyunsaturated fats

2. Part of the reason why the patient is underweight is due to _____.
   A. a lack of fats providing a concentrated source of energy for cells
   B. fats blocking digestion and absorption of carbohydrates as energy source to cells
   C. lipase not being able to break down proteins as an energy source for cells
   D. undigested fats accumulating and blocking cellular metabolism

3. This patient will tend to be deficient in _____ vitamins.
   A. water soluble
   B. all types of
   C. no
   D. fat soluble

Situation. A client has been found to have high levels of cholesterol and plaque development in arteries.

4. This client's diet will have to be lower in _____ in order to possibly lower his blood cholesterol level.
   A. egg yolks, butter, cream, cheese, and meat
   B. chicken, vegetables, and fruit
   C. fish, chicken, skim milk, and fruit
   D. bread, skim milk, fruit, and vegetables

5. A lipoprotein that is probably elevated in this client's blood and detrimental to his plaque development in arteries is _____.
   A. chylomicrons
   B. HDL (high density lipoproteins)
   C. IDL (intermediate-density lipoproteins)
   D. LDL (low-density lipoproteins)

6. Two exchange groups that this person will have to decrease in order to lower his blood cholesterol are _____.
   A. bread and fruit
   B. milk and bread
   C. meat and fat
   D. vegetable and fruit

7. The type of fat that this client will want to decrease and ways to do this are _____.
   A. saturated and use poultry, fish, and legumes in place of red meat
   B. unsaturated and eat cheese, meat, and butter
   C. polyunsaturated and eat luncheon meats, franfurters, and sausage
   D. saturated and consume whole milk, meat, and salad dressings

REFERENCES

1. Nieman, D. C., Butterworth, D. E., & Nieman, C. N. (1992). *Nutrition* (rev. 1st ed.) (p. 192). Dubuque: W. C. Brown.
2. Dietary guidance: A changing environment. (1991). *Dairy Council Digest, 62*(5), 28–29.
3. Christian, J. L., & Greger, J. L. (1991). *Nutrition for living* (3rd ed.) (p. 181). Redwood City, CA: Benjamin Cummings.
4. Robinson, C. H., Lawler, M. R., Chenoweth, W. L., & Garwick, A. E. (1990). *Normal and therapeutic nutrition* (17th ed.) (pp. 444–446). New York: Macmillan.

5 PROTEINS

OBJECTIVES

Upon completion of this chapter, you should be able to:

1. Describe the chemical building blocks of proteins.
2. Define essential and nonessential amino acids, peptide bonds, and complete and incomplete proteins.
3. Discuss denaturation of proteins in terms of what happens to proteins and two causative factors.
4. List and briefly discuss five functions of proteins.
5. Discuss digestion of proteins in the stomach and small intestine.
6. Describe deamination of proteins in terms of products and importance.
7. Define biological value (BV) and protein efficiency ratio (PER) and give three foods that have the highest BV and PER values.
8. Give the protein BV that can produce growth and the U.S. RDA for protein of this value, as well as for proteins with lower BV values.
9. Define and give examples of positive and negative nitrogen balance.
10. Give the protein RDA for adults.
11. Discuss protein-calorie malnutrition (PCM) problems such as marasmus and kwashiorkor in terms of causes and symptoms.
12. Analyze meals in terms of the grams and kilocalories contributed by proteins.

INTRODUCTION

protein The most fundamental constituent of living matter. Proteins are essential for the growth and repair of animal tissue.

The term **protein** comes from the Greek word *proteios*, meaning of prime importance or primary. This is a most appropriate name for this group, since proteins are the most fundamental constituents of living matter. Proteins function as major structural and functional components of every living cell.

CHEMISTRY OF PROTEINS

Proteins are organic compounds that are composed of carbon, hydrogen, oxygen, and nitrogen atoms. They differ from carbohydrates and lipids in that they contain nitrogen atoms in addition to carbon, oxygen, and hydrogen; some proteins also contain sulfur.

amino acid The fundamental building block of proteins.

The fundamental chemical building block of proteins is the **amino acid.** Figure 5-1 shows the amino and carboxyl acid groups that compose amino acids. These two groups form the core of each of the 20 different amino acids. What distinguishes one amino acid from another is the **R-group** (see Fig. 5-2). The R-group can be thought of as being "the rest of the molecule"; it varies from one hydrogen atom to a complicated group of carbons and hydrogens. The R-groups also vary in their electrical charge.

R-group The rest of the amino acid that is attached to the amine and acid portions of the molecule.

Essential and Nonessential Amino Acids

Twelve of the approximately 20 amino acids that are widely distributed, can be synthesized by the adult body from carbohydrates, lipids, and other amino acids. These 12 are designated **nonessential amino acids.** The other 8 are known as **essential amino acids** and must be present in the diet (see Table 5-1). It should be emphasized that "essential" and "nonessential" refer only to whether or not an amino acid needs to be present in the diet and is not related to its importance in body functions.

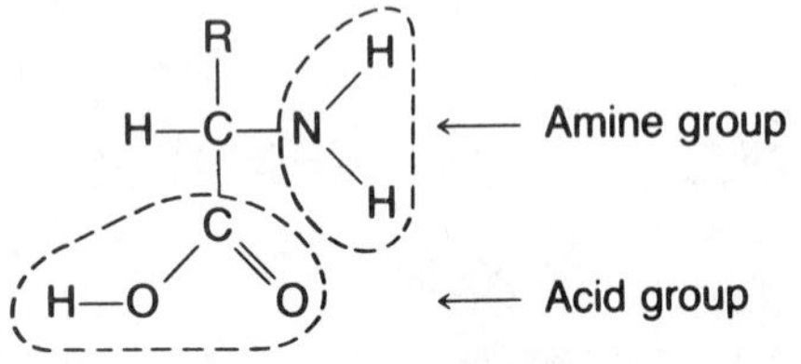

nonessential amino acids Amino acids that can be synthesized by the adult body from carbohydrates, lipids, and other amino acids.

essential amino acids Amino acids that must be present in the diet, since they cannot be synthesized by the body.

FIGURE 5-1 The core of an amino acid consists of amine and acid groups.

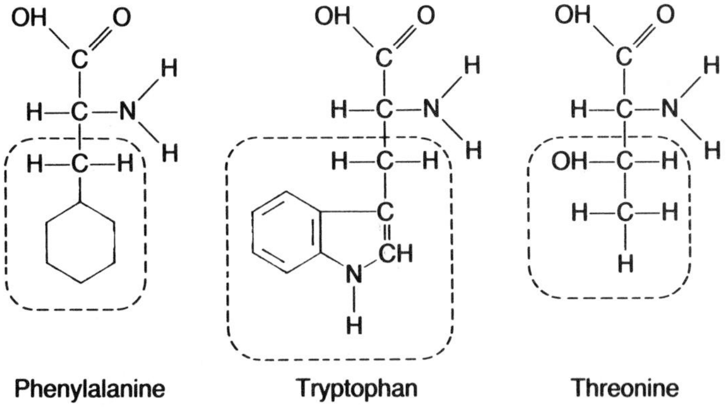

FIGURE 5-2 Three amino acids with their R-groups shown within the dashed lines.

Protein Structure

peptide bonds Chemical bonds that connect amino acids.

Proteins are very large molecules and frequently are composed of several hundred amino acids bonded together into long chains. **Peptide bonds** (see Fig. 5-3) join amino acids. Many proteins are composed of two or more connected chains that are twisted and folded into definite shapes (see Fig. 5-4).

TABLE 5-1 ESSENTIAL AND NONESSENTIAL AMINO ACIDS

Essential Amino Acids	Nonessential Amino Acids
Valine	Glycine
Leucine	Alanine
Isoleucine	Serine
Threonine	Aspartic Acid
Lysine	Glutamic Acid
Methonine	Tyrosine
Phenylanine	Proline
Tryptophan	Glutamine
	Asparagine
	Arginine
	Cysteine
	Histidine

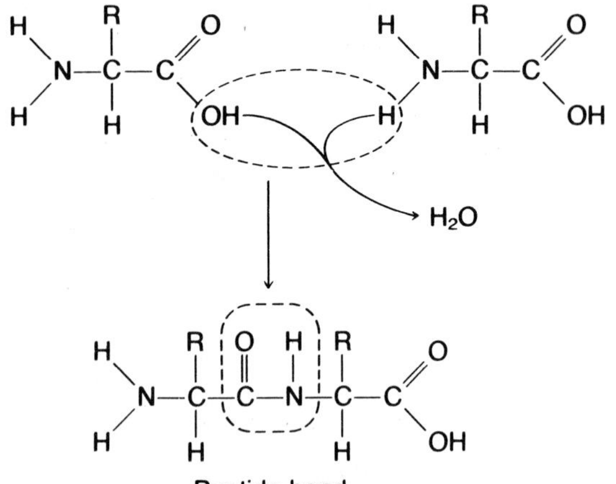

FIGURE 5-3 A peptide bond joins two amino acids together.

Complete and Incomplete Proteins

complete proteins Proteins
that contain all of the essential amino acids in amounts
needed by the body.

Complete proteins are found in animal products: meat, milk, cheese,
and eggs. **Incomplete proteins** are found in plant products: grains, kidney beans, garden peas, lima beans, seeds, and nuts.

incomplete proteins Proteins
lacking one or more of the
essential amino acids.

Sequence of Amino Acids in Proteins

The sequence in which amino acids are arranged in a protein is precise
and important. The body can synthesize so many different proteins because of the almost infinite number of ways the 20 amino acids can be
arranged. The function of each protein is directly related to its amino
acid sequence and to the shape of the molecule. To illustrate the importance of amino acid sequence to function, see the Clinical Application
"Sickle Cell Disease."

Sickle cell disease A disease
characterized by abnormal
hemoglobin that results in
sickle-shaped red blood cells.

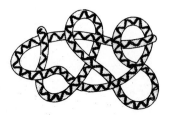

FIGURE 5-4 A twisted coiled shape of a protein is shown.

Clinical Application: Sickle Cell Disease

hemoglobin A protein molecule composed of four amino acid chains with one iron atom in each.

Sickle cell disease is characterized by abnormal **hemoglobin** in red blood cells (RBCs). Normal hemoglobin is composed of two kinds of amino acid chains. One chain in sickle cell hemoglobin is normal. In the other chain, the sixth amino acid should be *glutamine* but has been replaced by *valine.* This one alteration in the sequence of amino acids results in a hemoglobin molecule that cannot transport oxygen efficiently to the tissues. This condition is called *sickle cell disease* because the abnormal RBCs take on a stiff sickle shape (see Fig. 5-5 and Table 5-2). Due to their shape, the RBCs tend to become clogged in small capillaries, resulting in great pain and destruction of the cells. This problem is an inherited recessive trait and is seen almost exclusively in African Americans. Initial signs and symptoms are frequently seen in children under 2 years of age.[1]

denaturation A change in the chemical structure of a molecule; often occurs with protein molecules when certain conditions exist.

acidosis A condition in which the pH of blood is below 7.35; can result in the denaturation of proteins.

alkalosis A condition in which the pH of blood is above 7.45; can result in the denaturation of proteins.

Denaturation of Proteins

As stated previously, all proteins have a characteristic structure that determines their functions. If the structure of a protein is **denatured** (see Fig. 5-6), the functions of the protein are lost or altered. There are several factors that can cause proteins to be denatured in the body, such as high temperature and pH changes (**acidosis** or **alkalosis** conditions) in the blood. When these factors change, it is generally for a short period of time. As a result, the proteins are only temporarily denatured, resuming their normal shape once the condition is corrected. If the above changes

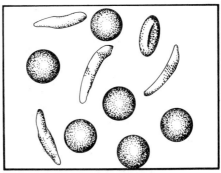

Normal RBCs and sickle cells

FIGURE 5-5 Normal red blood cells versus sickle cells.

**TABLE 5-2 NORMAL
VERSUS SICKLE CELL
SEQUENCE OF AMINO
ACIDS IN ONE CHAIN
OF HEMOGLOBIN**

Normal		Sickle Cell Disease
Valine	1	Valine
Histidine	2	Histidine
Leucine	3	Leucine
Threonine	4	Threonine
Proline	5	Proline
Glutamine	6	Valine
Glutamine	7	Glutamine
Lysine	8	Lysine

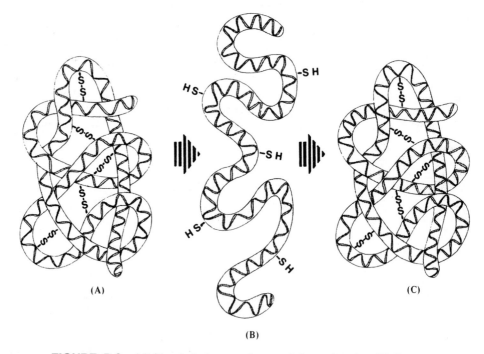

(A)

(B)

(C)

FIGURE 5-6 (*a*) Normal shape of a protein molecule. (*b*) Protein denatured or uncoiled. (*c*) Normal shape of protein restored.

persist, the proteins may be permanently denatured. An example of purposefully denaturing proteins is cooking an egg. Eggs are rich in complete proteins, but they are cooked or denatured before eating. Shampooing the hair is an example of temporary protein denaturation. The shampoo and water cause the **keratin** protein in hair to change shape temporarily, as indicated by the straightening of the hair. Once the hair is dried, the keratin protein molecules resume their normal shape, as evidenced by the appearance of the hair.

keratin A protein substance in hair and nails.

FUNCTIONS OF PROTEINS

Proteins have the greatest diversity of functions of the three energy nutrients. Several of the more important functions are discussed below.

Growth and Replacement (See Fig. 5-7)

As stated previously, proteins are the most fundamental constituent of living tissues; therefore, the growth and production of new tissues as well as replacement of old, worn-out cells require a constant input of essential and nonessential amino acids to the tissues. The cells then synthesize structural proteins such as **collagen** in connective tissue and *keratin* in hair. New tissue production occurs, for example, in a growing child and during pregnancy in both fetal and maternal tissues.

Examples of cell replacement include replacement of worn-out RBCs; replacement of **epithelial** cells that line intestinal tract and last for about

collagen Fibrous, insoluble protein found in connective tissue.

epithelial Cells that form the outer layer of the skin.

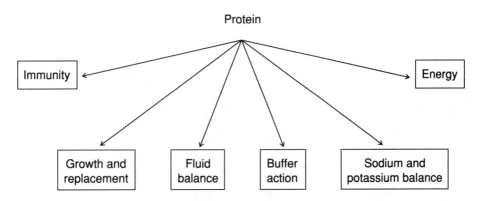

FIGURE 5-7 Functions of proteins.

a month; and constant loss and replacement of the outer layer of skin cells.

Immunity

antibodies Proteins formed by the body to combat antigens.

antigens Foreign substances (usually proteins) that invade the body; can cause infections and allergic reactions.

osmotic pressure Pressure on the cell membrane due to the inability of solutes to pass through it.

albumin A protein found in blood plasma that is important in maintaining fluid volumes in the blood.

One of the most important functions of proteins is to protect the body against infection from bacteria. **Antibodies** are the proteins that provide this protection. Specifically shaped antibodies are produced by white blood cells (WBCs) to inactivate **antigens.** Most of the time, the antibodies protect a person by destroying or inactivating a harmful antigen.

Fluid Balance

Proteins help to maintain levels of fluids in cells as well as in blood vessels. Proteins inside cells cannot diffuse across cell membranes and thereby create **osmotic pressure.** Osmotic pressure is very important in helping to maintain a balance of fluid between cells and tissues (see Fig. 5-8). Proteins in blood plasma, **albumin** for example, cannot move

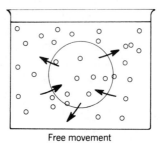

Free movement

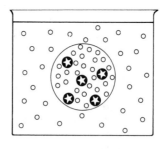

✪ = Protein
○ = Water molecule

FIGURE 5-8 Proteins inside cells help create intracellular osmotic pressure, which maintains the correct amount of water inside the cell.

across blood vessel walls and thereby help to maintain fluid volumes in blood.

Sodium and Potassium Balance

Sodium (Na^+) and potassium (K^+) ions are very important to the normal functioning of many cells. Sodium is concentrated outside cells (**extracellular**) and potassium is concentrated inside cells (**intracellular**). Cells maintain the position of these two ions by means of protein carriers in their membranes. Sodium and potassium ions tend to diffuse into and out of cells, respectively. The protein carriers transport the ions back to their original positions (see Fig. 5-9), a process often referred to as the **sodium-potassium pump.** The normal functioning of nerve and muscle cells requires the sodium-potassium pump.

Buffer Action

The normal pH of the blood, 7.35–7.45, is maintained by means of **buffers,** with blood proteins being one of the most important. Body processes constantly produce acids and bases that are transported by the blood to excretory organs. Negatively charged side chains of amino acids attract hydrogen (H^+) ions, thereby preventing the blood condition acidosis (pH below 7.35). If a large number of hydroxyl (OH^-) ions enters the blood, the condition alkalosis (pH above 7.45) exists. Protein buffers

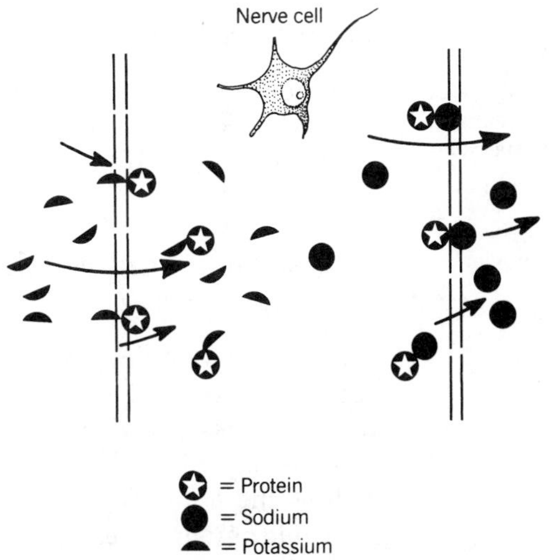

extracellular Fluid outside cells, such as plasma and interstitial fluid.

intracellular Fluid within cells.

sodium-potassium pump Protein carriers in cell membranes that transport sodium and potassium ions back to their original positions.

buffers Compounds in the blood that resist changes in pH with the addition of acids and bases.

Nerve cell

✪ = Protein
● = Sodium
◗ = Potassium

FIGURE 5-9 Proteins transport sodium out of and potassium into cells.

correct this imbalance by causing their positive side chains to release hydrogen ions, which combine with the hydroxyl ions to form water. This action prevents the pH of the blood from becoming too alkaline or increasing above 7.45. Ironically, proteins can be denatured by acids or bases, but they can absorb hydrogen ions in small quantities without causing their structure to change.

Energy

Proteins can be used as a source of energy (4 kcal/g), but at a high cost to the body. This high cost results from the fact that the previous functions of proteins are lost if they are used for energy. When the body does break down proteins for energy, the nitrogen atoms are not used, but rather are excreted. The nitrogen atoms are combined in the liver to form **urea,** which is excreted by the kidneys in urine.

urea A nitrogen waste product that results from the metabolism or deamination of amino acids and is excreted in the urine (see Chapters 17 and 20).

As the body decomposes amino acids for energy, approximately half of them are converted to glucose and then oxidized to release energy. This action is important because the brain normally uses only glucose as a source of energy.[2]

DIGESTION AND ABSORPTION OF PROTEINS

In order for all of the protein functions to be possible, the digestive tract must break down proteins into amino acids and absorb them.

Digestion in the Stomach

pepsin A gastric enzyme that breaks down proteins into short chain polypeptides, proteoses, and peptides.

The stomach secretes hydrochloric acid (HCl) and the enzyme **pepsin,** which break down proteins into smaller fragments, **proteoses** and **peptones** (see Fig. 5-10).

proteoses, peptones Intermediate-sized protein segments.

Digestion in the Small Intestine (see Fig. 5-10)

The proteoses and peptones move from the stomach into the duodenum region of the small intestine. Enzymes secreted by the pancreas break down proteoses and peptones into smaller fragments. This process is aided by secretion of sodium bicarbonate from the pancreas, which neutralizes the acidic fluid from the stomach.

dipeptides Molecules composed of two amino acid molecules.

A third group of enzymes secreted by the intestine function to break down the protein fragments into amino acids and **dipeptides.**

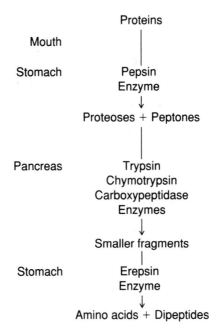

FIGURE 5-10   Digestion of proteins.

Absorption of Amino Acids, Dipeptides, and Tripeptides

ileum The terminal portion of the small intestine that is connected to the large intestine.

Amino acids, dipeptides, and tripeptides are absorbed by the jejunum and **ileum** regions of the small intestine. Once inside the intestinal cells, the dipeptides and tripeptides are broken down into amino acids, which are absorbed into the blood capillary vessels (see Fig. 4-12 for absorption of amino acids).

Actual absorption of amino acids occurs at specific sites by means of protein carriers. There is great competition for the carriers by the amino acids. If too many amino acids are present in the intestines at one time, their absorption will be hindered and many of them will not be absorbed but rather excreted in the feces. This condition is possible if a person ingests one of the liquid protein preparations. These preparations contain predigested amino acids and, since the material already contains amino acids, no digestion is required in order for them to be absorbed. However, because so many amino acids are competing for the absorption sites, many of them cannot be absorbed.

Following absorption, amino acids are transported by the blood to the cells, where they are metabolized or synthesized into proteins.

METABOLISM OF PROTEINS

■

Protein Synthesis

Cells absorb amino acids from the blood and synthesize proteins, decompose them for energy, or convert them into other molecules. Each cell has a need for specific proteins, the synthesis of which is controlled by **deoxyribonucleic acid (DNA)** in the nucleus. For details of this complicated process, you may consult a biochemistry or physiology textbook.

If, during protein synthesis, a nonessential amino acid is unavailable, the cell will synthesize the amino acid and attach it to the growing protein chain. However, if an essential amino acid is not present, synthesis of the protein ceases. One might think that the incomplete amino acid chain is held by the cell until it obtains the essential amino acid, but it is not. Instead, the chain is decomposed and the amino acids are returned to the blood, which contains the **amino acid pool.** It is important, then, to eat the eight essential amino acids within a 4-hour period. If they are not ingested during this period, many of the essential amino acids will be lost. People who eat foods such as meat, fish, poultry, cheese, eggs, or milk have no problems with this time frame, since these foods contain *complete proteins.* A strategy that vegetarians may wish to follow is one of *complementary protein* ingestion (mutual supplementation) (see Fig. 5-11). This strategy ensures that each food eaten supplies some amino acids that the others lack. By combining proper foods, one can get all of the essential amino acids. Some examples of complementary protein combinations are presented in Table 5-3.[3]

Deoxyribonucleic acid (DNA) A nucleic acid found in the cell nucleus. It contains genetic information for the synthesis of specific proteins.

amino acid pool A region in which large numbers of amino acids are maintained, such as in the liver. From the liver, the amino acids are distributed to the tissues.

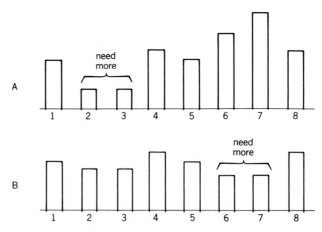

FIGURE 5-11 Example of protein mutual supplementation. Protein A lacks amino acids 2 and 3 but has sufficient quantities of amino acids 6 and 7. Protein B has sufficient quantities of amino acids 2 and 3 but lacks amino acids 6 and 7. Proteins A and B supplement each other.

TABLE 5-3 EXAMPLES OF COMPLEMENTARY PROTEIN COMBINATIONS

Complete protein: protein containing all of the essential amino acids.

Complementary protein combinations:
Peanut protein goes with wheat, oats, corn, rice, coconut
Soy protein goes with corn, wheat, rye, sesame
Legumes go with cereals
Leafy vegetables go with cereals

Traditional protein combinations:
Soybeans go with rice (Indochina)
Peas go with wheat (fertile Crescent)
Beans go with corn (Central and South America)

Catabolism of Amino Acids

catabolized Broken down.

deamination The removal of an amine group (NH_2) from each amino acid.

Amino acids are **catabolized** primarily in the liver. The most important catabolic reaction of amino acids is **deamination** (see Fig. 5-12). After an amino group is removed, it is converted to ammonia and then to urea, all in the liver. The rest of the amino acid molecule may be oxidized to release energy. If energy is not needed, the remains of the amino acids are converted to fat and stored in fat depots.

PROTEIN DIGESTIBILITY, QUALITY, AND RECOMMENDED DIETARY ALLOWANCE (RDA)

digestibility Pertains to the ease of digestion.

The amount of protein that is recommended per day depends upon such factors as **digestibility,** the completeness of the protein, and the individual's state of health.

Protein Digestibility

The ability of the body to digest and absorb proteins from various sources varies, as can be seen below:

Protein	% Absorbed
Animal	90
Legumes	80
Cereals and other plants	60–90

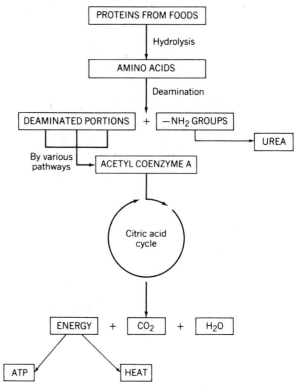

FIGURE 5-12   Deamination of a protein and metabolism of the remaining portion to release energy. (From Hole, John W., Jr., *Human Anatomy and Physiology*, 3d ed. © 1978, 1981, 1984 Wm. C. Brown Publishers, Dubuque, Iowa. All rights reserved. Reprinted by permission.)

As one can see from this list, if a person ate the same quantity of animal and cereal proteins, he or she would absorb considerably less cereal protein than animal protein.

Protein Quality

amino acid content   The number of essential amino acids present.

Biological value (BV) Measures the absorbed nitrogen that is retained for growth or maintenance and not excreted through the feces, urine, or skin.

Protein efficiency ratio (PER) Measures the growth of rats in relation to the amounts of protein eaten.

The quality of each protein is determined by its **amino acid content, biological value (BV),** and **protein efficiency ratio (PER).**

Amino Acid Content

A protein that contains all eight of the essential amino acids in exactly the right amounts is more completely used by the body than one that contains some of the essential amino acids in too small amounts.

Biological Value (BV)

The BV of a protein is defined as follows:

$$BV = \frac{\text{quantity of nitrogen retained by the body}}{\text{quantity of nitrogen absorbed from dietary protein}} \times 100$$

A BV of 70 is the minimum for a protein that contributes to tissue growth, assuming that an adequate number of calories are also ingested.

Protein Efficiency Ratio (PER)

Another criterion for evaluating protein quality is the protein efficiency ratio (PER), which is defined as follows:

$$PER = \frac{\text{weight gain of the animal}}{\text{protein intake of the animal}}$$

There is a wide range of BV and PER values for proteins. Animal proteins, such as eggs, milk, meat, poultry, and egg protein, have the highest BV. Plant proteins tend to have lower BV than animal proteins. However, they can provide an adequate supply of essential amino acids, but only if consumed in quantities greater than those of animal proteins needed to meet the body's requirements. Some of the more common foods and their BV and PER values are:

Food	BV	PER
Hen's egg, whole	94	3.92
Cow's milk	84	3.09
Fish	83	3.55
Beef	74	3.20
Soybeans	73	2.32

By these criteria, the best-quality protein is egg protein. Therefore, egg protein is generally regarded as the reference protein, and all other proteins are measured against it. As stated previously, a BV of 70 can produce growth. Therefore, if a person eats protein of this quality, the U.S. RDA is 45 g/day. However, if the BV of protein is less than 70, then the U.S. RDA is 65 g/day.

Recommended Dietary Allowance (RDA) for Protein

Protein is the first nutrient discussed that has an RDA. There are no RDA values for carbohydrates and fats. Nitrogen balance studies provide

nitrogen equilibrium
Conditions in which the amount of nitrogen consumed is equal to the amount excreted.

positive nitrogen balance   A state that occurs when more nitrogen is ingested than excreted.

negative nitrogen balance   A state that occurs when more nitrogen is excreted than ingested.

the basis for protein RDA values. These studies show that nitrogen lost by excretion must be replaced by nitrogen consumed in food. In other words, nitrogen in must equal nitrogen out. Most healthy adults are in **nitrogen equilibrium.** Some people ingest more nitrogen than they excrete, and vice versa. The former are in **positive nitrogen balance** and the latter are in **negative nitrogen balance.**

Growing children, pregnant women, and people recovering from serious wounds should be in positive nitrogen balance. The reason is that they need to synthesize new tissues to replace the damaged ones.

Negative nitrogen balance occurs frequently in people who are bedridden or go on reducing diets. Their protein tissues degenerate more quickly than new protein tissue is produced. Astronauts who spend several inactive days in space tend to suffer from a negative nitrogen balance. They are unable to exercise their muscles adequately and therefore suffer from a decrease in muscle mass.

The optimal amount of dietary protein varies. In establishing the amounts in Table 5-4, the Food and Nutrition Board of the National Research Council considered that the protein in a diet would be mixed (complete and incomplete), that not all proteins are used with 100% efficiency, and that individual needs vary. Most individuals can consume two-thirds of the RDA for protein listed in Table 5-4, and be assured of meeting their bodies' needs.

Note that the criterion of 0.8 g/kg for adults in Table 5-4 is based on ideal weight rather than actual weight. The reason is that the amino acids are needed by lean body tissues rather than fat tissues. Infants need more protein per body weight than any other age group, since they are growing rapidly and producing new blood, bone, muscle, and other tissues daily. In order for infants, children, and adolescents to maintain a

**TABLE 5-4 RDA
PROTEIN VALUES
FOR DIFFERENT
AGE GROUPS**

Age (yr)	RDA (g/kg)
0–½	2.2
½–1	1.6
1–3	1.1
4–10	1.0
11–14	1.0
15–18	0.9
19 and up	0.8

positive nitrogen balance, they need the amounts listed. Pregnant and lactating women also need a protein intake of 0.8 g/kg daily for their own body needs, as well as daily amounts of 10 and 12–15 g, respectively. During pregnancy, the increased protein provides for the needs of the developing fetus, as well as those of the mother.[4]

FOOD SOURCES OF PROTEIN

nitrogen-fixing bacteria
Bacteria that can take in nitrogen from the air and soil and convert it into proteins.

Two groups in the exchange system contribute large amounts of quality proteins: milk and meat (see Table 5-5). Vegetables and bread groups contribute small amounts of complete proteins and significant amounts of incomplete proteins. One plant family contains a large amount of complete high-quality proteins: legumes. These plants are rich in protein because their roots have nodules that contain **nitrogen-fixing bacteria.** Legumes, often called "poor man's meat," are an inexpensive source of protein. They are also low in fat and high in B vitamins and iron. A cup of cooked legumes supplies 31% of the U.S. RDA for protein and 42% of the iron.

PROTEIN-CALORIE MALNUTRITION (PCM)

Protein-calorie malnutrition (PCM) Malnutrition that is caused by deficits of calories, proteins, or both.

Protein-calorie malnutrition (PCM) may occur with deficits of calories, protein, or both. A calorie deficit results in a loss of body fat and, when either long-term or in the presence of depleted body fat stores, may result in decreased protein mass because the protein will be used as a source of calories. A protein deficit causes a loss of muscle or visceral protein mass regardless of the presence or absence of body fat. The

TABLE 5-5 PROTEIN CONTENT AND KILOCALORIES OF EXCHANGE GROUPS

Group	Serving Size	Carbohydrate (g)	Protein (g)	Fat (g)	Energy (kcal)
Milk (skim)	1 cup	12	8	Trace	90
Vegetable	½ cup	5	2	0	25
Fruit	1 serving	15	0	0	60
Bread	1 slice	15	3	Trace	80
Meat (lean)	1 oz	0	7	3	55
Fat	1 tsp	0	0	5	45

marasmus A type of protein-calorie malnutrition that results from a deficiency of proteins and calories.

kwashiorkor A type of protein-calorie malnutrition that results from a decreased protein intake.

hyperammonemia Excess ammonia in the blood.

hypophosphatemia A deficiency of phosphates in the blood.

deficit is due to the need for essential amino acids that the diet alone is not supplying. PCM is classified into two conditions: **marasmus** and **kwashiorkor.**

Marasmus

Marasmus usually occurs in infants 6 to 18 months of age when the mother's breast milk provides insufficient proteins and calories due to malnourishment of the mother. The infant is characterized by being grossly underweight, with an aged appearance (see Fig. 5-13). The cheeks and eyes are sunken. The abdomen may be swollen but the child's extremities are very thin, which is evidence of the wasting of muscle mass. Edema is minimal or absent and diarrhea is common. Body height is retarded and the child is apathetic, listless, and unable to cry.

Diagnosis of marasmus is based on physical findings of severe fat and muscle wastage as a result of prolonged calorie deficiency. Marasmus patients have a starved appearance, and frequently their weight and height are less than 80% of the standard values. Since marasmus is a chronic rather than an acute illness, it should be corrected gradually. An overly aggressive approach should be avoided, since it may result in metabolic imbalances such as **hyperammonemia** or **hypophosphatemia.**

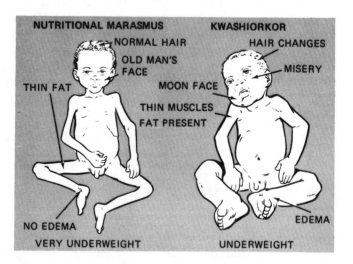

FIGURE 5-13 The appearance of children suffering from marasmus and kwashiorkor are shown. (From the U.S. Department of Health, Education and Welfare, Public Health Service Publication #1822, 1968.)

Kwashiorkor

In contrast to marasmus, kwashiorkor results from decreased protein intake for a short period of time. In children, this condition often occurs in the second child after he or she has been weaned after 1 year of age from breast milk to a starchy, low-protein diet of gruel or sugar water. A kwashiorkor child develops the following symptoms, which result from protein deficiencies (see Fig. 5-13):

- Edema—results from decreased synthesis of the protein albumin.
- Muscular wasting.
- Diarrhea—deterioration of the intestinal lining as a result of protein deficiency.
- Susceptibility to infections—these children are very susceptible to common childhood infections, which are often fatal. This extreme susceptibility results from the inability to synthesize antibodies that provide immunity.
- Depigmentation of hair and skin.
- **Hypoalbuminemia**
- Fatty infiltration of the liver.
- Decreased enzyme secretions of the pancreas.
- Severe vitamin A deficiency.
- Apathy—results from an inadequate amount of the protein hemoglobin, which carries oxygen to the cells, followed by release of energy.

hypoalbuminemia A low level of albumin in the blood.

In adults, kwashiorkor typically occurs in the hospitalized patient who is under acute stress from illness and surgery and is being supported with 5% dextrose solutions. Fat reserves and muscle mass tend to be normal or even above normal, which gives a deceptive appearance of adequate nutrition. Signs of kwashiorkor include easily pluckable hair, edema, and delayed wound healing. Characteristic laboratory values include severely depressed levels of proteins such as albumin, and the time of development may be as short as 2 weeks.

parenteral feedings Feedings that bypass the intestine and are infused directly into the veins.

Unlike the treatment of marasmus, **parenteral feedings** are often used in an attempt to restore normal metabolic homeostasis rapidly. One of the first objectives is to correct the diarrhea and electrolyte imbalances.[5]

Disease and Protein Requirements

In many disease states and with stress or trauma, protein requirements are increased because the body catabolizes large amounts of proteins for energy needs. As a result of the protein catabolism, the body is thrown into negative nitrogen balance and its weight declines.

In order to compensate for the protein losses, extra dietary protein together with calories must be provided. In severe cases, sometimes as much as 2–3 g of protein per kilogram of body weight may be necessary. However, in some disease states, particularly those involving the kidney or liver, protein intake must be decreased. The reason is that these two organs normally break down waste products of protein metabolism, but in a diseased state they cannot even handle normal amounts, much less increased amounts of waste products.

DISTRIBUTION OF PROTEIN KILOCALORIES IN BALANCED AND TYPICAL AMERICAN DIETS

As mentioned in Chapter 2, 10–15% of the total kilocalories in a balanced diet should come from proteins. This recommendation is for kilocalories only and is not specific for each individual. A much more formal recommendation for protein intake is the Recommended Dietary Allowance (RDA), which for an adult is 0.8 g of high-quality protein per kilogram of ideal body weight per day. If your ideal body weight is 55 kg, then $0.8 \times 55 = 44$ g of high-quality protein should be consumed each day. However, if you are consuming 1,500 kcal/day, then 10–15% is 150–225 kcal or 38–56 g. This example illustrates that the RDA for protein intake is based neither on the kilocalorie consumption nor on actual weight. Again, assume that your ideal body weight is 55 kg but that you actually weigh 65 kg. Your RDA for protein is still 44 g, since the recommendation is based on ideal and not actual weight.

Protein Content of the Exchange Groups and Typical American Meals

Table 5-5 gives the protein quality and content of the exchange groups. Using this information, we will calculate the protein content of some typical American meals. Let us assume that a 150-lb (68-kg) college student is at his ideal weight, his RDA for protein is $0.8 \times 68 = 54$ g, and he eats the meals listed in Table 5-6.

The RDA for protein for this student is 54 g, and as the calculations show, he consumes a total of 90 g for the three meals. Also, remember that the U.S. RDA for high-quality protein is 45 g. He actually consumed almost all of his RDA for protein at breakfast and lunch. Were the three meals balanced in regard to the distribution of kilocalories from protein?

TABLE 5-6 SAMPLE MENU

	Exchange(s)	Quality	g (kcal)/Protein	kcal
Breakfast				
2 eggs	2 medium fat meat	high	14 (56)	150
1 cup skim milk	1 milk	high	8 (32)	90
1 slice toast	1 bread	low	2 (8)	80
1 tsp margarine	1 fat	—	—	45
Lunch				
1 quarter-pound cheeseburger				
2 buns	2 bread	low	6 (24)	160
3-oz patty	3 high fat meat	high	21 (84)	300
1-oz low-fat cheese	1 low fat meat	high	7 (28)	55
Dinner				
4-oz hamburger steak	4 meat	high	28 (112)	400
½ cup mashed potatoes	1 bread	low	3 (2)	80
2 rolls	2 bread	low	6 (24)	160
2 tsp margarine	2 fat	—		90
			Total 96 (384)	1610

Kilocalories from protein = 360

Total kilocalories from all meals = 1,540

Percent of kilocalories from protein = $\dfrac{360}{1540} \times 100 = 23\%$

It is obvious that not only did the student consume (90 g) almost twice as much protein as is recommended (54 g), but the distribution of kilocalories (23%) from protein is almost twice as high as the recommended 10–15%. Unless the student's body is able to burn up the excess protein, it will be converted to fat and stored. In other words, in developed countries, people gain weight due to consumption not only of excess carbohydrates and fats but also of protein.

SUMMARY

- Amino acids are the chemical building blocks of proteins; each is composed of C, H, O, and N atoms and has an amine group along with an acid group. Amino acids differ in the structure of the R-groups.
- Essential and nonessential amino acids differ in that essential amino acids have to be provided by the diet since they cannot be synthesized, whereas the body synthesizes essential amino acids. Peptide bonds connect amino acids. Complete proteins contain all essential amino acids whereas incomplete proteins do not.
- Denaturation of proteins involves changing their shape and therefore their function; two causative factors are high body temperatures and pH changes (acidosis or alkalosis).
- Six functions of proteins include immunity, fluid balance, sodium and potassium balance, buffer action, energy, and growth-replacement of tissues.
- Digestion of proteins in the stomach involves pepsin breaking down proteins to peptides and proteoses; in the small intestine proteoses and peptides are broken down to dipeptides by pancreatic enzymes and to amino acids by intestinal enzymes.
- Deamination of proteins is important as the first step in oxidizing amino acids to release their energy; urea is the by-product of deamination of amino acids.
- Biological value (BV) is a measurement of the amount of nitrogen that is retained for growth and maintenance; protein effiency ratio (PER) measures the weight gain of rats in relation to the amount of protein eaten.
- A BV of 70 is the minimum value for producing growth or replacement; the U.S. RDA for this amount is 45 g/day whereas 65 g/day is the U.S. RDA for proteins of lower BV value.
- Positive nitrogen balance is when a person ingests more protein than excreted; a child undergoing growth is an example. Negative nitrogen balance is when a person ingests less protein than excreted; marasmus or kwashiorkor are examples.
- The adult RDA for protein is 0.8g/kg.
- Protein calorie malnutrition (PCM) is exemplified by marasmus and kwashiorkor. Marasmus results from prolonged calorie deficiencies; symptoms include a starved appearance, lack of energy, and low immunity. Kwashiorkor results from a rapid decline in proteins and involves muscular wasting, diarrhea, and susceptibility to infection.

REVIEW QUESTIONS

True (A) or False (B)

1. The amino acid is the chemical building block of proteins, and the carboxyl group varies from one amino acid to another.
2. Nonessential amino acids can be synthesized by the body, whereas essential amino acids have to be ingested in the diet.
3. A complete protein is defined as one that contains peptide bonds in several chains that are twisted around each other.
4. To increase the intake of complete proteins, one would consume more meat, milk, cheese, and egg products.
5. Denaturation of proteins is a condition that results from a change in the amino acid sequence.
6. Normal body temperature and pH of the blood can denature proteins.
7. Protein functions include growth and replacement, storage form of glucose, immunity, fluid balance, source of vitamins, buffer action, and energy source.
8. In the stomach, proteins are digested to amino acids and absorbed into the blood.
9. Absorption of amino acids occurs in the jejunum and ileum regions of the small intestine at specific sites and by protein carriers.
10. During protein synthesis, if essential amino acids are absent from a cell, the unfinished chain is broken down.
11. A person can avoid the problem in question 10 by eating more complete proteins.
12. Deamination of proteins involves the removal of urea and the oxidation of the remainder of the molecule to release energy.
13. The BV of a protein is a measurement of the quantity of nitrogen that is retained for growth and maintenance and not excreted.
14. The PER of a protein is a measurement of how many essential complete amino acids are present.

15. A protein BV of 70 is the minimum for growth, and the U.S. RDA for protein of this value is 45 g.
16. A person who consumes protein with a BV of less than 70 must eat about twice as much, or the U.S. RDA of 90 g.
17. All nutrients, including protein, have an RDA value.
18. The protein RDA for adults is 0.8 g per kilogram of ideal weight; if a person's ideal weight is 160 lb (73 kg), then he should consume 58 g of protein a day.
19. A person who consumes 75 g of protein a day and excretes 35 g would be in positive nitrogen balance.
20. In a balanced diet, 10–15% of the total kilocalories consumed per day should be contributed by proteins.
21. In a diseased state, consumption of protein should always be decreased in order to lessen the work of the kidneys and liver.

Multiple Choice

22. Amino acids that the body can synthesize are known as _____, and proteins that contain all of the essential amino acids needed by the body are _____.
    A. essential—complete proteins
    B. nonessential—incomplete
    C. nonessential—complete
    D. essential—incomplete
23. Denaturation of proteins involves:
    1. loss of protein structure
    2. loss of protein functions
    3. acidosis and alkalosis
    4. high temperature
       A. 1, 2, and 3   B. 1, 3   C. 2, 4   D. 4
       E. all of these
24. Which of the following protein functions and descriptions is (are) incorrectly paired?
    A. growth and replacement—collagen and keratin proteins.
    B. sodium and potassium balance—proteins block the movement of these ions into and out of cells.

C. buffer action—maintain blood pH of 7.35–7.45.
D. energy—proteins provide 4 kcal per gram of energy.
25. Which of the following correctly describes digestion of proteins in the stomach?
    A. proteins $\xrightarrow[\text{pepsin}]{\text{HCl}}$ amino acids
    B. proteins $\xrightarrow[\text{pepsin}]{\text{HCl}}$ proteoses and peptones
26. Which of the following is correct in regard to digestion and absorption of proteins in the small intestine?
    A. Enzymes in the small intestine break down protein fragments into amino acids, and dipeptides.
    B. The pancreas secretes no protein digestive enzymes.
    C. Absorption of amino acids and dipeptides occurs in the jejunum and ileum regions of the small intestine.
    D. A, C.
    E. B, C.
27. Synthesis of proteins is more efficient if _____ proteins are present in the body, and before proteins can be catabolized for energy they must be _____.
    A. complete—deaminated (removal of the NH_2 group)
    B. complementary—denatured
    C. incomplete—separated from urea
    D. essential—combined with DNA

Matching

___ 28. Biological value (BV)
___ 29. Protein efficiency ratio (PER)
___ 30. protein RDA for adult
___ 31. U.S. RDA for high-quality protein
___ 32. U.S. RDA for low-quality protein
    A. 0.8 g per kilogram of ideal weight
    B. amount of nitrogen retained for growth or maintenance
    C. 45 g/day
    D. 65 g/day
    E. measures growth in relation to amount of protein eaten

Match the following descriptions and symptoms with marasmus and kwashiorkor.

___ 33. chronic protein   A. marasmus
         deficiency
                              B. kwashiorkor
___ 34. exhibit severe fat and
         muscle wastage

___ 35. edema and easily pluckable hair

___ 36. fat reserves and muscle mass tend to be normal

___ 37. child exhibits an aged appearance

___ 38. increased susceptibility to infections

___ 39. can occur in patients who have been supported on 5% dextrose solutions for 2 weeks or longer

Questions 40–45 apply to the meals below. The information necessary to answer these questions is found in Table 5-5.

	Exchange(s)	g protein (kcal)	kcal
Breakfast			
1 egg	1 meat + ½ fat or medium-fat meat	___(28)	75
1 slice toast	1 bread	___(12)	80
1 tsp margarine	1 fat	0	45
Lunch			
1 cup skim milk	1 milk	___(32)	90
2 slices bread	2 bread	___(24)	160
1 oz cottage cheese	1 lean meat	___(28)	55
1 banana	2 fruit	0	120
Dinner			
6 oz fish	6 lean meat	___(168)	330
½ cup green beans	1 vegetable	___(8)	25
½ cup carrots	1 vegetable	___(8)	25
1 plain roll	1 bread	___(12)	80
1 tsp margarine	1 fat	0	45
1 cup skim milk	1 milk	___(32)	90
	Total	___(350)	Total 1220

40. The breakfast meal contains _____ g of protein and _____ total kcal contributed by carbohydrate, protein, and fat.
    A. 10–200   C. 28–195
    B. 16–32   D. 36–144

41. The lunch meal contains _____ g of protein and _____ kcal from all nutrients.
    A. 29–116   C. 22–76
    B. 21–425   D. 12–48

42. The dinner meal contributes _____ g of protein and _____ total kcal from all nutrients.
    A. 50–200   C. 57–595
    B. 42–725   D. 26–485

43. The three meals contribute a total of _____ g of protein and _____ total kcal from all nutrients.
    A. 89–1220   C. 350–1056
    B. 96–1678   D. 168–975

44. The number of kilocalories contributed by protein for all three meals is _____, which is _____ % of the total kilocalories for all three meals.
    A. 356–29   C. 198–21
    B. 543–10   D. 336–26

45. Using the information from question 43, did these three meals provide this person with an adequate number of kilocalories from protein?
    A. No; 30% is much higher than the recommended 10–15%.
    B. Yes; 10% is within the recommended range.

Completion

46. List and briefly discuss five functions of proteins.
47. Discuss protein-calorie malnutrition (PCM) problems such as marasmus and kwashiorkor in terms of causes and symptoms.

CRITICAL THINKING CHALLENGE

1. Calculate the RDA protein requirement for the following individuals (use the RDA table in this chapter):
   (NOTE: 1 kg = 2.2 lb)

   a. 6 month old, 14 pounds
   b. 6 year old, 46 pounds
   c. 12 year old, 100 pounds
   d. 65 year old, 170 pounds

2. Use the food label information below to answer the next several questions.

   Sirloin of beef in herb sauce with vegetables. Ingredients; beef sirloin, celery, chicken broth, mushrooms, onions, leeks, malt liquour, beef fat, honey, butter, beef base. Nutritional information per serving:

Calories	270
Protein	20 g
Carbohydrate	25 g
Fat	10 g

a. What percent of the total calories is from protein?

b. Which ingredients are providing complete proteins? Incomplete proteins?

3. Use the meal plan below to answer the next several questions.

   6 oz chicken (skin removed)
   1 cup pasta
   1/2 cup green peas
   2 whole-wheat dinner rolls
   1 cup skim milk

a. Calculate the total grams of protein.

b. Calculate the grams of complete protein or high-quality protein. List the foods.

c. Calculate the grams of incomplete protein or low-quality protein. List the foods.

d. What percent of total calories comes from proteins?

4. An acutely ill client has been admitted to the hospital with symptoms of protein calorie malnutrition (PCM) associated with complaints of 10 lb (4.5 kg) weight loss and nausea and vomiting during the past two weeks. Which of the following actions by the nurse is the most important aspect of the client's care?

a. Perform range of motion exercises daily.

b. Encourage oral fluid intake.

c. Have the client perform his own self-care activities.

d. Instruct the family and visitors on infection control measures.

REVIEW QUESTIONS FOR NCLEX

Situation. A 15-year-old client is a pregnant vegan vegetarian. She is very concerned about her pregnancy and what effect her vegan diet will have on her own body as well as the pregnancy.

1. This client's diet will _____ in _____ proteins.
   A. be deficient; incomplete
   B. not be deficient; complete
   C. not be deficient; complete or incomplete
   D. be deficient; complete

2. A strategy this vegetarian may want to follow is _____.
   A. complementary protein ingestion
   B. eating more quantities of vegetables and fruits
   C. eating more milk and vegetable exchanges
   D. consuming more fruits and vegetables

3. Which of the following protein functions, as regards the immediate needs of this client and her pregnancy, are lacking due to her vegan diet?
   A. immunity
   B. fluid balance
   C. buffer action
   D. growth and replacement

Situation. A client's ideal weight is 154 lb. (1 kg. = 2.2 lb). In one day he consumes the following exchanges: 10 lean meat, 1 skim milk, 6 bread, 3 fats.

4. What is the total amount of protein consumed by this client for the day?
   A. 46 g
   B. 56 g
   C. 76 g
   D. 96 g

5. What is the RDA protein amount for this client based on his ideal body weight?
   A. 37 g
   B. 45 g
   C. 56 g
   D. 63 g

6. What percent of the total kcal from these exchanges is due to protein?
   A. 31%
   B. 26%
   C. 11%
   D. 1%

7. If the total g of protein is excessive, compared to the client's body requirements, then the excessive amount is _____.
   A. converted to energy by cellular metabolism
   B. stored by the cells until the protein is required for growth

C. converted to fat and stored in fat storage areas of the body

D. excreted in the feces as undigested protein

REFERENCES

1. Whitney, E. N., Cataldo, C. B., & Rolfes, S. R. (1987). *Understanding normal and clinical nutrition* (2nd ed.) (p. 783). St. Paul: West.
2. National Research Council. (1989). *Diet and health implications for reducing chronic disease risk* (Report of the Committee on Diet and Health, Food and Nutrition Board) (pp. 1–750). Washington DC: National Academy Press.
3. Position paper on the vegetarian approach to eating. (1980). *Journal of the American Dietetic Association, 77,* 61–67.
4. National Research Council. (1989). *Recommended dietary allowances* (10th ed.) (pp. 92–93). Washington.
5. Soloman, N. W. (1985). Rehabilitating the severely malnourished infant and child. *Journal of the American Dietetic Association, 85*(1), 28–36.

6

VITAMINS

Upon completion of this chapter you should be able to:

1. Define and give a general description of vitamins.
2. Recognize the functions of vitamins A, D, E, and K.
3. Give the animal and plant food sources for vitamins A, D, E, and K.
4. Describe the deficiency and toxicity problems associated with vitamins A, D, E, and K.
5. Describe how the general characteristics of water-soluble vitamins differ from those of fat-soluble ones.
6. Recognize the functions of the vitamins thiamin, riboflavin, niacin, pyridoxine, cobalamin, folacin, and ascorbic acid.
7. Give the animal and plant food sources for the vitamins thiamin, riboflavin, niacin, pyridoxine, cobalamin, folacin, and ascorbic acid.
8. Describe the deficiency and toxicity problems associated with the vitamins thiamin, riboflavin, niacin, pyridoxine, cobalamin, folacin, and ascorbic acid.

INTRODUCTION
■

vitamins   A group of organic substances that are essential for normal metabolism, growth, and development of the body. They do not generate energy.

In the previous chapters, much information was presented concerning the nutritional importance of carbohydrates, lipids, and proteins in the body. The functions of these substances will not be performed, however, unless **vitamins** are also present. Their importance is so great that the *vita* part of the word *vitamin* comes from the fact that they are vital to cellular functions of the body.

GENERAL DESCRIPTION
■

noncaloric   Nonenergy-yielding.

coenzymes   A small non-protein molecule that combines with an inactive protein to make it an active enzyme.

fat soluble   Able to be dissolved in fats.

toxicity   The quality of being poisonous; a condition that can result from consumption of excess amounts of some vitamins.

hypervitaminosis A   An excess amount of vitamin A that results in a toxicity condition.

water soluble   Able to be dissolved in water.

Vitamins differ from carbohydrates, lipids, and proteins in that they are **noncaloric** nutrients. The molecular size of vitamins is quite small compared to that of the energy nutrients. For example, a molecule of vitamin C is about the size of a glucose molecule. They are never combined to form large molecules, unlike amino acids, for example. Many vitamins serve as helpers or, more accurately, as **coenzymes** in the metabolism of carbohydrates, lipids, and proteins. In carrying out this coenzyme function, they are not normally used up by body processes. Practically speaking, this means that the amount of vitamins the body can use is limited.

Consuming excessive amounts of vitamins is expensive, unnecessary, and may lead to unpleasant side effects. **Fat-soluble vitamins** can be stored in the body. This means that we do not need to consume them every day. In fact, an excessive accumulation of some vitamins leads to **toxicity; hypervitaminosis A** is an example.

Vitamins are divided into two groups according to their solubility: fat and **water soluble.**

Table 6-1 presents a summary of the food sources, functions, and deficiency/toxicity problems of each vitamin.

FAT-SOLUBLE VITAMINS
■

Vitamins, A, D, E, and K are soluble only in fats and are therefore absorbed into the blood together with dietary fats. They are stored in the body in adipose and liver tissues. Since they are insoluble in water, they can be transported by the lymphatic vessels or the blood only after they have attached to a protein carrier.

TABLE 6-1 SUMMARY OF WATER- AND FAT-SOLUBLE VITAMINS

Name	Food Sources	Functions	Deficiency/Toxicity
Vitamin A (retinol)	Animal Liver Whole milk Butter Cream Cod liver oil Plants Dark green leafy vegetables Deep yellow or orange fruit Fortified margarine	Dim light vision Maintenance of mucous membranes Growth and development of bones	Deficiency Night blindness Xerophthalmia Respiratory infections Bone growth ceases Toxicity Cessation of menstruation Joint pain Stunted growth Enlargement of liver
Vitamin D (cholecalciferol)	Animal Eggs Liver Fortified milk Plants None	Bone growth	Deficiency Rickets Osteomalacia Poorly developed teeth Muscle spasms Toxicity Kidney stones Calcification of soft tissues
Vitamin E (alpha-tocopherol)	Animal None Plant Margarines Salad dressing	Antioxidant	Deficiency Destruction of RBCs Toxicity Hypertension
Vitamin K	Animal Egg yolk Liver Milk Plant Green leafy vegetables Cabbage	Blood clotting	Deficiency Prolonged blood clotting Toxicity Hemolytic anemia Jaundice

(continued)

TABLE 6-1 SUMMARY OF WATER- AND FAT-SOLUBLE VITAMINS *(Continued)*

Name	Food Sources	Functions	Deficiency/Toxicity
Thiamin (Vitamin B₁)	Animal Pork, beef Liver Eggs Fish Pork Beef Plants Whole and enriched grains Legumes	Coenzyme in oxidation of glucose	Deficiency Gastrointestinal tract, nervous, and cardiovascular system problems Toxicity None
Riboflavin (Vitamin B₂)	Animal Milk Plants Green vegetables Cereals Enriched bread	Aids release of energy from food	Deficiency Cheilosis Glossitis Photophobia Toxicity None
Pyridoxine (Vitamin B₆)	Animal Pork Milk Eggs Plants Whole grain cereals Legumes	Synthesis of nonessential amino acids Conversion of tryptophan to niacin Antibody production	Deficiency Cheilosis Glossitis Toxicity Liver disease
Vitamin B₁₂	Animal Seafood Meat Eggs Milk Plants None	Synthesis of RBCs Maintenance of myelin sheaths	Deficiency Degeneration of myelin sheaths Pernicious anemia Toxicity None
Niacin (nicotinic acid)	Animal Milk Eggs Fish Poultry	Transfers hydrogen atoms for synthesis of ATP	Deficiency Pellagra Toxicity Vasodilation of blood vessels

Vitamin	Sources	Function	Deficiency / Toxicity
Folacin	Animal None Plants Spinach Asparagus Broccoli Kidney beans	Synthesis of RBCs	Deficiency Glossitis Macrocytic anemia Toxicity None
Biotin	Animal Milk Liver Plants Legumes Mushrooms	Coenzyme in carbohydrate and amino acid metabolism Niacin synthesis from tryptophan	Deficiency None Toxicity None
Pantothenic acid	Animal Eggs Liver Salmon Yeast Plants Mushrooms Cauliflower Peanuts	Metabolism of carbohydrates, lipids, and proteins Synthesis of acetylcholine	Deficiency None Toxicity None
Vitamin C (ascorbic acid)	Fruits All citrus Plants Broccoli Tomatoes Brussel sprouts Potatoes	Prevention of scurvy Formation of collagen Healing of wounds Release of stress hormones Absorption of iron	Deficiency Scurvy Muscle cramps Ulcerated gums Toxicity Raise uric acid level Hemolytic anemia Kidney stones Rebound scurvy

123

Vitamin A (Retinol)

Nature and General Characteristics

retinol A form of vitamin A that is found in food.

retinene A pigment that is derived from vitamin A and results from the breakdown of rhodopsin.

Most of the vitamin A we ingest exists in a form called **retinol.** Retinol is oxidized to **retinene,** which is the form that is functional in the response to vision in dim light (see Fig. 6-1).

Absorption, Storage, and Metabolism

Bile salts, along with fat, aid in the absorption of vitamin A through the intestinal mucosa into the blood. Vitamin A is transported to the liver, where 90% of it is stored and then distributed to the body tissues. Vitamin A is attached to a protein carrier in the liver before it is transported to the tissues to be metabolized. Therefore, if a person has a protein deficiency, transport of vitamin A and other fat-soluble vitamins is hindered.

Functions

retina The innermost layer of the eye that contains the visual receptors, rods, and cones.

rods Receptor cells in the retina of the eye that are sensitive to dim light.

cones Receptor cells in the retina of the eye that are sensitive to bright light and colors.

rhodopsin The compound secreted by the rods in the retina.

opsin A protein pigment that combines with retinene in the rods to form rhodopsin.

Vitamin A has three primary functions: dim light vision, maintenance of skin and mucous membranes, and normal bone and teeth development.

1. *Dim light vision.* The **retina** of the eye contains two different receptor cells, **rods** and **cones,** that are sensitive to light and transform it into nerve impulses. Rods secrete a compound called **rhodopsin,** which is composed of the protein **opsin** and retinene (a form of vitamin A). The reaction of rhodopsin with light and its resynthesis in dark are shown in Figure 6-1.

   As indicated in Figure 6-1, when dim light strikes rhodopsin, it is decomposed to opsin and retinene, with much of the retinene being destroyed. The destroyed retinene is quickly replaced by the rods oxidizing retinol. If an adequate amount of retinol is present, there is no problem with the rods changing retinol to retinene and then the resynthesis of rhodopsin in darkness. Rods are very sensitive to dim light; thus, vitamin A and rhodopsin are important in dim light vision

$$\text{Rhodopsin} \underset{\text{dark}}{\overset{\text{dim light}}{\rightleftarrows}} \text{opsin} + \underset{\text{(vit. A)}}{\text{retinene}} \rightleftharpoons \underset{\text{(vit. A)}}{\text{retinol}}$$

FIGURE 6-1 Role of retinene (vitamin A) and retinol (vitamin A) in dim light vision.

night blindness The inability to see well in dim light.

mucous membranes Membranes that line the cavities that open to the outside of the body.

keratinized To become hard or horny.

cornea The outer covering of the eye.

(see Fig. 6-1). However, if a deficiency of vitamin A exists, resynthesis of rhodopsin does not occur rapidly enough and the person experiences **night blindness.**

2. *Maintenance of mucous membranes.* **Mucous membranes** (see Fig. 6-2) are vitally important because they secrete mucus, which traps and removes invading bacteria, thereby protecting the body from infection. If the body is deficient in vitamin A, the mucous membranes lose their ability to secrete mucus and are transformed (**keratinized**) into a dry, hardened state. This condition reduces the ability of the membranes to resist infection. Two mucous membranes that often become keratinized are the respiratory mucosa and the **cornea** (see Fig. 6-3). Keratinization of the cornea can result in blindness and increased eye infections. Respiratory infections are increased when the respiratory mucosa is keratinized.

3. *Growth and development of bones.* Vitamin A is important, in some unknown manner, to the growth of bones in length and diameter (see Fig. 6-4).

Body Requirements

The amount of vitamin A a person needs is proportional to body weight. The amount required by the body is stated in terms of daily quantities; however, since it is stored in the liver, it is not necessary to ingest it daily. The Recommended Daily Allowances (RDA) for different people is given inside the front cover.

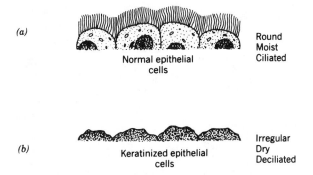

(a)

Normal epithelial cells

Round Moist Ciliated

(b)

Keratinized epithelial cells

Irregular Dry Deciliated

FIGURE 6-2 (*a*) Maintenance of the intestinal and respiratory linings by vitamin A. (*b*) Appearance of ciliated tissue with a vitamin A deficiency. (From Guthrie, Helen A.: *Introductory Nutrition*, ed. 5, St. Louis, 1983, The C.V. Mosby Co.)

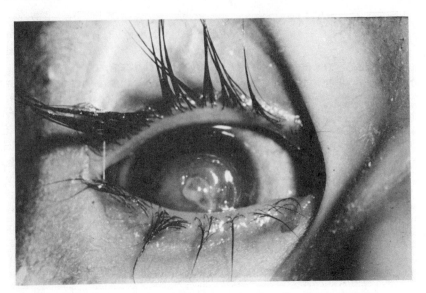

FIGURE 6-3 Keratinization of cornea due to vitamin A deficiency.
(Courtesy of Dr. D.S. McLaren, American University, Beirut, Lebanon.)

Food Sources

Sources of vitamin A are as follows:

Animal	Plant
Liver	Dark green leafy vegetables
Whole milk	Deep yellow or orange fruit and vegetables
Butter	Fortified margarine
Cream	
Egg yolk	
Cod liver oil	

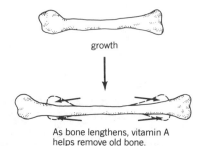

growth

As bone lengthens, vitamin A
helps remove old bone.

FIGURE 6-4 Role of vitamin A in the growth and development of bones.

carotene A precursor of vitamin A.

The vegetables and fruit mentioned above contain **carotene.** The body is able to convert carotene to vitamin A in the intestinal mucosa cells.

Vitamin A in food is fairly stable in the presence of light and heat but is easily destroyed by air (oxidized by reacting with oxygen) and sunlight (ultraviolet rays). Vitamin E is very helpful in that it is oxidized, instead of vitamin A, when they occur together. It is interesting that these two vitamins frequently occur together in foods.

Toxicity and Clinical Deficiency

Since vitamin A is a fat-soluble vitamin, it is stored in the body; therefore, the potential for toxicity problems exists. Some of the problems associated with vitamin A toxicity are joint pain, stunted growth, cessation of menstruation, and enlargement of the liver.

Toxicity frequency occurs in children because of parental overconcern about their getting the proper amounts of vitamins. These parents may inadvertently give their children too much vitamin A when they feed them breakfast cereals, milk, and chewable, candylike vitamins, all fortified with vitamin A. A daily dose of vitamin A in the amount of 5,000 retinol equivalents (RE) for a month has been reported as having toxic effects in infants. The ingestion of toxic levels of vitamin A may be a greater health hazard than a deficiency if one is consuming vitamin A in capsule form. Foods containing vitamin A can be eaten in large quantities without a toxicity problem, with the possible exception of liver.

A deficiency of vitamin A probably does not become clinically evident until after about a year of dietary deficiency. The reason is that the body can store about a year's supply of vitamin A in the liver. Clinical evidence of vitamin A deficiency is first seen in the eyes. Some examples of deficiency are summarized in Table 6-1 and below.

1. *Night blindness.* Since vitamin A is essential for the resynthesis of rhodopsin in the retina, this symptom is very common. It is difficult to detect in young children, and the doctor has to rely on the mother's noticing whether the child's vision at night is impaired.

xerophthalmia A condition in which the cornea becomes thickened and opaque.

2. **Xerophthalmia.** The cornea becomes thickened and opaque, resulting in blindness due to the decreased ability of light rays to enter the eye.
3. *Respiratory infections.* The mucosa of the respiratory tract also becomes keratinized (see Fig. 6-2) and therefore is not able to protect the individual from invading microorganisms.
4. *Cessation of bone growth.* Since vitamin A is important for normal bone growth and development, a deficiency can result in the failure of bones to grow and develop.

Vitamin A deficiency is widespread in India, South and East Asia, Africa, and Latin America. In the United States, it is most pronounced in Spanish-American and African-American children under 6 years of age.[1]

Vitamin D (Cholecalciferol)

Nature and General Characteristics

Vitamin D is a steroid compound that has hormonelike functions. Some people believe that it should be classified as a hormone, since it is synthesized in the skin. It is unique in another way: It occurs naturally in only a few common foods, but it can be formed in the body by the interaction of the skin and ultraviolet rays from the sun.

Absorption, Storage, and Metabolism

calcidiol The inactive form of vitamin D that is stored in the liver.

cholecalciferol Chemical name for vitamin D.

target organs Organs that are stimulated by hormones.

calcitriol The active form of vitamin D.

Vitamin D is absorbed through the small intestine with the aid of bile and is then carried into the general circulation by lymph. Vitamin D is removed from the blood and stored in the liver as **calcidiol.** It is also synthesized in the skin. Ultraviolet light rays from the sun convert cholesterol in the skin to **cholecalciferol,** or vitamin D_3 (see Fig. 6-5), which is transported from the skin and stored as calcidiol in the liver. Calcidiol is the most common form of vitamin D circulating in the blood but is an inactive form; therefore, it has little or no activity in **target organs. Calcitriol** is formed by the conversion of calcidiol in the kidneys (see Fig. 6-5), where the necessary enzyme is found. Calcitriol then travels through the blood to three primary target organs: the intestines, kidneys, and bones. Since calcitriol is secreted into the blood and travels to target organs, it is often described as a hormone.

Functions

The primary function of vitamin D is to aid the growth of bones (see Fig. 6-6). It does this in two ways. First, it increases the absorption of calcium and phosphorus from the small intestine. Second, it influences the deposition into and removal of calcium and phosphorus from bone tissue (see Fig. 6-6).

Body Requirements

The amount of vitamin D needed in the diet is difficult to establish, since the skin synthesizes some of it. However, the Food and Nutrition Board's recommended daily intakes are listed inside the front cover.

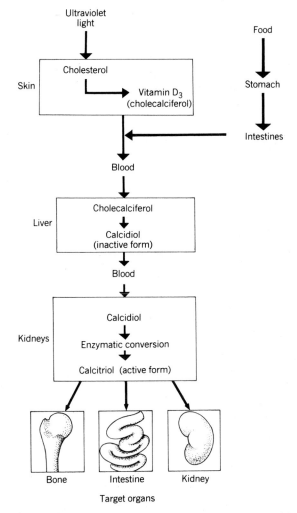

FIGURE 6-5 Synthesis of vitamin D (cholecalciferol) in skin, conversion to the inactive form (calcidiol) in the liver, and conversion to the active form (calcitriol) in the kidneys.

Food Sources

fortified The addition of nutrients to a food to make it richer than the unprocessed food.

As stated earlier, vitamin D is found naturally in only a few common foods: eggs, liver, butter, and cream. Therefore, we rely on **fortified** foods to make sure that we get our daily RDA. Milk is the best example of a food that is fortified with vitamin D. An adult who drinks two glasses of fortified milk daily can be assured of meeting the RDA even if he or she is not exposed to sunlight.[2]

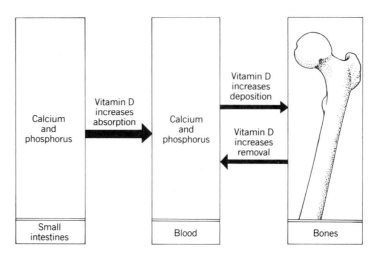

FIGURE 6-6   Role of vitamin D in the growth and development of bones.

hypercalcemia A condition in which the blood calcium level is elevated.

anorexia A loss of appetite.

calcification The hardening of soft tissues due to an accumulation of calcium.

Toxicity and Clinical Deficiency

Some of the problems associated with a toxic level of vitamin D are **hypercalcemia, anorexia, calcification** of soft tissues, head pain, and reduction in the growth rate of children (see Fig. 6-7). These toxic effects are summarized in Table 6-1, and hypercalcemia and calcification of soft tissues is discussed below.

1. *Hypercalcemia* (see Fig. 6-7). This condition results from an excessive amount of calcium being withdrawn from bones and absorbed into the blood from the intestines as a result of high levels of vitamin D. This condition can lead to other problems as follows:

   A. **Kidney stones** *and renal damage.* An excessive amount of calcium in the blood that circulates through the kidneys can result in the formation of kidney stones. Irreversible kidney damage can also result from excessive amounts of calcium being filtered by the kidneys.

   B. *Calcification of soft tissues.* Certain soft tissues (blood vessels, kidneys, and lungs) may calcify due to the accumulation of calcium in them (see Fig. 6-7). Kidney tissue is very prone to calcification, leading to kidney failure.

kidney stones The stones formed in the kidneys as a result of certain dietary and chemical changes (see Chapter 20).

osteomalacia The softening of the bones due to the loss of calcium or demineralization.

A deficiency of vitamin D can cause rickets in children, **osteomalacia** in adults, poorly developed teeth, muscle spasms, and involuntary twitching (see Fig. 6-8). These problems are summarized in Table 6-1 and on facing page.

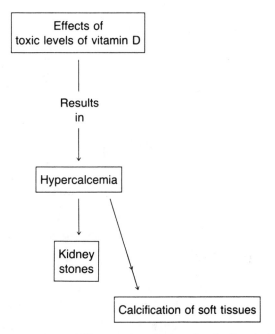

FIGURE 6-7   Effects of toxic levels of vitamin D.

1. *Rickets in children.* This problem has almost disappeared in the United States, primarily due to the fortification of milk. Cases are still seen in both Canada and Great Britain. Rickets is characterized by inadequate calcification of bones; as a result, the body weight causes the legs to bow (see Fig. 6-9). More serious bone deformities are bowed ribs and delayed closing of fontanels, which results in rapid enlargement of the head.

2. *Osteomalacia in adults.* This problem is also rare in adults unless the individuals have diseases that interfere with vitamin D absorption, such as **nontropical sprue,** obstruction of bile ducts, and pancreatic insufficiency. Osteomalacia is characterized by softening of bones due to the loss of calcium or demineralization. The limbs are deformed as well as the thorax, vertebral column, and pelvis. Bone fractures are also quite common.

nontropical sprue An alternative term for adult celiac disease (malabsorption disorder) (see Chapter 16).

3. *Poorly developed teeth.* Calcium is important for proper development of teeth. A deficiency causes slow eruption, improper development, and a greater tendency for tooth decay.

4. *Muscle spasms and twitching.* The blood calcium level is low in vitamin D deficiency, resulting in muscle twitches and spasms.[3]

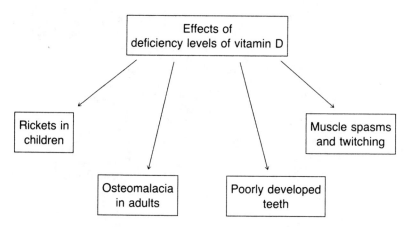

FIGURE 6-8   Effects of vitamin D deficiency.

Vitamin E (Alpha-Tocopherol)

Nature and General Characteristics

Vitamin E is chemically known as alpha-tocopherol (Greek: to bear off-spring). This name is derived from its function as an antisterility compound in rats. However, this function, as well as other nutritional roles of vitamin E (increasing male sexual potency and reducing heart problems) in humans, has not been substantiated after many years of research. There are four forms of the vitamin, but alpha-tocopherol is the most active form.

Absorption and Metabolism

Vitamin E is absorbed into the blood, as are other fat-soluble vitamins, with bile salts and fat being required.

Functions

antioxidant A compound that prevents oxidation.

The only documented nutritional role of vitamin E in humans is that of an **antioxidant.** Compounds such as vitamin A or polyunsaturated fatty acids (PUFA) cannot be used as well by the body after they have been oxidized. However, some compounds react more readily than others in the oxidation process. When such a compound is present in a mixture of compounds, it probably will be oxidized rather than the others. Vitamin E acts as an antioxidant for vitamin A and PUFA because it is more readily oxidized, thereby protecting them.

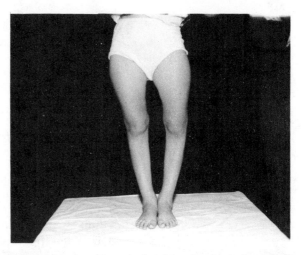

FIGURE 6-9 Rickets is characterized by inadequate calcification of the bones. As a result, the body weight causes the legs to bow.

Body Requirements

The RDA for different people for vitamin E is given in the RDA table (inside front cover).

Food Sources

The major food sources are fats and oils, particularly unsaturated fat products. This is a very fortunate coincidence, since the vitamin requirement apparently increases with the PUFA intake. Approximately 60% of the vitamin E we ingest comes from margarines, salad dressings, and shortenings. Ten percent comes from fruits and vegetables, and a small percentage comes from grains such as soybeans and wheat. Soybean oil and wheat germ oil contain very high concentrations of vitamin E. Green leafy vegetables are moderate sources, as are liver and eggs. Animal foods other than the two just mentioned are generally poor sources of the vitamin.

erythrocytes Red blood cells.

hemolyzed Broken down.

A deficiency of vitamin E in humans has been shown to be detrimental to **erythrocytes** when blood levels of vitamin E drop below 100 mg/dl. The red blood cells (RBCs) are **hemolyzed** and spill out hemoglobin. This serious problem is thought to result from the oxidation of PUFA in the RBC membranes. One way that oxidation occurs is by the addition of oxygen to a compound. PUFA in RBCs are very susceptible to this condition when the RBCs pass through capillaries in the lungs, where they exchange CO_2 for O_2. As described previously, normal amounts of vitamin E act as an antioxidant to protect PUFA and thereby prevent RBC hemolysis.

Vitamin K

Nature and General Characteristics

quinones A group of chemical compounds that includes vitamin K.

There are several forms of vitamin K, all of which belong to a chemical group called **quinones.** Bacteria in the large intestine produce vitamin K in quantities that are usually adequate for the body's needs. However, the intestine of a newborn infant is sterile. Therefore, no vitamin K production occurs until about the third or fourth day of life, when the bacteria have colonized the intestine.

Absorption and Metabolism

Vitamin K is absorbed with the aid of bile. Then chylomicrons transport the molecule to the liver, where most of it is stored and used. Any disorders that interfere with secretion of bile (such as cholecystitis) or absorption of fat (such as celiac sprue or cystic fibrosis) will interfere with absorption and transport of vitamin K. Water-soluble or water-miscible forms of vitamin K are available in these cases.

Functions

prothrombin A blood protein that contributes to blood clotting.

Vitamin K plays a role in blood clotting when a person is hemorrhaging by aiding in the synthesis of the protein **prothrombin** (see Fig. 6-10). Vitamin K aids in the synthesis of other blood-clotting factors as well.

Body Requirements

placenta A structure present within the uterus of a pregnant woman that is connected to the developing fetus and exchanges wastes and nutrients.

The recommended amount of vitamin K is presented in the inside back cover which gives the estimated safe and adequate daily dietary intakes (ESADDI). The amounts for adults are small, since intestinal bacteria generally synthesize enough for daily needs. Newborn infants and especially premature infants, however, are a special case, since only a limited amount of the vitamin is transported across the **placenta** into the infant's body during pregnancy. Also, as previously mentioned, the intestinal bacteria are not established for a few days after birth. Therefore, many authorities suggest that a newborn term or premature infant receive 1 mg of vitamin K in order to prevent hemorrhage problems.

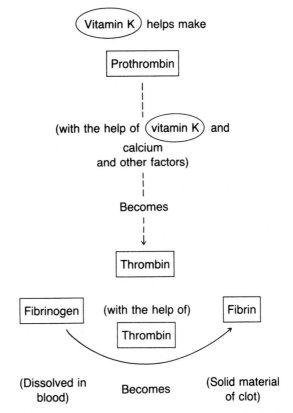

FIGURE 6-10 Role of vitamin K in blood clotting.

Food Sources

Green leafy vegetables, cabbage, and milk are good sources of vitamin K. Egg yolk and some types of liver (pork) contain moderate amounts.

Toxicity and Clinical Deficiency

hemolytic anemia A condition that results in the destruction of red blood cells (RBCs) at a faster than normal rate.

jaundice Yellow discoloration of the whites of the eyes and the skin.

Large amounts of vitamin K given to an infant over a prolonged period of time may produce **hemolytic anemia** and **jaundice.**

A deficiency of vitamin K normally is rare unless a person has difficulty in absorbing it, such as in a deficiency of bile. Another example is a person who has been taking large amounts of antibiotics (sulfonamides and tetracycline). These compounds either kill the intestinal bacteria or depress vitamin K synthesis. As a result, if an artery or vein is cut, the person will hemorrhage, since the blood-clotting process has been hindered.[4]

WATER-SOLUBLE VITAMINS

Certain vitamins are soluble in water and easily absorbed into blood. Excessive quantities of them are excreted rather than stored, unlike fat-soluble vitamins. Since water-soluble vitamins are readily excreted, it is unlikely that a person would store them to the point of developing toxicity problems. Water-soluble vitamins include B complex vitamins and ascorbic acid.

B Complex Vitamins

There are six major B complex vitamins and six minor ones. RDAs have been established for thiamin (B_1), riboflavin (B_2), B_6, B_{12}, niacin (nicotinic acid), and folacin (folic acid).

Several of the B vitamins function as coenzymes. The coenzymes have several specific functions, but they all have one thing in common: They are necessary for enzyme function.

Thiamin (Vitamin B_1)

General Characteristics, Absorption, and Metabolism

Vitamin B_1 is called *thiamin* because it contains a sulfur molecule and an amine group. It is absorbed from the duodenum into the general circulation, which carries it to the tissues. Alcohol and barbiturates hinder its absorption.

Functions

The principal function of thiamin is that of a coenzyme in the process of oxidizing glucose to form adenosine triphosphate (ATP), which is the basic energy molecule of the body. Thiamin prepares compounds (see Fig. 6-11) to enter the Krebs (citric acid) cycle, which is very important in the synthesis of ATP molecules.

Body Requirements

The need for thiamin increases with the need for calories. Thus, increased thiamin is quite important during growth periods, pregnancy and lactation, infections, and chronic illness.

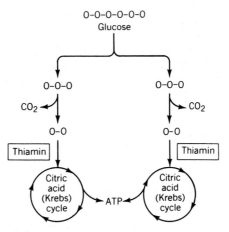

FIGURE 6-11 Role of thiamin in the synthesis of ATP.

The basic RDA is 0.5 mg/1,000 kcal/day. For example, if a 1-year-old child ingested 1,300 kcal/day, the RDA would be about 0.7 mg. A 19-year-old boy who ingested 3,000 kcal/day would need about 1.5 mg.

Food Sources

Good sources of thiamin are lean pork, beef, liver, whole or enriched grains, and legumes. Eggs, fish, and a few vegetables are fair sources. Thiamin is not as widely found in foods as are some of the other vitamins, such as A and C. Therefore, a person on an average diet, especially one low in calories, may have a thiamin deficiency.

Clinical Deficiency

Deficiencies of thiamin produce clinical disorders in the gastrointestinal, nervous, and cardiovascular systems. *Beriberi* is the term often used to describe this condition. The underlying cause of the symptoms is a decrease in the amount of energy released. Thiamin deficiency is most often seen in chronic alcoholics, since their diets are often inadequate in the proper amounts and types of foods. The nervous system is most dramatically affected. The earliest symptom indicating deterioration of the nervous system is heaviness of the legs. A burning sensation in the feet is often followed by progressive weakness of the toes, feet, legs, and thighs. In the cardiovascular system, the heart may weaken, followed by heart failure. The peripheral blood vessels are often weakened, resulting in **peripheral edema.** If the thiamin deficiency is persistent, an alcoholic

peripheral edema Excess accumulation of interstitial fluids within the extremities.

Wernicke-Korsakoff disease
A mental disorder caused by
a thiamin deficiency.

can ultimately develop a mental disorder called **Wernicke-Korsakoff disease.**

Riboflavin (Vitamin B₂)

General Characteristics

flavins A group of chemicals
that are fluorescent.

Vitamin B_2 is a member of a group of chemicals called **flavins,** which are fluorescent. Attached to the flavin part of the molecule is the five-carbon sugar, ribose, hence the name *riboflavin.*

Absorption of riboflavin occurs in the upper portion of the gastrointestinal tract by a specific transport system. The amount absorbed is higher in older compared to younger people. More riboflavin is absorbed when eaten with food than when taken separately.

Several drugs affect the metabolism of riboflavin, with tetracycline antibiotics and the thiazide diuretics increasing urinary excretion.

Functions

**Flavin adenine dinucleotide
(FAD)** An electron transfer
compound that transfers electrons and hydrogen atoms
from the Krebs cycle through
the cytochrome system to
oxygen.

cytochrome A molecule in
the electron transport system.

Similar to thiamin, riboflavin functions in the release of energy from food. Riboflavin is a component of the electron transfer compound called **flavin adenine dinucleotide (FAD).** FAD transfers electrons and hydrogen atoms from the Krebs cycle through the **cytochrome** system to oxygen. It is this transfer process that produces the majority of ATP or energy molecules for the body. Riboflavin also participates in the first step of the decomposition of fatty acids for the production of energy.

Body Requirements

The RDA for riboflavin are based on energy intake and are given on the inside front cover. As with thiamin, increased riboflavin intake is important during pregnancy and lactation, growth periods, infections, and chronic illness.

Food Sources

It is ironic that riboflavin is widely distributed in food, but only in small amounts in foods that we commonly eat. Examples of foods that are rich in riboflavin are milk, green leafy vegetables, cereals, and enriched bread.

Riboflavin is destroyed by ultraviolet rays (sunlight). This is one of the reasons why milk is no longer sold in transparent glass bottles. Transparent plastic bottles filter out more light and help to reduce the destruction of riboflavin.

Toxicity and Clinical Deficiency

There is no known toxicity from vitamin B_2. A deficiency of this vitamin can cause the following problems and is summarized in Table 6-1: **cheilosis, glossitis,** and **photophobia.** A riboflavin deficiency rarely occurs in isolation, but rather with other vitamin deficiencies.[5]

cheilosis Cracks at the corner of the mouth due to a deficiency of vitamin B_2.

glossitis Smooth, purplish appearance of the tongue due to a deficiency of vitamin B_2.

photophobia Sensitivity of the eyes to light and strain.

Niacin (Nicotinic Acid)

General Characteristics, Absorption, and Metabolism

Two forms of niacin exist: niacin and nicotinamide adenine dinucleotide (NAD) (see Fig. 6-12). The body converts niacin to nicotinamide, which is the active functional form of the vitamin. Niacin is absorbed in the upper part of the small intestine and is stored in very small quantities. The metabolism of niacin also includes its synthesis from the amino acid tryptophan. Research has shown that approximately 60 mg of **tryptophan** is converted to 1 mg of niacin.

tryptophan An amino acid.

Functions

Niacin is part of a coenzyme (NAD) that is vital in obtaining energy from glucose. NAD transfers hydrogen atoms and their energy to the electron transport system in cells for the purpose of synthesizing high-energy ATP molecules.

Body Requirements

The RDA for niacin, given on the inside front cover, is based on kilocalorie intake due to its role in obtaining energy from glucose.

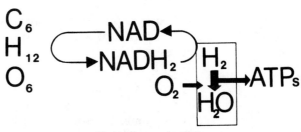

Electron transport system

FIGURE 6-12 The role of niacin (as a component of NAD) in transferring hydrogen (H_2) atoms in the electron transport system and synthesis of ATP.

Food Sources

Good sources of tryptophan are milk and eggs. Good sources of niacin are meat, poultry, and fish.

Toxicity and Clinical Deficiency

vasodilation   Increased diameter or size of blood vessels.

pellagra   A condition that is caused by a niacin deficiency.

dementia   A severe mental disorder involving impairment of mental ability.

Large amounts of niacin may result in **vasodilation** of blood vessels in the skin. **Pellagra** is a disease that may result from a niacin deficiency. It is characterized by the three Ds—diarrhea, **dementia,** and dermatitis. Diarrhea occurs when the intestinal mucosa becomes inflamed, excreting large amounts of watery feces.

A person suffering from dementia may exhibit mental confusion, anxiety, and depression. These problems occur when the nervous system does not get enough energy.

Dermatitis occurs on parts of the skin exposed to the sun, with the neck being a common location.

Most pellegra has been eliminated in the United States. It is still found, however, in some Third World countries where protein malnutrition is rampant.[6]

Pyridoxine (Vitamin B₆)

General Characteristics, Absorption, and Metabolism

Vitamin B_6 actually refers to several related compounds that are interconvertible and biologically active. Like the other water-soluble vitamins, vitamin B_6 is readily absorbed into the blood together with water from the small intestine. A small amount is stored in muscle tissue.

Functions

Pyridoxine is primarily involved with reactions involving the synthesis and catabolism of amino acids and, therefore, is important for protein synthesis.

1. *Synthesis of nonessential amino acids.* Vitamin B_6 aids in changing amino acids that occur in abundance to forms that the cells need at a given time. In other words, it aids in the synthesis of nonessential amino acids (see Fig. 6-13).
2. *Conversion of amino acid tryptophan to the vitamin niacin.* Vitamin B_6 converts **tryptophan** into the vitamin niacin (see Fig. 6-13) (discussed shortly).

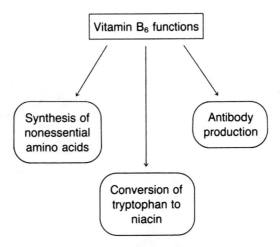

FIGURE 6-13   Functions of vitamin B_6.

3. *Antibody production.* Vitamin B_6 aids in the production of antibodies (see Fig. 6-13) that protect the body against the invasion of foreign antigens.

Food Sources

The best food sources of vitamin B_6 are bananas, baked potatoes, and chicken. Milk and eggs provide small amounts.

Toxicity and Clinical Deficiency

Deficiencies can result in cheilosis (see Fig. 6-14) and glossitis (see Fig. 6-15). The nervous system shows the deficiency by conducting an abnormal number of nerve impulses, which can result in **convulsions** and abnormal brain wave patterns.

convulsions Involuntary spasms or contractions of groups of muscles.

In addition to dietary deficiencies of vitamin B_6, several drugs interfere with its metabolism. Some examples are isoniazid (INH), levodopa (L-dopa), chloramphenicol, and particularly oral contraceptives.[7]

Cobalamin (Vitamin B_{12})

General Characteristics, Absorption, and Metabolism

Vitamin B_{12} is a complicated molecule that contains the mineral cobalt, hence the name *cobalamin.*

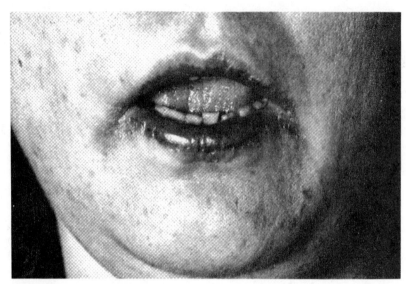

FIGURE 6-14 Cracking of skin at the corners of the mouth (cheilosis) due to deficiency of pyridoxine. (Courtesy of R.H. Kampmeier, M.D., Vanderbilt University.)

intrinsic factor A protein that is secreted by the gastric mucosa and combines with vitamin B_{12}, thereby making its absorption possible.

extrinsic factor A compound that refers to vitamin B_{12} and is formed outside the body.

gastritis Inflammation of the stomach lining.

Absorption of vitamin B_{12} is difficult due to its large size. To facilitate absorption, it combines with an **intrinsic factor** synthetized by the stomach mucosa. Vitamin B_{12} is called the **extrinsic factor,** since its source is outside the body. The intrinsic and extrinsic factors combine in the stomach to form a complex (see Fig. 6-16) that enables vitamin B_{12} to be absorbed from the small intestine.

The rate of vitamin B_{12} absorption tends to decrease with age, with pyridoxine deficiency, with **gastritis,** and in people who have congenital intrinsic factor deficiency. Interestingly, pregnancy enhances its absorption.

Functions

myelin sheath A sheath, composed of fatty material, that surrounds and insulates some nerve fibers.

Vitamin B_{12} interacts with the cardiovascular and nervous systems to help maintain homeostasis. It also interacts with the red bone marrow in the synthesis of RBCs (see Fig. 6-17). The importance of this function cannot be overemphasized, since RBCs carry oxygen gas molecules to the cells, resulting in the release of energy. Vitamin B_{12} is important to the nervous system, since it helps to maintain the **myelin sheath** that surrounds and insulates some nerve fibers.

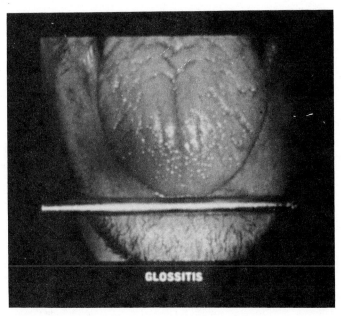

GLOSSITIS

FIGURE 6-15 A deficiency of vitamin B₆ (pyridoxine) may cause the tongue to become smooth (glossitis). (From Sandstead, H.H., Carter, J.P., and Darby, W.J. "How to diagnose nutritional disorders in daily practice," *Nutrition Today*, 4, 2 (Summer) 1969.)

Body Requirements

The body needs very little vitamin B₁₂ to be effective, as indicated in the RDA table (inside front cover).

Food Sources

Vitamin B₁₂ occurs in animal products only; none is found in plants. Seafood, meat, eggs, and milk are good sources. Strict vegetarians may become deficient in this vitamin and should consider vitamin supplements.

Toxicity and Clinical Deficiency

Toxicity problems are rare, since vitamins B₁₂ is stored in the liver and muscle tissues in small amounts. The amount stored, however, is often adequate to last for 3 to 5 years. This is evidenced by the fact that when a subtotal gastrectomy (partial removal of the stomach) is performed (see Chapter 16), it takes 3 to 5 years before a vitamin B deficiency occurs.

A vitamin B₁₂ deficiency may cause degeneration of myelin sheaths, resulting in numbness in the limbs, difficulty and poor coordination in

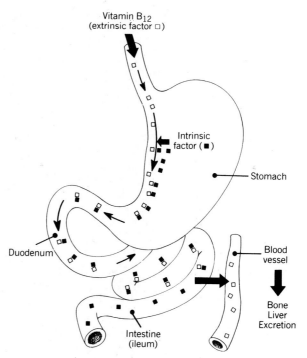

FIGURE 6-16 Combination of vitamin B$_{12}$ (extrinsic factor) and intrinsic factor to aid the absorption of vitamin B$_{12}$.

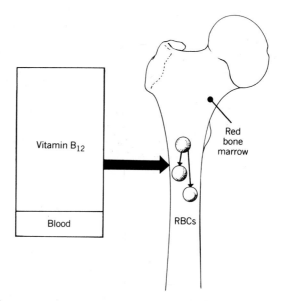

FIGURE 6-17 Role of vitamin B$_{12}$ in the synthesis of red blood cells (erythropoiesis) in red bone marrow.

walking, and coldness of the extremities. In severe deficiencies, the person may suffer from mental deterioration.

People who inherit the inability to synthesize the intrinsic factor cannot absorb adequate amounts of vitamin B_{12} and therefore suffer from **pernicious anemia.** In addition, people who have undergone **gastrectomies** face potential pernicious anemia. The reduced number of RBCs is frequently much larger than normal (**macrocytic anemia**) (see Fig. 6-18). Early detection of pernicious anemia is important to avoid the nervous system problems mentioned above.

Pernicious anemia, in relation to the two problems discussed above, cannot be prevented by increasing the intake of foods high in vitamin B_{12} or by taking supplements. The person must receive vitamin B_{12} by **intramuscular injections** or by parenteral infusion (see Chapter 14 for details of parenteral infusion of nutrients).

pernicious anemia Anemia that results from a deficiency of vitamin B_{12} because of a lack of the intrinsic factor.

gastrectomy Surgical removal of the stomach.

macrocytic anemia A type of anemia in which red blood cells are larger than normal.

intramuscular injections Injections of substances into muscles.

Folacin

General Characteristics, Absorption, and Metabolism

Folacin is actually a group of related compounds that have the same basic functions. It is absorbed into the blood from the upper intestine. Alcoholics have a decreased ability to absorb folic acid, since alcohol interferes with its absorption.

Functions

The most important function of folacin is the synthesis of the heme portion of hemoglobin molecules that are located in RBCs. Since hemoglo-

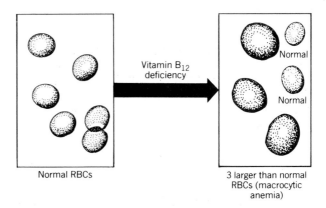

Normal RBCs

3 larger than normal RBCs (macrocytic anemia)

FIGURE 6-18 Normal red blood cells and larger than normal red blood cells (macrocytic anemia) due to vitamin B_{12} deficiency.

erythropoiesis The synthesis of red blood cells.

bin molecules are the main constituent of RBCs, **erythropoiesis** (see Fig. 6-19) is dependent upon an adequate amount of folacin in addition to vitamin B_{12}.

Body Requirements

The RDAs for folacin are given on the inside front cover. Notice the increased amount recommended during pregnancy. The reason is that a pregnant woman produces more RBCs in order to furnish oxygen gas and other nutrients not only for herself but also for the fetus.

Food Sources

Vegetables are an excellent source of folacin. In fact, the terms *folacin* and *foliage* are derived from the same root word. A strict vegetarian will obtain more than an adequate amount of folacin but may be deficient in vitamin B_{12}. Vegetables that are high in folacin are kidney beans, spinach, asparagus, and broccoli.

Toxicity and Clinical Deficiency

Toxicity from folacin is very rare, since it is water soluble and therefore not stored in great quantities in the body.

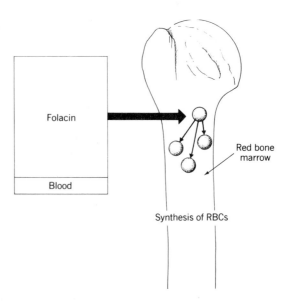

FIGURE 6-19 Role of folacin in the synthesis of red blood cells in red bone marrow.

Clinical deficiencies of folacin primarily affect the gastrointestinal tract and blood. The surface of the tongue may become smooth (glossitis), and the person may experience diarrhea.

A deficiency of folacin may result in a deficiency of RBCs or macrocytic anemia. Since these conditions are identical to a deficiency of vitamin B_{12}, what may appear to be a folacin deficiency may actually be a vitamin B_{12} deficiency. Also, a strict vegetarian may consume more than an adequate amount of folacin but not enough vitamin B_{12}. The deficiency of vitamin B_{12} may be masked because the folacin allows the RBCs to develop to their proper size and number, but this deficiency can lead to degeneration of myelin sheaths and thus to nerve damage.

Biotin

General Characteristics, Absorption, and Metabolism

Biotin is a sulfur-containing molecule and is absorbed in the upper part of the small intestine. Most of the biotin used by humans is synthesized by bacteria in the large intestine. Little is known about the metabolism and storage of biotin.

Functions

Biotin functions as a coenzyme in several biochemical reactions; carbohydrate and amino acid metabolism are examples. Other possible functions are niacin synthesis from tryptophan, formation of antibodies, and synthesis of pancreatic amylase. Research shows that the functions of biotin appear to be closely related to those of vitamin B_{12} and folic acid.

Body Requirements

The estimated safe and adequate daily dietary intake for biotin is given on the inside back cover. A normal American diet contains at least this much, and intestinal bacteria secrete a substantial amount of biotin.

Food Sources

Milk, liver, egg yolks, mushrooms, and legumes all contain biotin. Many foods have not been analyzed for their biotin content.

Toxicity and Clinical Deficiency

No toxicity or clinical deficiency problems in humans have been documented. Some deficiencies have been produced in experimental animals by dietary means.

Pantothenic Acid

General Characteristics, Absorption, and Metabolism

The name *pantothenic acid* is derived from the Greek word *pantos*, meaning everywhere. It is found extensively in all plants and animals. Little is known about where and how it is absorbed. It is stored in the liver, brain, kidney, and heart.

Functions

acetylcholine A neurotransmitter substance that is secreted at the axion ends of many neurons.

Pantothenic acid has two basic functions: metabolism of carbohydrates, lipids, and proteins and synthesis of **acetylcholine.**

Body Requirements

The estimated safe and adequate daily dietary intake is given on the inside back cover.

Food Sources

The best sources of pantothenic acid are eggs, liver, yeast, and salmon. Good sources are mushrooms, cauliflower, molasses, and peanuts. Fruits and milk are poor sources. Grains are a good source of pantothenic acid, but approximately 50% is lost in the milling process.

Toxicity and Clinical Deficiency

Research has yet to find any problems in humans with excessive quantities or deficiencies of pantothenic acid. Problems with the nervous system and eyes, as well as a decrease in growth, have been observed with deficiencies of pantothenic acid in experimental animals.

Summary of Important Points About B Vitamins

When one reviews the functions and deficiencies of the B vitamins, some general facts stand out:

1. *Nervous system malfunctions.* The nervous system depends heavily on glucose metabolism and therefore on thiamin. A deficiency of thiamin often causes nervous system disorders.
2. *Deficiency in RBC synthesis.* Erythropoiesis is especially important

upon vitamins such as folic acid and cobalamin (vitamin B_{12}). Anemia is one of the first symptoms of a deficiency of these two vitamins.

3. *Abnormal appearance of the tongue.* The tongue frequently shows signs of vitamin deficiencies and is readily observable. Since the tongue is part of the gastrointestinal tract, its abnormal appearance may be an indication of other gastrointestinal problems.

Vitamin C (Ascorbic Acid)

General Characteristics, Absorption, and Metabolism

spleen   A large glandular organ composed of lymphatic tissue.

adrenal gland   A gland located on top of the kidneys that secretes several different hormones.

scurvy   A disease that is characterized by weakness, skin degeneration, ulcerated gums, loss of teeth, and hemorrhages in the skin.

The term *ascorbic acid* is a derivative of the word *antiscorbutic,* meaning without scurvy. This term indicates that ascorbic acid is important in preventing scurvy. Vitamin C has a structure similar to that of monosaccharides. It is water soluble, absorbed from the small intestine into blood, and transported to the liver and **spleen.** Even larger amounts are stored in the **adrenal gland.**

Functions

1. *Prevention of* **scurvy** (see Fig. 6-20). This disease is characterized by weakness, skin degeneration, ulcerated gums (see Fig. 6-21), loss of

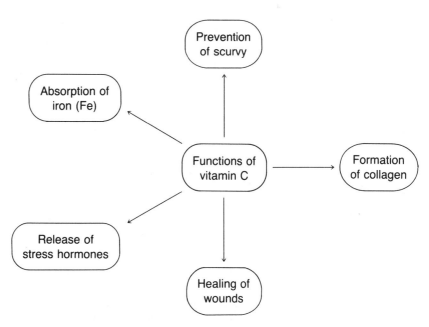

FIGURE 6-20   Functions of vitamin C.

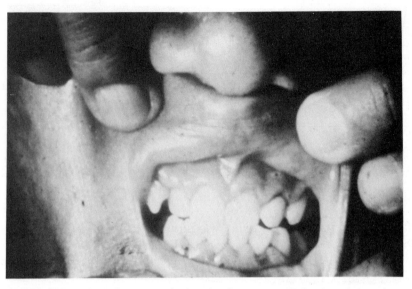

FIGURE 6-21   A deficiency of vitamin C can result in deteriorated or ulcerated gums. (Courtesy of the Centers for Disease Control, Atlanta, Ga.)

teeth, and skin hemorrhages. The symptoms of scurvy are related to breakdown of collagen.

2. *Formation of collagen.* Ascorbic acid aids in the synthesis of **collagen,** which is important in the structure of the skin, teeth, bones, and muscle.

3. *Healing of wounds.* Vitamin C aids in the healing of wounds. It does this by moving to the site of injury, where it promotes the formation of collagen in scar tissue. Vitamin C is often prescribed in large quantities for burn patients and patients who have had surgery to enhance the healing process.

4. *Release of stress hormones.* Vitamin C levels decrease in times of stress because it aids in the release of epinephrine and **norepinephrine** from the adrenal gland. These hormones prepare the body to overcome stress conditions.

5. *Absorption of iron.* Iron (Fe) exists in two states in the body: **ferric** (Fe^{3+}) and **ferrous** (Fe^{2+}), with the ferrous form being more readily absorbed. Vitamin C and hydrochloric acid (HCl) function to keep iron in the more absorbable form.

Since iron is the mineral that is present in RBCs, vitamin C is indirectly involved in the synthesis of RBCs.

collagen A protein that is important in the structure of skin, teeth, bones, and muscle.

norepinephrine A neurotransmitter secreted by the sympathetic nerves and as a hormone secreted from the adrenal gland.

ferric Chemical form of iron, Fe^{3+}; a less absorbable form than ferrous iron.

ferrous Chemical form of iron, Fe^{2+}; more absorbable form than ferric iron.

Body Requirements

The RDA for ascorbic acid is given on the inside front cover. These normal amounts must be increased for people who are under stress or are heavy cigarette smokers, or who are ill and have a fever. The amount of vitamin C needed for wound healing and formation of scar tissue following major operations or extensive burns may be as high as 1,000 mg/day or even more.

Food Sources

Ascorbic acid is found in all citrus fruits, cantaloupe, and strawberries. Vegetable sources include broccoli, tomatoes, brussel sprouts, greens, and potatoes (each potato contains only a small amount of vitamin C, but people eat potatoes so often).

Ascorbic acid is one of the vitamins most easily destroyed by heat, air, light, prolonged storage, copper and iron cookware, and the use of baking soda to preserve food color. Some suggestions for obtaining the maximum amount of ascorbic acid from preparation of foods are:

- Use the water that vegetables are cooked in. Since vitamin C is water soluble, some of it will be lost from vegetables when they are cooked.
- Quick-freeze foods that are being preserved.
- Refrigerate fresh foods containing the vitamin.
- Boil cooking water for at least 1 minute before adding food. Boiling rids the water of dissolved oxygen, which oxidizes vitamin C.
- Place frozen foods directly in boiling water (do not thaw in advance).

Toxicity and Clinical Deficiency

gout A metabolic disease characterized by an inability to metabolize purines and an elevated uric acid level in the blood.

In recent years, many people have advocated the ingestion of large doses of vitamin C to prevent the common cold. As a result, there have been many cases of toxicity, which have allowed scientists to study vitamin C toxicity. Some of the problems with vitamin C toxicity include raising the uric acid level in urine (see Fig. 6-22) and thereby increasing the chances of **gout** development in people who are already so predisposed. The toxic level of vitamin C may also cause hemolytic anemia in some ethnic groups such as African Americans, Jews, and Orientals. High vitamin C levels have also been found to impair the ability of white blood cells to give immunity to the body. An increase in kidney stones has been found to occur in some people. One of the most interesting problems with vitamin C toxicity is rebound scurvy. This condition also occurs in adults who stop taking megadoses of vitamin C abruptly as opposed to decreasing their intake gradually.[8]

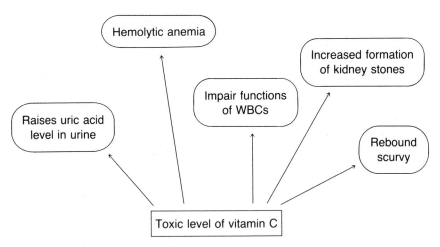

FIGURE 6-22 Effects of toxic levels of vitamin C.

Deficiencies can result in scurvy, muscle cramps, aching bones, dry, rough skin, and ulcerated gums (see Fig. 6-20).

Can Vitamin C Really Prevent Common Colds?

There has been much controversy regarding vitamin C since Linus Pauling's book *Vitamin C and the Common Cold* was published in 1970. Pauling advocated the use of massive doses (1,000–2,000 mg/day) of vitamin C in order to prevent colds. Numerous studies have been conducted to determine whether vitamin C does have these effects. A summary of some of the results from these studies is as follows:

1. The decrease in the number of colds averaged 0.1 per year in one study, which is not statistically significant.
2. The massive doses possibly decrease the duration of colds very slightly.
3. Whatever beneficial effects the massive doses of vitamin C have on colds, there is a danger of toxic side effects (described above).

The results of the studies do not support the claims made by Pauling and others that massive doses of vitamin C can prevent colds. However, this is a controversial subject, and research will continue.

Suggestions for Obtaining the Maximum Amount of Vitamins When Harvesting, Storing, and Cooking Foods

Harvest vegetables immediately before they are to be cooked or stored

Vitamin C especially and other vitamins are lost the longer vegetables are held before they are eaten or properly stored (see below for proper storage).

Store vegetables and fruits properly

While the best source of vitamins is fresh vegetables and fruits, the vitamin content can be decreased significantly by not storing them properly. The best ways to store foods, in decreasing order, are:

Frozen

This method preserves the vitamin content best because it stops the enzyme activity that destroys the vitamins.

Fresh

If a person harvests vegetables or fruits from a home garden and allows them to remain at room temperature before eating, the enzyme activity that destroys the vitamins continues with great losses.

If a person cannot eat fruits and vegetables immediately after harvesting them, but plans to do so within a few days, they should be kept in the refrigerator.

To reduce evaporation of water, fresh vegetables and fruits should be stored in covered containers or plastic bags.

Canned

This method causes the greater nutrient loss of the three because of the high temperatures required. In addition, water-soluble vitamins are lost in the water in which they are prepared.

Reduce preparation and cooking of vegetables

The more preparation and cooking of vegetables is required before eating, the greater the nutrient loss. To reduce the losses:

- Avoid soaking vegetables in water.
- When possible, cook vegetables in their skins.
- Cook in as little water as possible.
- Bake, steam, or broil vegetables.

- When boiling, uses tight-fitting lids to diminish evaporation of water.
- Cook vegetables in as short a time as possible. Long cooking times destroy more vitamin C, folacin, and vitamin B_6 than short ones.

Cook frozen vegetables in the frozen state

This practice reduces the loss of vitamins compared to thawing the vegetables before cooking.

Avoid cutting vegetables and fruits before cooking

The more vegetables and fruits are cut up before cooking, the more exposure to air they receive and the greater the loss of vitamins, especially vitamin C.

Avoid adding soda to vegetables

If soda is added to green vegetables to preserve their color, an alkaline medium is created that will destroy more vitamin C than an acid medium.

SUMMARY

- Vitamins are important as coenzymes for many enzymatic reactions; they are organic noncaloric compounds required in small amounts since they are not altered by chemical reactions.
- Vitamin A (retinol) functions in dim light vision, and maintenance of mucous membranes; vitamin D functions in growth of bones, and calcium and phosphorus absorption; vitamin E functions as an antioxidant for vitamin A; vitamin K functions in blood clotting.
- Vitamin A food sources are liver, whole milk, butter, egg yolk, and cream. Vitamin D food sources are eggs, liver, fortified milk, and butter. Vitamin E food sources are fats and oils, margarines, and salad dressings. Vitamin K food sources are egg yolks, liver, milk, green leafy vegetables, and cabbage.
- Vitamin A toxicity includes joint pain, stunted growth, cessation of menstruation; vitamin A deficiency includes night blindness, xerophthalmia, and cessation of bone growth. Vitamin D toxicity includes hypercalcemia, anorexia, kidney stones, and renal damage; vitamin D deficiency includes rickets in children, osteomalacia in adults, and muscle spasms. Vitamin K toxicity includes hemolytic anemia, and jaundice in infants; vitamin K deficiency includes prolonged clotting time.
- Fat-soluble vitamins require fats or bile to be absorbed whereas water-soluble vitamins only require water.
- Thiamin (vitamin B_1) functions as a coenzyme in oxidizing glucose to ATP, and prepares compounds to enter the citric acid cycle. Riboflavin (vitamin B_2) functions as a component of FAD (flavin adenine dinucleotide), which transfers hydrogens from citric acid cycle to the electron transport system. Niacin (nicotinic acid) functions as a component of NAD (nicotinamide adenine dinucleotide), which transfers hydrogens from glucose to electron transport system. Pyridoxine (vitamin B_6) synthesizes nonessential amino acids, converts amino acid tryptophan to niacin, and produces antibodies. Cobalamin (vitamin B_{12}) synthesizes RBCs and maintains myelin sheath on nerves. Folacin synthesizes RBCs. Ascorbic acid prevents scurvy, forms collagen, heals wounds, releases stress hormones, and aids in absorption of iron.
- Thiamin food sources include pork, liver, enriched grains, and legumes. Riboflavin food sources include milk, green vegetables, cereals, enriched bread. Pyridoxine food sources include baked potato, chicken, and bananas. Cobalamin food sources include seafood, meat, eggs, and milk. Folacin food sources include kidney beans, spinach, asparagus, and broccoli. Ascorbic acid food sources include all citrus fruits, cantaloupe, tomatoes, broccoli, potatoes, and greens.
- Thiamin deficiency problems include disorders of the gastrointestinal, nervous, and cardiovascular systems, often called beriberi. Riboflavin deficiency problems include cracks at corners of mouth (cheilosis), glossitis, photophobia. Niacin deficiency problems include diarrhea, dementia, and dermatitis (pellagra). Pyridoxine deficiency problems include cheilosis, glossitis, and abnormal brain waves. Cobalamin deficiency problems include degeneration of myelin sheath and pernicious anemia. Foalcin deficiency problems include glossitis and anemia. Ascorbic acid deficiency problems include scurvy, muscle cramps, aching bones, dry, rough skin, and ulcerated gums. Toxicity problems include raising uric acid, hemolytic anemia, rebound scurvy, tendency to form kidney stones.

REVIEW QUESTIONS

True (A) or False (B)

1. Vitamins are caloric compounds needed in large quantities.
2. Vitamin A functions in dim light vision, maintenance of mucous membranes, and synthesis of collagen.
3. Dark green vegetables or orange fruit are good sources of vitamin A.
4. Vitamin D is important for bone development by increasing the synthesis of protein molecules.
5. A deficiency of vitamin E can result in hemolysis of RBCs due to the destruction of polyunsaturated fatty acids (PUFA).
6. Since bacteria in the large intestine can synthesize vitamin K, a newborn infant has immediate protection against hemorrhaging.
7. Good food sources of thiamin are pork, beef, liver, and enriched grains.

8. Riboflavin is important in the development of bones.
9. A deficiency of pyridoxine may result in macrocytic anemia.
10. Vitamin B_{12} is important for the development of collagen and immunity.
11. Ascorbic acid is important for prevention of scurvy, formation of collagen, healing of wounds, and absorption of iron.
12. Vitamin E and A are often found together in foods, since vitamin E helps to protect vitamin A from being oxidized.
13. Carrots are an excellent source of carotene, which can be converted to vitamin D by the body.
14. Vitamin D aids the growth of bones by stimulating division of new bone cells.
15. A toxic level of vitamin D can result in osteomalacia, poorly developed teeth, and muscle spasms.
16. A deficiency of vitamin K is rare, since bacteria in the large intestine synthesize it.
17. The principal function of thiamin is to oxidize glucose for the formation of high-energy ATP molecules.
18. The best food sources of pyridoxine are milk and eggs.
19. A person who cannot synthesize the intrinsic factor is vitamin B_6 deficient and may exhibit macrocytic anemia.
20. Niacin is an example of a vitamin that the body can make from the amino acid tryptophan.
21. Pellagra is a niacin-deficiency disease and is characterized by diarrhea, dementia, and dermatitis.
22. A strict vegetarian is likely to have an adequate intake of folacin but may be deficient in cobalamin.
23. A deficiency of vitamin B_{12} may mask a folacin deficiency and, over a long period, lead to nerve damage.
24. Deficiencies of the B vitamins frequently result in nervous system malfunctions, RBC deficiency, and an abnormal appearance of the tongue.
25. Megadose levels of ascorbic acid increase its ability to form collagen, heal wounds, and absorb iron.

Multiple Choice

26. Toxicity problems with vitamin A include:
    1. joint pain.
    2. xerophthalmia.
    3. enlargement of the liver.
    4. night blindness.
       A. 1, 2, 3   B. 1, 3   C. 2, 4   D. 4
       E. all of these.
27. The RDA for vitamin D can easily be satisfied by consuming:
    A. 6 oz of beef.
    B. green vegetables.
    C. two glasses of fortified milk.
    D. legumes.
    E. potatoes.
28. The major food sources of vitamin E are:
    A. fats.
    B. carbohydrates
    C. proteins.
    D. oils.
    E. A, D.
29. Vitamin K aids the blood-clotting process by:
    A. the synthesis of collagen.
    B. the conversion of fibrinogen to prothrombin.
    C. the synthesis of prothrombin.
    D. the breakdown of platelets.
    E. none of these.
30. The principal function of thiamin is to:
    A. act as a coenzyme in the oxidation of glucose to form ATP.
    B. aid the conversion of amino acids.
    C. convert iron into a more absorbable form.
    D. act as an antioxidant.
31. _____ is a good food source of riboflavin, but this vitamin can be easily destroyed by _____.
    A. Meat—oxygen.
    B. Corn—cold temperatures.
    C. Fruit—sunlight.
    D. Liver—cooking.
    E. none of these.
32. Which of the following is (are) functions of pyridoxine?
    A. synthesis of nonessential amino acids.
    B. conversion of tryptophan to niacin.
    C. antibody production.
    D. A, C.
    E. A, B, C.

33. Which of the following is (are) *not correct functions* of cobalamin?
    A. synthesis of collagen.
    B. conversion of tryptophan to niacin.
    C. release of stress hormones.
    D. aid in blood clotting.
    E. all of these.
34. Which of the following foods is (are) good sources of vitamin C?
    A. citrus fruit, beef, eggs, milk.
    B. citrus fruit, broccoli, tomatoes, potatoes.
    C. strawberries, bread, meat, legumes.
    D. cantaloupe, corn, bananas, liver, milk.

Matching

Answers to Questions 35–41 may be used more than once.

___ 35. osteomalacia
___ 36. hypercalcemia
___ 37. xerophthalmia
___ 38. respiratory infections
___ 39. RBC hemolysis
___ 40. prolonged blood-clotting time
___ 41. kidney stones

A. vitamin D toxicity
B. vitamin A deficiency
C. vitamin K deficiency
D. vitamin E deficiency
E. vitamin D deficiency

Answers may be used only once.

___ 42. folic acid
___ 43. thiamin
___ 44. riboflavin
___ 45. niacin
___ 46. cobalamin

A. pernicious anemia
B. aids oxidation of glucose
C. pellagra
D. megaloblastic anemia
E. cheilosis

Completion

47. Explain why the amounts of riboflavin, niacin, and thiamin should be increased during growth periods, pregnancy and lactation, and infectious and chronic illness.
48. Give the animal and plant food sources for vitamins A, D, E, and K.
49. Give the animal and plant food sources for the vitamins thiamin, riboflavin, niacin, pyridoxine, cobalamin, folacin, and ascorbic acid.

CRITICAL THINKING CHALLENGE

1. Mrs. Smith has great trouble seeing well enough to drive at night. Her eyes also take a long time to adjust to the dark in a theater.
   a. What vitamin is possibly missing? List foods that can supply this vitamin.
   b. A severe deficiency of this vitamin could cause what problem?
2. Before grain enrichment, many people who ate large amounts of corn and cornmeal developed a dermatitis condition that was especially sensitive to sunlight. If the condition was not diagnosed and treated, it could lead to diarrhea and dementia (mental confusion, anxiety, and depression).
   a. What is the disease and vitamin at cause? Why would a diet high in corn cause this disease?
   b. What foods need to be increased to correct this problem?
3. A person recovering from third-degree burns over 35% of his body is on a high-calorie, high-protein, and high-vitamin diet.
   a. What two water-soluble vitamins need special attention in this case? Give reasons for your answer.
   b. List foods that will supply these two vitamins.
4. Discuss why a person suffering from chronic bronchitis, chronic obstructive pulmonary disease (COPD), or cystic fibrosis should consume large amounts of vitamins A and C.

REVIEW QUESTIONS FOR NCLEX

Situation. An assessment is done on a client as regards physical examination and diet history with the following results being discovered: skin hemorrhages, aching bones, dry rough skin, and ulcerated gums. Nutriton history indicated the client consumed almost no citrus fruits for several years.

1. The examination and diet history indicate the client may be deficient in vitamin _____.
   A. A
   B. B1
   C. C
   D. E

2. The functions of the deficient vitamin are _____.
   A. formation of collagen, healing of wounds, and release of stress hormones
   B. dim light vision, maintenance of mucous membranes, and growth of bones
   C. coenzyme in oxidation of glucose and aids release of energy from foods
   D. antioxidant, bone growth, and blood clotting
3. Foods that will have to be increased in order to provide adequate amounts of this vitamin are _____.
   A. eggs, liver, milk, spinach
   B. green leafy vegetables, cabbage, egg yolk
   C. deep yellow vegetables and fruits, fortified margarine, and spinach
   D. citrus fruits, broccoli, tomatoes, and potatoes

Situation. A client, who has been a chronic alcoholic for 10 years, is assessed with the following results—heaviness of the legs, burning sensation of the feet, and weakness of the toes. Nutritional history indicates a poor diet with little consumption of meat, grains, and vegetables.

4. The assessment and diet history of the client indicates he may be deficient in _____.
   A. thiamin
   B. folacin
   C. riboflavin
   D. niacin
5. The functions of the vitamin are _____.
   A. coenzyme in oxidation of glucose and release of energy
   B. synthesis of RBCs, maintenance of myelin sheaths
   C. conversion of tryptophan to niacin, and antibody production

   D. transfers hydrogen atoms for synthesis of ATP and synthesis of RBCs
6. Foods that need to be increased in order to provide adequate amounts of the vitamin are _____.
   A. green vegetables, cereals, enriched bread
   B. milk, eggs, fish, poultry
   C. pork, beef, fish, enriched grains
   D. seafood, milk, vegetables, citrus fruits

REFERENCES

1. Bendich, A., & Langseth, L. (1989). Safety of vitamin A. *American Journal of Clinical Nutrition, 99,* 358–371.
2. National Research Council. (1989). *Recommended dietary allowances* (10th ed.) (pp. 92–93). Washington.
3. DeLuca, H. E. (1988). Vitamin D and its metabolites. In M. E. Shils and V. R. Young (Eds.), *Modern nutrition in health and disease* (7th ed.). Philadelphia: Lea and Febiger.
4. Suttie, J. W., & Greger, J. L. (1988). Vitamin K deficiency from dietary vitamin K restriction in humans. *American Journal of Clinical Nutrition, 47,* 475–480.
5. McCormack, D. B. (1988). Riboflavin. In M. E. Shils and V. R. Young (Eds.), *Modern nutrition in health and disease* (7th ed.) (pp. 362–369). Philadelphia: Lea and Febiger.
6. Carpenter, K. J., & Lewin, W. J. (1985). A reexamination of the composition of diets associated with pellagra. *Journal of Nutrition, 115,* 543–552.
7. Bamji, M. S., Prema, K. et al. (1985). Vitamin supplements to Indian women using low-dosage oral contraceptives. *Contraception, 32,* 405–416.
8. Brown, J. E. (1990). *The science of human nutrition* (pp. 277–278). San Diego: Harcourt Brace Jovanovich.

7 MAJOR AND TRACE MINERALS

Upon completion of this chapter, you should be able to:

1. Distinguish between major and trace minerals.
2. Give the functions and food sources and describe the deficiency diseases of calcium.
3. Discuss the dietary factors that affect calcium absorption.
4. List the functions and food sources of phosphorus.
5. Describe the functions and food sources of potassium.
6. Discuss elevated blood potassium (hyperkalemia) and decreased blood potassium (hypokalemia).
7. List the functions and food sources of sodium
8. Discuss hypertension and sodium intake.
9. Give the functions, food sources, and imbalances of chloride ions.
10. Describe the functions and food sources of magnesium.
11. List the functions and food sources of sulfur.
12. Name the four forms of iron in the body and give their functions.
13. Discuss the four factors that increase the absorption of iron in the body.
14. Describe the four factors that decrease the absorption of iron in the body.
15. Give the food sources of heme and nonheme iron.
16. Describe iron-deficiency anemia in terms of the appearance of RBCs, high-risk groups, and treatment.
17. Describe the functions of iodine and name good food sources.
18. Describe goiter and cretinism.
19. Give the functions and food sources of zinc.

INTRODUCTION

minerals Small, inorganic elements that yield no energy.

acid-base balance A balance of the amount of acid and base ions so that blood pH is within the normal range, 7.35–7.45.

cations Minerals that are positively charged.

anions Minerals that are negatively charged.

major minerals Minerals that are present in the body in quantities greater than 5 g and are required at levels of 100 mg/day.

trace minerals Minerals that are present in the body in quantities of less than 5 g.

Minerals are small inorganic elements that yield no energy. They constitute only about 4% of the body weight but are essential as structural components and in many vital processes, such as regulation of the **acid-base balance** of body fluids and osmotic pressure. Even though minerals are inorganic, they are often combined with organic molecules as iron in hemoglobin and as iodine in thyroxin. Some minerals are found in the body as salts, such as calcium salts in bone. **Cations** include calcium, magnesium, potassium, and sodium ions. **Anions** include chlorine, fluorine, and iodine.

Minerals are divided into two groups:

Major minerals. Minerals present in the body in quantities greater than 5 g (1 tsp) and are required at levels of 100 mg/day or more. Examples are calcium (Ca), phosphorus (P), potassium (K), sulfur (S), sodium (Na), chlorine (Cl), and magnesium (Mg).

Trace minerals. Minerals present in quantities of less than 5 g. Examples are iron (Fe), iodine (I), fluoride (F), zinc (Zn), manganese (Mn), copper (Cu), selenium (Se), molybdenum (Mo), and chromium (Cr).

RDA values have been established for calcium, phosphorus, iodine, iron, magnesium, zinc, and selenium (for RDA values, see inside front cover).

Table 7-1 presents a summary of the food sources, functions, and deficiency/toxicity problems of each major mineral.

MAJOR MINERALS

Calcium (Ca²⁺)

General Characteristics

Calcium (Ca) is the most abundant mineral in the body, and 99% is stored in the bones and teeth. The remaining 1%, present in the blood and other tissue fluids, has several important functions, which will be discussed shortly.

Absorption

The amount of calcium absorbed into the blood depends upon the needs of the body. Normally, in adults, 10–30% of dietary calcium is absorbed;

TABLE 7-1 SUMMARY OF MAJOR MINERALS

Name	Food Sources	Functions	Deficiency/Toxicity
Calcium (Ca)	Milk exchanges Milk, cheese Meat exchanges Sardines Salmon Vegetable exchanges Green vegetables	Development of bones and teeth Permeability of cell membranes Transmission of nerve impulses Blood clotting	Deficiency Osteoporosis Osteomalacia Rickets
Phosphorus (P)	Milk exchanges Milk, cheese Meat exchanges Lean meat	Development of bones and teeth Transfer of energy Component of phospholipids Buffer system	(Same as calcium)
Potassium (K)	Fruit exchanges Oranges, bananas Dried fruits	Contraction of muscles Maintaining water balance Transmission of nerve impulses Carbohydrate and protein metabolism	Deficiency Hypokalemia Toxicity Hyperkalemia
Sodium (Na)	Table salt Meat exchanges Beef, eggs Milk exchanges Milk, cheese	Maintaining fluid balance in blood Transmission of nerve impulses	Toxicity Increase in blood pressure
Chlorine (Cl)	Table salt Meat exchanges	Gastric acidity Regulation of osmotic pressure Activation of salivary amylase	Deficiency Imbalance in gastric acidity Imbalance in blood pH
Magnesium (Mg)	Vegetable exchanges Green vegetables Bread exchanges Whole grains	Synthesis of ATP Transmission of nerve impulses Activator of metabolic enzymes Relaxation of skeletal muscles	
Sulfur (S)	Meat exchanges Eggs, poultry, fish	Maintaining protein structure Formation of high-energy compounds	

161

however, growing children and pregnant women absorb 50–60%. Dietary factors that influence calcium absorption are (see Figure 7-1):

Presence of an acid environment. Foods that are acid-forming increase the absorption of calcium. Cereals and protein foods are examples of acid-forming foods.

Intake of calcium and phosphorus in a ratio of 1 : 1 to 2 : 1. Absorption of calcium is increased when the diet contains a calcium: phosphorus ratio of 1 : 1 to 2 : 1. The average ratio of calcium to phosphorus in American diets is 1 : 1.6, which obviously is the reverse of what it should be for maximum calcium absorption. Apparently, part of the reason for the high level of phosphorus is the large number of soft drinks, rich in phosphorus, consumed by Americans. The end result of consuming this much phosphorus is less calcium absorption.

Increased intake of vitamin D. Vitamin D increases the absorption of calcium. Since milk contains large amounts of calcium, one can understand why milk is vitamin D fortified.

Presence of lactose. The lactose (sugar) in milk increases the absorption of calcium, as does vitamin D.

Functions

The reason 99% of the calcium is stored in the bones is that calcium is essential for the proper development and maintenance of bones and teeth (see Fig. 7-2).

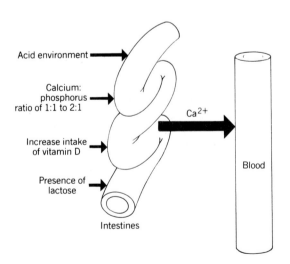

Acid environment

Calcium: phosphorus ratio of 1:1 to 2:1

Increase intake of vitamin D

Presence of lactose

Ca^{2+}

Blood

Intestines

FIGURE 7-1   Factors that influence calcium (Ca^{2+}).

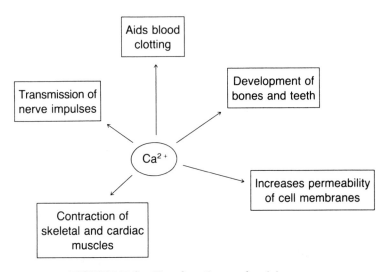

FIGURE 7-2 The functions of calcium.

permeability A state of being permeable, or allowing the passage of materials.

ions Atoms or molecules that have either a positive or a negative charge.

synapse The junction between two neurons where an impulse is transmitted.

Calcium is important to the **permeability** of cell membranes. Apparently it functions in the transport of certain **ions** into and out of cells through their membranes.

The contraction of skeletal and cardiac muscle tissues is dependent upon a certain level of calcium ions.

Transmission of nerve impulses at **synapses** between nerves and between nerve and muscle tissue depends upon calcium.

Blood clotting depends upon several cofactors, one of which is calcium. There are approximately 14 cofactors in blood clotting; calcium, vitamin K, and plasma proteins are examples.[1]

Food Sources

binder compounds Substances that inhibit absorption of calcium.

oxalic acid An acid found in some foods such as cocoa, rhubarb, and spinach. It inhibits the absorption of calcium, iron, and magnesium.

phytic acid A binder compound that forms an insoluble calcium complex.

The best food sources of calcium are found on the milk exchange list, 1. Lactose and vitamin D in milk increase its absorption. The meat exchange list, 5L, contains an excellent source of calcium—canned fish with bones; canned sardines and salmon are examples. The vegetable exchange list, 2, includes foods that contain calcium, such as dark green vegetables, but they also contain **binder compounds.** The binder compound in dark green vegetables is **oxalic acid,** which combines with calcium to form complexes that are insoluble (see Fig. 7-3). Cereal grains also contain **phytic acid,** which forms an insoluble calcium complex (see Fig. 7-3). Children who have milk allergy or lactose intolerance can obtain calcium from sources such as fortified soy milk and from calcium

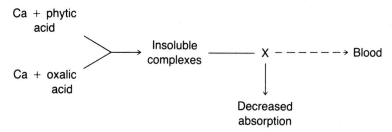

FIGURE 7-3   Binder compounds, oxalic and phytic acids, form insoluble complexes with calcium.

salt supplements such as calcium gluconate, lactate, sulfate, and carbonate.

The calcium RDA for men (25–50 years old) is 800 mg/day (one glass of milk contains 300 mg of calcium) and women (25–51+) 800 mg/day. Pregnant women are advised to consume 1,200 mg/day in order to protect the skeleton from loss of calcium to the developing fetus. It is recommended that postmenopausal women consume 1,500 mg/day in order to reduce **osteoporosis,** which will be discussed in more detail next.

osteoporosis A progressive demineralization of bones that results in the reduction of bone tissue.

Calcium Deficiency Diseases: Rickets and Osteoporosis

Osteoporosis. The ultimate result of osteoporosis is that bones become so fragile that they fracture quite easily. This condition is very prevalent in women after **menopause.** The reasons why osteoporosis is more common in women and the possible causes are (see Table 7-2):

menopause A permanent cessation of menstruation when ovaries, fallopian tubes, uterus, vagina, and breasts atrophy.

Hormonal changes following menopause. Osteoporosis occurs more frequently in women after they have undergone a decrease in sex hormones (primarily estrogen). The exact mechanism by which a decrease in estro-

TABLE 7-2 CAUSES OF OSTEOPOROSIS AND OSTEOMALACIA

Osteoporosis	Osteomalacia
Decreased hormone (estrogen) levels after menopause	Prolonged malabsorption
Impaired calcium absorption	Renal failure
Low calcium intake over many years	Inadequate intake of calcium during pregnancy

gen results in loss of calcium from bones is unknown. However, research shows that the loss of total body calcium increases from an average of 0.22% per year for premenopausal women to an average of 1.5% per year after menopause.

Low calcium intake over many years. Apparently osteoporosis is not caused by a low calcium intake only as an adult, but rather by a low intake starting in childhood and continuing into the adult years.

Impaired calcium absorption. Prolonged impairment of calcium absorption possibly can result in osteoporosis.[2]

The pelvic bone and vertebrae exhibit the fragility characteristics of osteoporosis more than any other bones. It is very common for elderly people to fall and fracture a hip into so many small fragments that it cannot be repaired and must be replaced with an artificial hip.

It is very important for postmenopausal women to be informed about the need to consume large amounts of calcium, approximately 1,500 mg/day (1.5 g/day).[3] Consumption of 5 glasses of milk per day will satisfy this amount or consumption of **calcium supplements.** This increased intake is needed not only to offset the losses from bone but also to offset the decreased amount of calcium that is absorbed by the intestines. The efficiency of calcium absorption decreases after age 45 in women and age 60 in men.[3]

calcium supplements
Calcium supplements vary as to the amount of calcium that is present. Calcium carbonate tablets are 40% calcium, or a 600 mg tablet contains 240 mg of calcium. Calcium lactate contains 13% and calcium gluconate 9% calcium.

Rickets. The clinical signs of rickets include stunted growth, bowing of the legs, enlargement of the wrists and ankles, and a hollow chest.

Osteomalacia. Factors that commonly cause osteomalacia in the United States (see Table 7-2) are as follows:

Prolonged malabsorption. Long periods of malabsorption and decreased calcium intake will result in removal of calcium stored in bones for use in various physiological functions (clotting of blood, transmission of nerve impulses) (see Fig. 7-2). Sprue and steatorrhea (see Chapter 16 for details of these two diseases) are two malabsorption problems that may result in osteomalacia.

Renal failure. The kidneys are important for calcium absorption because vitamin D is activated by the kidneys; therefore, kidney failure will result in a decreased amount of vitamin D, decreasing the absorption of calcium.

Inadequate intake of calcium during pregnancy. Women are susceptible to osteomalacia due to an increased need for calcium. Women who have undergone several pregnancies and had a diet inadequate in vitamin D and calcium are especially susceptible.[4]

Phosphorus (P)

General Characteristics

Phosphorus is the second most important mineral in the body. Approximately 85% of phosphorus is combined with calcium in bones to form calcium phosphate, $Ca(PO_4)_2$. The rest of the phosphorus is located in body cells as the phosphate ion (PO_4).

Absorption

The absorption of phosphorus is closely related to that of calcium, and the factors that influence its absorption also affect phosphorus. However, approximately 70% of dietary phosphorus is absorbed compared to 10–30% of dietary calcium.

Functions

The functions of phosphorus (see Fig. 7-4) are as follows:

Development of bones and teeth. Phosphorus combined with calcium is very important in the proper development of teeth and bones.

Transfer of energy in cells. Phosphorus is an important component of adenosine triphosphate (ATP) molecules, which store and transfer en-

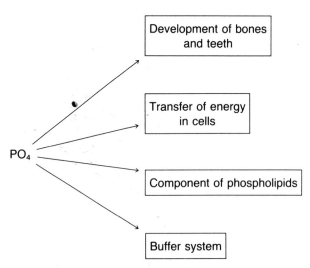

FIGURE 7-4 The functions of phosphorus.

ergy in cells. Phosphorus must also combine with B vitamins before they can play major roles in energy metabolism.

Component of phospholipids. Phospholipids are a major component of cell membranes, in which they help regulate what enters the cells. Phospholipids also help to transport other lipids in the blood, since they are normally insoluble in water.

Buffer system. One of the buffer systems in the blood that helps to maintain its acid-base balance contains phosphorus.

Food Sources

As with calcium, the milk exchange list 1 is the best source of phosphorus. Since muscle tissue contains a high level of ATP for metabolism, lean meat on the meat exchange list 5 is a good source of phosphorus. Some foods are high in phosphorus as a result of the addition of phosphorus-containing compounds in their processing. Some examples are carbonated beverages, cheeses, and processed meats.

Phosphorus Imbalance Diseases

A deficiency of phosphorus (hypophosphatemia) can result from various problems. End-stage renal disease can result in a phosphorus deficiency due to a decreased level of activated vitamin D, thereby reducing its absorption. Malabsorption diseases such as sprue can cause phosphate deficiency due to a decreased ability to absorb vitamin D and phosphate. In addition, people who chronically take large amounts of antacids may have a low phosphate level and may experience weakness, anorexia, bone pain, and bone demineralization.

An excess of phosphorus (hyperphosphatemia) often results from renal disorders where decreased urination occurs. Since the level of phosphorus is inversely related to that of calcium, a hyperphosphatemic condition also results in a low blood calcium level. The end result can be muscle tetany.

Potassium (K^+)

General Characteristics

Potassium is the most abundant cation in the intracellular fluid of cells (see Fig. 7-5). Approximately 98% of the potassium in the body is located in the cells. However, the small amount in the blood has some very important functions, as described below. The level of potassium in the blood is regulated by the hormone aldosterone.

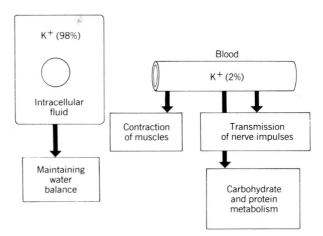

FIGURE 7-5 The roles of potassium in the blood.

Contraction of muscles. Potassium is very important in the contraction of skeletal and especially cardiac muscle tissue.

Maintenance of water balance. The osmotic pressure inside cells is due to the concentration of potassium ions; therefore, the shifting of water into cells is due to the pressure created primarily by potassium ions. Imbalances in the amount of potassium and the resultant shifting of fluids will be discussed later in this section.

Transmission of nerve impulses. Transmission of nerve impulses through muscles and along nerves is strongly dependent upon the concentration of potassium as well as sodium ions.

Carbohydrate and protein metabolism. Potassium is important in glycogenesis. It functions as a catalyst in the synthesis of proteins.

Food Sources

The best sources of potassium are foods on the fruit exchange list 4. Fruits that are high in potassium are oranges, bananas, and dried fruits. Foods from the meat exchange list 5 and the vegetable exchange list 2 contain smaller amounts. Specific amounts of potassium in various foods are given in Appendix E.

hyperkalemia Elevated blood potassium levels.

hypokalemia Decreased blood potassium levels.

Diseases Related to Potassium Deficiencies and Excesses

Most problems related to potassium are grouped under **hyperkalemia** and **hypokalemia**.

Hyperkalemia. Potassium excess frequently results from oral or intravenous overdosages when potassium is given for the correction of electrolyte imbalances. Other common causes of potassium excess are renal failure and severe dehydration.

The previously mentioned functions of potassium that are affected by hyperkalemia are weakness of heart contractions and of respiratory muscles. The nervous system is also affected, with the patient displaying mental confusion.

Hypokalemia. Potassium deficiency may result from the chronic use of **diuretics,** surgery, diarrhea, and vomiting. A major problem of low blood potassium is that it produces **tachycardia.** With prolonged use of diuretics in certain medical situations, foods high in potassium or supplements should be given to help eliminate hypokalemia.[5]

diuretics Agents that promote urine excretion and are used to alleviate edema (see chapters 17 and 20).

tachycardia Rapid and irregular heartbeat.

Sodium (Na$^+$)

General Characteristics

Sodium is the most abundant cation in extracellular fluid, with about two-thirds being located in the blood. The other one-third is located in bones.

Absorption and Excretion

Sodium is easily absorbed into blood from the intestines. The blood level of sodium is controlled by the kidneys; they excrete excess quantities in urine, and when the blood level is low they conserve it. The hormone **aldosterone** controls the activities of the kidneys; an increase in the aldosterone level results in greater sodium absorption, and a decrease results in reduced absorption. A person can also lose sodium via perspiration, from gastric secretions lost as a result of vomiting, and from the repeated use of diuretics.

aldosterone A hormone secreted from the adrenal gland that regulates the levels of sodium and potassium.

Functions

The functions of sodium are similar to those of potassium. They include (see Fig. 7-6) the following:

Maintenance of fluid balance in the blood. Sodium is the major ion in the blood and therefore plays a major role in maintaining the osmotic pressure and fluid level of the blood. Whenever the level of sodium in the blood is normal, so is the level of water. Likewise, whenever the level of sodium is high or low, the level of water will be adversely affected.

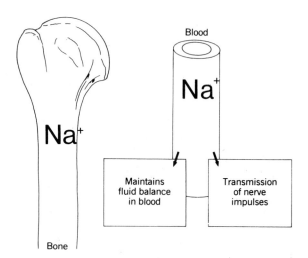

FIGURE 7-6   Sodium and its roles in the body.

More details about this condition will be presented at the end of this section.

Transmission of nerve impulses. The transmission of impulses along nerves and muscles is dependent upon a normal concentration of sodium ions.

Maintenance of acid-base balance. Two of the buffer systems that help maintain the normal pH of the blood are sodium monohydrogen phosphate (Na_2HPO-[4]) and sodium dihydrogen phosphate (NaH_2PO_4).

Food Sources

The most predominant source of sodium in the daily diet is table salt ($NaCl$), 40% of which is sodium. Generally speaking, animal foods contain more sodium than plant foods. Good sources of sodium include cheese, milk, processed meat, poultry, shellfish, fish, and eggs. Cereals, fruits, and vegetables are lower in sodium unless it is added during processing. Other foods high in salt are those that have been preserved with salt, such as cured ham and bacon. Specific amounts of sodium in various foods are given in Appendix E. Processed foods generally have salt added to them for taste; however, food companies have recently started marketing some processed foods with no added salt.

An often overlooked source of sodium is the public water supply. The sodium standard for public water is 20 mg/liter, but the water may contain more or less depending on the geographic location. Water containing over 100 mg per liter of sodium could have an effect on hypertensive persons, who should probably consider using bottled, distilled water for drinking and cooking.

There is no RDA value for sodium, since it is so readily abundant in our diet and drinking water. Also, since the kidneys regulate the level of sodium in the blood very effectively, a person could consume large amounts but have a normal concentration in the blood. The average American diet contains 10 g table salt and 4 g sodium (40% of 10). For adults with no hypertension, an intake of about 500 mg is estimated to be the amount needed to replace the daily losses. Hypertension and its relationship to sodium is discussed next.

Hypertension and Sodium Intake

Hypertension is related to many factors—obesity, genetic predisposition, smoking, personality type, and stress. It may be helped or hindered by the level of sodium in the diet. If a person with hypertension has a high level of blood sodium, this condition will result in a high osmotic pressure, pulling a large volume of water into the blood. This increased blood volume causes the person's already high blood pressure to rise even higher. The relationship between the level of blood sodium, blood volume, and blood pressure is shown in Figure 7-7. Likewise, if a hypertensive person decreases the intake of sodium, this will generally help to decrease the blood pressure. It is recommended that people with hypertension consume no more than 1–2 g sodium per day. Low-sodium diets and specific foods will be discussed in Chapter 18.[6] Sodium deficiency in the blood is uncommon but can be caused by inadequate monitoring when using diuretics, severe vomiting, very heavy perspiring, and certain diseases such as cystic fibrosis and **Addison's disease.** Deficiency symptoms include nausea, vomiting, acid-base imbalance, and diarrhea.

Addison's disease A disease caused by insufficient secretion of adrenal hormones.

Chlorine (Cl⁻)

General Characteristics

Chloride (Cl^-) is the form in which chlorine is present in the body. This anion is found primarily in the extracellular fluid, with gastric secretions

High level of Na^+ in blood = High blood osmotic pressure = Increased movement of H_2O into blood = Increased blood volume = Increased blood pressure

FIGURE 7-7 The relationship between the level of blood sodium, blood volume, and blood pressure.

and cerebrospinal fluid being the two most common examples. Chloride ions in gastric secretions are combined with hydrogen ions to form hydrochloric acid.

Absorption

Chloride ions are absorbed readily into the blood from the intestines, and the kidneys control this level by either excreting the excess or conserving chloride ions. The body can also lose chloride ions by excessive perspiration, diarrhea, and vomiting.

Functions

The functions of chlorine in the extracellular fluid are the following (see Fig. 7-8):

Gastric acidity. Chloride ions combine with hydrogen in the stomach to form hydrochloric acid, which is essential for digestion of protein and for conversion of iron into a more absorbable form.

Regulation of osmotic pressure. Chloride ions combine with sodium ions in the blood to help maintain the osmotic pressure, thereby helping to maintain a normal blood volume.

Activation of salivary amylase. Chloride ions in the saliva function to activate salivary amylase, which is an enzyme that begins the breakdown of starch.

Food Sources

The most common dietary source of chlorine is table salt, or sodium chloride (NaCl). Foods that are high in sodium typically are high in chlorine; meats, seafood, milk, and eggs are examples.

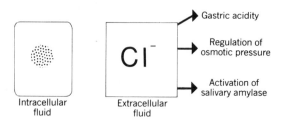

FIGURE 7-8 Chloride ions in extracellular fluid and its roles.

Chlorine Deficiency Diseases

Prolonged vomiting results in the loss of chlorine that is in the hydro-chloric acid of gastric secretions. These losses can cause the pH of the stomach to shift from the acid to the alkaline range, interfering with protein digestion and iron absorption. Diarrhea can cause losses of chlorine from the intestinal tract, resulting in an acid-base imbalance in the blood.

High levels of chlorine in the body are rare, since the kidneys will remove any excess and excrete it in the urine.

Magnesium (Mg^{2+})

General Characteristics

Magnesium is the second most important cation in the cells or intracellular fluid. However, approximately 70% of it is located in the bones, where it is combined with calcium and phosphorus salts. The other 30% is in the cells of the soft tissues and in body fluids, where its functions are described next.

Functions

The most important roles of magnesium (see Fig. 7-9) are as follows:

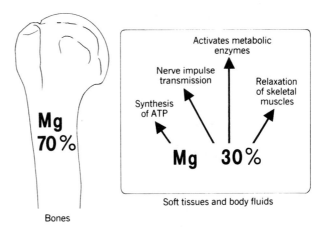

FIGURE 7-9 Magnesium in soft tissues and body fluids and its functions.

Synthesis of ATP. Magnesium activates the enzymes necessary to add the third phosphate group to ADP to form ATP.

Transmission of nerve impulses. Magnesium interacts with sodium and potassium to allow the transmission of impulses along nerves and muscles.

Activator of enzymes necessary for metabolism of carbohydrates, proteins, and fats. The metabolic pathway that results in the release of energy from carbohydrates, fats, and lipids involves many enzymes and magnesium helps to activate them.

Relaxation of skeletal muscles. The relaxation of muscles after contraction involves magnesium.

Food Sources

The exchange lists and examples of foods that are high in magnesium are:

chlorophyll The green pigment found in most plant cells that is important for photosynthesis.

Vegetable list 2. Magnesium is a component of **chlorophyll**; therefore, most green vegetables are good sources.

Bread list 4. Whole grains are a good source of magnesium. Whole-wheat bread, bakery products, and cereals rich in whole grains are excellent sources of magnesium.[7]

Magnesium Deficiency and Effects on the Body

Magnesium is widely available in the diet; therefore, a deficiency is rare. Some conditions that can result in magnesium deficiency are alcoholism, prolonged diarrhea, vomiting, and intestinal malabsorption. A prolonged deficiency can result in **tetany** and an increased startle response to sound and touch. Magnesium deficits in alcoholics are thought to be the cause of the hallucinations from which they often suffer.

tetany Continuous, forceful muscle contraction.

Sulfur (S)

General Characteristics

Sulfur is present in all cells in the body, usually as a part of cell proteins. Keratin is the most common protein that contains sulfur. It is found predominantly in hair, skin, and nails.

heparin An anticoagulant or substance that prevents blood clotting.

Three amino acids are composed of sulfur—cystine, cysteine, and methionine. Sulfur is also found in other organic compounds such as **heparin,** insulin, thiamin, and biotin.

Functions

The structure of protein molecules is maintained by disulfide (—S—S—) linkages that help to hold amino acid chains together in a distinct shape (see Fig. 7-10). The rigid structure of keratin protein in hair, skin, and nails is the result of its high sulfur content.

Another important function of sulfur is the formation of some high-energy compounds in the energy metabolism pathways. Some enzymes in the energy pathway are activated by the presence of sulfur.

Food Sources

Proteins are the main source of sulfur in the diet, specifically proteins that contain cystine, cysteine, and methionine. Examples of foods that are rich in these amino acids are cheeses, eggs, poultry, and fish.[7]

TRACE MINERALS

basal metabolic rate The rate at which the body uses energy for maintenance of homeostasis at rest.

As mentioned earlier in the chapter, trace minerals are those present in the body in quantities of less than 5 g. Despite their small amounts, these minerals are involved in some very important functions—transport of oxygen and regulation of the **basal metabolic rate.** Four trace minerals—iron, iodine, zinc—have been studied extensively enough so that recommended dietary allowances (RDAs) have been established for them. In 1980 the Committee on RDA published estimated safe and adequate daily dietary intakes (ESADDI) for five other trace minerals—

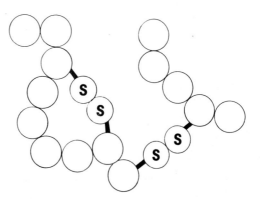

FIGURE 7-10   The role of sulfur in maintaining the structure of protein molecules.

manganese, fluoride, chromium, molybdenum, and copper. Only those trace minerals for which RDAs or ESADDI have been established will be discussed in this chapter. Table 7-3 presents a summary of the food sources, functions, and deficiency/toxicity problems of trace minerals.

IRON (Fe)

Iron is the best-known micromineral due to its important role in transporting oxygen to the cells. It is unusual in that there is no known mechanism that regulates its excretion. Iron balance is regulated at the intestinal site of absorption and will be discussed in detail later.

Forms in the Body

Iron is found in the body in five different forms with different functions.

TABLE 7-3 SUMMARY OF TRACE MINERALS

Name	Food Sources	Functions	Deficiency/Toxicity
Iron (Fe)	Meat exchanges Meat, fish, poultry	Transport oxygen and carbon dioxide	Iron deficiency anemia
Iodine (I)	Meat exchanges Seafood Iodized salt	Regulates basal metabolic rate	Deficiency: goiter, cretinism
Zinc (Zn)	Meat exchanges Eggs, oysters Milk exchange	Formation of collagen Component of insulin Component of many vital enzymes	
Selenium (Se)	Meat exchanges, liver, seafood	Antioxidant	
Copper (Cu)	Meat exchanges Oysters, liver	Oxidation of glucose	
Manganese (Mn)	Meat exchanges Nuts, peas, and beans	Component of metabolic enzymes	
Fluoride (F)	Drinking water, seafoods	Reduces dental caries	
Chromium (Cr)	Meat exchanges Eggs, meats	Binds insulin to cell membranes	
Molybdenum (Mo)	Meat exchanges Liver, legumes Bread exchanges Whole grains	Metabolism of nucleic acids to uric acid	

Transport Iron

transferrin (nonheme iron)
A combination of iron and a globulin protein; important as the transport form of iron.

Most iron is combined with other molecules in the body, but one form, **transferrin (nonheme iron),** is found circulating in the plasma (see Fig. 7-11). This form is important since it is the one that carries iron throughout the body to all cells.

Hemoglobin and Myoglobin

myoglobin (heme iron) A protein molecule composed of four amino acid chains, with one iron atom in each that is found in muscle tissue.

Approximately 70% of iron is found in red blood cells (RBCs) as hemoglobin (heme iron) (see Fig. 7-11). Another 5% of the iron is in the form of **myoglobin (heme iron).** Hemoglobin is the most important form, since it transports oxygen to all of the cells, where it is used in the metabolism of glucose for energy. Myoglobin is important as a reservoir of oxygen in the muscles. It holds onto oxygen until the muscles need it during sustained muscle contractions.

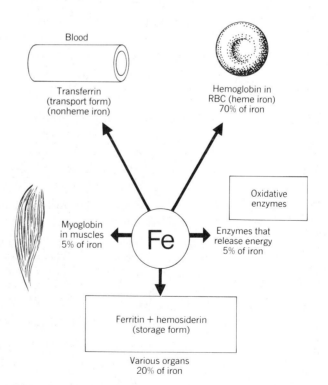

FIGURE 7-11 The five forms of iron and the percentage of each in the body.

Storage Iron

ferritin A form of iron that is stored in the liver, spleen, and bone marrow.

hemosiderin An insoluble form of iron that is stored in the liver.

About 20% of the total body iron is stored in various organs as **ferritin** and **hemosiderin** (see Fig. 7-11). Iron that is not taken up by RBCs and muscle tissue to form hemoglobin and myoglobin is stored as ferritin in the liver, spleen, and bone marrow. Hemosiderin is stored in the liver.

Enzymatic Iron

The remaining 5% of the iron in the body is found as a component of oxidative enzymes (see Fig. 7-11) that are vital to the release of energy from glucose.[8]

In summary, the majority of iron in the body exists in an active functioning form, hemoglobin. This form is vital in that it transports oxygen to the cells, where it is involved in the metabolism of glucose with the release of energy.

Absorption, Use, and Excretion

As mentioned earlier, there is no mechanism to control the excretion of iron; rather, it is controlled by the amount that is absorbed and stored. There are several factors that control the amount of iron absorbed. These factors are described and illustrated in some detail next.

Factors Affecting Absorption

Chemical form of iron. Iron usually enters the body in food as ferric iron (Fe^{3+}), which cannot be readily absorbed. The hydrochloric acid (HCl) in the stomach changes iron to the ferrous iron (Fe^{2+}) form, which can be easily absorbed (see Fig. 7-12). Ascorbic acid in the diet along with iron enhances its conversion to the ferrous state. This is one reason why the 1980 RDA for ascorbic acid for adults was raised from 45 to 60 mg.[2]

Physiological need for iron. When there is a greater need for iron in the body, as during growth periods and pregnancy, more iron is absorbed. Actually, what increases iron absorption during these periods is the amount of ferritin present in the cells of the mucosa lining the duodenum (see Fig. 7-12). The relationship between the amount of ferritin and absorption of iron is an inverse one, as shown below:

$$\frac{\text{Decreased}}{\text{ferritin}} = \frac{\text{increased}}{\text{absorption of iron}}$$

$$\frac{\text{Increased}}{\text{ferritin}} = \frac{\text{decreased}}{\text{absorption of iron}}$$

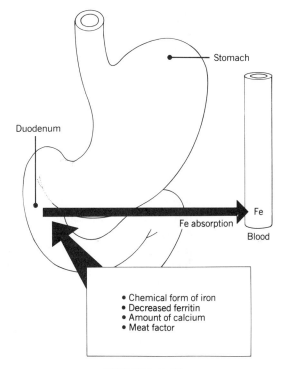

Stomach

Duodenum

Fe
Fe absorption
Blood

- Chemical form of iron
- Decreased ferritin
- Amount of calcium
- Meat factor

FIGURE 7-12

During periods of growth and pregnancy, mucosal ferritin levels decrease; during other periods they increase. Therefore, less iron is absorbed and excreted.

This relationship is important, since it increases the absorption of iron when the body actually needs it but prevents excess storage in tissues to the point of causing an iron toxicity problem.

Amount of calcium. Calcium binds to phosphate and phytate, which prevents them from inhibiting the absorption of iron (see Fig. 7-12).

Presence of "meat factor." Research results show that nonheme iron is absorbed better if meat, fish, or poultry (MFP) is present along with nonheme foods (see Fig. 7-12).

These factors increase the absorption of iron into the blood through the duodenum and jejunum regions of the small intestine, where the number of villi is greatest.

Factors that decrease the absorption of iron are:

High-fiber diet. A diet that is high in fiber tends to move food through the intestines so quickly that it reduces iron absorption.

Surgical removal of stomach. When the stomach or a portion if it is surgically removed, the amount of hydrochloric acid is decreased; therefore, the ability to convert iron from the ferric form to the ferrous form is reduced.

Diets high in cereals and grains. Phytic and oxalic acids tend to combine with iron and hinder its absorption.

ulcerative colitis A disease of the large intestine that is characterized by inflammation of the intestinal mucosa and ulcers (see Chapter 16).

Malabsorption problems. Celiac sprue, **ulcerative colitis,** and diarrhea are examples of malabsorption problems that hinder iron absorption.

Generally, about 10% of iron in a mixed diet is absorbed, or about 1 mg out of 10 mg ingested. Absorption of iron from the heme iron pool (hemoglobin and myoglobin) is distinctly better than from the nonheme iron pool (ferritin and hemosiderin). Specifically, iron absorption from liver and other meats can be as high as 10–30%, whereas absorption of iron from nonheme sources such as grains and vegetables is usually less than 5%.[8] A true vegetarian who consumes no meat products at all should be aware of this very low absorption rate of iron.

The 1989 RDA for iron in adult men is 10 mg and for adult women 15 mg. Women have a higher value since they lose greater amounts of iron due to blood loss from menstruation.

Function

As mentioned earlier, most of the iron is removed from the blood and used by the bone marrow in the synthesis of hemoglobin to form RBCs (see Fig. 7-13). After about 120 days, RBCs are broken down, but approximately 90% of the iron is conserved and reused in their synthesis.

cytochrome enzyme systems An iron-containing protein molecule that is important for the synthesis of adenosine triphosphate (ATP) molecules.

The other major way that the body actively uses iron is in the **cytochrome enzyme systems** that oxidize glucose with the release of energy (see Fig. 7-13).

Excretion

Very little iron is lost from the body. As mentioned earlier, when RBCs are destroyed in the liver and bone marrow, 90% is conserved and reused in the synthesis of new RBCs. A small amount of iron is lost daily in sweat, hair, shed skin cells, and urine (see Fig. 7-13).

Food Sources

The best food sources of iron (40% heme iron, 60% nonheme iron) are meat, fish, and poultry (meat exchanges). Good sources (nonheme iron)

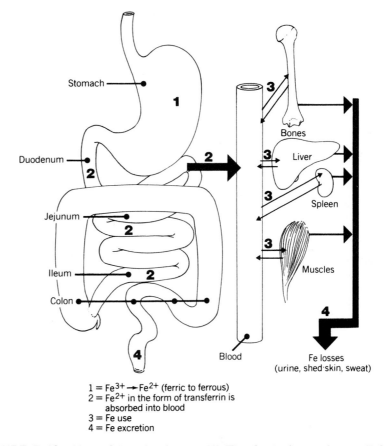

1 = $Fe^{3+} \rightarrow Fe^{2+}$ (ferric to ferrous)
2 = Fe^{2+} in the form of transferrin is
    absorbed into blood
3 = Fe use
4 = Fe excretion

FIGURE 7-13 Use of iron is shown. (1) The ferric form of iron (Fe^{3+}) is converted to the ferrous form (Fe^{2+}) in the stomach. (2) The ferrous form of iron is shown being absorbed into the blood, where 70% of iron will be in the hemoglobin molecules of red blood cells. Transferrin is the transport form in the blood. (3) Iron is shown moving into bones, where it is incorporated into red blood cells, stored in the liver and spleen, and functions as a component of myoglobin within muscles.

are fortified breads and cereals (bread exchanges), dark green vegetables (vegetable exchanges), and raisins, prunes, and apricots (fruit exchanges).

Vegetables, bread, and fruit are not as good sources as meat because they contain only nonheme iron, which cannot be absorbed as well as heme iron in meat exchanges. Also, vegetables and fruit that are high in fiber tend to interfere with iron absorption. The absorption of nonheme foods can be improved by combining these foods with ascorbic acid or

MFP. Apparently each 1 g of ascorbic acid or 1 g of MFP can enhance the absorption of nonheme iron. A meal containing nonheme iron could be iron enchanced if the following were incorporated:

(1) 4 fl oz orange juice (60 mg ascorbic acid)
2 oz sliced beef (60 mg MFP)

or

(2) 1 large sliced tomato (30 mg ascorbic acid) plus
1 oz beef (30 mg MFP)[8]

Iron Deficiency Anemia

anemia A reduction in the number of RBCs.

Iron deficiency **anemia** is the most common nutritional deficiency in the United States and is the leading cause of anemia. **Iron deficiency anemia** is characterized by a low number of RBCs, and the cells are **microcytic.** In addition, the RBCs are **hypochromic.** Since iron deficiency anemia is characterized by a low number of RBCs that are small in size and pale in color, this problem is often described as **hypochromic microcytic anemia.**

iron deficiency anemia A reduced number of RBCs that are smaller than normal.

microcytic An RBC that is smaller in size than normal.

hypochromic Pale in color.

hypochromic microcytic anemia Anemic condition characterized by RBCs that are smaller in size and pale in color.

Laboratory Indicators

There are several biochemical laboratory determinations that can indicate iron deficiency anemia. Some determinations are:

Serum ferritin
Total iron-binding capacity
Hemoglobin/**hematocrit**

total iron-binding capacity A measurement of the percentage of saturation of transferrin. It evaluates the amount of extra iron that can be carried.

Symptoms

hematocrit A percentage of RBCs in a sample of whole blood.

Iron deficiency anemia can result in a variety of abnormal changes in the body. Most of these changes are related to the fact that the anemic person's tissues must function with less oxygen and therefore have less energy. Fatigue followed by decreased work performance are two common symptoms. The risk of infection is also increased. Impairment of growth in infants can occur when their diets are iron deficient.

High-Risk Groups

There are four groups who are quite susceptible to the development of iron deficiency anemia.

Infants. Infants between the ages of 4 months and 3 years are vulnerable. During this period the child's iron stores are depleted, and the body size more than doubles; however, his or her diet is often composed almost exclusively of milk, which is a poor iron source.

Infants that are born to mothers who are iron deficient and low-birthweight infants are very susceptible to iron deficiency anemia.

Adolescents. During adolescence, teenagers undergo rapid growth spurts and their blood volume expands tremendously. Their diets often do not contain enough iron for the body's increased needs.

Pregnant Women. During pregnancy the iron needs of the woman increase as her blood volume and tissues expand. In addition, iron is needed for the development of the fetus. It is common today for physicians to prescribe an iron supplement during pregnancy to prevent iron deficiency.

Menstruating Women. When women menstruate, their iron stores decrease due to the loss of blood. **Intrauterine devices (IUDs)** increase menstrual blood loss, whereas oral contraceptives decrease it.[5]

Intrauterine devices (IUDs) Objects inserted into the uterus for contraceptive purposes.

Iron Deficiency: Treatment

Treatment of iron deficiency can take two forms—dietary management and iron supplementation. Dietary management involves increasing animal products—MFP. In addition, foods high in vitamin C should be increased, since they can double the absorption of iron from a meal. Likewise, milk and milk products should not be increased, since they can decrease the amount of iron absorbed from the same meal. Bottle-fed infants should receive iron-fortified formula. When solid foods are introduced, iron-fortified cereals and vitamin C–enriched apple juice are good choices. Iron supplementation involves the use of oral **ferrous sulfate.** The iron in the usual 300-mg tablets is absorbed best when taken between meals but is poorly tolerated. Iron is better tolerated if taken immediately after meals.

ferrous sulfate An oral iron supplement that is often given to correct iron deficiency anemia.

IODINE (I)

thyroid gland An endocrine gland located below the larynx and in front of the trachea. Secretes thyroxine and triiodothyronine hormones.

Iodine is a trace mineral that is present in the body in very small quantities—20–50 mg. Approximately 75% of it is concentrated in the **thyroid gland.**

Functions

thyroxine (T₄) A thyroid
hormone that regulates the
body's metabolism. Each thyroxin molecule contains four
iodine atoms; therefore, it is
designated as T₄.

Iodine functions as a component of two thyroid hormones, **thyroxine
(T₄)** and triiodothyronine (T₃). As Figure 7-14 shows, thyroxine contains
four iodine molecules and triiodothyronine three. These hormones are
secreted from the thyroid gland and regulate the basal metabolic rate,
the rate at which the body uses energy for maintenance of homeostasis.
As a result of this function, iodine is very important to the growth and
development of the body tissues, especially the nervous system.

Requirement and Food Sources

The adult RDA for iodine is only 150 μg/day. The RDA for pregnant
and lactating women is 175 and 200 μg, respectively. The meat exchange
list with seafood specifically is the best food source of iodine. However,
the average diet does not provide an adequate amount of iodine unless it
includes iodized table salt, which is the main dietary source of iodine.
This situation is especially true in noncoastal geographic locations.

goitrogens Substances that
block the absorption or use of
iodine.

Some foods contain a substance, **goitrogens,** which block the absorption or utilization of iodine. Foods of the cabbage family, such as rutaba-
gas, turnips, and cabbage, contain goitrogens.

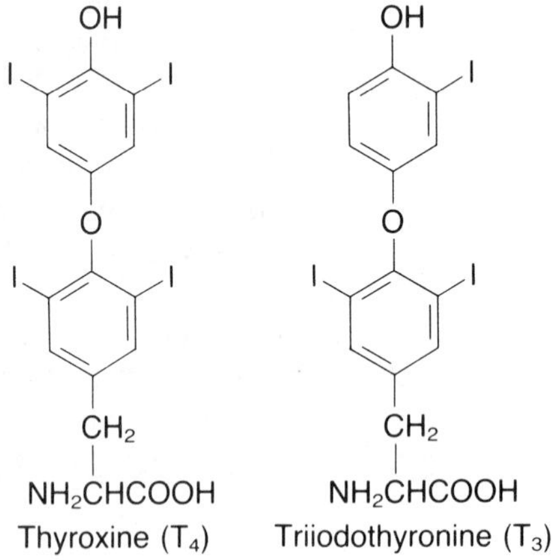

FIGURE 7-14 The two hormones, thyroxine (T₄) and triiodothyronine
(T₃), in which iodine functions as a component are shown. (From
Hole, John W., Jr., *Human Anatomy and Physiology*, 3d ed. (c) 1978,
1981, 1984 Wm. C. Brown Publishers, Dubuque, Iowa. All rights reserved. Reprinted by permission.)

Diseases Related to Deficiency and Excess

goiter An enlargement of the thyroid gland.

People who are deficient in iodine may develop a **goiter** (see Fig. 7-15). The gland enlarges in order to capture the small amount of iodine present. These people exhibit a low metabolic rate, body temperature, and sluggishness. **Cretinism** (see Fig. 7-16) is a condition in which an infant is born with an iodine deficiency and is characterized by stunted growth, dwarfism, and varying degrees of mental retardation. These problems occur because the metabolic rate of the infant is inadequate for nervous system development and growth of tissues. Cretinism in the United States is rare but can occur in an infant whose mother was severely iodine deficient. Early detection and treatment with thyroid extracts can avoid much of the mental retardation and improve growth.[9]

cretinism A condition caused by an iodine deficiency in an infant.

Excessive iodine intake may also result in the formation of a goiter. These people have high levels of thyroxin and triidothyronine, and exhibit a high metabolic rate, nervousness, and weight loss.

ZINC (Zn)

Zinc is second to iron in the amount present in the body. It is located in the eyes, reproductive organs, liver, muscle, and bones.

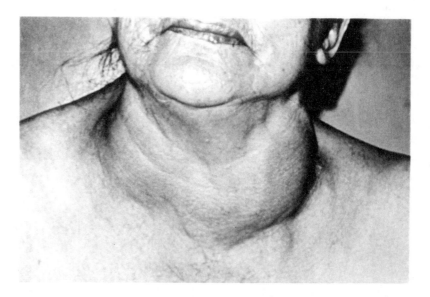

FIGURE 7-15 A goiter may develop as a result of an iodine deficiency.

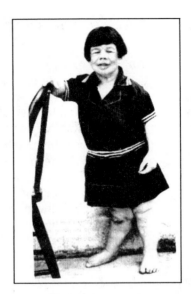

FIGURE 7-16 Cretinism is characterized by stunted growth, dwarfism, and varying degrees of mental retardation. (From Chaffee, E.E., and Lytle, I.M., *Basic Physiology and Anatomy,* 4th ed. Philadelphia, J.B. Lippincott Co., 1979. Reprinted with permission.)

Functions

Some important functions of zinc (see Fig. 7-17) are as follows:

Formation of collagen. The formation of collagen is dependent upon zinc. It is not surprising that a zinc deficiency can hinder wound healing and tissue repair.

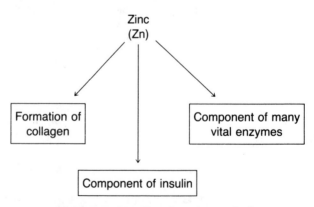

FIGURE 7-17 The functions of zinc.

Component of insulin. Insulin is a protein molecule with zinc as a component. It apparently increases the duration of insulin action after injection.

Component of many vital enzymes. It is a component of many enzymes that are involved in metabolic activities such as the release of carbon dioxide from tissues to lungs; protein digestion and synthesis; and carbohydrate metabolism.

Food Sources

The best food sources of zinc are those on the milk list and, on the meat list, eggs and seafood, especially oysters. Poor food sources are those on the vegetable list. Oxalic acids hinder the absorption of zinc in vegetables. Foods on the bread list are also poor in zinc. Phytic acid and fiber hinder absorption of zinc from grains.

Selenium (Se)

Functions

Selenium is a trace mineral that is known to function as an antioxidant to prevent damage to cell structures. Various studies have shown that selenium can have a protective effect against certain cancers.

Availability of selenium in soils and water varies considerably. For example, in China almost no selenium is present in the soil and water. Therefore, its effects vary considerably depending upon its availability.

Food Sources

The best food sources of selenium are grains, seafood, and meats. Since selenium content in soils and water varies, therefore, the amount found in grains varies tremendously. Meats are the best source of selenium because it attaches to amino acids, and meats contain more amino acids than do plants.

Deficiency and Toxicity

Studies have shown that selenium deficiencies can result in increased risk of cancer and possibly a type of heart disease. In China, a disease of the heart muscle has been found in many children due to selenium deficiency. Increasing selenium in these children's diets has been found to prevent development of this disorder.

Selenosis is the term for selenium toxicity. Toxicity problems in humans can result in hair and nail loss plus liver damage.[10]

TRACE MINERALS WITH ESTIMATED SAFE AND ADEQUATE DAILY DIETARY INTAKE

As mentioned at the beginning of the chapter, only four trace minerals have RDAs. Five trace minerals in 1980 were assigned ESADDI values (see inside back cover for the values for these minerals). Their essential nature has long been established, but is was not until 1980 that they were assigned values. The values for these five minerals appear as ranges of intake rather than as detailed, age-specific recommendations because of the uncertainty of the nutrient requirements.

Copper (Cu)

Copper and iron are metabolized in much the same ways and, in addition, share some functions. Copper is involved with iron in the enzymatic reactions that oxidize glucose and release energy. Copper, along with iron, is involved in the synthesis of hemoglobin. It aids in the synthesis of collagen and the maintenance of the myelin sheath around nerve fibers.

The meat list is the best source of copper, with oysters, shellfish, liver, and legumes as examples. Fresh foods in general are better sources of copper than processed foods. Cow's milk is a poor source of copper, but human breast milk contains a large amount.

Manganese (Mn)

Manganese is a component of many enzymes that are involved in metabolic reactions. The site of most of the reactions include bones, reproductive organs, and liver.

Manganese is especially abundant in foods such as bran, coffee, tea, nuts, peas, and beans.

Fluoride (F)

Fluoride ions are found primarily in bone and the enamel of teeth. Research indicates that fluoride ions reduce the incidence of caries when fluoride ions are present in the drinking water, applied topically to teeth, or included in toothpaste. Fluoride acts by enhancing the ability of teeth to withstand the effects of acid formed by cavity-causing bacteria. Numerous studies have shown a reduction of dental caries by 50–70% when public water is fluoridated.[3]

The main dietary sources of fluoride are drinking water, tea, and seafoods.

Excess Intake

Excessive intake of fluoride, such as in areas where fluoride is naturally high in the drinking water, can cause **tooth mottling.** Skeletal deformities can also occur with prolonged high fluoride intake. Fluoride toxicity is rare, since artificially fluoridated water levels are kept within a safe narrow range.

tooth mottling Brown discoloration of the teeth.

Chromium (Cr)

Chromium is associated with an increase in glucose tolerance. It is found in the body as a part of the **glucose tolerance factor.**

Chromium levels tend to decrease with age, which leads some researchers to believe that chromium deficiency is related to maturity-onset diabetes (**non-insulin-dependent diabetes**).[3]

Dietary sources of chromium are egg yolks, meats, cheeses, beer, and whole grains.

glucose tolerance factor A compound that helps to bind insulin to cell membranes.

non-insulin-dependent diabetes Also known as *type II diabetes.*

Molybdenum (Mo)

Molybdenum is a component of enzymes involved in the metabolism of nucleic acids to uric acid. It is an important enzyme in the uptake of nitrogen in legume plants. The highest amounts are found in the liver and kidneys.

A good food source is the meat list, with legumes and organ meats (liver and kidneys) being examples. The bread list with grains is another good source.

SUMMARY

- Major minerals are present in the body in amounts greater than 5 g and are needed in the body at levels of 100 mg/day or more; trace minerals are also present but are required in smaller amounts than major minerals.
- Calcium aids in the development of bones and teeth, permeability of cell membranes, and contraction of cardiac and skeletal muscles. Food sources of calcium include milk and foods on the milk list. Calcium deficiency diseases include rickets and osteoporosis.
- Dietary factors that affect calcium absorption are an acid environment in the gastrointestinal tract, a phosphorous ratio of 1 : 1 to 2 : 1 in the diet, and an increase in intake of vitamin D and lactose in the diet.
- Functions of phosphorous include development of bones and teeth, transfer of energy in cells, component of phospholipids, and buffer system. Food sources of phosphorous include milk, meat, carbonated beverages, cheeses, and processed meats.
- Potassium aids in the contraction of muscles, maintenance of water balance, transmission of nerve impulses, and carbohydrate and protein metabolism. Food sources of potassium include oranges, bananas, and dried fruits.
- Hyperkalemia (elevated blood potassium) results from oral or intravenous overdosages of potassium, renal failure, and dehydration; symptoms include weakness of heart contractions and respiratory muscles. Hypokalemia (decreased blood potassium) results from chronic use of diuretics, surgery, diarrhea, and vomiting; symptoms include tachycardia.
- Sodium maintains fluid balance in blood and transmits nerve impulses. Food sources of sodium include table salt, cheese, milk, processed meat, poultry, shellfish, and eggs.
- Hypertension is aggravated by high sodium intake and hypertensives are advised to consume no more than 1–2 g (400–800 mg) of sodium per day.
- Chloride ions maintain gastric acidity, regulate osmotic pressure of blood, and activate salivary amylase. Food sources of chloride ions are table salt and foods high in salt. Imbalances of chloride ions include problems with digestion of proteins and iron absorption.
- Functions of magnesium include the synthesis of ATP, nerve impulse transmission, activation of metabolic enzymes, and relaxation of muscles; food sources of magnesium include green vegetables and whole grains.
- Sulfur helps maintain structure of proteins and forms high-energy compounds.
- Four forms of iron in the body and functions include: transferrin—(transport form); hemoglobin and myoglobin, which transport oxygen; ferritin and hemosiderin (storage form); enzymatic iron, which is a component of oxidative enzymes.
- Four factors that decrease iron absorption in the body are a high fiber diet, surgical removal of the stomach, a diet high in cereals and grains, and pre-existing malabsorption problems.
- Food sources of heme iron include meat, fish, and poultry; food sources of nonheme iron include fortified breads, cereals, dark-green vegetables, raisins, prunes, and apricots.
- Iron deficiency anemia is characterized by RBCs being very small in size and few in number (hypochromic microcytic anemia). High-risk groups include infants, adolescents, and pregnant women. Treatment includes increasing MFP and iron supplementation.
- Iodine functions as a component of the thyroid hormones triiodothyronine and thyroxine; good food sources include iodized salt and seafood.
- Goiter is described as an enlarged thyroid gland due to a deficiency of iodine; cretinism is a deficiency of iodine in an infant.
- Functions of zinc include the formation of collagen, and as a component of insulin and many vital enzymes; good food sources of zinc include eggs, seafood, and milk.

REVIEW QUESTIONS

True (A) or False (B)

1. Major minerals differ from trace minerals in that major minerals are present in quantities greater than 5 g.
2. More calcium is absorbed when the calcium: phosphorus ratio in the diet is close to 2 : 1.
3. The greater the amount of lactose and vitamin D in the diet, the greater the amount of calcium that will be absorbed.

4. The functions of calcium include healing of wounds, maintaining osmotic pressure in blood, and maintaining the structure of protein molecules.

5. The best sources of calcium are foods that are on the milk exchange list.

6. Canned sardines and salmon are excellent sources of calcium, but absorption is hindered due to the presence of the binder compounds oxalic and phytic acids.

7. Osteoporosis is a calcium deficiency disease that is common in young women before menopause.

8. As the level of the sex hormone (estrogen) decreases, the absorption of calcium increases.

9. Women over 45 years of age need to consume 1,500 mg of calcium (5 glasses of milk per day) in order to offset the losses due to decreased estrogen and decreased calcium absorption by the intestines.

10. Two factors that can result in osteomalacia are renal failure and prolonged malabsorption.

11. Even though the same basic factors that affect calcium absorption affect phosphorus, approximately 70% of dietary phosphorus is absorbed compared to 10–30% of dietary calcium.

12. The majority of phosphorus is located in the blood, where it is a component of phospholipids and certain buffer systems.

13. Foods from the milk and meat exchange lists are the best sources of phosphorus.

14. Approximately 98% of potassium is found in extracellular fluids, where it functions in contractions of muscles, maintenance of water balance, and transmission of nerve impulses.

15. Foods from the meat and vegetable exchange lists are very high in potassium.

16. Sodium is an anion that is predominantly located inside cells, where it is quite important in the proper development of bones and teeth.

17. Forty percent of table salt (NaCl) is sodium, and the average American diet contains 10 g.

18. The average American diet contains about twice as much sodium (4 g) as is recommended.

19. A person with high blood pressure needs to increase the intake of sodium, since this will reduce the blood volume and thereby lower the blood pressure.

20. Sulfur is important in maintaining the structure of protein molecules.

Multiple Choice

21. Which of the following dietary factors influence calcium absorption?
    1. presence of lactose
    2. increased intake of vitamin D
    3. intake of calcium and phosphorus in a 2 : 1 ratio
    4. alkaline environment in the gastrointestinal tract

    A. 1, 2, 3. B. 1, 3. C. 2, 4. D. 4
    E. all of these.

22. The _____ exchanges have some foods that are good sources of calcium, but they contain the 'binder compounds' _____, which inhibit its absorption.
    A. meat—ascorbic and lactic acids.
    B. fruit—sulfate and phosphate.
    C. vegetable and bread—oxalic and phytic acids.
    D. milk and meat—carbonate and sulfate.
    E. none of these.

23. Osteoporosis is more common in postmenopausal than premenopausal women because of _____.
    A. low calcium intake.
    B. impaired calcium absorption.
    C. renal failure.
    D. reduced level of estrogen.

24. Which of the following are functions of phosphorus?
    1. development of bones and teeth
    2. contractions of muscles
    3. component of phospholipids
    4. maintaining water balance

    A. 1, 2, 3. B. 1, 3. C. 2, 4. D. 4
    E. all of these.

25. Which of the following foods are the best sources of potassium?
    A. meat, green vegetables, bread.
    B. oranges, bananas, dried fruits.
    C. oranges, milk, whole wheat bread.
    D. green vegetables, milk, cottage cheese.

26. Sodium is the most abundant _____ in _____ fluid.
    A. anion—intracellular.
    B. cation—extracellular.
    C. anion—extracellular.
    D. cation—intracellular.

27. The functions of sodium are _____ and _____.
    A. contractions of muscles—transmission of nerve impulses.
    B. blood clotting—development of bones and teeth.
    C. Component of phospholipids—maintain the structure of protein.
    D. maintenance of fluid balance—transmission of nerve impulses in blood.

Indicate in each of the following paired items whether the nutrient content of A is (a) appreciably higher, (b) appreciably lower, or (c) approximately the same as that of B.

		Column A	Column B
28.	__ calcium	milk	yogurt
29.	__ potassium	green beans	oranges
30.	__ magnesium	spinach	beef
31.	__ sodium	milk	eggs
32.	__ calcium	skim milk	whole milk
33.	__ phosphorus	meat	milk
34.	__ potassium	bananas	meat

True (A) or False (B)

35. The transport form of iron is transferrin, which carries iron through the blood to all of the tissues.
36. Approximately 70% of iron is stored in RBCs as ferritin and hemosiderin.
37. The chemical form of iron that is most readily absorbed is ferric (Fe^{3+}) iron.
38. Iron absorption is constant despite the needs of the body.
39. Nonheme iron absorption is increased if meat, fish, or poultry (MFP) are included with nonheme foods.
40. Three factors that decrease the absorption of iron are a high-fiber diet, surgical removal of stomach, and diets high in cereals and grains.
41. In a mixed diet, about 50% of iron is absorbed, whereas a diet high in MFP increases iron absorption up to 70%.
42. The most common form of iron is hemoglobin, which transports oxygen and carbon dioxide in RBCs.
43. Iron deficiency anemia is characterized by RBCs

that are small in size, pale in color, and few in number.
44. Groups that are most likely to develop iron deficiency anemia are the elderly, postmenopausal women, and women taking oral contraceptives.
45. Iodine is important in regulating the body's metabolic rate.
46. Seafoods and vegetables in the cabbage family, such as turnips and cabbage, are good sources of iodine.
47. An excess of iodine can cause cretinism and goiter.
48. Zinc is important in the formation of collagen, as a component of insulin, and as a component of many vital enzymes.
49. The vegetable and bread lists are good sources of zinc.

Multiple Choice

50. Which of the following is correct?
    A. transport iron—transferrin
    B. hemoglobin—where 70% of the iron in the body is found
    C. ferritin—form of iron found in oxidative enzymes
    D. B, C
    E. A, B
51. Factors that increase the absorption of iron are:
    1. a change from ferric to ferrous iron
    2. a high-fiber diet
    3. presence of MFP in the diet
    4. a diet high in cereals and grains

    A. 1, 2, 3   B. 1, 3   C. 2, 4   D. 4
    E. none of these
52. The percentage of iron generally absorbed in a mixed diet is _____, and in a diet high in nonheme sources such as grains and vegetables, the percentage of iron absorbed is _____.
    A. 50—30
    B. 10—5
    C. 30—10
    D. 70—50
    E. none of these
53. Dietary management of iron deficiency anemia includes:

A. increasing animal products
B. taking more ferrous sulfate
C. increasing the intake of foods high in vitamin C
D. A, C
E. B, C

54. The function(s) of iodine is (are) _____.
   A. formation of collagen
   B. a component of insulin
   C. as a component of hormones that regulate the basal metabolic rate
   D. a component of many metabolic enzymes

55. The average diet will be deficient in iodine unless _____ is (are) included.
   A. iodized salt
   B. green leafy vegetables
   C. cabbage
   D. vitamin C

56. Which of the following food lists are the best sources of zinc?
   1. vegetable   3. bread
   2. meat   4. milk
   A. 1, 2, 3   B. 1, 3   C. 2, 4   D. 4
   E. none of these

57. A diet that is low in iron and _____ can result in decreased synthesis of RBCs or anemia.
   A. manganese
   B. fluoride
   C. chromium
   D. selenium
   E. copper

58. Chromium is important in the body as a (an) _____.
   A. component of enzymes that metabolize nucleic acids to uric acid
   B. component of the Glucose Tolerance Factor
   C. compound that reduces the incidence of dental caries
   D. none of these

Matching

___ 59. chromium   A. aids oxidation of glucose and release of energy

___ 60. fluoride   B. component of many enzymes involved in metabolic reactions

___ 61. selenium   C. reduces the incidence of dental caries

___ 62. manganese   D. helps bind insulin to cell membranes

___ 63. copper   E. functions as an antioxidant

Completion

64. Discuss four dietary factors that influence calcium absorption.
65. Describe osteoporosis and discuss three reasons why this condition is more prevalent in women between 40 and 60 years of age.
66. Discuss four factors that increase the absorption of iron in the body.

CRITICAL THINKING CHALLENGE

Dinner	Ca mg	Fe mg	Na mg	Zn mg
3 oz flounder, baked with margarine	14	.3	151	.7
1/2 cup corn, cooked from raw	1.6	.5	14	.4
1/2 cup broccoli, cooked	47	.6	22	.6
2 whole-wheat rolls	50	.2	434	1.2
1 tsp margarine, soft, 40% fat	2.5	0	136	0
1 cup skim milk	302	.1	126	.9
1 cup peaches, fresh	9	.2	1	.3

Use the information above to answer the following questions.

1. The total number of mg for Ca, Fe, Na, and Zn compose what percent of the total RDA for each of these minerals? Assume that the person consuming the food is a 30-year-old male. (Use RDA table on inside front cover, except for Na value which is in the chapter.)
2. Using the information above, determine what specific foods (that would be commonly eaten for breakfast and lunch) should be consumed to achieve the RDA balance for each mineral (if more

of the mineral is required). (Consult Appendix C for a specific food and quantities of the minerals.)

3. Mary is a pregnant 15-year-old. Give the iron RDA for her and discuss the best way for Mary to achieve this level of iron.

4. A postmenopausal woman wants to take calcium carbonate tablets (a house brand) to help prevent osteoporosis. Using information in this chapter, calculate how many tablets (600 mg per tablet) she will need to take to meet the recommended amount for a postmenopausal woman.

REVIEW QUESTIONS FOR NCLEX

Situation. Mr. A has recently been diagnosed as having hypertension. His doctor put him on a diet to try to lower his blood pressure.

1. The mineral in Mr. A's diet that will have to be limited in order to control his blood pressure is _____.
   A. calcium
   B. magnesium
   C. potassium
   D. sodium

2. The exchange, that potentially contains the most of the mineral, that Mr. A really has to watch in his daily diet is _____.
   A. bread
   B. meat
   C. fruit
   D. vegetable

3. Examples of foods, from the exchange in the question above, that specifically have to be limited are _____.
   A. freshly baked bread
   B. processed meat (ex. bacon, ham, cheeses)
   C. fresh fruits (ex. apples, bananas, oranges)
   D. fresh vegetables (ex. green beans, corn, and lima beans)

4. The relationship between the causative mineral and Mr. A's hypertension is _____.
   A. calcium—excessive permeability of cell membranes
   B. magnesium—contraction of smooth muscles in blood vessels

C. potassium—excessive water retention inside cells
D. sodium—excessive fluid retention in blood vessels

Situation. Jane, a 13 year old, has recently been diagnosed as having iron deficiency anemia. Jane's doctor is treating her condition by dietary management and iron supplementation.

5. The exchange that has to be increased the most in her daily diet, in order to increase her intake of iron is _____.
   A. vegetable
   B. fruit
   B. bread
   D. meat

6. Specific foods that have to be increased, in relation to the exchange above, in order to increase iron in Jane's diet are _____.
   A. vegetables (ex. green beans, lima beans, corn, and sweet potatoes)
   B. fruit (ex. fresh oranges, apples, and bananas)
   C. bread (ex. white or wheat and polyunsaturated margarine)
   D. meat (ex. meat, fish, poultry, and citrus fruits)

7. The functions of iron in Jane's body are _____.
   A. synthesis of hemoglobin for RBCs and cytochrome enzyme systems
   B. formation of muscle tissue and increase hematocrit level
   C. to increase absorption of calcium and increase production of ATP
   D. to increase blood ferritin and to increase acidity of stomach

REFERENCES

1. Nieman, D. E., Butterworth, D. E., & Nieman, C. N. (1992). *Nutrition* (rev. 1st ed.) (pp. 279–280). Dubuque: W. C. Brown.

2. National Institutes of Health Consensus Conference. (1986). Osteoporosis. *Journal of the American Medical Association, 252,* 799–1685.

3. Walden, O. (1989). The relationship of dietary and supplemental calcium intake to bone loss

and osteoporosis. *Journal of American Medical Dietetic Association, 89,* 397.

4. National Research Council. (1989). *Recommended dietary allowances* (10th ed.) (pp. 92–93). Washington.

5. Whelton, P. K., & Klag, M. J. (1987). Ventricular ectopy, diuretics, and hypokalemia. *Clinical Nutrition, 6,* 59–64.

6. Kaplan, N. M. (1986). Dietary aspects of the treatment of hypertension. *Annual Review of Public Health 7,* 503–519.

7. Brown, J. E. (1990). *The science of human nutrition* (pp. 324–325). San Diego: Harcourt Brace Jovanovich.

8. Monsen, E. R. (1988). Dietary factors which impact iron bioavailability. *American Dietetic Association, 88,* 786.

9. Hetzel, B. S. (1988). Iodine deficiency disorders. *Lancet* (June 18), p. 1386.

10. Diplock, A. T. (1987). Trace elements in human health with special reference to selenium. *American Journal of Clinical Nutrition, 45,* 1313–1322.

8

WATER

Upon completion of this chapter, you should be able to:

1. Give the percentage of total body weight composed of water and in the extracellular and intracellular compartments.
2. List and describe the five functions of water.
3. Define osmosis and describe its importance in the body.
4. Define osmolality and describe the two criteria that determine its level.
5. Define isotonic, hypertonic, and hypotonic fluids and their effects on the shift of fluids through membranes.
6. Determine in which direction water will shift, given specific osmolalities of fluids.
7. Describe how diarrhea results in a shift of fluids through membranes until dehydration occurs.

INTRODUCTION

Of all the nutrients in the body, water is one of the most important. This statement is evidenced by the fact that the body can survive a deficiency of all the other nutrients for long periods (months, even years), but can survive for only a few days without water. This fact is a strong indicator of how important water is to the maintenance of homeostasis.

PERCENTAGE OF BODY WEIGHT AS WATER AND LOCATION

Water makes up 60% of the total body weight of an adult[1] and 75% of that of an infant. The reason for this difference is that an infant has a higher body surface area and metabolic rate than an adult. Another interesting point is that body water tends to decrease as body fat increases. Notice the following relationships:

	Percentage of Total Body Weight Composed of Water
Normal-weight person	60
Obese person	50
Lean person	70

One might think that an obese person has a greater percentage of body weight as water than a lean person, but this is not true. The reason is due to the fact that adipose tissue does not contain much water, but muscle tissue does. An interesting point in this regard is that 1 lb of protein tissue retains 4 lb of water. Therefore, if an obese person has struggled to lose 25 lb and then gains 1 lb of protein tissue, the result is the retention of 4 lb more of water.[1] It is easy to see why many obese people say that the smallest amount of food tends to make them gain weight and therefore that dieting is futile.

Water is located in fluid compartments throughout the body. These compartments, and the percentage of total body weight consisting of water in each, are (see Fig. 8-1):

Compartment	Percentage of Body Weight
Extracellular	20
Intracellular	<u>40</u>
	Total: 60

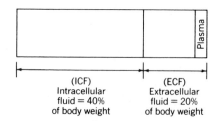

FIGURE 8-1 The fluid compartments and the percentage of water according to body weight. (From T. Randall Lankford, *Integrated Science for Health Students,* 3rd ed. 1984. Reprinted by permission of Reston Publishing Company, a Prentice-Hall Company, 11480 Sunset Hills Road, Reston, Va. 22090.)

Water shifts back and forth between these compartments as a result of changes in osmotic pressure, which will be discussed shortly.

FUNCTIONS OF WATER IN THE BODY

Water has several important functions in the body (see Fig. 8-2).

reactant A substance that interacts with other substances to produce products.

ionize Chemical process by which substances break apart into ions.

Reactant

Water is a **reactant** in various chemical reactions. Ionic compounds **ionize** to electrolytes as a result of water molecules:

$$NaCl + H_2O \rightarrow Na^+ + Cl^- + H_2O$$

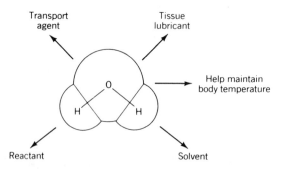

FIGURE 8-2 The functions of water in the body.

Several of the minerals discussed in Chapter 7 actually exist as electrolytes as a result of ionization in water. Carbohydrates, lipids, and proteins are broken down into their basic chemical components by water and enzymes, breaking chemical bonds.

Solvent

solvent   A fluid that causes a solute to dissolve and form a solution.

A **solvent** is a fluid that causes a **solute** to dissolve, forming a solution. Water serves as the solvent for most chemical reactions in the body.

solute   A substance that dissolves in a solvent.

Transport Agent

Blood, urine, and sweat are extracellular fluids composed primarily of water. They transport nutrients and wastes to and from cells.

Helps Maintain Body Temperature

Celsius (C)   A unit of temperature measurement on the Celsius scale.

specific heat   The amount of heat required to raise the temperature of 1 g of liquid 1°C (Celsius).

synovial   A fluid that lubricates bones articulating in joints.

More heat is required for water than any other liquid to raise its temperature. The amount of heat required to raise the temperature of 1 g of liquid 1°C (**celsius**) is called **specific heat.** The high specific heat characteristic of water is the reason that it is slow to change from cold to hot or hot to cold. In other words, water does not change temperature very readily, which explains why it is used in hot-water bottles and cold compresses. The high specific heat of water benefits the body by preventing rapid cooling or heating. As a result, body temperature is maintained at a fairly constant level.

Tissue Lubricant

serous   A fluid that lubricates body walls and organs that are coated with the fluid.

Water is the major constituent of **synovial** and **serous** fluids.[2]

MOVEMENT OF WATER BETWEEN FLUID COMPARTMENTS

edema   Accumulation of water in tissues.

dehydration   An excess loss of fluids from tissues.

As stated previously, water shifts back and forth between the fluid compartments. This shifting of fluids is a normal process and helps to maintain homeostasis. However, the shifting of the fluids between compartments is sometimes excessive, causing **edema** or **dehydration.** The mechanism responsible for the shifting of fluids between compartments and the conditions that can initiate the shift will be discussed next.

Osmosis

osmosis The movement of water from a low-solute concentration to a high-solute concentration through a membrance permeable to water only.

The mechanism responsible for shifting of fluids back and forth between compartments is **osmosis.** Solutes are substances that dissolve in water. In order for osmosis to occur, a cellular membrane must be impermeable to the majority of solutes but permeable to water. Since solutes cannot pass across a membrane, they create a pressure called *osmotic pressure,* which varies directly with the concentration of solutes.[3] Osmotic pressure pulls water through the membrane from the low- to the high-solute concentration. As water moves through the membrane, it lowers the solute concentration on the more concentrated side, since only water is in motion. Likewise, the solute concentration on the less concentrated side increases as water moves to the other side of the membrane. In other words, one side of the membrane becomes more concentrated as it loses water alone and no solute, whereas the other side of the membrane is diluted as water alone moves to that side and the number of solute particles remains the same.

These changes occur until the concentrations of the solutions on both sides of the membrane are equal or an equilibrium is established. The underlying importance of osmosis is that it maintains or restores equal solute concentrations on both sides of a cell membrane, which is essential for maintenance of homeostasis.

Osmolality

osmolality The number of osmoles per kilogram of solvent.

osmole The standard unit of measure of osmotic pressure.

milliosmole (mOsm) Equals 1/1,000th of an osmole.

The concentration of a solute, and likewise of a solution, can be expressed in terms of **osmolality.*** An **osmole** is the standard unit of measure for osmotic pressure. Generally, the osmole is too large a unit for satisfactory use in expressing the osmotic activity of a solution in the body. Therefore, the term **milliosmole** (mOsm) is commonly used.

Two criteria determine the osmolality of a solution. One criterion is the number of solute particles in a solution; the greater the concentration of a solution, the higher the osmolality or osmotic pressure. The second criterion is the size of the particles. The smaller the particles, the higher the osmolality or osmotic pressure. The reason is that more particles are hitting the membrane and therefore increasing the osmotic pressure.[3] The importance of the second criterion is illustrated by comparing two solutions with equal concentrations but different-sized particles, as shown on facing page.

---

*The term *osmolarity* is commonly used by health professionals in expressing the osmotic activity of a solution. Osmolarity refers to the number of osmotically active particles per liter of solution (solvent plus solute). Clinical differences between the two terms are slight.

5% glucose	5% glycogen
5 g/dl	5 g/dl
Small particles	Large particles
High osmotic pressure	Low osmotic pressure

As shown above, the 5% glucose solution has a higher osmotic pressure than the 5% glycogen solution. The reason is that glucose particles are much smaller than glycogen particles.

Whole-protein molecules are very large and have little or no osmotic effect. However, individual amino acids are smaller particles that have an osmotic effect similar to that of low molecular weight carbohydrates.

Fats are not water soluble and thus have no osmotic effect.

Electrolytes such as sodium and potassium are comparatively small particles that have a great effect on the osmolality of a solution.

In summary, foods that contain high concentrations of simple sugars, electrolytes, and amino acids have the greatest effects on osmolality. See the Clinical Application "Osmotic Pressure."

Clinical Application: Osmotic Pressure

Tube Feeding

elemental formulas
Liquid formulas that contain simple sugars and amino acids.

Some commercial tube formulas used in tube feeding are known as **elemental formulas** (see Chapter 16 for details on tube feeding and elemental formulas). These formulas create a very high osmotic pressure in the intestines; thus, if infused at full strength, they cause a large amount of water to shift into the intestines, resulting in diarrhea. To prevent this problem, the formulas are generally started at half strength, which reduces their osmotic pressure by half, and are gradually increased to full strength as the body adapts to the solution.

Cathartic Drugs

cathartic   Laxative drugs.

Many of the **cathartic** drugs used in treating constipation contain large amounts of salts that ionize into electrolytes when dissolved in intestinal fluids. This action creates a high osmotic pressure in the intestines, causing water to shift into and soften the feces. Some examples of these drugs are milk of magnesia (magnesium hydroxide), epsom salts (magnesium sulfate), and Fleet enema (sodium phosphate and sodium biphosphate).

Osmolality of Body Fluids

The osmolality of normal body fluids is approximately 300 mOsm/kg. The body attempts to maintain the osmolality of its fluids by osmosis. Various problems can cause the osmolality of body fluids to become higher or lower than the norm. Intravenous (IV) fluids as well as food and drink may be higher or lower than this value, which can result in a shift of fluids from one compartment to another.

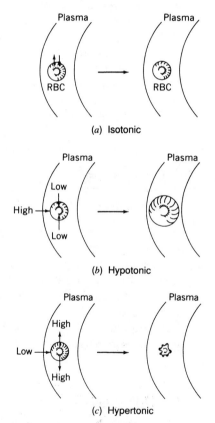

(a) Isotonic

(b) Hypotonic

(c) Hypertonic

FIGURE 8-3 Isotonic, hypertonic, and hypotonic solutions and their effects on cells. (*a*) Isotonic: The osmolarities of the plasma and the RBC are equal. As a result, the movement of water into and out of the RBC is equal, and no net change occurs in the RBC. (*b*) Hypotonic: The osmolarity of the plasma is lower than that of the RBC. The result is a net movement of water into the RBC, as indicated by the arrows. (*c*) Hypertonic: The osmolarity of the plasma is higher than that of the RBC. The result is a net movement of water out of the RBC, causing the RBC to shrink or become crenated.

isotonic A food or solution that has the approximate osmolality of body fluids: 300 mOsm.

hypertonic A food or solution that has an osmolality of at least 340 mOsm or higher.

hypotonic A food or solution that has an osmolality of 240 mOsm or lower.

physiological solutions Solutions in which the osmotic pressure exerted by the solutions is equal to that of body fluids.

The osmolality of foods and body fluids can be **isotonic, hypertonic,** or **hypotonic.** These osmolalities are discussed below.

Isotonic. Figure 8-3 shows that isotonic osmolality has no net effect on the amount of water in fluid compartments or cells. Water does shift through membranes in this condition; however, the amount that shifts into a cell is equal to the amount that shifts out.

Two solutions that are isotonic to normal body fluids are 5% glucose and 0.9% sodium chloride (NaCl). Since the osmotic pressure exerted by these two solutions is equal to that of body fluids, they are known as **physiological solutions.** These two physiological solutions are frequently used in IV solutions, injections, and others.

Hypertonic. Figure 8-3 shows the effects of a hypertonic solution on compartments or tissue cells. Since this solution has a higher osmolality than adjacent fluid compartments or cells, it tends to pull fluids out of these regions. This action can result in shrinkage of cells and fluid compartments or dehydration.

Hypotonic. Figure 8-3 shows the effect of a hypotonic solution on fluid compartments or cells. Since the osmotic pressure of this solution is lower than that of adjacent cells or compartments, water tends to move from the solution into cells or fluid compartments.[3] See the Clinical Application "Disorders That Can Cause Hypertonic, Hypotonic, and Fluid Imbalances."

WATER CONTENT OF FOODS

Fluids are the main source of water in the body. Some foods contain a considerable amount of water. Table 8-1 shows the approximate percentage of water in the different exchanges.

Osmolality of Certain Foods

The approximate osmolality of common foods and beverages is as follows:

Food	mOsm/liter
Whole milk	275
Tomato juice	595
Cola	680
Apple juice	870
Ice cream	1150
Grape juice	1170[4]

TABLE 8-1 WATER CONTENT OF EXCHANGE GROUPS

Exchange	Approximate % of Water	Approximate Amount of Water Per Exchange Serving
Milk	85	1 cup = 204 ml
Vegetables	70–95	½ cup = 70–95% × wt. of vegetables (See Appendix C for weights of specific vegetables)
Fruit	70–95	½ cup = 70–95% × wt. of fruit (See Appendix C for weights of specific fruits)
Bread	35	1 slice = 11 ml
Cooked cereals	80–90	½ cup = 98–110 ml
Dry cereal	3	¾ cup = 0.5–1.0 ml
Meat		
Cooked rare	75	1 oz = 23 ml
Cooked well done	40	1 oz = 12 ml

Source: Adapted from D. F. Tver, *Nutrition and Health Encyclopedia.* New York: Van Nostrand Reinhold Co., 1981. All rights reserved.

Some of these foods and beverages, such as ice cream and grape juice, are extremely hypertonic. They cause fluids to shift from the various compartments into the intestines, as shown in Figure 8-4. As a result of this shift, a person may experience the following:

Feeling of fullness

Increased peristaltic activity of the intestines

Nausea

Diarrhea

Dehydration

The dehydration effect is the reason why one generally becomes thirsty after eating ice cream. Obviously, a food or beverage that has a lower osmolality will cause less water to be shifted into the intestines and should therefore be better tolerated than one of higher osmolality. Hospitalized patients who are receiving nutritional formulas, either orally or by tube, can tolerate a wide range of osmolalities if the formulas are administered slowly and additional fluids are given. However,

Clinical Application: Disorders That Can Cause Hypertonic, Hypotonic, and Fluid Imbalances

Illnesses that result in prolonged vomiting or diarrhea can cause dehydration. This condition is due to a hypertonic imbalance that initially begins in the intestines (see p. 206 and Figure 8-4 for details on diarrhea).

Edema is an abnormal accumulation of extracellular fluid within the interstitial spaces. One factor that can cause edema is a hypotonic condition in the blood due to a low protein concentration, such as protein-calorie malnutrition.

Examples of Intravenous Solutions That Are Isotonic, Hypertonic, and Hypotonic

Some examples of solutions that are administered intravenously are as follows:

Isotonic. D_5W, a 5% dextrose solution that is commonly administered intravenously.

Hypertonic. $D_{10}W$ and $D_{20}W$ are 10 and 20% dextrose solutions, respectively. They are frequently used in **total parenteral nutrition (TPN)** (see Chapter 14 for details on these solutions and TPN). These solutions contribute more kilocalories than a 5% solution but are also hypertonic, thereby creating a potential for more fluid to be shifted into the vessels.

Total parenteral nutrition (TPN) Solutions that are composed of dextrose for energy, amino acids for tissue synthesis, fats for energy, and essential fatty acids plus vitamins and minerals.

Hypotonic. 2.5% dextrose in 0.45% sodium chloride is an example of a hypotonic solution. This solution can be used to shift fluids into cells when the body is dehydrated.

---

certain patients are more likely to develop symptoms of intolerance when receiving formulas of high osmolality. These include:

Debilitated (very weak) patients

Gastrointestinal disorder patients

Pre- and postoperative patients

Gastrostomy patients

Jejunostomy patients

gastrostomy Feeding directly into the stomach through a specially created opening.

DIARRHEA: EXAMPLE OF THE SHIFT OF WATER OUT
OF FLUID COMPARTMENTS

An example of how a change in one fluid compartment can result in compensatory changes in all the compartments is diarrhea (see Fig. 8-4). Prolonged diarrhea results in large losses of fluids from the intestines or gastrointestinal tract fluid compartment. The large losses of fluids compared to the loss of minerals causes the gastrointestinal tract to become hypertonic (see Fig. 8-4). Water shifts from the intestinal wall cell compartment into the gastrointestinal tract (water moving from the low-solute concentration in the intestinal cell compartment to the high-solute concentration in the gastrointestinal tract) in a compensatory move to dilute the high-solute concentration in the gastrointestinal tract. This original hypertonic condition and shift of fluids progresses until the body cell compartment finally becomes dehydrated (see Fig. 8-4).

In summary, prolonged diarrhea initially results in a hypertonic condition in the gastrointestinal tract. The initial compensatory shift of fluids causes each fluid compartment to be affected, in turn, by a change in the concentration of fluids in adjacent compartments until dehydration results.

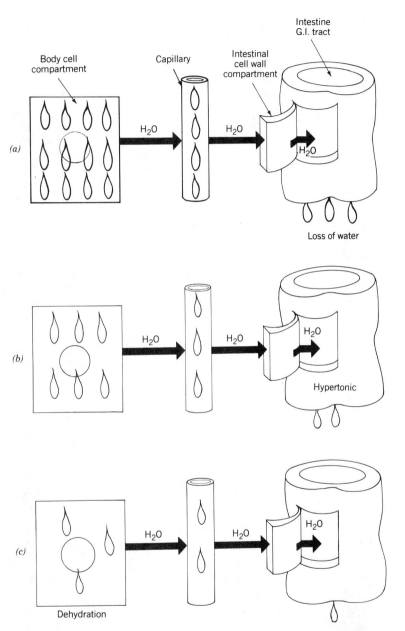

FIGURE 8-4 (*a*) The gastrointestinal tract and the adjacent compartments are shown, with H_2O loss from the gastrointestinal tract. (*b*)
H_2O loss from the gastrointestinal tract causes it to become
hypertonic, which results in a shift of water from each compartment
toward the gastrointestinal tract. (*c*) The final result of this shift is
that the body cell compartment becomes dehydrated.

SUMMARY

- Water composes approximately 60% of total body weight in adults and 75% in infants; approximately 20% of water is in the extracellular body compartment and 40% in the intracellular compartment.
- Water acts as a reactant, solvent, transport agent, and tissue lubricant, and helps to maintain body temperature.
- Osmosis is the movement of water from a low-solute concentration to a high-solute concentration through a membrane permeable to water only; it is important in the body in that it shifts water from one compartment to another.
- Osmolality is the concentration of a solution; two criteria that affect osmolality are the number of solute particles dissolved in water and the size of the particles.
- Isotonic fluid is a fluid with an osmolality of 300 mOsm, or osmolality equal to normal osmolality of body fluids, and will have no effect on shifting water into or out of cells. Hypertonic is a fluid with an osmolality of at least 340 mOsm or higher; the effect is to pull water out of cells or dehydration. Hypotonic is a fluid with an osmolality less than 240 mOsm; the effect is to shift water into cells.
- Diarrhea causes a hypertonic condition in the gastrointestinal (G.I.) tract due to loss of water from the body; this causes a shifting of water from body compartments toward the G.I. tract until dehydration occurs.

REVIEW QUESTIONS

True (A) or False (B)

1. Obese people have a greater percentage of their body weight as water than lean people.
2. The majority of water in the body is located in the extracellular fluid compartment.
3. Water is a solvent and causes solutes to dissolve, forming solutions.
4. The high specific heat characteristic of water is the reason why body temperature remains fairly constant.
5. Osmosis is the mechanism responsible for the shift of solutes through membranes.

6. Osmosis is defined as the movement of water from a low-solute concentration to a high-solute concentration through a membrane permeable to water only.
7. If the concentration of a solution inside a cell is 2.0% NaCl and that outside the cell is 0.9%, water will tend to move into the cell.
8. Two criteria, the number of solute particles and the size of the particles, determine the osmolality of a solution.
9. A fluid such as grape juice that has an osmolality of 1,170 mOsm is hypotonic and causes fluids to shift out of the intestines into other body compartments.
10. A 0.9% NaCl solution and a 5% glucose solution are isotonic fluids and have osmolalities of about 300 mOsm.
11. The two fluids mentioned in question 10 will result in the net movement of water into the bloodstream when they are given in IVs.

Multiple Choice

12. Which of the following is incorrect?
    1. Water composes 60–75% of the total body weight.
    2. Obese people have a smaller percentage of their body weight as water than lean people.
    3. Water composes about 75% of the total body weight of an infant.
    4. Less water is in the intracellular than in the extracellular compartment.

    A. 1, 2, 3,   B. 1, 3   C. 2, 4   D. 4
    E. all of these

13. Which of the following functions of water is (are) correct?
    1. reactant
    2. solvent.
    3. transport agent
    4. tissue lubricant

    A. 1, 2, 3   B. 1, 3   C. 2, 4   D. 4
    E. all of these

14. Osmosis is defined as the
    A. movement of water through a membrane from a low-water concentration to a high-water concentration.

B. movement of water from a high-solute concentration to a low-solute concentration through a membrane permeable to water only.

C. movement of water from a low-solute to a high-solute concentration through a membrane permeable to water only.

D. none of these

15. Which of the following would cause a solution to have a high osmolality?
   A. very small particles
   B. very large particles
   C. large number of particles
   D. B, C
   E. A, C

16. Which of the following solutions has the highest osmolality?
   A. 5% glycogen
   B. 5% NaCl
   C. 5% protein
   D. 5% fat

17. If a person eats ice cream with an osmolality of 1,150 mOsm/liter, this food is _____ and will result in a shifting of fluids _____ the intestines.
   A. isotonic—equally into and out of
   B. hypotonic—out of
   C. hypertonic—out of
   D. hypotonic—into
   E. hypertonic—into

18. Hospitalized patients who might develop symptoms of intolerance when fed nutritional formulas of high osmolality, either orally or by tube, are _____ patients.
   A. debilitated (very weak)
   B. gastrointestinal disorder
   C. gastrostomy
   D. pre- and postoperative
   E. all of these

19. Diarrhea can result in dehydration because a (an) _____ condition is initially formed in the gastrointestinal tract that ultimately results in a shift of water _____ the intestines.
   A. hypotonic—out of
   B. hypertonic—into
   C. isotonic—out of
   D. hypotonic—into
   E. none of these

Matching

Each answer may be used more than once.

___ 20. fluid or food with an osmolality of less than 240 mOsm

___ 21. physiological solution

___ 22. solution that, in the gastrointestinal tract, can cause dehydration

___ 23. 5% glucose, 0.9% NaCl

___ 24. solution that, in a cell, would cause a shift of fluids into it

A. hypotonic solution

B. hypertonic solution

C. isotonic solution

Completion

25. Describe five functions of water.
26. Describe the basic osmotic balance problem that may occur with elemental tube formulas if they are not started at half strength.
27. Describe diarrhea in terms of the initial osmotic imbalance that starts the shift of water and which fluid compartment is ultimately affected.

CRITICAL THINKING CHALLENGE

1. Calculate the amount of water in the following foods: (use information in Table 8-1). Show calculations. (1 q of water = 1 ml)
   a. 1/2 cup green beans, fresh, cooked wt. 63 g
   b. 1 slice whole-wheat bread   wt. 35 g
   c. 1 banana (peeled wt.)   wt. 114 g
   d. 1 oz chicken, light meat, well done wt. 28 g
2. If a normal-weight person weighs 185 pounds, calculate approximately how many pounds are due to water.
3. Give the osmolalities of isotonic, hypertonic, and hypotonic IV fluids and a clinical example of each.
4. You are caring for a client admitted with dehydration. Which of the following orders can be carried out without questioning the physician?
   a. Start an IV (intravenous) of D10W (10% dextrose in water).
   b. Start an IV of 2.5% dextrose in 1/2 strength (0.45) normal saline.

c. Start an IV of D5NS (5% dextrose in normal saline).
d. Start an IV of D20W (20% dextrose in water).

REVIEW QUESTIONS FOR NCLEX

Situation. A client has had diarrhea for several days and is hospitalized with dehydration.

1. The loss of fluids from the gastrointestinal tract causes it to become _____.
   A. isotonic
   B. hypertonic
   C. hypotonic
   D. no change in tonicity
2. The dehydrated condition of this client means that the _____ compartment is finally affected by the shifting of water from one compartment to another.
   A. extracellular fluid
   B. gastrointestinal tract
   C. body cell
   D. intestinal wall cell
3. An intravenous solution that could be used to help reverse this dehydrated condition is _____.
   A. D50W-dextrose (glucose) 50% in water solution
   B. D10W-dextrose (glucose) 10% in water solution
   C. D20W-dextrose (glucose) 20% in water solution
   D. D2.5%, NaCl .45%-2.5% dextrose (glucose), .45% in saline solution

Situation. A client has been suffering from constipation and decides to take milk of magnesia to eliminate this problem.

4. The milk of magnesia has a(an) _____ osmotic pressure which will function to shift water into the _____ compartment.
   A. isotonic—body cell
   B. hypotonic—intracellular
   C. hypertonic—gastrointestinal
   D. isotonic—extracellular

REFERENCES

1. Vokes, T. (1987). Water homeostasis. *Annual Review of Nutrition, 7,* 383–406.
2. Nieman, D. C., Butterworth, D. E., & Nieman, C. N. (1992). *Nutrition* (rev. 1st ed.) (pp. 314–315). Dubuque: W. C. Brown.
3. Marieb, E. N. (1992). *Human anatomy—Physiology* (p. 71). Redwood City, CA: Benjamin Cummings.
4. *Osmolality* (Monograph). Minneapolis: Doyle Pharmaceutical Co.

PART II

NUTRITION THROUGHOUT THE LIFE CYCLE

9. ENERGY, OBESITY, AND UNDERWEIGHT

10. NUTRITION DURING PREGNANCY AND LACTATION

11. NUTRITION DURING INFANCY, CHILDHOOD, AND ADOLESCENCE

12. NUTRITION AND THE ELDERLY

9

ENERGY, OBESITY, AND UNDERWEIGHT

OBJECTIVES

Upon completion of this chapter, you should be able to:

1. Define and give the unit for measurement of energy in nutrition.
2. Distinguish between positive and negative energy balance and the results when there is a deficit or surplus of 3,500 kcal.
3. Give the percentage of body weight from fat that indicates obesity and the percentages above suggested weight that indicate overweight and obesity.
4. Discuss the three metabolic or internal causes of obesity.
5. Name the three critical periods when the number of fat cells can increase dramatically and therefore result in juvenile obesity.
6. Name and describe the three theories in terms of how the hypothalamus knows when the person is hungry or satiated.
7. Discuss the three external causes of obesity.
8. Describe the five nonrecommended diets for the treatment of obesity.
9. Describe the three recommended methods for the treatment of obesity.
10. Define underweight and describe anorexia nervosa as well as bulimia and bulimarexia.

INTRODUCTION

energy The capacity to do work.

In Chapter 1, we mentioned that carbohydrates, fats, and proteins are designated as energy nutrients. They release energy when oxidized, which is used by the body to maintain homeostasis. The maintenance of homeostasis depends upon continual input of **energy.**

In this chapter, we will discuss energy in more detail, including energy balance and the results of imbalance: obesity and underweight.

MEASUREMENT OF ENERGY

Kilocalorie (kcal) The amount of heat required to raise the temperature of 1,000 g of water 1°C.

Calorie (cal) The amount of heat required to raise the temperature of 1 g of water 1°C.

Examples of how the body uses energy to accomplish work are contractions of the heart to move blood, movement of food along the digestive tract, and contraction of respiratory muscles in moving air into and out of the lungs. In other words, almost all body activities involve work and thereby require an expenditure of energy.

Energy is measured and expressed in nutrition in terms of heat units called **kilocalories (kcal)** (see Fig. 9-1). Chemists and physicists measure energy in terms of a **calorie (cal),** which is defined as the amount of heat required to raise the temperature of 1 g of water 1° Celsius (C) (see Fig. 9-1).

Recall that carbohydrates, proteins, lipids, and alcohol provide different amounts of energy; carbohydrates and proteins yield 4 kcal/g and triglycerides (fats) yield 9 kcal/g. Alcohol provides 7 kcal/g when oxidized.

ENERGY BALANCE

energy balance The amount of energy remaining in the body when energy output is subtracted from energy input.

positive energy balance A situation in which energy input is greater than energy expenditure.

Energy balance refers to the amount of energy remaining in the body when energy output is subtracted from energy input:

Energy balance = energy input − energy output

A **positive energy balance** will result in weight gain. For example:

Energy balance = 2,500 kcal − 2,000 kcal
　　　　　　　　　input　　　　expenditure
　　　　　　　　= +500 kcal

If this positive 500-kcal energy balance continues every day for 1 week, the person will gain 1 lb, since a 3,500-kcal surplus equals 1 lb of weight gain. A positive energy balance results in weight gain and is the

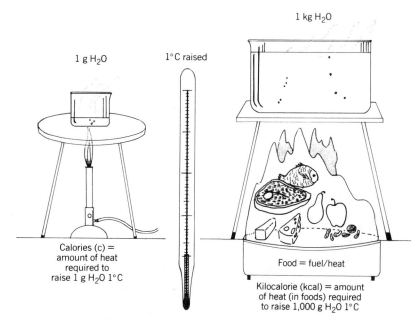

FIGURE 9-1 The two kinds of calories.

overweight Body weight that is more than 10% above ideal weight.

obesity Body weight that is 15–25% above ideal weight.

negative energy balance A situation in which energy expenditure is greater than energy input.

type of balance that can result in **overweight** and ultimately **obesity**.[1] Overweight and obesity will be discussed later in the chapter.

A **negative energy balance** occurs when an adult has a greater energy expenditure than input:

$$\text{Energy balance} = \underset{\text{input}}{2{,}000 \text{ kcal}} - \underset{\text{expenditure}}{2{,}500 \text{ kcal}}$$
$$= -500 \text{ kcal}$$

If this negative 500-kcal energy balance continues every day for 1 week, the person will lose 1 lb, since a 3,500-kcal deficit equals 1 lb of weight loss. A negative energy balance is necessary for weight loss, which will be discussed later in the chapter.

If energy intake equals energy expenditure, the person's current weight will be maintained.

Energy Intake

energy intake Energy supplied by the three energy nutrients: carbohydrates, fats, and proteins.

Foods from the three energy nutrients, carbohydrates, fats, and proteins, compose the **energy intake**. The Recommended Dietary Allowance (RDA) for energy for various age groups is given in Table 9-1.

TABLE 9-1 MEDIAN HEIGHTS AND WEIGHTS AND RECOMMENDED ENERGY INTAKE

Category	Age (years) or Condition	Weight (kg)	Weight (lb)	Height (in.)	Average Energy Allowance (kcal)[a] Per kg	Average Energy Allowance (kcal)[a] Per day[b]
Infants	0.0–0.5	6	13	24	108	650
	0.5–1.0	9	20	28	98	850
Children	1–3	13	29	35	102	1,300
	4–6	20	44	44	90	1,800
	7–10	28	62	52	70	2,000
Males	11–14	45	99	62	55	2,500
	15–18	66	145	69	45	3,000
	19–24	72	160	70	40	2,900
	25–50	79	174	70	37	2,900
	51+	77	170	68	30	2,300
Females	11–14	46	101	62	47	2,200
	15–18	55	120	64	40	2,200
	19–24	58	128	65	38	2,200
	25–50	63	138	64	36	2,200
	51+	65	143	63	30	1,900
Pregnant	1st trimester					+0
	2nd trimester					+300
	3rd trimester					+300
Lactating	1st 6 months					+500
	2nd 6 months					+500

[a]In the range of light to moderate activity, the coefficient of variation is ±20%.
[b]Figure is rounded.
Source: Adapted from *Recommended Dietary Allowances,* 10th edition, 1989, with permission of the National Academy Press, Washington, DC.

ENERGY EXPENDITURE

Energy is expended by the body to maintain organ systems when at rest, during physical activity, and specific dynamic action. Total energy expenditure is the sum of these three components.

Resting Energy Expenditure (REE)

The expenditure of energy for the maintenance of body systems when at rest is known as resting energy expenditure (REE). Basal metabolic rate (BMR) is more precisely defined as REE measured soon after awakening in the morning and at least 12 hours after the last meal. REE is not usually measured under resting conditions. In practice, BMR and REE are used interchangeably.

Several factors that influence REE (see Fig. 9-2) are discussed below.

Body Surface Area

body surface area Total surface area of an individual, which can be determined from charts based on the person's height and weight.

The greater the **body surface area,** the higher the REE. If a short, fat person and a tall, thin person both weighed 170 lb, the latter would have the higher REE. The reason is that this individual has a greater skin surface area through which heat is lost; therefore, the REE must be higher to replace the lost heat.

Sex

Men generally have a faster REE than women. One reason is that men have a greater proportion of muscle tissue compared to fat tissue than women. Muscle (lean) tissue is more metabolically active than fat tissue. A lean man has a higher REE than a man who is fatter and has a greater percentage of less active adipose tissue.

Fever

fever Elevation of body temperature above normal.

Fever is an example of increased expenditure of energy by the cells to destroy the bacteria or viruses that are causing the infection. In order to provide this increased energy as well as the basal energy, the BMR will

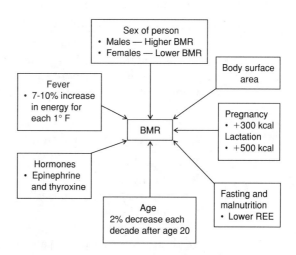

FIGURE 9-2 Factors that influence the REE.

rise. Generally, the body needs approximately 7–10% more energy for each 1°F rise in temperature to maintain the REE.[2] This increase can be accomplished only by increasing the amount of calories in the diet of the individual.

Hormones

Two hormones that influence REE are epinephrine and thyroxine (T_4). Epinephrine is released from the adrenal glands in times of stress. In order to overcome the stress, many body activities are activated, raising the REE.

Thyroxine influences the REE at all times by increasing the rate at which carbohydrates are catabolized or oxidized to produce energy. **Hyperthyroidism** usually results in elevated thyroxine levels (described in Chapter 7), which can increase the REE by as much as 80% whereas **hypothyroidism** may reduce it by as much as 30%.

hyperthyroidism Excessive activity of the thyroid gland, which results in increased secretion of thyroxine.

hypothyroidism Decreased activity of the thyroid gland, which results in an underproduction of thyroxine.

Age

The REE increases from birth to age 2 and then begins to drop slightly until puberty, when it increases again as the person goes through a growth spurt. After age 20 the REE decreases by about 2% every 10 years. In many adults, this decrease in REE may be greater than 2% because of decreased physical activity, decreased muscle tone, and increased body fat.

Pregnancy and Lactation

Pregnancy is a period when the mother's REE increases because of the rapid growth and development of the fetus. Lactation also increases the REE as the mother's body produces breast milk. The RDA for energy tables show 300 kcal more than the normal energy needs for a pregnant woman and 500 kcal more for a lactating woman (see Table 9-1).

Fasting and Malnutrition

Fasting and malnutrition lower the REE as a result of loss of muscle tissue and decrease in body functions. In reality, this REE decrease is a homeostatic response to conserve energy, since the body is not receiving an adequate amount.

As stated previously, REE is the minimum amount of energy the body needs to expend to maintain homeostasis when it is at rest. However, REE accounts for about 50–70% of the total kilocalorie requirement for people who are sedentary or moderately active. Since this description fits most people in the United States, unless a person is very physically active, his or her energy requirements do not exceed the basal metabolism requirement. Physical activity and its influence on energy expenditure will be discussed next.

Physical Activity

physical activity The amount of energy expended by the body to contract the skeletal muscles in voluntary activities.

A second component of energy expenditure is **physical activity.** The actual amount of energy expended for a physical activity depends on muscle involvement, on body weight, and on the length of the activity period. Table 9-2 gives some examples of the kilocalories expended per hour.

TABLE 9-2 AMOUNT OF ENERGY EXPENDED FOR VARIOUS ACTIVITIES

Activity	Calories expended per hour[a]	
	Man[b]	Woman[b]
Sitting quietly	100	80
Standing quietly	120	95
Light activity:	300	240
Cleaning house		
Office work		
Playing baseball		
Playing golf		
Moderate activity:	460	370
Walking briskly (3.5 MPH)		
Gardening		
Cycling (5.5 MPH)		
Dancing		
Playing basketball		
Strenuous activity:	730	580
Jogging (9 min./mile)		
Playing football		
Swimming		
Very strenuous activity:	920	740
Running (7 min./mile)		
Racquetball		
Skiing		

[a]May vary depending on environmental conditions.
[b]Healthy man, 175 lb; healthy woman, 140 lb
Source: McArdle, WD Katch, FI and Katch, VL: (1986) *Exercise Physiology: Energy, Nutrition and Human Performance,* 2nd ed. Philadelphia, Lea & Febiger

For any physical activity, the actual expenditure of energy depends upon the person's physical condition and the efficiency with which the exercise is carried out or its form. In other words, a person who is in good physical condition and is close to the ideal weight will actually expend less energy per hour for a particular physical activity than a person who is heavier and not in good physical condition.

A simple method of estimating the amount of energy expended on muscular activities is to classify the person's lifestyle and then add to the REE a percentage for his or her particular classification, as shown below and discussed on pages 220–222.

Sedentary: REE + 40–50%

Lightly active: REE + 55–65%

Moderately active: REE + 65–70%

Very active: REE + 75–100%[3]

Typically, physical activity decreases as the person ages. On the average, the person's total energy needs (REE + physical activity) decrease by about 5% per decade after the age of 20. Do not confuse this decrease with the 2% per decade for REE only that was discussed earlier.

Specific Dynamic Effect

specific dynamic effect The expenditure of energy when food is consumed.

When a person consumes food, energy is expended. This energy is used in the digestion, absorption, and transport of nutrients in the body. This expenditure of energy is known as the **specific dynamic effect** or specific dynamic action of food. The amount of energy needed for specific dynamic action is calculated at 10% of the total kilocalories used for REE and physical activity.[2]

CALCULATING TOTAL ENERGY REQUIREMENTS

The total energy needs of a person can be estimated or calculated by several short methods. One formula that can be used to estimate the resting energy expenditure (REE) or the basal energy expenditure (BEE) of resting individuals who are not under stress is as follows:[3]

Men:

$$REE = 66 + (13.7 \times wt) + (5 \times ht) - (6.8 \times age)$$

Example: A 47-year-old, 5 ft 9 in. (69 in.) man who weighs 145 lb.

$$REE = 66 + (13.7 \times 145 \text{ lb}) + (5 \times 69 \text{ in.}) - (6.8 \times 47)$$
$$66 + (1{,}987) + (345) - (320) = 2{,}078 \text{ kcal}$$

Women:

$$REE = 655 + (9.6 \times wt) + (1.7 \times ht) - (4.7 \times age)$$

Example: A 35-year-old, 5 ft 2 in. (62 in.) woman who weighs 115 lb

$$REE = 655 + (9.6 \times 115) + (1.7 \times 62) - (4.7 \times 35)$$
$$655 + (1,104) + (105) - (165) = 1,699 \text{ kcal}$$

Once the REE has been calculated, then the amount of energy expended for physical activity can be calculated using the percentages given on p. 220. As an example, using our 47-year-old man from above, and assuming he is moderately active:

$$REE \times 65\text{–}70\% = \text{kcal expended for physical activity}$$
$$2,078 \times .65\text{–}.70 = 1,350 \text{ kcal}$$

In order to calculate REE + physical activity, these figures are added together:

$$2,078 + 1,350 = 3,428 \text{ kcal}$$

The last step to calculate our 47-year-old man's total energy requirements is to determine how many kcal are required for specific dynamic effect of food. This can be calculated by:

$$REE + \text{physical activity} \times \text{specific dynamic effect of food}$$
$$3,428 \times .10 = 343 \text{ kcal}$$
$$3,428 + 343 = 3,771 \text{ kcal}$$

In summary, the total energy requirements for a person can be calculated by the formula below:

REE kcal + physical activity kcal + specific dynamic effect of food kcal

Again using our moderately active 47-year-old man:

$$2,078 \text{ kcal} + 1,350 \text{ kcal} + 343 \text{ kcal} = 3,771 \text{ kcal}$$

Another method involves multiplying the suggested body weight by a factor that takes into consideration BMR + energy for light activity + specific dynamic effect.

The energy factors for men and women, according to the age range, are:

Men (age)	kcal/kg/day	kcal/lb/day
23–50	39	18
51–75	34	16
76+	29	13

These values allow for a 2% decrease in REE per decade and a reduction in activity of 200 kcal/day for men and women between 51 and 75 years, 500 kcal for men over 75, and 400 kcal for women over 75. These factors also estimate the energy needs only for light activity.

Women (age)	kcal/kg/day	kcal/lb/day
23–50	36	17
51–75	33	15
76+	29	13

SUGGESTED WEIGHTS FOR ADULTS AND BODY COMPOSITION

Suggested Weights for Adults

The perfect weight for individuals just does not exist. The table below presents suggested weights for people based on their age and height. The table also shows that people over age 35 can be heavier than 19–34-year-olds. The ranges in weights allow for frame size and different amounts of bone and muscle for the same height.

Body Composition and Determination of Overweight and Obesity

Body composition is important in determining whether a person is overweight or obese. A certain percentage of a person's body weight must be composed of fat due to its important functions (heat insulation, protection of vital organs, reserve energy source). Research has shown that the following percentages are ideal in terms of fat as a percentage of body weight and the percentages that indicate obesity:

	Normal percentage of body weight	Percentage of body weight from fat that indicates obesity
Men	15–20	25
Women	20–25	30[7]

anthropometric measurements Measurements of the size, weight, and proportions of the human body.

Anthropometric measurements constitute the most common method for measuring body composition.

TABLE 9-3 SUGGESTED WEIGHTS FOR ADULTS

Height[a]	Weight in pounds[b]	
	19 to 34 years	35 years and over
5'0"	97–128[c]	108–138
5'1"	101–132	111–143
5'2"	104–137	115–148
5'3"	107–141	119–152
5'4"	111–146	122–157
5'5"	114–150	126–162
5'6"	118–155	130–167
5'7"	121–160	134–172
5'8"	125–164	138–178
5'9"	129–169	142–183
5'10"	132–174	146–188
5'11"	136–179	151–194
6'0"	140–184	155–199
6'1"	144–189	159–205
6'2"	148–195	164–210
6'3"	152–200	168–216
6'4"	156–205	173–222
6'5"	160–211	177–228
6'6"	164–216	182–234

[a]Without shoes.
[b]Without clothes.
[c]The higher weights in the ranges generally apply to men, who tend to have more muscle and bone; the lower weights more often apply to women, who have less muscle and bone.
Source: National Research Council. (1989). *Recommended dietary allowances* (10th ed.) (pp. 92–93). Washington.

Anthropometric Measurements

calipers An instrument with two bent or curved legs. It is frequently used for measuring skinfold thickness.

triceps A muscle located on the back of the upper arm.

overfat Disproportionately high percentage of fat tissue.

A trained individual can use **calipers** to measure the thickness of a fold of skin (see Fig. 9-3). This skinfold measurement is usually made on the **triceps** midway between the shoulder and elbow, with the arm hanging freely.

A general guideline is that a skinfold measurement above the 95 percentile is indicative of obesity (see Table 9-4).

One major advantage of measuring obesity by body composition is that it allows one to distinguish overweight from **overfat.** For example, a muscular athlete who is active in strenuous sports may be overweight according to height-weight tables but not overfat. This overweight situation

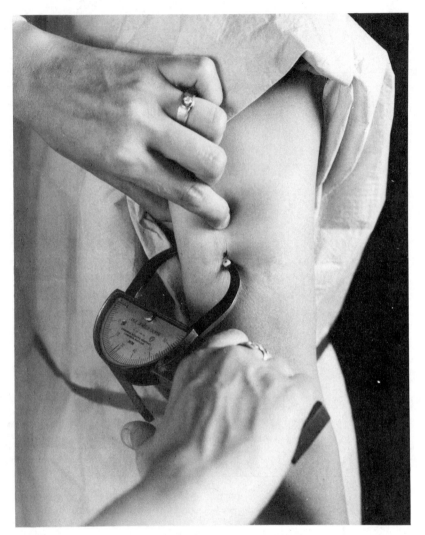

FIGURE 9-3 Measurement of a skinfold on the back of the upper arm with calipers. (Photo by Pilar A. Garcia.)

is not a nutritional problem, as is overfat, since the excess weight is due to a disproportionately high amount of muscle tissue.

OVERWEIGHT AND OBESITY

Overweight is defined as body weight that is more than 10% above the suggested weight. *Obesity* is defined as body weight that is 15–25%

TABLE 9-4 TRICEPS SKINFOLD PERCENTILES (MILLIMETERS) FOR MALES AND FEMALES

Age	Male					Female				
	5th	25th	50th	75th	95th	5th	25th	50th	75th	95th
1–1.9	6	8	10	12	16	6	8	10	12	16
2–2.9	6	8	10	12	15	6	9	10	12	16
3–3.9	6	8	10	11	15	7	9	11	12	15
4–4.9	6	8	9	11	14	7	8	10	12	16
5–5.9	6	8	9	11	15	6	8	10	12	18
6–6.9	5	7	8	10	16	6	8	10	12	16
7–7.9	5	7	9	12	17	6	9	11	13	18
8–8.9	5	7	8	10	16	6	9	12	15	24
9–9.9	6	7	10	13	18	8	10	13	16	22
10–10.9	6	8	10	14	21	7	10	12	17	27
11–11.9	6	8	11	16	24	7	10	13	18	28
12–12.9	6	8	11	14	28	8	11	14	18	27
13–13.9	5	7	10	14	26	8	12	15	21	30
14–14.9	4	7	9	14	24	9	13	16	21	28
15–15.9	4	6	8	11	24	8	12	17	21	32
16–16.9	4	6	8	12	22	10	15	18	22	31
17–17.9	5	6	8	12	19	10	13	19	24	37
18–18.9	4	6	9	13	24	10	15	18	22	30
19–24.9	4	7	10	15	22	10	14	18	24	34
25–34.9	5	8	12	16	24	10	16	21	27	37
35–44.9	5	8	12	16	23	12	18	23	29	38
45–54.9	6	8	12	15	25	12	20	25	30	40
55–64.9	5	8	11	14	22	12	20	25	31	38
65–74.9	4	8	11	15	22	12	18	24	29	36

Source: From *Understanding Normal and Clinical Nutrition* (p. 251) by E. N. Whitney, C. B. Cataldo, and S. R. Rolfes, 1987, St. Paul, MN: West.

underweight Body weight that is more than 10% below the ideal weight.

severe obesity Body weight that is 30–100% above the ideal weight.

massive (morbid) obesity Body weight that is more than 100% above the ideal weight.

above the suggested weight, with 20% being the most common percentage. Likewise, a person who is more than 10% below the table weight is considered **underweight.**

Weights that are 30–100% above suggested weight are classified as **severe obesity; massive** or **morbid obesity** refers to weights that are more than 100% above normal.[4]

In summary, obesity can be determined by two different methods—measuring body composition, and comparing a person's body weight with suggested weight tables. The specific measurements that indicate overweight or obesity for each method given on page 226.

Overweight and obesity are examples of a positive energy balance, in which more kilocalories are being consumed than used.

	Overweight	*Obesity*
Body composition		
Anthropometric measurements		Triceps skinfold measurement greater than 95th percentile in Table 9-4.
Ideal weight tables	10% above ideal weight	15–25% above ideal weight, with 20% being most common

Incidence of Obesity

Various studies have been conducted to determine the incidence of obesity in the United States. These studies estimate that 25–30% of adults and at least 10% of children are either overweight or obese. They also show that obesity is more common among women than men. It is greatest among African American women between the ages of 45 and 74 and those below the poverty level.[5]

Causes of Obesity

Some experts consider obesity to be America's number one malnutrition problem and believe that the problem has been expanding to epidemic proportions rather than diminishing in recent years.

Obesity, as stated earlier, is a problem of positive energy balance, in which more kilocalories are consumed than expended, resulting in the storage of fat and weight gain. The question, then, is, why do so many people overeat and create a positive energy balance? Research has found that the factors that lead to obesity can be placed into two major categories—**metabolic** (internal) and **regulatory** (external).

metabolic factor (internal) An internal factor that can lead to obesity.

regulatory factor (external) An external factor that can lead to obesity.

Metabolic (internal). Some of the metabolic factors that will be discussed in more detail are genetic, physiological, and hormonal.

Regulatory (external). Psychological, social, and cultural factors and lack of exercise are regulatory factors that will be discussed in more detail.

Metabolic (Internal) Factors

genetic Congenital or inherited.

Genetic Factors. A considerable body of data suggests that a predisposing factor in obesity is **genetic** background. Figure 9-4 shows that if both

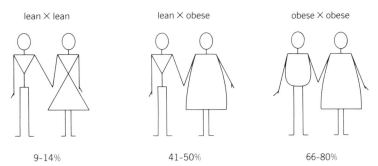

lean × lean   lean × obese   obese × obese

9-14%   41-50%   66-80%

FIGURE 9-4 Genetic chances of a child's developing obesity. (Reprinted with permission from Weinsier, Roland L., and Butterworth, C.R., Jr.: *Handbook of Clinical Nutrition*, St. Louis, 1981, The C.V. Mosby Co.)

parents are lean, the incidence of obesity in their children is about 9–14%. If one parent is obese, the incidence rises to 41–50%. If both parents are obese, it rises to 66–80%. The research done on obesity as an inherited trait shows that if a person inherits genes from obese parents, he or she has simply inherited the potential for being obese; however, the environment actually determines whether or not this potential is expressed. In studies done with identical twins in which both inherited genes from obese parents, but were raised by different families, in some cases one twin became obese because of the poor eating habits learned from his parents. The other twin remained lean because of positive eating behaviors learned from his parents. In summary, the evidence that people can be genetically predisposed to obesity is strong; however, the environment can inhibit or enhance this predisposition.

hunger An inborn instinct that causes a physiological response to the body's need for food.

appetite A learned psychological response to food that is initiated for reasons other than the need for food.

satiety A sensation of fullness that follows a meal.

hypothalamus An area at the base of the brain that contains centers of hunger and satiety and secretes the antidiuretic hormone.

Physiological Factors. Obesity is often the result of an inability to respond adequately to **hunger** and **appetite** as well as satiety sensations. For example, the smell of frying bacon can make a person want to eat even though he or she may already be full. **Satiety** is the sensation of fullness that follows a meal, and is thought to be a combination of physiological and psychological responses.

The **hypothalamus** (see Fig. 9-5) region of the brain receives nerve impulses from various regions of the body concerning the body's energy needs. It can interpret these impulses as either hunger or satiety sensations.

How does the hypothalamus know when the body needs food or is full? This has long been an intriguing question for nutritionists, especially since the answer might help to explain why people become obese. Three

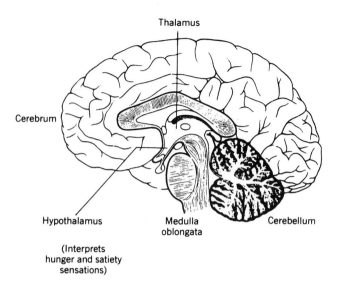

Thalamus

Cerebrum

Hypothalamus

Medulla
oblongata

Cerebellum

(Interprets
hunger and satiety
sensations)

FIGURE 9-5   The hypothalamus region of the brain, where interpretation of hunger and satiety signals occurs. (From T. Randall Lankford, *Integrated Science for Health Students*, 3rd ed., 1984. Reprinted by persmission of Reston Publishing Company, a Prentice-Hall Company, 11480 Sunset Hills Road, Reston, Va. 22090.)

glucostatic theory   The theory that when the blood glucose level is high, a person will feel full, and when it is low, the person will feel hungry.

lipostatic theory   The theory that the tissues, especially the fat tissues, signal the brain when the level of fat is increased above or decreased below a certain level.

set point theory   The theory that the body is programmed to maintain a certain amount of fat.

widely accepted theories that attempt to answer this question are the **glucostatic, lipostatic,** and **set point theories.**

Glucostatic theory. Figure 9-6 shows that the brain (the hypothalamus apparently being the primary site) is able to monitor the blood glucose level; when it is low (below 70 mg/dl), the hunger sensation is the result. Figure 9-6 also shows that when the blood glucose level is high (above 120 mg/dl), a satiety sensation is produced.

In other words, this theory states that there is an inverse relationship between blood glucose level and hunger; that is, as the blood glucose level decreases, the sensation of hunger increases. The relationship between blood glucose and satiety is direct; as the blood glucose level increases, so does the sensation of satiety. This mechanism monitors short-term needs as the blood glucose level varies from hour to hour.

Lipostatic theory. The lipostatic theory states that the tissues, especially the fat tissues, signal the brain when they are satiated (see Fig. 9-7). Likewise, when fat decreases below a certain level, the brain interprets this action as a need for food and a hunger sensation is created. People with more fat cells have to eat more food before they experience satiety.

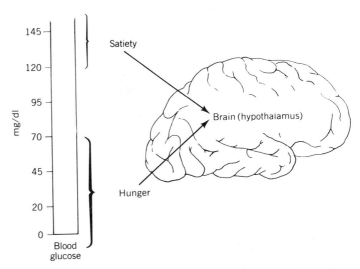

FIGURE 9-6 Glucostatic theory. The hunger sensation results from a drop in the blood glucose level below 70 mg/dl, and a satiety sensation results from a blood glucose level above 120 mg/dl.

This mechanism involves long-term regulation, since the content of fat cells changes slowly.

Set point theory. Since the number of fat cells is theorized to be fixed by adulthood, an obese person has a greater number of fat cells and thus a greater amount of fat to maintain. According to this theory, each person has a body weight that functions as a "set point" (which may be an obese weight in some people) (see Fig. 9-8); when this weight is exceeded, the hypothalamus recognizes the need to lose weight. Likewise, when the body weight is below the set point, the hypothalamus recognizes the need to gain weight. People who try to lose weight below their set point may actually lose lean tissue rather than fat tissue, as shown in rat studies.[6]

Whether the hypothalamus recognizes hunger and satiety according to the glucostatic, lipostatic, or set point theories or combinations of them, obesity results from their malfunctions. The obese person may have a defective monitoring system, so that the hypothalamus does not recognize when the blood glucose level is back to normal; therefore, food may be consumed beyond the satiety level. Likewise, since an obese person has to consume more food to fill the fat cells than a lean person, the hypothalamus may not recognize when the obese person has reached a satiety level. Finally, it may be that some people are destined to be overweight and obese due to their set point; therefore, losing and maintaining the weight loss may be impossible for them.

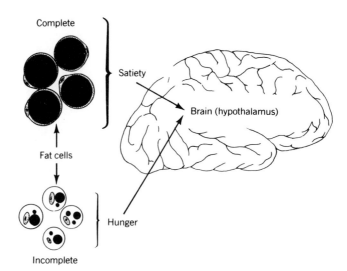

FIGURE 9-7 Lipostatic theory. Satiety sensations result from the fat tissues being "full" of fat. Hunger sensations result from emptiness of the fat tissues.

Hormonal Factors. In rare cases, obesity may be caused by hormonal imbalances. The most common example is a decreased level of thyroxine, which results in a lowering of the REE. If the person continues to consume food in the same quantities as before the lowering of the REE, weight gain is inevitable. Likewise, an increased level of thyroxine will result in an increased REE and weight loss if there is no change in the quantity of food consumed.

In summary, internal factors are not related to the environment (except for the role that the environment plays in hindering or enhancing the predisposition to be obese); rather, the problems originate internally and are influenced by internal physiological changes. A very small percentage of obese cases are due to these internal physiological factors. The majority are due to regulatory or external factors, which are discussed next.

Regulatory (External) Factors

Regulatory factors that can result in obesity are independent of physiological factors and instead are related to the environment. People who become obese due to external factors are not very sensitive to internal cues such as hunger and satiety sensations. Instead, they are very sus-

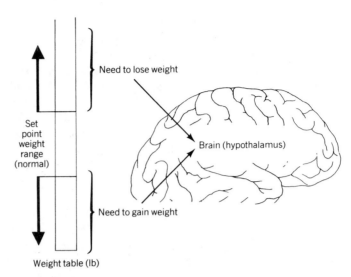

FIGURE 9-8 Set point theory. When the set point weight is exceeded, the hypothalamus interprets this condition as a need to lose weight. When body weight drops below the set point, the hypothalamus recognizes a need to gain weight.

ceptible to external cues such as the time of day and the availability, sight, and taste of food.

Psychological Factors. Some people eat to satisfy needs other than hunger. These needs form the basis of psychological factors that can lead to obesity.

The inability of some individuals to recognize and express emotions such as anger, fear, frustration, rejection, and anxiety may lead to abnormal eating patterns. **Binge eating** is an example of an eating pattern that may result in obesity.

People who are under emotional or physical stress often find relief by overeating. In addition to overeating, stress results in the release of large amounts of epinephrine and **adrenocorticotrophic (ACTH) hormones,** which increase the amount of energy used to overcome the stress situation. These hormones can increase energy by stimulating the release of large amounts of glucose, fatty acids, and amino acids. If the stressed individual does not metabolize all of these energy nutrients, the body will convert them to fat. In addition, if stress results in the lowering of the blood glucose level, a hunger sensation is created and the person may overeat soon after the situation is over. Lean and overly thin people respond in an opposite manner; they tend to reject food and metabolize their energy nutrients more efficiently.

binge eating Consumption of large amounts of food in a short period of time.

Adrenocorticotrophic hormone (ACTH) A hormone that is secreted by the anterior pituitary gland.

Psychotherapy has been found, in some cases, to be a successful treatment for obesity that results from basic psychological disorders.

Social Factors. Social and cultural habits are external factors that can result in obesity in children and adults. Some cultures view a fat baby as healthy and obese adults as wealthy and powerful individuals.

Cultural norms (see Chapter 1 for more details on cultural influences on food habits) determine acceptable foods, attitudes toward eating, and obesity. It is very important for medical personnel to have knowledge of or access to the food patterns of major cultures in the United States in order to assess responses to diets more efficiently and to teach nutrition concepts to patients.

Socioeconomic factors also influence attitudes toward obesity, as evidenced by data that show that poor African American women have higher rates of obesity than white women. However, African American men have lower rates than white men.

Lack of Exercise. Probably the single most important causative factor in obesity is inactivity. This conclusion is partially validated by recent food consumption data showing that people are consuming fewer kilocalories today than they did a few years ago. This inconsistency is partially explained by people's reduced physical activity due to the availability of convenience appliances in the home, machines at work, and modern transportation to carry them back and forth. Little exercise is required in today's society to carry out daily activities. Therefore, to increase energy expenditure today, a person has to make a constant effort to exercise.

Two other points about lack of exercise and obesity concern the consumption of fewer kilocalories by obese compared to normal-weight people and the role of exercise in regulating the physiological appetite. Studies show that obese people often consume fewer kilocalories than lean ones; however, these obese people were so inactive that they still managed to have a positive energy balance. Other studies have shown that active people are better able to regulate their physiological appetite mechanism and are less influenced by external cues. Apparently, the more sedentary a person is, the greater the chance of failure of the hunger-satiety mechanism and the greater the chance the person will be influenced by the environment.[7]

NONRECOMMENDED TREATMENTS OF OBESITY

Many methods have been used to treat obesity; some are recommended by nutritional experts and others are not. Table 9-5 presents a summary of the nonrecommended methods.

TABLE 9-5 NONRECOMMENDED METHODS FOR TREATING OBESITY

Method	Comments
A) Drugs	
Diet pills	Diminish appetite
	Can cause serious side effects (nervousness and insomnia)
	Danger of addiction if used over a long period
Hormones	Hormone injected along with a 400- to 500-kcal diet.
HCG (human chorionic gonadotropin)	Claim that HCG suppresses appetite has not been substantiated; side effects are unknown and possibly dangerous
Thyroid	Increases REE but may result in loss of lean tissue
	May cause adverse effects on heart if not medically controlled
Diuretics	Causes water loss, not loss of fat tissue
	Long-time use can lead to dehydration and potassium deficiency
B) Fasting	May be used in hospital settings for morbid obesity when the patient is allowed noncaloric fluids, vitamins, and mineral supplements
	Rapid weight loss at first, but declines as REE decreases
	Does not teach new food behavior patterns
	Loss of lean tissue and ketosis may occur
C) Surgery	
Intestinal bypass surgery	Surgical removal or tying off of a large portion of the small intestine to decrease the absorption of food
	Generally used only on patients who are 100 lb or more overweight in whom the risks to health from obesity are greater than those from surgery
	Can result in severe side effects: liver failure, kidney stones, and malnutrition; mortality reports range from 2 to 10%
D) Diets	

Approach	Characteristics	Potential Problems	Examples[a]
Moderate kcaloric restriction (the only method likely to lead to healthy, maintainable fat loss)	Usually 1200–1800 kcal per day Reasonable balance of macronutrients Encourages exercise May employ behavioral approach	Loss of motivation because there are no dramatic, immediate results	The Setpoint Diet Slim Chance in a Fat World Weight Watcher's Diet The American Heart Association Diet Mary Ellen's Help Yourself Diet Plan
Extremely low carbohydrate	Fewer than 100 gm carbohydrate per day	Initial loss of water weight primarily—which is often quickly regained Fatigue Headaches May predispose to subsequent binging	Atkin's Diet Revolution Calories Don't Count Drinking Man's Diet Woman Doctor's Diet for Women The Doctor's Quick Weight Loss Diet (Stillman's)

(continued)

TABLE 9-5 NONRECOMMENDED METHODS FOR TREATING OBESITY *(Continued)*

Approach	Characteristics	Potential Problems	Examples[a]
Extremely low carbohydrate *(continued)*			The Complete Scarsdale Medical Diet
Extremely low fat	Less than 20% of calories from fat Limited (or elimination of) animal protein sources, all fats, nuts, seeds	May be inadequate in protein and certain minerals May decrease absorption of fat-soluble vitamins Low satiety value	The Rice Diet Report The Macrobiotic Diet The Pritikin Diet
Novelty diets	Promote certain nutrients, foods, or combination of foods as having unique, magical, or previously undiscovered qualities	Usually severely limit or eliminate certain food groups, thereby making diet nutritionally inadequate Difficult to adapt to normal lifestyle	Dr. Berger's Immune Power Diet Fit for Life Diet The Rotation Diet The Beverly Hills Diet
Very low kcalorie diets	Fewer than 800 kcal per day Also known as protein-sparing modified fasts	Likely to result in body protein losses if used by other than severely obese Requires close medical supervision Usually weight is regained after program is ended Difficult to adapt to normal lifestyles May cause dry skin, thinning hair, constipation	Optifast Cambridge Diet The Rotation Diet Genesis
Formula diets	Based on formulated or packaged products Many are very low calorie diet regimens (see above)	Weight regain when person resumes eating regular food Often very low in kcalories, potentially leading to additional problems described above, including electrolyte imbalance	U.S.A. (United Sciences of America), Inc. Optifast Genesis Cambridge Diet Herbalife Slimfast

[a]Diets may be listed in more than one category if multiple characteristics apply.
Note: From *Nutrition for Living* (3rd ed.), by J.L. Christian and J.L. Greger, 1991. Redwood City, CA: Benjamin Cummings.

One writer has estimated that there are about 2,000 weight reduction diets, and more than 50% of them are unsafe.[8] A logical question to ask is, "How can I distinguish a fad diet from a recommended weight loss diet?" Below are some of the typical claims made by fad diets; these diets should be avoided:

The diet promises ease and comfort in weight loss. Successful weight loss takes a great deal of work and sometimes involves discomfort in regard to exercise.

The diet promises extremely rapid weight loss. Claims such as a loss of 5–8 lb/week are impossible except on starvation or very-low-carbohydrate diets. The early weight loss is almost totally water, not fat, and the rate of loss decreases the longer one remains on such a diet.

The diet restricts or includes only a few foods. Examples are the grapefruit or egg diet. The results are inadequate nutrient intake, boredom, and quick abandonment of the diet.

The diet requires you to purchase a "secret formula" or "magic pill." Most of the claims made for these aids have not been scientifically verified and are frequently quite expensive.

The diet is published in a book or magazine. In a free society, anyone can publish anything, true or not, if he or she can find someone who will publish it.

RECOMMENDED TREATMENTS OF OBESITY

The recommended and proven treatments of obesity are:

- A nutritionally balanced caloric diet
- A reasonable increase in physical activity
- An understanding of behavior modification

Nutritionally Balanced Diet

As stated earlier, weight loss cannot occur unless a person has a negative energy balance, that is, expending more energy than he or she is consuming. The starting point, then, is to estimate the person's specific energy needs (the methods for doing so were presented earlier in this chapter). This estimate should be based on the person's suggested weight, not on the actual caloric intake.

Once the person's energy needs have been determined, one can calculate how many kilocalories must be cut in order to achieve a negative energy balance. Let us assume that Jane is overweight and needs 2,500 kcal to maintain her suggested ideal weight. She wants to lose weight only at the recommended rate, which is 1–2 lb/week. In order to reach this goal, Jane has to reduce her daily intake by 500–1,000 kcal. Remember that to lose 1 lb a person has to have a 3,500-kcal deficit. Let us assume that Jane wants to lose 2 lb/week:

2,500	Kilocalories needed to maintain her recommended ideal weight
− 1,000	Daily kilocalorie deficit needed to lose 2 lb/week
1,500	Jane cannot consume more than 1,500 kcal/day in order to lose up to 2 lb/week. Table 9-6 presents an example of a 1,500-kcal diet.

It is important to emphasize that nutritional adequacy cannot be maintained on fewer than about 1,200 kcal/day—1,000 at the very least. After the total kilocalories that can be consumed per day is determined, the specifics of the diet need to be planned. They should include the following factors:

Adequacy. As pointed out in regard to the fad diets in Table 9-5, most of them are not adequate in nutrients. It is important that the diet have the proper amounts of servings from the four food groups but stay within kilocalorie limits.

Emphasis on nutrient density. To achieve an adequate diet, foods that are high in nutrients but low in kilocalories have to be emphasized. Refer to Chapter 1 for examples of skim milk as opposed to whole milk or lean meat as opposed to medium- or high-fat meat. This will require familiarizing the person with the six exchange lists (discussed in Chapter 1 and presented in Appendix A). Refer to Table 9-6 for specific examples in a 1,500-kcal diet.

Emphasis on balance. Remember from Chapter 1 that a nutritious diet needs to be balanced—55–60% of kilocalories from carbohydrates, 30% from fat, and 10–15% from protein. Fad diets are frequently negligent in that they are often extremely low in carbohydrates and sometimes in protein. It is important to include some fat in each meal, since fat will increase satiety and prolong the onset of hunger pains.

Readily adaptable to family meals or public eating places. It is very important that the diet be practical or include foods that are readily available and exclude foods that are exotic or that the person does not like. Fad diets frequently consist of foods that are not readily available or are exotic.

plateaus Periods during weight reduction in which the person is not losing weight.

In addition to planning the diet, it should be emphasized that the dieter will reach **plateaus** in the weight loss period. It might help the dieter get through these periods if he or she understands why they occur

TABLE 9-6 SAMPLE MEAL PLAN FOR A 1,500-KCAL DIET

	Exchange	Total kcal
Breakfast		
Skim milk, 1 cup	1 milk	90
Eggs, 2	2 meat + 1 fat	150
Orange juice, ½ cup	1 fruit	60
Bagel, 1	2 bread	160
Coffee/tea	free	0
Lunch		
Tuna, ½ cup	2 meat	110
Onions, celery, ½ cup	1 vegetable	25
Mayonnaise, 1 teaspoon	1 fat	45
Rye bread, 2 slices	2 bread	160
Lettuce, pickle	free	0
Peach, medium	1 fruit	60
Tea	free	0
Snack		
Yogurt, 2% milk, 1 cup	1 milk + 1 fat	120
Banana, small, ½	1 fruit	60
Dinner		
Chicken, baked, no skin, 4 ounces	4 meat	220
Green beans, 1 cup	1 vegetable	25
Salad: tomatoes, onions, celery, radishes, ½ cup total	1 vegetable	25
Lettuce, wine vinegar	free	0
Corn, ⅓ cup	1 vegetable	25
Potato, small	1 bread	80
Wine, dry white, 3 ounces	1 bread	80
Total kilocalories for day:		1495

Source: Patricia J. Long and Barbara Shannon, *Focus on Nutrition,* © 1983, p. 177. Reprinted by permission of Prentice-Hall, Inc., Englewood Cliffs, N.J.

in the first place. Essentially, plateaus result from the temporary increase and retention of water in the tissues. The increase in water results from the oxidation, or burning up, of fat tissue. Retention results because it takes water a long time to move from the tissues into the lymph and blood before it can be excreted by the kidneys.

Increase in Physical Activity

An important accompaniment to a nutritional diet in losing weight is increasing physical activity. It is much easier to achieve a negative energy balance if one exercises rather than remaining sedentary. It is important to dispel the common myth that increasing exercise stimulates the appetite, making it more difficult to create a negative energy balance. Studies show that people who engage in moderate exercise such as running, swimming, or calisthenics for 1 hour/day do not experience an increase in appetite.[9] In fact, as mentioned earlier, the active individual is more sensitive to the appetite mechanism than the more sedentary person.

What kind of exercise is the most productive of weight loss? The answer is, many kinds. However, in deciding what exercise to engage in, the person should choose one that can be incorporated into the daily routine. Preferably, the exercise should employ large muscle groups and should be rhythmic. Walking, riding a bicycle, swimming, and running are ideal. The minimum length of time that exercise should be engaged in is 20–30 minutes at least three times per week.[9]

Behavior Modification

The third and final component of a successful weight loss program is to identify unhealthy eating habits and then help the obese person to learn constructive behaviors. This component is critical to the long-term success of the weight loss program. Almost any person can diet for a period of time and lose a few pounds, but it is much more difficult to maintain the weight loss for an extended period of time.

Three steps are often involved in **behavior modification** for weight control:

Keeping a food diary. Many obese people do not realize that they have a tendency to eat foods at certain times when they are in various moods. Also, they do not realize that they frequently eat too fast and are not sensitive to satiety signals. In order to identify these factors, a person needs to keep a **food diary** (see Fig. 9-9). It enables the dieter to judge whether eating occurs because of hunger or in response to cues from the environment. Ultimately, the diary provides clues concerning what prompts the person to overeat.

Controlling the stimuli associated with eating. The second step involves designing the environment so that there is a decrease in the **stimuli** that prompt the person to eat. Examples are restricting meals to certain rooms at certain times and requiring the person to eat slowly and consume bulky foods first.

Reinforcement for appropriate behavior. This step involves a formal reward for appropriate behavior and should be something the individual prizes or enjoys doing.

The dieter may find that peer support is very helpful in behavior modification. Groups such as Weight Watchers and Take Off Pounds

behavior modification An approach to the correction of undesirable eating habits. This procedure involves the manipulation of environmental and behavioral variables.

food diary A record of what a person eats, the mood he or she is in while eating, and the circumstances in which eating occurs.

stimuli Changes in an environmental condition that cause a response.

Food diary

FOOD EATEN Quantity Type	TIME Circle time if food was part of meal	SOCIAL Alone? With whom?	WHERE EATEN Home Work Restaurant Recreation	MOOD WHEN EATING A—Anxious B—Bored C—Tired D—Depressed E—Angry
1 C. Coffee	2 pm	with Kate	espresso house	tired
2 TBs. half & half Creamer half	"	"	"	"
croissant	"	"	"	"
butter - 1 TBs.	"	"	"	"
Jam 1 TBS.	"	"	"	"

FIGURE 9-9   An example of a food diary, which is important in behavior modification. (From Patricia J. Long, Barbara Shannon, *Focus on Nutrition*, ©1983, p. 173. Reprinted by permission of Prentice-Hall, Inc., Englewood Cliffs, N.J.)

Sensibly (TOPS) offer weekly meetings at which the person can receive support, evaluate the progress, and become educated.

UNDERWEIGHT, ANOREXIA NERVOSA, BULIMIA, AND BULIMAREXIA

Underweight

Underweight is defined as a body weight that is 15–20% below the ideal weight tables. People generally do not consider underweight to be a problem in the United States. Despite the view that underweight is not a problem and may even be healthy, research shows that underweight persons have decreased resistance to infection, tend to become easily fatigued, and are often sensitive to a cold environment.[6]

Anorexia Nervosa

Anorexia nervosa A self-starvation disease that is characterized by severe disruption of the person's eating behavior.

Anorexia nervosa is actually a misnomer, since the person actually does not have a loss of appetite. Most anorexics are girls in their mid-teens and typically exhibit these characteristics:

- They are well educated.
- They have been raised in a middle- to upper-class family.
- They are preoccupied with thinness and exercise.
- They are highly competitive and perfectionistic.

Why would a girl with all these characteristics go on a starvation diet to the point where she might weigh only 65–70 lb and be on the verge of death? The answer is that this is a complicated psychological disorder. Psychologically, anorexics have a distorted perception of their body image and view themselves as fat even though they may have reached the lower end of their recommended weight range. This disorder is not a problem because of the mortality but rather because of the size of the population at risk. According to the American Psychiatric Association, as many as 1 out of every 250 girls between the ages of 12 and 18 may become anorectic every year.[10]

Bulimia and Bulimarexia

bulimia An enormous appetite that is satisfied by eating binges.

bulimarexia Purging of food.

Two complications of anorexia are **bulimia** and **bulimarexia.** An anorexic may eat several pounds of sweet, fattening foods. These binges are followed by bulimarexia, in which an attempt is made to remove the food from the body by inducing vomiting, taking large doses of laxatives, or using enemas. Bulimia is not as life-threatening as anorexia, but it can cause disturbances in electrolyte balance and dehydration.[3]

The treatment of an anorexic is a three-stage process. The first stage is restoration of normal nutrition. This step is often a problem, since the anorexic is not very receptive to voluntary eating. Hospitalization may be required, with either IV feeding by **hyperalimentation** or nasogatric tubes into the stomach. The advantage of these methods is that the patient cannot get rid of the nourishment by vomiting.[11]

hyperalimentation Injection of hyperosmolar fluids directly into the superior vena cava vein.

The second stage begins when the person's weight starts to return to normal and involves **psychotherapy.** This stage is critical to the long-term success of reversing anorexia nervosa. The individual and her family must be cooperative, must acknowledge the problem, and must motivate themselves to overcome it. Behavior modification and group therapy have been shown to be effective.

psychotherapy Any of a number of related techniques for treating mental illness by psychological methods. It is often used in the second stage of treating anorexia nervosa.

The third stage involves teaching the anorectic and her family proper nutritional concepts, as well as helping them eliminate misconceptions about nutrition.

SUMMARY

- Kilocalorie, the unit of measurement in nutrition, is defined as the amount of heat required to raise the temperature of 1 kg of water 1 degree Celsius.
- Positive energy balance equals energy input being greater than energy expenditure; if it continues, a person will gain weight. Negative energy balance is where energy expenditure is greater than energy consumption; if it continues, a person will lose weight.
- Percentage of body weight from fat that indicates obesity is 25% for males and 30% for females; 10% above suggested weight is indicative of overweight and 15–25% above suggested weight is indicative of obesity.
- Three metabolic or internal causes of obesity are genetic, physiological, and hormonal.
- Three critical periods that can result in an increase in fat cells for juveniles (that is, juvenile obesity) are the last three months of fetal development, the first three years of life, and adolescence.
- Three theories on how the hypothalamus senses when a person is hungry are the glucostatic, lipostatic, and set point theories.
- External causes of obesity are psychological and social factors plus lack of exercise.
- Five nonrecommended diets for treatment of obesity are: a diet that promises ease and comfort; a diet that promises extremely rapid weight loss; a diet that restricts or includes only a few foods; one that requires the purchase of a secret formula or magic pill; or one published in a book or magazine.
- The three recommended methods for treatment of obesity are a nutritionally balanced weight loss diet, increase in physical activity, and behavior modification.
- Underweight is defined as 15–20% below the suggested weight. Anorexia nervosa is a self-starvation disease; bulimia and bulimarexia involve an anorexic engorging large amounts of food followed by purging.

REVIEW QUESTIONS

True (A) or False (B)

1. Energy in nutrition is measured by the kilocalorie (kcal).
2. If a person consumed 2,300 kcal/day and expended 3,000 kcal/day, he would have a positive energy balance and could gain weight.
3. The total expenditure of energy involves maintaining the REE, physical activity, and specific dynamic action.
4. If two people each weigh 180 lb but Mr. A is 6 ft tall and Mr. B is 5 ft 8 in. tall, Mr. A would have a higher REE.
5. After age 20 a person's REE is stable and does not change.
6. If a person had a temperature of 102.6°F, his or her REE will increase by about 10%.
7. The energy required to maintain the BMR in sedentary or moderately active people is very low (10–15%).
8. Ideally, a person's body weight should consist of as little fat as possible.
9. The body weight of a man is composed of 30% fat; therefore, he is obese.
10. One advantage of determining obesity by body composition (what percentage of the body weight is composed of fat) is that it allows one to distinguish overweight from overfat.
11. When using suggested weight tables, a person is classified as obese if his or her weight is 10% above suggested weight.
12. The factors that can lead to obesity are placed into two categories—metabolic and internal.
13. Children who inherit genes from obese parents are doomed to become obese despite their environment.
14. Three periods when the potential for fat cells to increase in number (hyperplasia) are the last 3 months of fetal development, the first 3 years of life, and adolescence.
15. Hunger is a physiological response to the body's need for food, and appetite is a learned psychological response to food.
16. The majority of obese cases are the result of malfunction of the physiological factors.
17. Most cases of obesity result from insensitivity to internal cues and susceptibility to external cues.
18. A decrease in people's physical activity has been accompanied by better control of the appetite mechanism.
19. The three recommended and proven methods for treatment of obesity are a diet that restricts or includes only a few foods, promises a slow, steady

weight loss, and stresses the ease of losing weight.

20. If one needs 2,800 kcal to maintain suggested weight and reduces consumption to 1,800 kcal/day, one will be able to lose 4 lb/week.

21. Anorexia nervosa is a self-starvation disease that is typically found in well-educated, middle- to upper-class girls.

22. Two complications of anorexia nervosa are bulimia (eating large quantities of food) and bulimarexia (purging by vomiting or taking laxatives or enemas).

23. The treatment of anorexia nervosa involves restoration of normal nutrition, psychotherapy, and teaching proper nutritional concepts to the anorectic and her family.

Multiple Choice

24. Which of the following is (are) correct?
    1. The kilocalorie is the amount of energy required to raise the temperature of 1 kg of water 1°C.
    2. The calorie is the amount of energy required to raise the temperature of 1 g of water 1°C.
    3. The kilocalorie is the correct unit of energy measurement in nutrition.
    4. The calorie is the energy measurement used by chemists and physicists.
       A. 1, 2, 3   B. 1, 3   C. 2, 4   D. 4
       E. all of these

25. If a person had an energy intake of 2,900 kcal/day and an energy expenditure of 2,400 kcal/day, the person would _____ per week.
    A. lose 1 lb
    B. gain 2 lb
    C. be in energy balance and gain no weight
    D. gain 1 lb
    E. none of these

26. Which of the following increase the REE?
    1. increased surface   3. pregnancy and
       area   lactation
    2. increasing age   4. fasting
       after 30
       A. 1, 2, 3   B. 1, 3   C. 2, 4   D. 4
       E. all of these

27. The energy expenditure of the body involves three components: _____.

1. appetite   3. physical activity
2. REE   4. specific dynamic
                          action
   A. 1, 2, 3   B. 1, 3   C. 2, 3, 4   D. 4
   E. all of these

28. The percentage of body weight from fat that indicates obesity for men is _____ and for women is _____.
    A. 15–20
    B. 25–15
    C. 10–30
    D. 25–30

29. The incidence and causes of obesity are:
    1. 25–30% in adults (obese or overweight).
    2. metabolic factors (genetic, physiological, and hormonal).
    3. regulatory (psychological, social, cultural, and lack of exercise).
    4. more common among women than among men.
       A. 1, 2, 3   B. 2, 4   C. 1, 3   D. 4
       E. all of these

Matching

___ 30. juvenile-onset obesity

___ 31. adult-onset obesity

___ 32. appetite

___ 33. hunger

___ 34. hypothalamus

A. physiological response to body's need for food

B. region of the brain that interprets hunger and satiety signals

C. learned psychological response to food

D. obesity beginning during any of three critical periods

E. results from hypertrophy of fat cells only

Completion

35. Discuss the four metabolic or internal causes of obesity.

36. Describe the three recommended treatments of obesity.

37. Define underweight. Describe anorexia nervosa, bulimia, and bulimarexia.

CRITICAL THINKING CHALLENGE

1. Calculate the total energy requirements for a 50-year-old male (5'9", 162 lbs.) who is moderately active. Show all calculations.
2. If a person decreases his daily kcal intake by 600 kcal per day, how long will it take him to lose 35 pounds? Show calculations.
3. If a person has a positive energy balance of 200 kcal per day, how long will it take him to gain 10 pounds?
4. Which of the following statements supports the glucostatic theory?
   a. "When I eat six small meals throughout the day, I don't ever feel really hungry."
   b. "The more I eat, the hungrier I feel."
   c. "I have to eat a large meal before I feel satisfied."
   d. "No matter what I eat, I seem to maintain the same weight."

REVIEW QUESTIONS FOR NCLEX

Situation. A male client is 45 years old, 5'8" tall, weighs 215 lb. and is sedentary.

1. Using Table 9-3 the client is _____.
   A. at suggested weight
   B. overweight
   C. obese
   D. severely obese
2. Assume the client's total energy requirements per day to be 3800 kcal and he is placed on a 1500 kcal per day diet. How long will it take him to lose 10 pounds?
   A. 15 days
   B. 25 days
   C. 35 days
   D. 45 days
3. Which combination of exchanges will allow this client to achieve the 1500 kcal per day diet?
   A. 3 milk, 5 vegetable, 5 fruit, 6 bread, 8 meat, and 2 fat
   B. 2 milk, 5 vegetable, 3 fruit, 4 bread, 6 meat, and 2 fat

C. 4 milk, 4 vegetable, 4 fruit, 4 bread, 4 meat, and 4 fat
   D. 1 milk, 6 vegetable, 5 fruit, 6 breads, 3 meats, and 7 fats
4. This client mentions that he has been a body builder for 15 years and does not feel that he is obese, despite his scale weight. A health professional decides to determine if he is overweight, overfat, or obese by measuring _____.
   A. his frame size
   B. his wrist size
   C. his waist size
   D. his body composition
5. A specific test that can be done, in relation to the question above, is determining his _____.
   A. frame size by his shirt size (small, medium, and large)
   B. wrist size in centimeters
   C. waist size in inches
   D. triceps skinfold measurement in millimeters

REFERENCES

1. Suitor, C. J. W., & Crowley, M. F. (1984). *Nutrition: Principles and application in health promotion* (2nd ed.) (pp. 79–81). Philadelphia: J. B. Lippincott.
2. Hamilton, E. M., Whitney, E. N., & Sizer, F. S. (1985). *Nutrition: Concepts and controversies* (3rd ed.). St. Paul: West.
3. Whitney, E. N., Cataldo, C. B., & Rolfes, S. R. (1987). *Understanding Normal and clinical nutrition* (2nd ed.). St. Paul: West.
4. Manson, J. E. et. al. (1987). Body weight and longevity: A reassessment. *Journal of the American Medical Association, 257,* 353–358.
5. Stunkard, A. J., Foch, T. T., & Hrubec, Z. (1986). A twin study of human obesity. *Journal of the American Medical Association, 256,* 51–54.
6. Berdanier, C. D., & McIntosh, M. K. (1991). Weight loss—weight regain: A vicious cycle. *Nutrition Today, 26*(5), 6–12.
7. Vasselli, J. R., & Maggio, C. A. (1988). Mechanisms of appetite and body-weight regulation. In *Obesity and weight control.* Rockville: Aspen Publishers.
8. Rock, C. L., & Coulston, A. M. (1988). Weight-control approaches: A review by the California

Dietetic Association. *Journal of the American Dietetic Association, 88,* 44–48.

9. Wilmore, J. H. (1983). Appetite and body composition consequent to physical activity. *Research Quarterly Exercise Sport, 54,* 415–425.

10. Healy, K., Contry, R. M., & Walsh, N. (1985). The prevalence of binge-eating and bulimia in 1063 college students. *Journal of Psychiatric Research, 19,* 161–166.

11. Dalvit-McPhillips, S. A. (1984). Dietary approach to bulimia treatment. *Physiology and Behavior, 33,* 769–775.

10

NUTRITION DURING PREGNANCY AND LACTATION

Upon completion of this chapter, you should be able to:

1. Give the RDA values for the following during pregnancy and lactation: energy (kilocalories) protein, iron and folacin, calcium, and phosphorus, plus vitamin D and other minerals.
2. State the function or importance of the above nutrients and energy in pregnancy and lactation.
3. Describe the symptoms of the fetal alcohol syndrome (FAS) and the typical woman who is most likely to have a FAS child.
4. Describe the causes, symptoms, and dietary treatment for nausea and vomiting and pregnancy-induced hypertension.

INTRODUCTION

miscarriage (spontaneous abortion) Interrupted pregnancy before the seventh month.

There is no period of a woman's life when nutrition is more important than during pregnancy. The fetus is totally dependent upon the nutritional status of the mother for its development. In addition to the development of the fetus, an optimum diet is important for the mother. Pregnancy brings about many physiological and psychological changes in the mother's body. An inadequate diet during pregnancy may not allow the mother's body to adapt to these changes, which could result in the following problems:

premature (preterm) baby Birth of a baby prior to the 38th week of pregnancy.

Miscarriage (spontaneous abortion). Interrupted pregnancy before the seventh month.

low birth weight (LBW) baby A baby that weighs less than 5.5 lb (2500 g).

Premature (preterm) baby. Birth of a baby before the 38th week of pregnancy.

Low birth weight (LBW) baby. A baby that weighs less than 5.5 lb (2,500 g).

stillborn infant A baby dead at birth.

Stillborn infant. A baby dead at birth.

Pregnancy-induced hypertension (PIH) Formerly called *toxemia of pregnancy* and characterized by proteinuria, hypertension, and edema.

Pregnancy-induced hypertension. Formerly called *toxemia of pregnancy* and characterized by proteinuria, hypertension, and edema.

Fetal alcohol syndrome (FAS) Characterized by growth retardation, physical deformities, behavioral defects, and mental retardation in a baby born to an alcoholic mother.

Fetal alcohol syndrome (FAS). Characterized by growth retardation, physical deformities, behavioral defects, and mental retardation in a baby born to an alcoholic mother.

Nutrition is important not only during but also before pregnancy. If a woman has been well nourished from childhood through adolescence, she will need to make few changes in her diet during pregnancy, as discussed below.

NUTRITIONAL REQUIREMENTS DURING PREGNANCY AND LACTATION

lactation Production of milk by the mammary glands.

The nutrient needs of a mother during pregnancy and **lactation** are higher for many nutrients than those of the nonpregnant woman. Table 10-1 presents the Recommended Dietary Allowances (RDAs) for pregnancy and lactation.

Energy (Kilocalories)

Requirements during Pregnancy

The energy needs of the mother during pregnancy are increased by about 300 kcal/day. Actually, this increase is not really required during

TABLE 10-1 THE REVISED 1989 RECOMMENDED DIETARY ALLOWANCES[a]

Category	Age (years) or Condition	Weight[b] (kg)	Weight[b] (lb)	Height[b] (cm)	Height[b] (in)	Protein (g)	Fat-Soluble Vitamins Vitamin A (μg RE)[c]	Vitamin D (μg)[d]	Vitamin E (mg α-TE)[e]	Vitamin K (μg)	Water-Soluble Vitamins Vitamin C (mg)	Thiamin (mg)	Riboflavin (mg)	Niacin (mg NE)[f]	Vitamin B6 (mg)	Folate (μg)	Vitamin B12 (μg)	Minerals Calcium (mg)	Phosphorus (mg)	Magnesium (mg)	Iron (mg)	Zinc (mg)	Iodine (μg)	Selenium (μg)
Infants	0.0–0.5	6	13	60	24	13	375	7.5	3	5	30	0.3	0.4	5	0.3	25	0.3	400	300	40	6	5	40	10
	0.5–1.0	9	20	71	28	14	375	10	4	10	35	0.4	0.5	6	0.6	35	0.5	600	500	60	10	5	50	15
Children	1–3	13	29	90	35	16	400	10	6	15	40	0.7	0.8	9	1.0	50	0.7	800	800	80	10	10	70	20
	4–6	20	44	112	44	24	500	10	7	20	45	0.9	1.1	12	1.1	75	1.0	800	800	120	10	10	90	20
	7–10	28	62	132	52	28	700	10	7	30	45	1.0	1.2	13	1.4	100	1.4	800	800	170	10	10	120	30
Males	11–14	45	99	157	62	45	1,000	10	10	45	50	1.3	1.5	17	1.7	150	2.0	1,200	1,200	270	12	15	150	40
	15–18	66	145	176	69	59	1,000	10	10	65	60	1.5	1.8	20	2.0	200	2.0	1,200	1,200	400	12	15	150	50
	19–24	72	160	177	70	58	1,000	10	10	70	60	1.5	1.7	19	2.0	200	2.0	1,200	1,200	350	10	15	150	70
	25–50	79	174	176	70	63	1,000	5	10	80	60	1.5	1.7	19	2.0	200	2.0	800	800	350	10	15	150	70
	51+	77	170	173	68	63	1,000	5	10	80	60	1.2	1.4	15	2.0	200	2.0	800	800	350	10	15	150	70
Females	11–14	46	101	157	62	46	800	10	8	45	50	1.1	1.3	15	1.4	150	2.0	1,200	1,200	280	15	12	150	45
	15–18	55	120	163	64	44	800	10	8	55	60	1.1	1.3	15	1.5	180	2.0	1,200	1,200	300	15	12	150	50
	19–24	58	128	164	65	46	800	10	8	60	60	1.1	1.3	15	1.6	180	2.0	1,200	1,200	280	15	12	150	55
	25–50	63	138	163	64	50	800	5	8	65	60	1.1	1.3	15	1.6	180	2.0	800	800	280	15	12	150	55
	51+	65	143	160	63	50	800	5	8	65	60	1.0	1.2	13	1.6	180	2.0	800	800	280	10	12	150	55
Pregnant						60	800	10	10	65	70	1.5	1.6	17	2.2	400	2.2	1,200	1,200	320	30	15	175	65
Lactating	1st 6 months					65	1,300	10	12	65	95	1.6	1.8	20	2.1	280	2.6	1,200	1,200	355	15	19	200	75
	2nd 6 months					62	1,200	10	11	65	90	1.6	1.7	20	2.1	260	2.6	1,200	1,200	340	15	16	200	75

[a]The allowances, expressed as average daily intakes over time, are intended to provide for individual variations among most normal persons as they live in the United States under usual environmental stresses. Diets should be based on a variety of common foods in order to provide other nutrients for which human requirements have been less well defined. See text for detailed discussion of allowances and of nutrients not tabulated.

[b]Weights and heights of Reference Adults are actual medians for the U.S. population of the designated age, as reported by NHANES II. The median weights and heights of those under 19 years of age were taken from Hamill et al. (1979) (see pages 16–17). The use of these figures does not imply that the height-to-weight ratios are ideal.

[c]Retinol equivalents. 1 retinol equivalent = 1 μg retinol or 6 μg β-carotene. See text for calculation of vitamin A activity of diets as retinol equivalents.

[d]As cholecalciferol. 10 μg cholecalciferol = 400 IU of vitamin D.

[e]α-Tocopherol equivalents. 1 mg d-α tocopherol = 1 α-TE. See text for variation in allowances and calculation of vitamin E activity of the diet as α-tocopherol equivalents.

[f]1 NE (niacin equivalent) is equal to 1 mg of niacin or 60 mg of dietary tryptophan.

Source: National Research Council. (1989). Recommended dietary allowances (10th ed.) (pp. 92–93). Washington.

mammary glands
Specialized glands in the breasts that secrete milk during pregnancy.

trimester A period of 3 months.

the first 2 months of pregnancy.[1] During the first 2 months, the fetal and maternal changes are not as dramatic as they are from the third month through the rest of the pregnancy. The extra 300 kcal are important for the growth of the mother's uterus and **mammary glands,** and increasing blood volume. During the last **trimester,** the extra kilocalories are necessary for the growth of the placenta and fetus.

The National Academy of Sciences recommends the following guidelines for weight gain for pregnant females[2]:

1. Normal-weight women: 25–35 lb
2. Underweight women: 28–40 lb
3. Overweight women: 15–25 lb

A weight gain of over 1 lb/week is a clue that the woman is getting more kilocalories than she needs for healthy development of the baby. If this excess weight gain continues, the woman could have a postpregnancy overweight problem.

Requirement during Lactation

The recommended amount of energy for a woman who is lactating is +500 kcal/day compared to +300 kcal/day for pregnancy. The metabolic needs of a mother are actually higher during lactation than during pregnancy, hence the need for the recommended higher level of kilocalories.

The mother's breasts produce about 850 ml (3¾ cups) of milk per day for her nursing infant. The +500 kcal/day is actually not enough to produce the milk; approximately 750 kcal are required. The extra 250 kcal come from the body metabolizing fat that was stored during pregnancy. This stored fat will be used up in about 3 months; therefore, women who breast-feed may need to increase their kilocalorie intake at this point.[1]

Protein

Requirement during Pregnancy

The protein requirement during pregnancy is 60 g/day. The increased protein is required for the increased blood volume, enlarged uterus and breasts, and, most important, for the synthesis of new tissues in the developing fetus.

Requirement during Lactation

During lactation the protein requirement is 65 g/day. The extra protein is important as a normal constituent in milk. Human milk has an average protein content of 1.2 g/dl.

Iron and Folacin

Requirement during Pregnancy

Pregnancy results in an increased synthesis of red blood cells (RBCs) (erythropoiesis) in the mother; the fetus produces its own. These changes require increased amounts of iron, with some estimates being as high as 1,000 mg per pregnancy. Many women are iron deficient when they become pregnant. In addition, the average woman absorbs only about 1–2 mg iron per day from her diet, while needing about 3 mg. In order to compensate for the deficiency and the increased needs during pregnancy, the RDA is 15 mg of supplemental iron. As indicated, the iron should be in the form of supplementation, since nutritional experts do not feel that diet alone can supply this high level of iron.

Pregnancy requires more folacin than nonpregnancy primarily for increased RBC synthesis. The RDA for folacin during pregnancy is 400 µg, more than double the 180 µg recommended in nonpregnancy. As with iron, this recommended increase should come from supplements. The reason is that folacin is found primarily in liver, leafy green vegetables, and legumes, which usually cannot be consumed in large enough quantities to supply this high level of folacin.

Requirement during Lactation

Iron supplementation of 15 mg is recommended during lactation, primarily for replacement of iron stores lost during pregnancy. After birth, erythropoiesis, and therefore the need for folacin, decreases. The increased folacin during lactation is needed primarily to compensate for the amount secreted in breast milk.

Calcium, Phosphorus, and Vitamin D

Requirement during Pregnancy

Calcium, phosphorus, and vitamin D are needed in increased amounts for bone formation in the fetus. Since calcium and phosphorus are deposited together in bones, the RDA of +400 mg/day is the same for both of them. Likewise, a level of 10 μg of vitamin D is recommended, since it is important for absorption and deposition of calcium and phosphorus.

These nutrients are important not only for the development of the fetal skeleton but also to prevent demineralization of the mother's bones. If the woman's diet is calcium deficient, calcium will be removed from her bones and used by the fetus.

Requirement during Lactation

Notice that in Table 10-1 the requirements for calcium, phosphorus, and vitamin D during lactation are the same as those during pregnancy. The increased amounts after birth are needed to replace these nutrients that are secreted in breast milk. If the replacement is not accomplished during lactation, demineralization of the mother's skeleton will occur.

Other Vitamins and Minerals

Requirement during Pregnancy

Vitamins B_6 and B_{12} are needed in increased amounts. Vitamin B_6 is important for increased protein synthesis in the fetus and mother. Vitamin B_{12} is important for increased RBC production and for the development and maintenance of the nervous system in the fetus and mother.

Increased amounts of vitamin C are important for absorption of iron and for the development of connective tissues and the walls of blood vessels in the fetus and mother. Niacin, thiamin, and riboflavin are required in increased amounts to help provide the increased kilocalories.

Vitamin A is needed in increased amounts for cell development and bone formation in the fetus. Vitamin E is important to help preserve tissue integrity and prevent the breakdown of RBCs.

Zinc in increased amounts is important, since it functions in many important enzyme reactions. The +3 mg of zinc is a higher amount than actually needed during pregnancy, but one must take into account the fact that it is poorly absorbed.

Iodine is needed in increased amounts of +25 μg for the production of extra thyroxine, which is important for the increased metabolic rate of the mother.

Requirement during Lactation

The RDA of vitamin B_6, like that of folacin, is lower during lactation than during pregnancy. Vitamins A, E, and C, thiamin, riboflavin, niacin, zinc, and iodine are all required in larger amounts during lactation than during pregnancy. The primary reason is their inclusion in breast milk. In addition, the increases in thiamin, riboflavin, and niacin are important for the increased energy needs during lactation.[3]

PROPER DIET FOR PREGNANCY AND LACTATION

The RDAs for most of the previously discussed nutrients can be achieved by following a variation of the Food Guide Pyramid as shown in Table 10-2.

Alcohol Use During Pregnancy

Much research has been done concerning the effects of alcohol on the development of the fetus during pregnancy. These studies indicate that chronic excess alcohol consumption during pregnancy can result in the fetal alcohol syndrome (FAS). A child diagnosed as having FAS exhibits many abnormalities, such as mental retardation, poor coordination, hyperactivity, facial abnormalities, and abnormal bone formation. FAS children typically are born to women who have had a history of alcoholism for about 7 years.

TABLE 10-2 DAILY FOOD GUIDE FOR PREGNANCY AND LACTATION

	Number of Servings		
Food Choices	Nonpregnant Woman	Pregnant Woman	Lactating Woman
Meat and meat substitutes	1	2	2
Milk and milk products	2	3 to 4	4 to 5
Fruits and vegetables			
Vitamin C and vegetables	1 to 2	1 to 2	1 to 2
Dark green vegetables	1	1	1 to 2
Other fruits and vegetables	2	4 to 6	4 to 6
Grains (breads and cereals)	6	10	10
Other foods	Foods from other groups can be added when above foods have been included. Foods from other groups help achieve the recommended daily kilocalorie level and add variety to meals.		

Source: Adapted from National Research Council. (1989). *Recommended dietary allowances* (10th ed.) (pp. 92–93). Washington.

Much controversy exists about how much alcohol, if any, is safe for a pregnant woman to consume. No absolutely safe level has yet been established. However, consumption of alcohol by pregnant women is common. Moderate drinking (fewer than two drinks weekly) has been shown in some studies to have no measurable adverse outcome of pregnancy.[4]

Many nutritionists believe that since no absolutely safe level of alcohol consumption has been established, a pregnant woman should avoid alcohol totally during pregnancy.

PROBLEMS AND COMPLICATIONS OF PREGNANCY

Nausea and Vomiting (Morning Sickness)

morning sickness Nausea and vomiting experienced by pregnant women.

The occurrence of nausea and vomiting is often called **morning sickness;** however, it can occur at any time. It is almost unavoidable, since it results from hormonal increases that take place early in the first trimester. Unlike most nausea, relief from morning sickness is achieved by keeping a small amount of food in the stomach. One suggestion is that the meals be small and low in fat content. In addition, eating a few soda crackers or melba toast 15–30 minutes before getting out of bed and confining liquids to between-meal periods help to relieve morning sickness.

Pregnancy-induced Hypertension (PIH)

proteinuria The loss of protein in the urine.

PIH is characterized by hypertension, **proteinuria** (loss of protein in urine), edema, and, in severe cases, convulsions or coma. The traditional term for this condition, *toxemia of pregnancy,* is being phased out, since there are no toxins in the blood. There are two stages of PIH:

preeclampsia Sudden high blood pressure or an increase of 20–30 mmHg in systolic pressure and 10–15 mmHg in diastolic pressure.

Preeclampsia. Characterized by proteinuria in excess of 5 g in 24 hours and sudden edema in many parts of the body. It usually occurs during the last 20 weeks of pregnancy.

Eclampsia. Symptoms of preeclampsia, but also accompanied by convulsions and possibly coma.

eclampsia High blood pressure accompanied by convulsions and coma.

Preeclampsia often occurs in women who have diabetes or hypertension. In addition, it is often seen in pregnant teenage girls and women from lower socioeconomic groups. The cause of preeclampsia is unknown, but possible nutritional reasons are low calcium intake, high sodium intake, decreased protein and kilocalorie intake, and general malnutrition.[5]

Preeclampsia problems result from vasoconstriction of arteries, which reduces blood flow through the placenta to the fetus. Decreased blood flow can hinder proper growth and development of the fetus, with an increased risk of premature and stillborn births. This condition can generally be prevented by following an optimum diet for pregnancy.

Dietary treatment for preeclampsia in the acute phase involves parenteral solutions or intravenous infusion of nutrients. Women not in an acute phase have been found to benefit from a well-balanced diet somewhat high in protein, plus a high intake of calcium.

SUMMARY

- During pregnancy, RDA values are as follows: kcal, +300 kcal/day; protein, 60 g/day; iron, 15 mg/day; folacin, 400 µg/day; calcium and phosphorous, +400 mg/day; vitamin D, +5 µg/day.
- During lactation, RDA values are as follows: kcal, +500 kcal/day; protein, 65 g/day; iron, 30 mg/day; folacin, 400 µg/day; calcium and phosphorous, same as pregnancy; vitamin D, same as pregnancy.
- The above-mentioned nutrients are important to a pregnant woman in the following ways: kcal—growth of mother's uterus, mammary glands, and increasing blood volume; protein—mother's increased blood volume, enlarged uterus and breasts, and synthesis of new tissues in the developing fetus; iron—increased synthesis of RBCs; folacin—increased synthesis of RBCs; calcium and phosphorous—development of fetal skeleton; vitamin D—absorption of calcium into fetal skeleton.
- Symptoms of fetal alcohol syndrome (FAS) include mental retardation, poor coordination, hyperactivity, facial abnormalities, and abnormal bone formation.
- Causes for pregnancy-induced hypertension (PIH) are not known but low calcium intake, high sodium intake, decreased protein and kcal intake, and general malnutrition are possible nutritional reasons. Symptoms of PIH include sudden high blood pressure, proteinuria, and possibly convulsions and a coma. A well-balanced diet will prevent the problem, and parenteral or intravenous solutions are used when the condition exists.

REVIEW QUESTIONS

True (A) or False (B)

1. An ideal pattern of weight gain for a pregnant woman is to gain most of her weight during the first trimester, when the fetus is growing rapidly. B
2. A weight gain of over 1 lb/week indicates that a woman is consuming more kilocalories than needed for healthy development of the baby. A
3. The recommended kilocalorie intake during lactation is higher than during pregnancy, since the mother's metabolism is higher in order to produce milk. A
4. The RDA for energy (+500 kcal) during lactation is more than adequate for the production of 850 ml of breast milk per day. B
5. The purpose of the +30 g of protein per day in the daily diet of a pregnant woman is for the synthesis of new tissues in the fetus. B
6. Nutritionists do not feel that a pregnant woman should take iron pills if she consumes a large amount of iron-rich foods. B
7. An increased intake of folacin is recommended during pregnancy due to its importance for increased RBC synthesis by the mother and fetus. A
8. Increased intake of folacin during lactation is recommended primarily to compensate for the amount the mother secretes in breast milk. A
9. Calcium, phosphorus, and vitamin D in increased quantities during pregnancy and lactation help to prevent demineralization of the mother's skeleton. A
10. A pregnant teenager who is a vegetarian and does not believe in taking any vitamin tablets should be able to achieve an adequate diet. B
11. A proper diet for pregnancy should contain both animal and plant proteins to provide folacin, iron, magnesium, and zinc. A
12. In a diet for pregnancy, more servings of milk and milk products are recommended than in a diet for nonpregnant women. A
13. Morning sickness (nausea and vomiting) is unavoidable, since it results from hormonal increases in the first trimester of pregnancy. A
14. PIH is always a result of excessive sodium and low protein intake. B

Multiple Choice

15. The recommended increase of +300 kcal/day for a pregnant woman is important for:
    1. growth of the uterus
    2. growth of the fetus
    3. growth of the placenta
    4. increasing the strength of the mother's abdominal muscles

    A. 1, 2, 3   B. 1, 3   C. 2, 4   D. 4
    E. all of these

16. Since the pattern of weight gain is more important than the total amount gained, at the end of the first trimester (3 months) a pregnant woman should have gained _____.
    A. ¾ to 1 lb/week, therefore 12 lb
    B. one-third of 22–27 lb, or 7–9 lb
    C. 2–4 lb
    D. as little as possible

17. The recommended protein increase in a pregnant woman's diet is +30 g, which can be partially achieved by __3__ servings of protein foods.
    A. +20 g—two
    B. +50 mg—three
    C. +400 µg—four
    D. +30 g—three

18. Iron and folacin should be increased in the diet of a breast-feeding mother for the purpose of _____ and are best supplied by _____.
    A. replacing the amounts lost during pregnancy and secreted in breast milk—taking iron and folacin supplements
    B. increasing RBC synthesis in the mother and fetus—consuming foods that are rich in iron and folacin
    C. increasing the blood volume in the mother—eating liver and leafy green vegetables
    D. none of these

19. A proper diet for a pregnant woman is _____.
    A. milk—four servings
       meat—two servings
       fruits and vegetables—five servings
       breads and cereals—ten servings
       other foods—enough servings to achieve kilocalorie requirements
    B. milk—two servings
       protein foods—two servings
       fruits and vegetables—four servings
       breads and cereals—four servings
       other foods—should not consume foods other than those above

20. FAS children exhibit abnormalities such as _____.
    A. mental retardation
    B. hyperactivity
    C. facial abnormalities
    D. all of these

21. The preeclampsia stage of PIH is characterized by:

1. convulsions   3. coma
2. proteinuria   4. sudden high
                         blood pressure
    A. 1, 2, 3   B. 1, 3   C. 2, 4   D. 4
    E. all of these

22. Dietary treatment for preeclampsia involves _____.
    A. parenteral solutions and a balanced diet high in carbohydrate and fats
    B. parenteral solutions and a balanced diet high in protein and calcium
    C. a low-carbohydrate, high-liquid, high-vitamin diet
    D. none of these

Completion

23. Give the RDA values during pregnancy and lactation and the function or importance of energy, protein, iron, and folacin.

24. Describe the causes, symptoms, and dietary treatment of pregnancy-induced hypertension (PIH).

CRITICAL THINKING CHALLENGE

1. Using the number of servings in Table 10-2, write a suggested menu for a pregnant woman that will have 2,500 kcal.

2. Give the nutrients that are increased for a pregnant woman. Describe their importance and two food sources of each.

3. Ms. A is in her 25th week of pregnancy. She was transported to the clinic after experiencing convulsions. On exam, her blood pressure was elevated and she had proteinuria.
   a. These symptoms are characteristic of what complication?
   b. Prepare a teaching plan to identify for Ms. A the possible causes of this complication and the dietary interventions she should implement.

REVIEW QUESTIONS FOR NCLEX

Situation. A normal weight 23-year-old pregnant woman is referred to you for nutritional counseling.

1. She wants to know about how much weight she should gain and your RDA recommendation is _____.
   A. 15–25 lb
   B. 25–35 lb
   C. 28–40 lb
   D. 40–50 lb
2. An increase in protein to 60 g/day is important for _____.
   A. increased blood volume
   B. enlarged uterus and breasts
   C. synthesis of new tissues in developing fetus
   D. all of the above
3. Increased daily amounts of iron (15 mg) and folacin (400 µg) are both primarily important for _____.
   A. increased RBC synthesis
   B. increased milk production
   C. increased tissue syntesis
   D. increased energy needs
4. The increased amounts of iron and folacin can only be obtained by _____.
   A. eating large amounts of vegetables
   B. eating large amounts of fruits
   C. eating large amount of meats, fish, and poultry
   D. taking supplements
5. Increased daily amounts of calcium and phosphorous (400 mg) and 10 µg of vitamin D is important for _____.
   A. development of fetal skeleton and prevent demineralization of mother's bones
   B. muscle contractions and nerve impulse conduction in the fetus and mother
   C. tissue integrity and prevent breakdown of RBCs

   D. increased metabolic activity and release of ATP for tissue synthesis
6. Recommendations of the number of servings of food choices to accomplish the above discussed nutrients are _____. (See Table 10.2)
   A. meat 2; milk 3 to 4; fruits and vegetables 5 to 8; breads 10
   B. meat 6; milk 2 to 3; fruits and vegetables 2 to 3; breads 4
   C. meat 3; milk 4 to 6; fruits and vegetables 4 to 6; breads 6
   D. meat 4; milk 1 to 3; fruits and vegetables 1 to 3; breads 2

REFERENCES

1. National Research Council. (1989). *Recommended dietary allowances* (10th ed.) (pp. 92–93). Washington.
2. The latest on eating for two. (1990). *Tufts University and Dietetics Nutrition Letter 8*, 7.
3. National Academy of Sciences, Committee on Nutritional Status During Pregnancy and Lactation, Food and Nutrition Board. (1990). *Nutrition during pregnancy.* Washington, DC: National Academy Press.
4. Halmesmaki, E., Raivio, K. O., & Ylikarkala, O. (1987). Patterns of alcohol consumption during pregnancy. *Obstetrics and Gynecology, 69*, 594.
5. Marya, R. K., Rathee, K.L.S., & Monrow, M. (1987). Effect of calcium and vitamin D supplementation on toxemia of pregnancy. *Gynecologic and Obstetric Investigation, 24*, 38.

11

NUTRITION DURING INFANCY, CHILDHOOD, AND ADOLESCENCE

OBJECTIVES

Upon completion of this chapter, you should be able to:

1. Discuss the advantages of breast feeding compared to bottle feeding.
2. Describe changes in cow's milk (used in formulas) to resemble breast milk more closely.
3. Give two reasons for adding solid foods to a baby's diet and a possible schedule for introduction of solid foods.
4. Discuss food allergies, colic, PKU, and diarrhea in terms of the possible causes and dietary treatment of each.
5. Describe the changes and dietary needs of toddlers, preschoolers, and school-age children.
6. Discuss how kilocalories, protein, and minerals are important in the diet of adolescents.
7. Describe the relationship of acne and diet in adolescents.
8. Discuss obesity and anorexia nervosa, in terms of possible causes and dietary treatment in adolescents.

NUTRITION DURING INFANCY

infancy The period from time of birth through the first year.

Infancy is the period from the time of birth through the first year. An infant grows at a fantastic rate, with the weight usually doubling at 6 months of age and being triple the birth weight by 1 year. In other words a child who weighed 7 lb at birth should weigh 14 lb at 6 months and 21 lb by 1 year. Nutrition is essential for an infant to grow at these rates.

First Foods for the Infant

Whether a woman breast-feeds or bottle-feeds the infant, the initial source of nutrients is milk. Many authorities recommend breast feeding as the best means of feeding the infant. Breast milk contains most of the important nutrients in appropriate amounts to support the growth and development of the infant (see Fig. 11-1). Proteins and carbohydrates in breast milk are in a form that allows easier digestion and absorption. Cholesterol is higher in breast milk than cow's milk, which is important for the production of nerve tissue and bile. Vitamin C is higher in breast milk than cow's milk. However, vitamin D is usually less than the Recommended Dietary Allowance (RDA) in breast milk. This deficiency can usually be overcome by exposing the infant to sunlight for short periods of time. However, if the infant is rarely exposed to sunlight because of climate or clothing, a vitamin D deficiency is possible. Vitamin B_{12} can be deficient in breast milk, especially if the mother is a true vegetarian or vegan and is not supplementing her diet.

Calcium and phosphorus are present in breast milk in the more desirable calcium : phosphorus ratio of 2 : 1 compared to 1 : 1 to 1 : 1.5 in many formulas. This ratio is beneficial to the infant's bone and teeth growth, normal cellular functions, and enzymatic reactions.

Besides vitamin D, four other nutrients that are lower in breast milk compared to cow's milk are sodium, potassium, chloride, and iron. Sodium, potassium, and chloride are approximately three times lower in breast milk compared to cow's milk. The advantage is that there is less stress on the infant's kidneys in regulating their level. The lower level of iron in breast milk may seem to be a detriment; however, approximately 49% of this iron is absorbed compared to about 1% of the iron in cow's milk.

One of the most important advantages of breast feeding is the immunologic effects it offers. Breast milk contains antibodies that protect the infant against many infections that invade through the gastrointestinal tract. In addition to having fewer infections, breast-fed infants have fewer allergic reactions even if there is a family history of such disorders.[1]

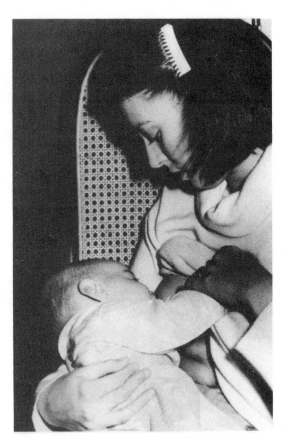

FIGURE 11-1 Breast feeding. (From McFarlane, J.M., Whitson, B.J., and Hartley, L.M. *Contemporary Pediatric Nursing: A Conceptual Approach.* New York: John Wiley & Sons, Inc., © 1980. Reprinted with permission.)

Some studies indicate that breast feeding prevents infantile obesity. One reason is that a breast-fed baby feeds only when he or she is hungry, whereas parents often require a bottle-fed baby to consume all of the bottle even though the infant may be already full.

One nonnutritional benefit of breast feeding is the promotion of **bonding** between the mother and child. This psychological value is beneficial to both the mother and the child. However, parents who elect to bottle-feed their infant can also achieve this bonding by holding, kissing, touching, and talking to the infant (see Fig. 11-2).

Breast feeding offers the following advantages to the mother:

bonding The formation of an emotional link between the mother and the infant.

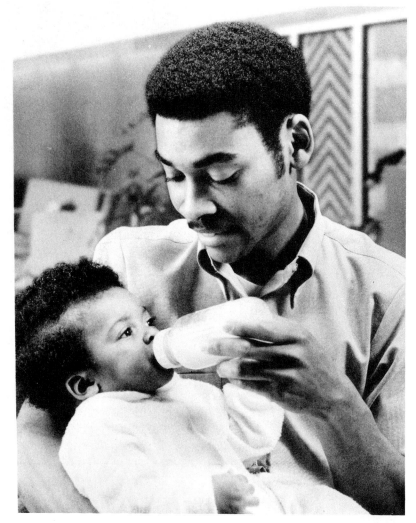

FIGURE 11-2   Bottle feeding. (Courtesy of Gerber Foods.)

involution   The contraction of the enlarged uterus after birth.

oxytocin   A pituitary hormone that stimulates uterine contractions.

Uterine contraction. The enlarged uterus will undergo **involution** more rapidly because breast feeding stimulates the release of **oxytocin,** which promotes uterine contraction.

Weight loss. The loss of weight gained during pregnancy is increased by breast feeding, assuming the mother does not consume too many kilocalories, since her metabolic needs are high.

Lower cost. Breast feeding is more economical than buying commercial formulas, despite the fact that the mother must consume more food for milk production.

DDT (dichloro diphenyl trichloroethane) An insecticide that is toxic to insects and humans. It has been found in human breast milk.

Polychlorinated biphenyls (PCBs) Chemicals used in the manufacture of plastics. They are not biodegradable and have been found in breast milk.

psychotherapeutics Drugs used in the treatment of manic-depressive illness.

While breast feeding has many advantages for both the mother and the child, there are some conditions in which it is not advisable. If the mother has a poor nutritional status, her ability to form milk with the proper level of nutrients is hindered.

If a mother is exposed to large amounts of environmental chemicals, such as **DDT** and **polychlorinated biphenyls (PCBs),** she should consider bottle feeding. The reason is that these chemicals have been found in breast milk. In addition, if a lactating woman is on a crash diet, increased fat metabolism and possibly increased release of PCBs from fat tissues will occur.

Women who drink alcohol or consume large amounts of caffeine, nicotine, and **psychotherapeutic** drugs (e.g., lithium) should be aware that these substances will be transmitted in breast milk.

If a mother is overanxious, has no desire, or cannot conveniently breast feed because she is employed outside the home, she may transmit feelings of hostility and anxiety, rather than love, to the infant.

As discussed above, there are certain conditions in which formula feeding is better than breast feeding. Each formula contains cow's milk that has been modified to closely resemble breast milk. For example, proteins have been altered so that they can be more easily digested. In addition, saturated butterfat is replaced by unsaturated vegetable oil. All brands are fortified with vitamins and are available with or without iron fortification.

Some infants are sensitive to protein in formulas; therefore, milk-substitute formulas such as soybean preparations are available.

Skim milk should not be used in infant feeding, since it lacks the essential fatty acid linoleic acid and kilocalories.

Introduction of Solid Foods (Beikost)

Adding solid foods to a baby's diet should be based on two considerations:

- Supplying increasing amounts of nutrients that milk alone cannot supply.
- Supplying the foods in a form the baby is physically able to handle.

Some parents want to introduce solid foods when an infant is only 1 month old. This early introduction of solid food presents several problems. One problem is that babies do not develop voluntary swallowing movements until they are about 3–4 months old. Also, with early introduction of solid foods, salivary amylase for digestion of starches is not present until the second or third month, and the ability of the kidneys to handle an increased level of wastes is not developed until the end of the second month.

Most physicians recommend that solid foods not be introduced until the infant is 4–6 months of age. The Nutrition Committee of the American Academy of Pediatrics recommends that solid foods not be introduced before 3 months of age. One possible schedule for introduction of solid foods is as follows[2]:

Month	Food
4	Cereal
5–6	Strained vegetables
6–7	Strained fruits
6–8	Finger foods (crackers, bananas, etc.)
7–8	Strained meat
10	Strained or mashed egg yolk
10	Bite-sized cooked foods

Cereals are usually introduced first because of their ease of digestion. They are an excellent source of B vitamins and iron (see Fig. 11-3). Rice cereal is a good first choice, since it usually does not cause food allergies.

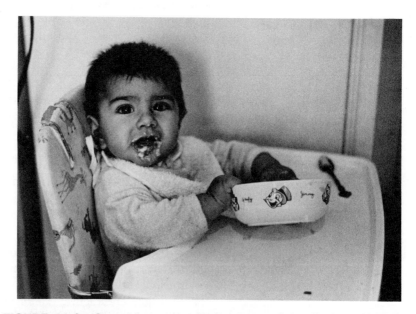

FIGURE 11-3 Cereal is an excellent source of the B vitamins and iron for an infant. (Courtesy of Barbara Rios.)

Vegetables are frequently introduced before fruits because they are harder to "learn" to like than the sweeter fruits. When fruits are introduced first, mothers often complain that the baby will not eat vegetables. The reason is that all babies like the sweet taste of fruits and frequently do not care for the taste of vegetables when they are introduced second.

Egg whites are generally not recommended until after 1 year of age. The reason is that infants are frequently allergic to egg whites but not to egg yolks.

While some parents want to introduce solid foods too early, others delay introduction past the age of 6 months. This situation is more common with breast-fed than bottle-fed children. There are two problems with this delay. First, breast milk is low in iron, especially in comparison to what the infant needs by 6 months of age. Second, breast milk may not contain enough protein for the needs of the infant after 6 months.

Infant Problems Related to Nutrition

Food Allergy

An infant who is allergic to a food develops antibodies to that food. The antibodies are formed by the body to attack and destroy the food, which is the equivalent of an antigen.

Unfortunately, this antigen–antibody response causes serious symptoms in the infant, including **hives** (itching and burning swelling of the skin), **eczema** (redness and small blisters on the skin), **bronchitis, asthma,** coughing, sneezing, diarrhea, and **colic.** It is common for allergic symptoms to appear during the early months of life.

Some of the more common nutrients that infants are allergic to are cow's milk protein, egg protein, wheat protein, and compounds in orange juice. Treatment of allergies involves identification and elimination of the suspected food from the infant's diet. Infants from families with a history of allergies should be breast-fed for the first 4–6 months. Infants who are allergic to cow's milk can be given a milk-free formula such as a soybean formula. Sometimes children outgrow allergies; therefore, the offending food, especially cow's milk, should be reintroduced at a later time.

Colic

Colic, usually seen in infants less than 3 months old, is characterized by profuse crying after eating. Most often the cause is overfeeding with formula. Bacteria often ferment the excess milk, resulting in gas buildup. Dietary adaptations include diluting formula with water, avoiding the use of complex carbohydrates, burping the infant frequently, and experi-

hives Itching and burning swellings of the skin.

eczema Redness and small blisters on the skin.

bronchitis Inflammation of the bronchi, the passageways to the lungs (see Chapter 19).

asthma A respiratory condition, characterized by recurrent attacks of wheezing, that may be due to bronchitis.

colic A spasm in an organ accompanied by pain.

menting with the temperature of the formula, since an infant sometimes tolerates a cold formula better than a warm one.

Phenylketonuria

Phenylketonuria (PKU) A disorder in an infant caused by the absence of the enzyme phenylalanine hydroxylase, which oxidizes phenylalanine to tyrosine.

congenital metabolic disorder An inherited metabolic disorder that a child is born with, such as phenylketonuria (PKU).

inborn error of metabolism The same as a congenital metabolic disorder.

phenylalanine hydroxylase An enzyme that synthesizes tyrosine from phenylalanine.

tyrosine A nonessential amino acid.

phenylalanine An essential amino acid.

Phenylketonuria (PKU) is called a **congenital metabolic disorder** or **inborn error of metabolism.** This means that the infant is born with the problem, which consists of a lack of the enzyme **phenylalanine hydroxylase.** This enzyme functions in the synthesis of the amino acid **tyrosine** from **phenylalanine.** The resulting excess buildup of phenylalanine can result in hyperactivity, irritability, and ultimately mental retardation if left untreated.

The dietary treatment for PKU is a low-phenylalanine diet. Since phenylalanine is an essential amino acid important for tissue synthesis, it cannot be totally eliminated. However, foods rich in phenylalanine such as milk can be reduced in the infant's diet. A milk-substitute formula that is 95% free of phenylalanine (Lofenalac) is used in the treatment of PKU. Small amounts of milk are mixed with the formula to provide the needed amount of phenylalanine.

The introduction of solid foods to the diet is done according to phenylalanine exchange food lists. The foods, such as cereals, vegetables, and fruits, provide small amounts of phenylalanine. Meat, fish, poultry, and dairy products are high in phenylalanine and have to be restricted.[3]

Diarrhea

One of the most common causes of diarrhea is overfeeding. Inflammation of the intestinal wall accompanies diarrhea, along with temporary loss of the enzyme lactase, which digests lactose in milk. Because of the loss of lactase, consumption of milk when an infant has diarrhea will only worsen the problem. Dietary treatment of diarrhea in an infant consists of replacement of lost fluids and electrolytes (sodium, chloride, potassium), using a solution such as Pedialyte or Lytren. As the diarrhea subsides, the enzyme lactase reappears, and progression to a dilute formula and finally to a full formula should follow.

Diarrhea can result from many problems, such as allergies and intestinal infections in infants. They should never be taken lightly, since the infant can become dehydrated and even die. If an infant's diarrhea does not improve in approximately 24 hours, a physician should be consulted.

NUTRITION DURING CHILDHOOD

Childhood is the stage of the life cycle that extends from infancy to adolescence and can be subdivided into the toddler, preschool, and school-age periods.

Toddlers

toddlers Children from 1 to 3 years of age.

The growth rate of **toddlers** slows down, causing their appetite and consumption of food to decrease. Parents should be aware that these changes are normal and should not be overly concerned that the toddler does not seem to be eating enough.

Although the toddler is not growing as rapidly as during infancy, important muscle changes are occurring. The muscles of the back, buttocks, and thighs are enlarging and strengthening as the toddler begins to stand erect and walk. Much body fat is lost as the muscles increase in size and the bones become harder. The body shape changes from a rather chubby to a more lean appearance.

Muscle control continues to develop, especially fine motor movements. Handling of eating utensils increases, as well as a desire to become independent. As a result, toddlers want to feed themselves but may not be able to do so successfully. The desire for independence is often exhibited by avoiding nutritious foods (e.g., vegetables) and preferring nonnutritious foods such as sweets.

Toddlers tend to imitate adult behavior. Therefore, if parents observe good food habits, toddlers are likely to integrate them into their own behavior.

Diet

The Food Guide Pyramid plan is the basis of dietary planning for toddlers, with a recommended pattern being the following:

Food Group	Number of servings	Portion Size
Milk	3	Cup
Meat and meat substitutes	2	1–2 oz
Fruits/vegetables	4	$\frac{1}{2}$ cup for vegetables $\frac{1}{2}$ cup for fruits
Bread/cereal	4	$\frac{1}{2}$ to 1 slice of bread $\frac{1}{2}$ cup of ready-to-eat cereal $\frac{1}{4}$ to $\frac{1}{2}$ cup of spaghetti and macaroni
Fat	3	Pats of soft margarine
Nutrient-dense snacks		As desired for necessary kilocalories

milk anemia Anemia that results from feeding older infants only milk that is low in iron.

Milk consumption of more than three cups by toddlers can result in **milk anemia,** since this consumption excludes other foods that are higher in iron. Whole milk rather than skim milk should be consumed until the child is 2 years old, since it contains linoleic acid (essential fatty acid).

Consumption of meat or meat substitutes is important for this group, since their muscles are actively developing. However, if the toddler does not like meat, two glasses of milk and one serving of meat or a substitute will provide an adequate amount of protein.

As with adults, the fruit and vegetable servings should include one serving of a vitamin C–rich fruit or vegetable such as tomato. In addition, one serving of a leafy green or yellow vegetable should be consumed. Toddlers often like raw vegetables served as finger foods.

Iron is frequently low in the diet of toddlers; therefore, it is important that the child be offered iron-enriched cereals. Infant cereals are also a good source of iron. In selecting cereals, parents should consider the amount of sugar and fiber in addition to the amount of iron.

In addition to servings of the above foods, a toddler should get servings of margarine for vitamin A and fats for vitamin E. Since toddlers' stomachs are small, they will not be able to eat all these foods in three meals a day. Instead, they will want to eat food between meals. Parents should recognize that this is a normal pattern. Between-meal snacks can provide essential nutrients that are not necessarily rich in concentrated sweets. Some examples are as follows:

Fruits: apples and oranges cut into small wedges
Vegetables: raw carrots, cucumbers, and celery
Bread: unsalted whole grain crackers
Cheese: small pieces of natural cheese
Peanut butter: spread on small pieces of bread
Sweets: oatmeal, bran, and raisin cookies

It is important for parents to remember that because the toddler's growth rate is slowing down, his or her appetite will be decreased. In addition, the desire to become more independent will cause the toddler to be erratic in his eating habits. If parents are too rigid with the child, serious appetite problems and nonacceptance of foods could result.

Preschoolers

preschoolers Children from 3 to 6 years of age.

Preschoolers have the same dietary requirement as toddlers. Their growth continues to be slow, and they have little appetite. Permanent food habits are developing during this period; therefore, parents should strive to set a good example by eating the appropriate foods. A pre-

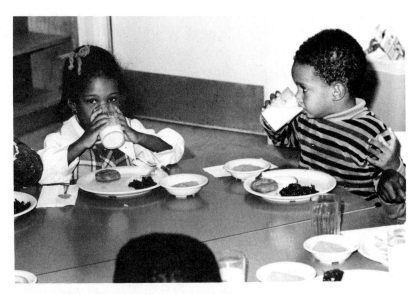

FIGURE 11-4 Preschoolers' eating habits are influenced by their nursery or preschool peers. (U.S. Department of Agriculture photo.)

schooler's eating habits are often influenced by those of nursery or preschool peers (see Fig. 11-4).

School-age Children

school-age children Children from 6 to 12 years of age.

School-age children tend to grow at a slow, steady rate. A child's body type should be established by now. Some children are athletic and burn up many kilocalories, whereas others are more sedentary.

Dietary habits are formed by this stage. Snacking is common now, especially after school; therefore, it is important for nutrient-dense snacks to be provided. Breakfast is a very important meal for this age group, since it provides the energy and nutrients for the learning activities that occur before lunch. Since the snacking opportunities for a hungry child before lunch are nonexistent, breakfast should be adequate to last until lunch. Good dietary habits are very beneficial to the child, since parental supervision at lunch is impossible. School lunch programs offer children a nourishing meal and encourage them to consume foods that they might not normally be offered (see Fig. 11-5).

The diet for this group, in terms of the number of servings and portion sizes, is essentially the same as for the preschool child, with modifications based on the child's appetite. Protein intake continues to be important for muscle development. Vitamin A and C deficiencies are common in this group; therefore, emphasis on vegetables and fruits to supply these nutrients or a multivitamin supplement is important.

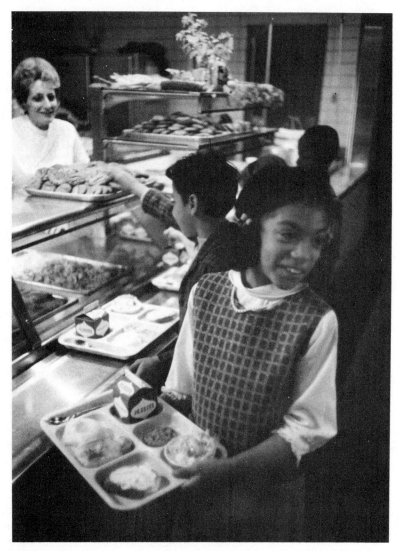

FIGURE 11-5 School lunch programs offer the school-age child a nourishing meal. (Courtesy of the National Dairy Council.)

NUTRITION DURING ADOLESCENCE

Diet for Adolescence

adolescence The period of life from 12 to about 20 years of age.

Adolescence is the period that bridges childhood and adulthood. It extends from the onset of puberty to the achievement of adult size, or the years from 12 to about 20.

The rate of growth during adolescence is greater than that of any other period of life except infancy. It is common for boys to grow 4 in. in a year and gain 20 lb. Girls may increase over 3 in. in height and gain somewhat less weight. The growth spurt is accompanied by increased appetite and nutrient needs.

Kilocalories. The RDA for energy of boys during adolescence is, on average, 2,500–2,900 kcal. For girls the average is 2,200 kcal. These are average figures and may be considerably higher for some adolescents.

Protein. An increase in protein during this period is important in boys for increased muscle mass. During puberty, increased levels of the hormone **testosterone** result in the extensive use of protein for the synthesis of lean muscle tissue and long bone growth. In girls the increased protein, under the influence of the hormone **estrogen,** is used in the synthesis of increased fat tissues in the abdominal area, breasts, and hips. In addition, protein is important in the widening of the **pelvic girdle.** Before the start of puberty, protein is important in girls for long bone growth; this is when most of their increase in height occurs.

Minerals. The RDA for calcium and phosphorus during adolescence is 50% higher than it is during childhood for the increase in bone growth. Teenage girls who diet often eliminate milk and therefore are calcium deficient. Iron requirements are high for both boys and girls. High levels of iron are needed for menstruating girls to replace what they lose in menstrual fluid. In boys, the extra iron is important for expanded blood supply and increased muscle mass.

The Food Guide Pyramid is the basis of dietary planning for adolescents. The only modification in the number of servings compared to that of adults is an increase in milk from two to four servings. This increase is essential if adolescents are to achieve the high level of calcium they need.

Acne is a problem that affects about 80% of adolescents. The reason it is so prevalent is not related to diet but rather to an increased level of sex hormones that begins at puberty. The **sebaceous glands** are stimulated to secrete more **sebum** by the high level of these hormones. Pores are often blocked by dirt, which causes the sebum to accumulate and form **blackheads** and **pimples.** Bacterial infection of the glands sometimes follows. Diet has no effect on causing or improving acne, despite the myth that foods such as chocolate, fried foods, milk, and sweets cause this condition. While adolescents may wish to restrict their intake of these foods, it should be emphasized that this practice will not necessarily prevent acne.

---

testosterone The male sex hormone secreted by the testes. It stimulates the development of male secondary sex characteristics.

estrogen The female sex hormone secreted by the ovaries. It stimulates the development of the female secondary sex characteristics.

pelvic girdle A ring of bones in the pelvic region composed of two hip bones joined to the sacrum.

sebaceous glands Glands in the skin that secrete the oily substance sebum.

sebum An oily secretion of the sebaceous glands. It lubricates and waterproofs the skin and hairs.

blackheads A plug of sebum within a hair follicle.

pimples Small, elevated areas of pus containing lesions of the skin. They are often called blackheads.

CHILDHOOD AND ADOLESCENT PROBLEMS
RELATED TO NUTRITION

Obesity

A common nutritional problem in adolescence is obesity, which affects about 10–20%.[4] Generally, the cause of the problem is lack of exercise rather than excess consumption of kilocalories.

It is very important that adolescents try to lose excess weight before the end of adolescence, since those who do not tend to be obese throughout adult life. Dietary management consists of decreasing the consumption of kilocalories while consuming adequate amount of the essential nutrients. This can generally be accomplished by decreasing the number of snacks, desserts, and second portions. Equally important is encouraging the adolescent to become more physically active.

Anorexia Nervosa and Bulimia

The opposite of obesity is anorexia nervosa and bulimia, which are states of self-induced starvation and overeating followed by vomiting, respectively. These disorders are seen in adolescent girls and are described in detail in Chapter 10.

SUMMARY

- Advantages of breast feeding compared to bottle feeding are: 1) nutrients are either in increased amounts or in a form that makes them more absorbable or useable; 2) possibly prevents infantile obesity; and 3) strengthens bonds between mother and child.
- Cow's milk (used in formulas) is modified to make it more like breast milk in the following ways: proteins are altered to make them more digestible; saturated butterfat is replaced by unsaturated vegetable oil; and the milk is fortified with vitamins and sometimes iron.
- When adding solid foods to a baby's diet, supply increased amounts of nutrients that milk alone cannot supply, and supply foods in a form the baby is physically able to handle.
- Causes of colic include overfeeding or is secondary to allergies. To treat, dilute formula, avoid feeding baby complex carbohydrates, burp baby often, and feed cold formula to baby instead of hot. Causes of PKU include lack of the enzyme phenylalanine hydroxylase, which causes buildup of phenylalanine and results in hyperactivity, irritability, and ultimately mental retardation; treatment involves low phenylalanine diet with Lofenalac. Diarrhea can be caused by overfeeding and creates an inflammation of the intestinal wall; treatment involves replacing lost fluids and electrolytes and diluting formula.
- The dietary needs of toddlers, preschoolers, and school-age children are based on the Food Guide Pyramid given in Chapter 2.
- Nutrient needs for adolescents are as follows: kcal—2,500–2,900 for males and 2,200 for females; increased protein for growth; increased calcium and phosphorous for growth of skeleton; increased iron needs for boys to meet their expanding blood volume and for girls to replace iron lost during menstruation.
- There is no relationship between diet and acne. Acne is caused by increased levels of sex hormones and sebum.

REVIEW QUESTIONS

True (A) or False (B)

1. Not only is breast milk the best source of nutrients for an infant, but the proteins and carbohydrates are in a form that is more easily absorbable.
2. An important advantage of breast milk is the immunologic feature of increased resistance to infections and fewer allergies.
3. A mother who breast-feeds does not have to worry about the infant's diet being deficient in any nutrients.
4. Formulas contain cow's milk that has been modified to make it more absorbable.
5. A mother who bottle-feeds her infant should consider using skim milk rather than whole milk in order to reduce the amount of cholesterol and saturated fat in the infant's diet.
6. A major consideration regarding when to introduce solid foods into the diet of an infant is age, and at 2 months is a good time.
7. Since breast milk is such a good food for infants, a mother should breast-feed the infant until at least the age of 1 year.
8. When introducing solid foods into the infant's diet, one should introduce vegetables before fruits, since vegetables are harder to like.
9. Although whole eggs are an excellent source of nutrients, only the yolk should be introduced before the infant is 1 year old due to a possible allergic reaction to egg white.
10. Allergic reactions in infants usually do not occur until after 1 year of age, and the symptoms are minor ones such as diarrhea and bronchitis.
11. Dietary treatment of PKU consists of complete elimination of the offending amino acid phenylalanine.
12. Dietary treatment for diarrhea consists of feeding milk to the infant in order to replace the lost nutrients as quickly as possible.
13. The growth rate and therefore the appetite of toddlers is greater than during infancy.
14. Milk consumption by toddlers should not exceed about three cups, since excess amounts may lead to milk anemia.
15. Enriched cereals are an excellent source of iron for toddlers.
16. In order to have toddlers develop good eating habits, parents should prevent them from consuming between-meal snacks.
17. Often a preschooler's rate of growth is slow, and there is little appetite.
18. Increased protein intake is important for adolescent boys due to a great amount of fat deposition.

19. Increased protein intake is important for adolescent girls for protein synthesis in the abdomen and hip regions.
20. There is no relationship between acne and diet in adolescents; rather, acne is a result of increased levels of sex hormones and sebum production.

Multiple Choice

21. Potential advantages of breast feeding compared to bottle feeding an infant is (are):
    1. immunologic
    2. lower level of cholesterol
    3. possible prevention of infantile obesity
    4. greater amount of iron intake
    A. 1, 2, 3   B. 1, 3   C. 2, 4   D. 4
    E. all of these
22. Adding solid foods to a baby's diet should be based on which of the following considerations?
    A. helping the infant sleep through the night
    B. supplying the foods in a form the baby is physically able to handle
    C. supplying increasing amounts of nutrients that milk alone cannot supply
    D. A, B
    E. B, C
23. Which of the following infant problems and dietary adaptations are correct?
    A. PKU—shift from whole milk to skim milk
    B. colic—substitution of soybean formula for the one causing the problem
    C. diarrhea—increase the feeding of whole milk to get more fat into the gastrointestinal tract
    D. all of these
    E. none of these
24. Which of the following correctly describe the diet during childhood?
    1. toddlers—emphasis on protein for muscle changes but not high levels of kilocalories, since the appetite is decreased
    2. preschoolers—much higher intake of proteins and kilocalories than toddlers due to rapid growth
    3. school-age children—dietary habits formed at this time, and breakfast is very important for good performance in classes before lunch
    A. 1, 2, 3   B. 1, 3   C. 2, 3   D. 3
    E. all of these

25. Nutrient needs and their importance during adolescence are:
    1. kilocalories:—boys average 1,700–1,900 kcal; girls average 1,500 kcal
    2. protein—increased amount is important in girls for the synthesis of fat tissues in the breasts, abdomen, and hips.
    3. minerals—same amounts of calcium and phosphorus are needed as in adults for bone growth
    4. increased iron intake—important in girls to replace the amounts lost during menstruation
    A. 1, 2, 3   B. 1, 3   C. 2, 4   D. 4
    E. all of these

Completion

26. Describe four nutrient advantages of breast feeding. Describe three other advantages of breast feeding.
27. Give two reasons for adding solid foods to a baby's diet and a possible schedule for introduction of solid foods.

CRITICAL THINKING CHALLENGE

1. A new mother tells the nurse, "I'm breast feeding because I know that my milk is better than formula and will give my baby everything he needs." What statement by the nurse is important to prevent a potential vitamin deficiency?
   a. "You need to talk with your doctor about your baby's needs."
   b. "Most babies need to take a vitamin supplement."
   c. "You will need to monitor your baby's intake carefully."
   d. "When the weather is nice, spend short periods of time with your baby in the sunlight."
2. Which statement by a healthy toddler's mother indicates a need for teaching?
   a. "Billy's appetite is so poor now. He doesn't eat like he used to."
   b. "Billy sure is changing. He doesn't look so chubby anymore."
   c. "Billy tries to feed himself but he gets more on the floor than in his mouth."

d. "Billy doesn't seem to like meat but he does drink his milk and eats a little meat each day."

3. Identify the recommended level of kcal, protein, and minerals for adolescents.
   a. Explain the rationale for these needs.
   b. Identify food choices the adolescent can make to meet these needs.

REVIEW QUESTIONS FOR NCLEX

Situation. A woman in her third trimester of pregnancy asks you about some of the advantages of breast feeding versus bottle feeding. Each response that follows is comparing advantages of breast milk in relation to cow's milk.

1. Proteins and carbohydrates in breast milk are in a form that _____.
   A. requires no digestion
   B. is in the simple building block state
   C. allows easier digestion and absorption
   D. can be stored more easily

2. Cholesterol is higher in breast milk than cow's milk which is _____.
   A. detrimental since high levels of cholesterol are not good
   B. important for production of nerve tissue and bile
   C. a disadvantage since it will predispose the infant to atherosclerosis
   D. important for building up levels of adipose tissue in the newborn

3. Calcium and phosphorus are present in _____.
   A. the more desirable ratio of 2 : 1 compared to 1 : 1 in cow's milk
   B. deficient amounts and therefore infant should be exposed to sunlight for short periods of time
   C. much larger amounts in cow's milk than breast milk
   D. a more desirable ratio of 1 : 1 in cow's milk compared to 0.5 : 1 in breast milk

4. Three nutrients that are low in breast milk compared to cow's milk are sodium, potassium, and chloride. This is a(an) _____.
   A. disadvantage because the functions they provide are decreased
   B. advantage because of less stress on the infant's kidneys
   C. disadvantage because these nutrients are crucial to the early development of the infant
   D. advantage because the enzymes necessary to digest these nutrients are not being secreted at birth

5. Iron and vitamin D are present in _____ amounts in breast milk compared to cow's milk.
   A. equal
   B. lower
   C. very large
   D. no appreciable

6. One of the most important advantages of breast feeding is the _____.
   A. immunologic effect
   B. high levels of iron and calcium
   C. balanced levels of the important nutrients
   D. high levels of sodium, potassium, and chloride ions

12 NUTRITION AND THE ELDERLY

Upon completion of this chapter, you should be able to:

1. Define the term *elderly* and describe their proportion in relation to the rest of the population.
2. Discuss the nutrient needs of the elderly.
3. Discuss why many authorities recommend increased calcium intake for the elderly.
4. Describe the importance of high-fiber diets for the elderly.
5. Describe dietary planning for the elderly.
6. Differentiate between nutrition programs for the elderly.

INTRODUCTION

elderly People who are 65 years of age or older.

The **elderly** are a rapidly increasing age group in the United States as well as worldwide. The proportion of elderly persons in the United States increased from 6.8% in 1940 to almost 13% in 1990. Many researchers predict that by the year 2030 the number of elderly persons will be 20% of the total population.[1] These percentages indicate that the elderly are a small percentage of the population; the following figures indicate that they use a considerably higher percentage of the health services provided in the United States. In 1984 the elderly accounted for:

29% of the country's health care costs

34% of all days in short-stay hospitals

87% of the occupants in nursing homes

25% of the prescription drugs used

15% of all visits to doctor's offices[2]

There are various reasons why the elderly use a much higher percentage of the health care services compared to their proportion of the population. One reason may be nutrition.

It is important for health care professionals to understand nutritional needs and deficiencies of the elderly, especially since their number and their use of health care facilities are increasing.

NUTRIENT NEEDS OF THE ELDERLY

Little scientific evidence exists on the nutritional needs of the elderly. Table 12-1 shows that their nutrient needs are included in the 51+ age group.

Kilocalorie Needs

The 1989 RDA values given in Table 12-1 show that men and women in the 51+ age group need a 600 kcal and 300 kcal decrease, respectively. This reduction is recommended because of a reduction in the basic metabolic rate (REE) and the activity level. The reduction in REE is primarily due to a decrease in muscle and organ tissues. Due to aging, an increased proportion of the body weight is adipose tissue and a decreased proportion is muscle and organ tissues. Elderly people tend to reduce their physical activity. This reduction, combined with the decreased REE, indicates that their kilocalorie intake should be reduced.

TABLE 12-1 MEDIAN HEIGHTS AND WEIGHTS AND RECOMMENDED ENERGY INTAKE

Category	Age (years) or Condition	Weight (kg)	Weight (lb)	Height (cm)	Height (in.)	REE[a] (kcal/day)	Multiples of REE	Average Energy Allowance (kcal)[b] Per kg	Average Energy Allowance (kcal)[b] Per day[c]
Infants	0.0–0.5	6	13	60	24	320		108	650
	0.5–1.0	9	20	71	28	500		98	850
Children	1–3	13	29	90	35	740		102	1,300
	4–6	20	44	112	44	950		90	1,800
	7–10	28	62	132	52	1,130		70	2,000
Males	11–14	45	99	157	62	1,440	1.70	55	2,500
	15–18	66	145	176	69	1,760	1.67	45	3,000
	19–24	72	160	177	70	1,780	1.67	40	2,900
	25–50	79	174	176	70	1,800	1.60	37	2,900
	51+	77	170	173	68	1,530	1.50	30	2,300
Females	11–14	46	101	157	62	1,310	1.67	47	2,200
	15–18	55	120	163	64	1,370	1.60	40	2,200
	19–24	58	128	164	65	1,350	1.60	38	2,200
	25–50	63	138	163	64	1,380	1.55	36	2,200
	51+	65	143	160	63	1,280	1.50	30	1,900
Pregnant	1st trimester								+0
	2nd trimester								+300
	3rd trimester								+300
Lactating	1st 6 months								+500
	2nd 6 months								+500

[a] Calculation based on FAO equations then rounded.
[b] In the range of light to moderate activity, the coefficient of variation is ±20%.
[c] Figure is rounded.
Source: From *Recommended Dietary Allowances* (10th ed.), 1989, Washington, DC: National Academy Press. Reprinted by permission of the National Academy of Sciences.

Protein

Table 12-1 shows that the RDA for protein for the elderly is the same as that of their younger counterparts: 65 g for men and 50 g for women, or 0.8 g per kilogram of ideal body weight. However, the elderly frequently have chronic illnesses that require medications. To counteract these illnesses and the effects of medications, they frequently require increased protein intake.

Carbohydrates and Fat

The consumption of carbohydrates by the elderly should be the same as that of younger people in that it should compose about 50% of the total kilocalories consumed. The majority of the carbohydrates should come from complex carbohydrates, as opposed to concentrated sweets, which are the major source for many elderly.

Fat intake for the elderly should be basically the same as that for younger people: 30% of total kilocalories, with emphasis on intake of polyunsaturated fats and decreased consumption of saturated fats.

Minerals

The RDA for calcium for the elderly is 800 mg/day. However, many authorities recommend that this be increased to 1,200 mg/day to decrease the potential development of osteoporosis (see Chapter 7 for details). Increasing consumption of high-calcium foods such as milk may not always be possible, since many elderly persons have a lactase deficiency. Therefore, calcium supplements may be required to reach these elevated levels.

Recommended intake of iron for the elderly is the same as that for younger people. Iron deficiency anemia in the elderly is often not due to dietary deficiency but rather to chronic blood loss, as from ulcers, and to decreased absorption as a result of reduced hydrochloric acid secretion.[3]

Vitamins

The elderly tend to have vitamin abuse as well as vitamin deficiencies. Many elderly persons consume a vitamin supplement and are predisposed to the various problems of vitamin toxicity.[4] They should be counseled about the unnecessary expense of consuming vitamin supplements if they eat an adequate diet and the problems with vitamin toxicity (see Chapter 6 for details).

The elderly may be deficient in B complex vitamins due to inadequate consumption of fruits and vegetables. Others are deficient because they overuse laxatives or have impaired secretion of bile. Thiamin and riboflavin are two B complex vitamins found in deficient amounts.[5]

Fiber

There are no RDA values for the amount of fiber in the diet. However, most elderly persons need to increase their fiber intake to help alleviate constipation and possibly to reduce the chance of developing colon cancer. As described in Chapter 3, the average American eats about 10–20 g of fiber per day; this must be increased to 25–35 g/day to be beneficial. The elderly should be encouraged to increase their fiber intake by consuming fruits, bread and cereal, and vegetables.

DIETARY PLANNING FOR THE ELDERLY

Dietary planning for the elderly is essentially the same as for younger people. It focuses on the Food Guide Pyramid and exchange lists. The elderly need to have a good understanding of these two food guides.

An essential component of dietary planning for the elderly is information about their living conditions (see Fig. 12-1), including whether they live alone, whether they have facilities to store perishable foods, and whether they cook only for themselves or others. Elderly persons who live alone are more likely to have an inadequate diet than those who live and eat with others. Determining the approximate amount of money spent each month on food is important before effective dietary planning can be done.

Once the above information has been obtained, the planning should not impose too many dietary restrictions, cooking restrictions, and changes in shopping habits. Too many restrictions and changes result in

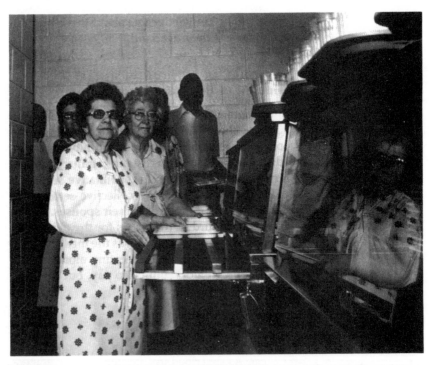

FIGURE 12-1 Elderly persons who live alone are more likely to have an inadequate diet than those who live and eat with others. (Courtesy Coordinating Council for Senior Citizens.)

less compliance of the elderly with the planning. The more active a role the person has in the dietary planning, the more likely he or she will be to follow the diet plan.

NUTRITION PROGRAMS FOR THE ELDERLY

Several programs have been established to help the elderly alleviate the problems of malnutrition and isolation. It is important for health professionals to be knowledgeable about these programs so that they can refer the elderly if they need aid.

Community Nutrition Programs (Title III of the Older American Act)

Community-based programs for the elderly are operated through state agencies. Major goals are to provide low-cost, nutritious meals, an opportunity for social interaction, nutritional education, shopping assistance, transportation, and counseling or referral to other social and rehabilitative services.

The meals are served in collective settings to individuals who are 60 years of age or older and to their spouses. They are designed to provide at least one-third of the RDAs for the elderly. The social atmosphere at the sites is almost as valuable as the meals. Elderly persons who associate with others, as opposed to eating alone, tend to be better nourished. The elderly are not required to pay, but they may contribute voluntarily to the meals.

Home-delivered Meals (Meals on Wheels)

In these programs, volunteers usually deliver hot noon meals to homebound elderly, feeble, or handicapped individuals. Frequently, a cold supper is left for those who cannot prepare their own meals.

SUMMARY

- Elderly are defined as people over the age of 65; in 1990 they encompassed percentage approximately 13% of the population in the United States; many experts predict that this will grow to 20% by 2030.
- Men and women in the 51+ age group should reduce their kcal intake by 600 kcal/day and 300 kcal/day, respectively, due to their reduction of REE; protein intake should be 0.8 g/kg/day; all the other nutrients remain the same as for younger people.
- Increased calcium is recommended for the elderly to reduce osteoporosis.
- High-fiber diets are recommended for the elderly to reduce constipation and possibly to reduce chances of colon cancer.
- Dietary planning for the elderly is built on the same basic guidelines as for younger people or utilizes the exchange system or the Food Guide Pyramid plan.
- Nutritional programs for the elderly include community nutrition programs, which are for people 60 years of age or older and provide at least one-third of the RDAs for the elderly; home-delivered meals (Meals on Wheels) are available for people who are homebound, feeble, or handicapped.

REVIEW QUESTIONS

True (A) or False (B)

1. The elderly are increasing in numbers as well as using a large percentage of health services. (T)
2. The RDA values for nutrient requirements for the elderly are very different from those of younger people. (F)
3. Most nutritional authorities recommend that the elderly decrease their protein consumption to approximately one-half that of the RDA value. (F)
4. Even though elderly persons' bones are not growing, it is recommended that they increase their calcium consumption to reduce the risk of osteoporosis. (T)
5. The elderly almost never exhibit vitamin excesses or vitamin toxicities. (F)
6. Increasing the fiber intake to 25–50 g/day may help the elderly avoid colon cancer and decrease constipation. (T)

Multiple Choice

7. Which of the following is (are) correct in regard to the elderly?
   1. decreasing in number
   2. many have poor diets
   3. have good diets
   4. use a high percentage of health care services

   A. 1, 2, 3   B. 1, 3   C. 2, 4   D. 4
   E. all of these

8. The nutrient needs of the elderly are _____.
   1. decreased kilocalories below RDA values
   2. carbohydrates should be 50% of daily kilocalories
   3. increased protein above RDA values
   4. reduction in calcium below RDA values

   A. 1, 2, 3   B. 1, 3   C. 2, 4   D. 4
   E. all of these

9. Increased protein intake in the elderly is important for _____ and _____.
   A. tissue synthesis—increased peristalsis
   B. counteracting illness—effects of medications
   C. increased metabolism—countering mental confusion
   D. none of these

10. Increased intake of calcium is recommended for the elderly to _____.
    A. improve the healing of bone fractures
    B. reduce senility
    C. decrease osteoporosis
    D. reduce edema

11. Dietary planning for the elderly involves _____.
    A. the Food Guide Pyramid exchange lists, and few restrictions
    B. extensive changes in nutrient intakes, shopping habits, and food preparation
    C. the Geriatic Food Plan, exchanges for the elderly, and dietetic foods
    D. none of these

Completion

12. Discuss why increased calcium intake is recommended for the elderly.
13. Describe the importance of high-fiber diets for the elderly.

CRITICAL THINKING CHALLENGE

1. Discuss the nutrient needs of the elderly and the impact social and financial constraints have on their ability to meet their needs.
2. Which statement by an elderly client best increases the rate of compliance with a dietary plan?
   a. "I live alone and I can still take care of myself."
   b. "I have a place to cook. A couple of us old folks share a kitchen."
   c. "I'm glad they've come out with all these canned products since my refrigerator isn't dependable."
   d. "Working with the diet lady has helped me understand what I need to eat."
3. Describe the community nutrition programs that are operated in your community by state and private agencies.

REVIEW QUESTIONS FOR NCLEX

Situation. A 65-year-old woman asks you to discuss her nutrient needs at this age. She tells you that she has always been concerned about her diet and wants to be sure that she is knowledgeable about the diet for an elderly person.

1. Elderly need fewer kcal than younger people and the main reason is _____.
   A. their digestive system cannot secrete adequate amounts of enzymes
   B. primarily due to a decrease in muscle and organ tissues
   C. their level of ATP is lower
   D. their appetite is lower
2. The calcium needs of the elderly is _____ younger people and the reason is _____.
   A. the same to higher than; to decrease chances of developing osteoporosis
   B. lower than; to decrease chances of forming kidney stones since their kidneys are less functional
   C. much higher than; to provide calcium for cellular membrane transport

   D. same as; that there is no difference in calcium needs between younger and elderly people
3. Iron intake in elderly is _____ that of younger people and iron deficiency is often _____.
   A. much higher than; due to diet
   B. much lower than; due to not eating enough meat, fish, and poultry
   C. the same as; due to chronic blood loss such as ulcers
   D. very much lower than; due to large losses from the gastrointestinal tract
4. Elderly are often deficient in B complex vitamins and two reasons why are: _____ and _____.
   A. inadequate consumption of fruits and vegetables; overuse of laxatives
   B. inadequate secretion of enzymes; digestive tract cant absorb adequate amounts
   C. inadequate secretion of hydrocholric acid; narrowing of gastrointestinal tract where absorption occurs
   D. impaired secretion of bile; inadequate secretion of digestive enzymes
5. Fiber in the diet of the elderly should be _____.
   A. decreased in order to reduce loss of nutrients
   B. increased in order to reduce constipation
   C. the same as when they were younger since there is no need to increase it
   D. very low since it will hinder the digestion and absorption of various nutrients

REFERENCES

1. U.S. Department of Health and Human Services, Public Health Service. (1990). *Healthy People 2000: National health promotion and disease prevention objectives.* Washington, DC. DHHS.
2. Lecos, C. (1984, September). Diet and the elderly. *FDA Consumer,* p. 22.
3. Manore, M. M., Vaughan, L. A., & Carroll, S. S. (1989). Iron status in the free-living, low income very elderly. *Nutrition Report International, 39,* 1.
4. Boyle, L. (1990). Brown bag vitamin review for elders. *Journal of Nutritional Education, 22*(6), 310b.
5. Suter, P. M., & Russell, R. M. (1987). Vitamin requirements of the elderly. *American Journal of Clinical Nutrition, 45,* 501–512.

P A R T

III

THERAPEUTIC NUTRITION

13   INTRODUCTION TO DIET THERAPY

Upon completion of this chapter you should be able to:

1. Give the principle and purposes of diet therapy.
2. Give the four key components of nutritional assessment.
3. State the importance of the anthropometric measurements—triceps skinfold thickness and midarm muscle circumference.
4. State what specific nutrients are measured by serum albumin, creatinine height index, serum transferrin, and hemoglobin-hematocrit laboratory tests.
5. Name the three ways in which a diet history is important to patients.
6. Discuss the advantages and disadvantages of the dietary methods—24-hour recall, usual intake pattern, food frequency record, and food diary.
7. Recognize and list the characteristics, underlying causes, anthropometric and laboratory measurements, and length of time to develop marasmus and kwashiorkor.
8. Give the four components of a problem-oriented medical record.
9. State and describe what the letters of the acronym SOAP stand for in relation to progress notes in a problem-oriented medical record.
10. Describe the four possible modifications of normal diets.
11. Name the four ways in which hospital diet manuals are important.
12. Name the steps involved in the implementation of a nutritional care plan.
13. Describe the components involved in the evaluation of a nutritional care plan.

INTRODUCTION

In Part I, we discussed the basic principles of nutrition in relation to the human body. We also examined changes in nutritional needs during the human life span. Part III covers the nutritional needs of people when they are ill.

The chapters discuss the application of basic nutritional principles in clinical care. Readers must comprehend normal nutrition and metabolism before the principles of **diet therapy** will be clear, so they may need to refer back to the chapters on normal nutrition.

diet therapy The use of modified diets to help a person overcome or cope with an illness or interrelated illnesses.

It should be emphasized that information in this chapter refers to hospitalized patients; however, these principles also apply to people in nursing homes, private practice, community centers, outpatient clinics, and their own homes.

PRINCIPLE AND PURPOSE OF DIET THERAPY

Principle

therapeutic nutrition Nutritional care that is used to help a person cope with an illness.

Therapeutic nutrition is based on modification of the nutrients in a normal diet to help a patient overcome or cope with a specific illness or interrelated illnesses. It is essential that a student have a good foundation in normal nutrition and metabolism.

Purpose

The basic purpose of therapeutic nutrition (diet therapy) is to help restore homeostasis in a patient. Diet therapy is used in three ways to achieve this purpose:

- As a major means of treatment
- To prevent further illness
- In conjunction with other treatments

The care of hospitalized patients takes into account five factors that can affect their nutritional status:

Physiological. Almost any illness affects the physiological functions of the body. A therapeutic diet is designed to help correct physiological malfunctions.

Psychological. Hospitalization itself is a psychological stress that may cause people to become depressed or withdrawn. Children (particularly very young ones who cannot communicate well) need special help in their psychological adjustment to a therapeutic diet.

Cultural. People's cultural, ethnic, and religious background directly affects their values and attitudes about food as well as their reaction to illness and medical treatment. All of these factors have to be considered if a therapeutic diet is to be successful.

Social. Hospitalization takes people away from their family and friends and the sociability of meals with them. The food pattern and time of meals in the hospital probably differ from what they normally experience. Input and support from family and friends for a therapeutic diet may play a major role in the patient's adjustment.

Economic. Worries about the cost of the hospital bill, lost income from the job, or concern about when he or she will be able to go back to work can affect a person's appetite and acceptance of a therapeutic diet.

By recognizing the many factors that affect a hospitalized patient, the health team and patient can work together to plan a therapeutic diet that meets his or her unique needs.

IDENTIFYING AND PROVIDING NUTRITIONAL CARE TO PATIENTS

Two tools are used most frequently in identifying and providing nutritional care to patients: the clinical care process and the problem-oriented medical record (POMR). In addition to these processes, there are many specific tools that can be used, such as food exchange tables, food composition tables, and height–weight charts.

CLINICAL CARE PROCESS

clinical care process A series of activities (assessment, planning, implementation, and evaluation) used by health professionals to identify and meet patients' needs.

The **clinical care process** is identical to the four steps described in Chapter 1: assessment, planning, implementation, and evaluation. Table 13-1 presents a summary of these four steps.

Assessment

Assessment, the first step in providing nutritional care, involves a determination of the nutritional status of the patient. It includes four key components: historical data, physical examinations, anthropometric measurements, and laboratory tests. The data from each component are

TABLE 13-1 SUMMARY OF THE FOUR STEPS IN THE CLINICAL CARE PROCESS

Assessment
Identification of the nutritional status of a patient
  Collection of data by historical data, physical examinations, anthropometric measurements, and laboratory tests
Statement of the problem/nursing diagnosis

Planning
Establishment of goals, objectives, and specific activities for correcting nutritional problems
Nutritional care plan

Implementation
Putting the nutritional care plan into action
Providing an adequate normal or modified diet
Providing nutrition education and counseling

Evaluation
Measurement of the patient's progress
Evaluation of the effectiveness of the nutritional care plan
Modification of the plan based on the evaluation

Source: Adapted from *Nutrition: Principles and Application in Health Promotion* (2nd ed.) (p. 298), by C.J.W. Suitor and M. F. Crowley, 1984, Philadelphia: J. B. Lippincott.

difficult to interpret, but when the components are put together, a complete picture of the person's nutritional status emerges. The individual components of nutritional assessment will now be discussed in detail.

Historical Data

The first component of nutritional assessment involves collecting subjective historical data. The person's medical, diet, and drug history, when combined with the other three components, helps to complete the picture of his or her nutritional status.

In this chapter, the only historical data that will be discussed in detail is diet.

Medical history. The person's medical history (for example, any recent major illness or surgery) basically consists of the medical record or chart. When an examiner reviews this history, he or she is looking for important risk factors that can have either long- or short-term effects on the patient's nutritional status. Risk factors can affect nutrition by interfering with ingestion, digestion, absorption, metabolism, or excretion of nutrients.

Drug history. In the last few years, the importance of drugs and their interactions with foods have been recognized. A professional performing an assessment should inquire whether the patient is or has been taking any drugs. The amount and length of time should be noted on the drug history portion of the patient's medical record.

Diet history. The patient's history is important for three reasons. First, it identifies the patient who is at high risk of having or developing a nutritional problem. Second, it reveals which foods are acceptable to the patient in order to plan a therapeutic diet he or she will follow. Third, it serves as a check on the findings of the clinical examination and laboratory tests.[1]

subjective Conditions or changes perceived by the patient rather than by a health examiner.

Assessing the patient's diet history involves gathering **subjective** data on the quality and quantity of the diet, indicating history inadequacies or excesses. The interviewing skill of the history taker and the cooperation and memory of the patient are critical to the accuracy of the data gathered.

Several methods are used to determine food intake:

24-hour recall A recounting of the kinds and amounts of food consumed during the 24 hours preceding the interview.

24-hour recall. This is the most commonly used method and involves the person, or parent of a child, remembering the kinds and amounts of food consumed during the 24 hours preceding the interview. Table 13-2 is an example of a 24-hour recall form that can be filled out by a patient or by an interviewer for an illiterate person.[2]

Advantages

- It can be done quickly
- It is less frustrating to the patient to recall the diet for only 24 hours as opposed to a longer period of time

Disadvantages

- It relies on the patient's memory; therefore, accuracy varies
- The previous day's intake may not be usual
- It does not provide a good estimate of the quantity of food eaten, since it is difficult for many people to estimate quantities

usual intake pattern A recounting of the foods that a person first eats or drinks during the day.

Usual intake pattern. This method is similar to the 24-hour recall in that a person is asked to recall the first thing he or she usually eats or drinks during the day. Similar questions are asked until a typical pattern is established.

Advantages

- It gives a more long-term picture of food intake
- It is useful in verifying food intake when the past 24 hours have been atypical

TABLE 13-2 A 24-HOUR RECALL FORM

24-Hour Recall

Name:
Date and time of interview:
Length of interview:
Date of recall:
Day of the week of recall:
   1-M 2-T 3-W 4-Th 5-F 6-Sat 7-Sun

I would like you to tell me everything you (your child) ate and drank from the time you (he/she) got up in the morning until you (he/she) went to bed at night and what you (he/she) ate during the night. Be sure to mention everything you (he/she) ate or drank at home, at work (school), and away from home. Include snacks and drinks of all kinds and everything else you (he/she) put in your (his/her) mouth and swallowed. I also need to know where you (he/she) ate the food. Now let us begin.

What time did you (he/she) get up yesterday?

Was it the usual time?

When was the first time you (he/she) ate or had anything to drink yesterday morning? (List on the form that follows.)

Where did you (he/she) eat? (List on form that follows.)

Now tell me what you (he/she) had to eat and how much?

(Occasionally the interviewer will need to ask):
When did you (he/she) eat again? or, Is there anything else?
Did you (he/she) have anything to eat or drink during the night?

Was intake unusual in any way?   Yes   No
(If answer is yes) Why?
                In what way?

What time did you (he/she) go to bed last night?

Do(es) you (he/she) take vitamin or mineral supplements?
     Yes   No
(If answer is yes) How many per day?
                Per week?

What kind? (Insert brand name if known.)
Multivitamins
Ascorbic acid
Vitamins A and D
Iron
Other

(continued)

TABLE 13-2 FOOD FREQUENCY RECORD *(Continued)*

Time	Where eaten	Food	Type and/or preparation	Amount	Food code*	Amount code*

Code
H = Home
R = Restaurant, drug store, or lunch counter
CL = Carried lunch from home
CC = Child-care center
OH = Other home (friend, relative, baby-sitter, etc.)
S = School, office, plant, or work
FD = Food dispenser
SS = Social center, eligible senior citizen, etc.
*Do not write in these spaces.

Source: Barbara Luke, *Principles of Nutrition and Diet Therapy*, pp. 369–370. Copyright © 1984 by Barbara Luke. Reprinted by permission of Little, Brown and Company.

Disadvantages

- The same as for 24-hour recall

food frequency record A method that is used to determine how many times per day, week, month, or year a person consumes certain foods from the Basic Four Food Groups.

Food frequency record. This method is used to determine how many times per day, week, month, or year a person consumes specific foods from the Food Guide Pyramid (Table 13-3).[1] The data are analyzed by a computer and translated into an average daily nutritional intake. The data can then be analyzed to determine whether the person is consuming the proper amounts of food from the four food groups or whether the diet is inadequate.

TABLE 13-3 FOOD FREQUENCY RECORD

Food Frequency Checklist

Directions: Indicate how often you eat each food item listed below, in terms of number of times consumed per week, number of times per month, seldom, or never. List the type of food, where appropriate.

Food Item	*Type*	*How often*
Meat		
Fish		
Poultry		
Eggs		
Lunch meats		
Pizza		
Peanut butter		
Dried peas and beans		
Nuts		
Milk		
Yogurt		
Cheese		
Milk desserts		
Citrus fruit or juice		
Dried fruit		
Other fruit		
Leafy green vegetables		
Dark yellow vegetables		
Potatoes		
Other vegetables		
Bread		
Cereal		
Pasta		
Rice		
Other grains		
Butter/margarine		
Oil/salad dressing		
Bacon and sausage		
Fried foods		
Cream (sweet or sour)		
Sweets		
Sugar/sugar substitute		
Snack foods		
Salt/salt substitute		
Carbonated beverages/fruit drinks		
Alcoholic beverages		
Coffee/tea		

Other foods not listed that you eat regularly

Source: Dudek, S. G. (1987) *Nutrition Handbook for Nursing Practice*, Philadelphia, Lippincott.

Advantages

- It helps pinpoint nutrients that are excessive or deficient in the diet

Disadvantages

- It is very time-consuming
- It requires a trained interviewer
- It requires a computer or hand-calculated analysis

Food diary. This method involves the person's keeping a written record of the food consumed for a specified period of time and the factors associated with intake (time of day, place eaten, mood, etc.) (Figure 9-9). A 3-day diary is usually appropriate for people whose intake does not vary significantly from day to day (infants, school-aged children, and most adults). A 7-day or longer diary may be needed for people whose intake is more variable (obese people and adolescents).

Advantages

- The diary keeper plays an active role and may begin to see and understand his or her own food habits
- Professionals get a good idea of the patient's lifestyle and factors that influence his or her diet
- It helps determine the foods to which the person has allergies

Disadvantages

- There is poor compliance with recording of information
- It yields qualitative rather than quantitative data
- The patient can unconsciously change his or her eating habits during the time the diary is kept

Analysis of Dietary Data. Once dietary information has been gathered, it has to be compared to standards such as laboratory and anthropometric data. The standards in this case are the recommended nutrient intakes, which in the United States are the recommended dietary allowance (RDA) and the Food Guide Pyramid (see Chapter 2 for details on these standards).

The easiest assessment is to compare the patient's food intake with the Food Guide Pyramid. It is more difficult to compare the person's intake with the RDA values, since this comparison frequently involves converting household portion sizes to a weighed amount. Failure of a person's diet to meet RDA standards does not necessarily mean that malnutrition exists. The reason, as discussed in Chapter 2, is that RDAs are calculated to be above-average physiological requirements for each nutrient except kilocalories. Remember, also, that nutritional standards were developed for healthy people and nutrient needs are sometimes different for people who are ill.

Physical Examinations

overt Open and observable.

A physical examination involves observing and examining a patient. The observations are carried out in an orderly manner, focusing on one area of the body at a time. The purpose is to detect **overt** nutritional deficiencies or potential difficulties with ingestion, absorption, digestion, or excretion.

An examiner looks for physical signs and symptoms associated with malnutrition. Examination of the skin, hair, mouth, and eyes is particularly important. The reason is that physical signs of malnutrition appear most rapidly in body structures with a rapid turnover of cells. Table 13-4 lists areas of the body, their normal appearance, and signs associated with malnutrition.[3]

If suggestive physical findings and historical data are recorded, they should be pursued further by laboratory tests, anthropometric measurements, and dietary assessments.

TABLE 13-4 PHYSICAL SIGNS INDICATIVE OR SUGGESTIVE OF MALNUTRITION

Body Area	Normal Appearance	Signs Associated with Malnutrition
Hair	Shiny; firm; not easily plucked	Lack of natural shine; hair dull and dry; thin and sparse; fine, silky, and straight; color changes; can be easily plucked
Face	Skin color uniform; smooth, pink, healthy appearance; not swollen	Skin color loss; skin dark over cheeks and under eyes; lumpiness or flakiness of skin of nose and mouth; swollen face; enlarged parotid glands; scaling of skin around nostrils
Eyes	Bright, clear, shiny; no sores at corners of eyelids; membranes a healthy pink and moist; no prominent blood vessels or mounds of tissue or sclera	Eye membranes are pale or red; redness and fissuring of eyelid corners; dryness of eye membranes; dull appearance of cornea; softness of cornea; scar on cornea; ring of fine blood vessels around cornea
Lips	Smooth; not chapped or swollen	Redness and swelling of mouth or lips, especially at corners of mouth

(continued)

TABLE 13-4 *(Continued)*

Body Area	Normal Appearance	Signs Associated with Malnutrition
Tongue	Deep red; not swollen or smooth	Swelling; scarlet and raw tongue; purplish color of tongue; smooth tongue; swollen sores; hyperemic and hypertrophic papillae; atrophic papillae
Teeth	No cavities; no pain; bright	May be missing or erupting abnormally; gray or black spots; cavities
Gums	Healthy; red; do not bleed; not swollen	"Spongy" and bleed easily; recede
Glands	Face not swollen	Thyroid enlargement (front of neck); parotid enlargement (cheeks become swollen)
Skin	No signs of rashes, swellings, dark or light spots	Dryness of skin; sandpaper feel of skin; flakiness of skin; skin swollen and dark; red swollen pigmentation of exposed areas; excessive lightness or darkness of skin; black and blue marks due to skin bleeding; lack of fat under skin
Nails	Firm; pink	Nails are spoon-shaped; brittle, ridged nails
Muscular and skeletal systems	Good muscle tone; some fat under skin; can walk or run without pain	Muscles have "wasted" appearance; baby's skull bones are thin and soft; round swelling of front and side of head; swelling of ends of bones; small bumps on both side of chest wall (on ribs)—beading of ribs; baby's soft spot on head does not harden at proper time; knock knees or bow legs; bleeding into muscle; person cannot get up or walk properly
Internal systems Cardiovascular	Normal heart rate and rhythm; no murmurs or abnormal rhythms; normal blood pressure for age	Rapid heart rate; enlarged heart; abnormal rhythm; elevated blood pressure
Gastrointestinal	No palpable organs or masses (in children, however, liver edge may be palpable)	Liver enlargement; enlargement of spleen (usually indicates other associated diseases)
Nervous	Psychological stability; normal reflexes	Mental irritability and confusion; burning and tingling of hands and feet; loss of position and vibratory sense; weakness and tenderness of muscles (may result in inability to walk); decrease and loss of ankle and knee reflexes

Source: From *Introductory Nutrition and Diet Therapy* by M. M. Eschleman, 1992, Philadelphia: Lippincott/Harper & Row. Reprinted by permission.

Anthropometric Measurements

body size Height and weight.

body composition The percentage of total body weight that is composed of fat, muscle, and water.

objective Observable or measurable phenomena.

Anthropometric measurements, the third component of nutritional assessment, involves measurements of **body size** (height, weight) and **body composition** (fat, muscle, water). These measurements are relatively **objective** and are simple and inexpensive methods of assessing, in particular, the patient's protein and calorie reserves. In order to determine whether or not anthropometric measurements for an individual are normal, they must be compared with standards specific for sex and age. Some of these standards are presented in this text.

Anthropometric measurements can be used in two ways:

- They can be used to compare an individual's nutritional status with that of the population as a whole.
- Repeated measurements over a period of time can provide record of changes in the individual's nutritional status.

Some of the more common measurements and what they measure are as follows:

Height and weight. These two measurements are the most useful indicators of nutritional status, especially underweight, overweight, and obesity (see Chapter 9 for standards).

Recent weight loss exceeding 10% of the usual weight indicates a need for extensive nutritional assessment and possibly aggressive measures of nutritional support. In order to determine this 10% weight loss, a valuable measurement is the percent **usual body weight (% UBW):**

Usual body weight (UBW) The normal or usual weight of a person.

$$\% \text{ UBW} = \frac{\text{actual weight}}{\text{usual weight}} \times 100$$

which determines what is normal for each individual. This is an especially important measurement for obese people, since malnutrition may be overlooked if weight measurements are based on ideal body weight only.[4]

In addition to measuring height and weight in children, head and chest circumference measurements are important in determining growth.

triceps skinfold thickness Measurement of skin thickness over the triceps brachii muscle, a good indicator of overall fatness.

Triceps skinfold thickness. This is an indirect measurement of body fat or calorie reserves. It is considered to be a good indicator of overall fatness, since about 50% of body fat is located subcutaneously. The technique involves the use of calipers and is illustrated in Figure 9-3. The measurements can be compared with standards to determine if a person is normal, overweight, or obese.

One important difference between the skinfold measurement and body weight is that it measures actual gain or loss of body fat. A change in body weight frequently is the result of water loss or retention, and not necessarily a change in the amount of body fat.

Midarm muscle circumference (MAMC) A measurement of the circumference of the arm. Usually done approximately midway between the shoulder and elbow. Using the formula, it is a good indicator of lean body or muscle mass.

Midarm Muscle Circumference (MAMC). This measurement is an indirect indicator of lean body or muscle mass. The contribution of the underlying fat tissue is then determined by using the following formula:

$$MAMC = arm\ circumference\ (cm) - (3.14 \times skinfold)\ (cm)$$

Again, these measurements should be compared to standard values or plotted on reference graphs.

Anthropometry in Children. Anthropometric measurements are especially useful in children to detect abnormal growth patterns. The rate of change in body stature or structure occurs more rapidly and makes detection of the problem easier.

In severely malnourished children, a radiographic examination of the hand and wrist aids in determining the biologic age of the child, since malnutrition can severely retard the biologic age.

Laboratory Assessment

intrinsic Functional substances in blood or urine.

Laboratory tests, the last component of assessment, provide current information about the nutritional status inside the body, whereas anthropometric measurements concern changes that have already occurred. Laboratory tests measure the level of nutritional, excretory, and **intrinsic** substances in blood and urine.

The main purpose of laboratory assessment is to detect marginal nutritional deficiencies before the onset of overt clinical signs. Laboratory tests today are very important in detecting protein-calorie malnutrition (PCM). Interpretation of test results must be done very carefully and can be used with more confidence when supportive information such as diet history, clinical symptoms, and anthropometric measurements are available.

Some of the more common laboratory measurements and comments about them are listed below.

Nutrient Measured	Test	Comments
Protein visceral	Serum albumin	Useful indicator of prolonged protein depletion
		Can decrease significantly in 10 days or less in patients in catabolic stress who are receiving only 5% dextrose
		Decreases in albumin levels can also occur in liver disease, renal disease, and congestive heart failure

Nutrient Measured	Test	Comments
Skeletal muscle mass	**Creatinine height index**	Reflects amount of skeletal muscle mass
		Reliable test assumes normal renal function, since renal disease lowers amount of creatinine excreted in urine
		Not a very practical test for nutritional screening, since a 24-hour urine collection is needed
		Decrease in creatinine with loss of lean body mass accompanies PCM
Protein that transports iron	**Serum transferrin**	Main function of this protein is transport of iron
		Considered to be a more sensitive indicator of PCM than the serum albumin test
		Elevated values occur in iron deficiency, pregnancy, **hypoxia**, and chronic blood loss
		Decreased values occur in pernicious anemia, chronic infection, liver disease, protein malnutrition, and iron overload[6,8]
Iron	Hemoglobin and hematocrit	Both measure the level of iron, with hemoglobin being a more direct measurement of iron deficiency than hematocrit
		Decreased values occur in hemorrhage, anemia, and PCM
		Elevated values occur in dehydration and polycythemia

creatinine height index A laboratory test that measures the amount of creatinine excreted in the urine. Creatinine results from muscle metabolism; therefore, it is indicative of the skeletal muscle mass.

serum transferrin test A test that measures the amount of globulin protein that transports iron; a sensitive indicator of PCM.

hypoxia A decreased amount of oxygen available to the tissues.

Other laboratory tests that can be used to assess nutritional status are as follows:

Minerals: iron, calcium, and iodine

Blood lipids: cholesterol, triglycerides

Enzymes implicated in heart disease and liver disease

Blood-forming nutrients: folic acid, vitamins B_6 and B_{12}

Water-soluble vitamins: thiamin, riboflavin, niacin, and ascorbic acid

Fat-soluble vitamins: A, D, E, and K

Stool tests for occult blood and fat

Tests for immunologic function

Laboratory assessment definitely has advantages in determining the nutritional status of a patient, but there are some disadvantages as well. One disadvantage is the high cost of laboratory tests. These expenses need to be considered in the context of maintaining a reduced cost of health care for the general population. Another disadvantage is the danger of a negative reaction by the patient to having blood drawn and possible infection.

Nutritional Status of Hospitalized Patients and Iatrogenic Malnutrition

iatrogenic malnutrition
Physician-induced malnutrition.

Practitioners over the years have not done a detailed assessment of their patients' nutritional status, nor have they considered the effect of nutrition in increasing recovery time. Therefore, many hospitalized patients have experienced **iatrogenic malnutrition.** This term should not be interpreted as malicious intent or as a disregard for the patient's welfare. It generally results from a reduced emphasis on principles of nutrition, with an accompanying overemphasis on medical technology or pharmacologic treatment.

Malnutrition may occur in hospitalized patients in as little as 2 weeks, as evidenced by a 20 to 79% decrease in vitamins A and C, serum albumin level, hemoglobin, hematocrit, weight loss, and midarm muscle circumference. Often patients have been found to have a decreased nutritional status at the time of hospital discharge.

Protein-Calorie Malnutrition (PCM)

Studies of hospitalized patients performed during the last 10 years have revealed the presence of PCM in one-fourth to one-half of the medical-surgical populations. The major complications produced by PCM include slow wound healing and increased chances of infection. If a high priority is placed on identification, treatment, and prevention of PCM, it is possible to prevent a long, unnecessary hospital stay. The characteristics of patients who are at a high risk of developing PCM are listed in Table 13-5.

Some factors contributing to PCM include the following:

- Surviving long trauma that contributes to exhausted nutritional reserves
- Failure to assess the patient's ability to heal and resist complications
- Premature dependence on antibiotics, discounting the body's ability to resist infections[5]

There are three main types of PCM (see Chapter 5 for details on the symptoms of these conditions):

TABLE 13-5 CHARACTERISTICS OF PATIENTS AT RISK OF DEVELOPING PCM

1. Below 80% or above 120% of standard body weight
2. Rapid weight loss of 10% or more
3. Long periods on simple intravenous solutions without oral nutrient intake
4. Alcoholism
5. Conditions contributing to nutrient loss, such as:
   Malabsorption syndromes
   Short-gut syndromes and fistulas
   Renal dialysis
   Draining abcesses
6. Hypermetabolic conditions such as:
   Burns
   Infection
   Trauma
   Prolonged fever
7. Drug/nutrient interactions, particularly with:
   Steroids
   Antitumor agents
   Immunosuppressants
8. Clear liquid diet for more than 5 days
9. Recent surgery/impending surgery
10. Obesity
11. Illness of 3 weeks' duration or more
12. Patient N.P.O. (nothing by mouth) restricted for diagnostic tests

Marasmus. This type generally takes months or even years to develop, since it involves both fat and muscle wasting. A long-term kilocalorie deficit is the underlying cause. This deficit initially results in depletion of the body's fat stores, followed by depletion of protein in order to supply enough kilocalories.

Laboratory findings are not altered significantly, and assessment is based primarily on decreases in anthropometric measurements such as triceps skinfold thickness (less than 3 mm) and MAMC (less than 15 cm).

Since this problem is more chronic than acute, the treatment needs to be started slowly in order to allow readaptation of the intestinal and metabolic functions. Mortality is low.

Kwashiorkor. This type of PCM is different from marasmus in that the primary underlying cause is a very low intake of protein but not necessarily a low intake of kilocalories. It frequently occurs in hospitalized patients with poor protein intake (such as those on intravenous, clear liquid, or full liquid diets for a long period) in the presence of stress such as illness or surgery. This protein deficiency condition is an acute problem and can develop in 2 weeks, as opposed to a chronic problem like marasmus (see Table 13-6 for a comparison of the characteristics of marasmus and kwashiorkor).

Unlike marasmus, with kwashiorkor laboratory tests are the primary component of assessment. Sharp declines in serum albumin levels (less than 2.8 g/dl) and lymphocyte count (less than 1,200 cells/mm^3) are two examples. The major reason why anthropometric measurements are not significant in assessing this condition is due to edema, which results from lowered serum albumin levels. Edema causes the person to have a fairly well-nourished appearance. Other signs indicating kwashiorkor include delayed wound healing and scalp hair that is easily pluckable.

Marasmic kwashiorkor. The combined state of marasmic kwashiorkor may occur when a malnourished patient is threatened by the stress of illness or surgery. This condition is life-threatening. The patient usually has a body weight that is less than 60% of the standard, edema, and a severely depleted weight-for-height standard. The patient runs a high risk of infection and other serious complications.[6]

Planning

As mentioned in Table 13-1, once assessment is completed, planning involves the establishment of goals, objectives, and specific activities for correcting nutritional problems. The end result of planning is a nutritional care plan.

TABLE 13-6 COMPARISON OF MARASMUS AND KWASHIORKOR

	Marasmus	*Kwashiorkor*
Underlying cause	Long-term kilocalorie deficits	Low protein intake
Time course of development	Months to years	Weeks
Anthropometric measurements	Triceps skinfold thickness <3 mm MAMC <15 cm	Not important, since person generally looks fairly normal
Laboratory measurements	Not important, since generally not changed from normal	Decreased serum albumin level, <2.8 g/dl Decreased lymphocyte count, <1,200 cells/mm^3
Physical signs	Starved appearance	Edema Easily pluckable hair
Mortality	Low	High

goal A statement of the desired outcome in a patient.

objective A statement of a short-term specific step to be used to help achieve a goal.

normal A diet that consists of any and all foods and provides the RDAs and adequacy by means of the Four Food Group Plan.

modified (therapeutic) A normal diet that has modifications of nutritional components.

high-fiber diet A diet that contains large amounts of fiber (greater than 40 g) such as fresh fruits, vegetables, and bran cereals.

clear liquid diet A diet limited to liquids such as broths, Jello, and strained fruit juices.

low-residue diet A diet low in residue and fiber; it is also called a *low-fiber diet.*

soft diet A diet modified in consistency that includes high-protein liquid foods and solid foods low in fiber.

high-potassium diet A diet that contains foods that are rich in potassium such as bacon, bran, instant coffee, and oatmeal.

low-sodium diet A diet that allows no salt in cooking or at the table; all cured and canned meats are also eliminated.

hiatal hernia A condition in which the stomach protrudes through an opening in the diaphragm through which the esophagus passes.

A **goal** is a statement of the desired outcome in a patient and is written in general terms. An **objective** is a statement of a specific short-term step to be taken to help achieve the goal. Examples of each are as follows:

Goal: gradual weight gain until desirable body weight is achieved

Objective: weight gain of 1 lb/week by increasing the patient's daily diet by 500 kcal/day.

The purpose of a goal is to provide a general direction to the health care team for correction of the patient's problems. Objectives, however, help the team to decide what specific steps need to be taken in order to accomplish the goal.

After the goal and objectives have been determined, the specific diet for meeting the patient's needs is written in the medical record.

Types of Diets

A physician will write a specific diet order based on assessment data. The diet will be one of two types:

Normal (regular, house, standard). This is the most frequently used diet. The only modification is a frequent reduction in kilocalories due to the patient's inactivity.

Modified (therapeutic). There are four possible modifications to normal diets:

- *Texture.* Consistency and fiber content are altered. **High-fiber, clear liquid, low-residue,** and **soft diets** are examples. The main purpose is to provide ease of chewing, swallowing, or digestion in order to rest affected organs. Gastrointestinal, postsurgery, and cardiovascular patients are examples of patients who commonly receive this diet modification.
- *Nutrient level.* Reduced or high-kilocalorie, low-fat, **high-potassium, low-sodium,** and high-protein diets are examples. Patients who commonly are prescribed a modified nutrient level diet are those with elevated serum lipid levels and kidney diseases.
- *Frequency of meals.* Three meals a day may be replaced by six small meals to reduce stress to the organ systems. Patients with ulcers and **hiatal hernia** receive this type of diet.
- *Exclusion of certain foods.* Foods containing lactose, wheat, and purines are examples. People who have lactose intolerance, gluten-induced enteropathy, and gout often receive this type of diet.

Initiation and Nomenclature of Diets

A physician orders a specific diet based on the assessment of the patient. The name of the diet should correspond to the name given in the hospital's diet manual. The diet order should describe exactly the nutrient modifications as opposed to being written in general terms. As an example, instead of a diet order reading "low sodium, high protein, and high kilocalories," it is much better if it reads "500 mg sodium, 120 g protein, and 3,000 kcal."

The actual formulation of the diet is done according to information in the hospital's diet manual. The manual generally describes which foods are allowed and not allowed together with the rationale for and adequacy of the diet. A sample menu is often included as well. In some hospitals the manual is compiled by the dietitians, physicians, and nurses and approved by the administrators. Other hospitals may adopt a manual from an association such as a state dietetic association. Hospital diet manuals are important in four ways:

- As a guide for the physician in prescribing a diet
- As a reference for the nurses
- As a procedural tool for the dietitian
- As a teaching tool for new health team members

Implementation

The next step in the clinical care process after planning is implementation. As Table 13-1 indicates, implementation involves putting the nutritional care plan into action, providing an adequate normal or modified diet, and providing nutritional education and counseling.

Providing an Adequate Normal or Modified Diet

Providing an adequate normal or modified diet is dependent upon the interaction of the patient, nurses, and dietary department of the hospital or health care facility. The success of any diet depends upon how well a patient accepts and eats it. In order to enhance success, it is very important that the nurses and dietitians determine what foods are acceptable to the patient within the guidelines of the prescribed diet. In large hospitals, this is frequently done by giving menus that allow patients to select food from three or more food items within the categories of appetizer, entree, vegetable, salad, bread, dessert, and beverage. Sometimes a diet may have to be individualized for a patient due to his or her social, cultural, religious, or ethnic background.

Providing Nutritional Education and Counseling

Education of a patient is an essential part of implementing the new diet. A dietitian is the most qualified person to provide nutritional education; however, the nurse has more contact with the patient and therefore plays a major role in education. There are many times when patient teaching can take place: at the bedside, during a treatment, or even in the community. Some important suggestions for educating a patient are as follows:

Treat the patient as an individual. Each person has different eating habits, knowledge about nutrition, and the ability to learn. The teacher must be a good listener and assess these points.

Help the patient see how the information is relevant to his or her goals. Most people will not learn nutrition information unless it is relevant to their daily or long-term goals. As an example, a boy who is active in sports may learn and accept his diet better if he understands it may improve his athletic performance.

Emphasize the patient's good food habits. Positive reinforcement of good eating behavior is more likely to be repeated than emphasis on bad eating habits.

Choose the right time to teach the patient. Patients cannot concentrate on teaching if they are under stress or upset. If possible, let patients decide when the teaching sessions will occur or tell them the schedule in advance so that they will be prepared.

Try to involve the patient actively. Nutritional information is retained better if a patient is actively involved in the learning as opposed to just listening to a lecture. As an example, a diabetic may learn more from being involved in the planning of an exchange diet as opposed to listening to a lecture.

Teach small amounts of material at a time. Most people can learn material better if only one or two points are covered in 15- to 30-minute sessions as opposed to several points in an hour-long session.

Teaching Aids and Materials

A patient generally will learn more if the teaching is enhanced with nutrition education materials or teaching aids. Many health agencies have printed and audiovisual materials that present nutritional information at different age and education levels.

The printed material often includes meal plans, exchange lists, diet teaching sheets, and schedules that are valuable to patients not only in the hospital but especially when they go home. It is particularly important for a patient who is receiving a therapeutic diet to be able to take home a written diet plan prepared by a health agency or the hospital.

Evaluation

Evaluation is the last of the four steps in the clinical care process. As mentioned in Table 13-6, this step involves measurement of a patient's progress, evaluation of the effectiveness of the nutritional care plan, and modification of the plan based on the evaluation.

Measurement of a Patient's Progress

Measurement of a patient's progress involves essentially many of the same anthropometric, laboratory, and physical measurements that are performed during assessment. An evaluation of how much a patient has learned about his or her diet and condition can also be made. Some examples are as follows: Has the patient lost the amount of weight that was prescribed? Is a diabetic's blood sugar under control, and does this person have a general understanding of the prescribed exchange diet and injection of insulin? Has a sodium-restricted diet lowered blood pressure, and does the patient show a knowledge of foods that are low in sodium?

PROBLEM-ORIENTED MEDICAL RECORD (POMR)

Problem-oriented medical record (POMR) A communication tool that focuses on a patient's health problems and the structuring of a cooperative health care plans to cope with the identified problems.

The **POMR** is the second general tool used by many hospitals and professionals in identifying nutritional problems and providing nutritional care to patients. This type of medical record provides a logically organized method for recognizing a patient's problems. It provides a patient-centered problem-solving approach to care, one that all health disciplines contributing to the care of the patient can use together.

There are four basic components of a POMR:

Defined data base. This includes the nursing history, assessment, physician's history, and physical examination.

Problem list. This list consists of problems that demand attention of a diagnostic, therapeutic, or educational nature. The problems can be socioeconomic, **demographic,** psychologic, and physiologic in nature.

demographic The study of human populations in terms of size, growth, density, and other vital statistics.

Plans. A care plan is established for each problem and should include further data that need to be collected, therapeutic measures to be implemented, and education of the patient and his or her family.

Progress notes. These are narrative notes made by all members of the health team that describe the patient's progress in dealing with his or her problems. The format for writing progress notes is known as **SOAP**, which stands for Subjective, Objective, Assessment, and Planning.

SOAP Subjective, objective, assessment, and planning. This is a format in which progress notes are written.

- Subjective data: record of how the patient feels, his or her concerns and his symptoms.
- Objective data: facts such as physical findings, laboratory data, and the patient's response to treatments and education.
- Assessment: professional interpretation of the subjective and objective data.
- Plans: revision of the initial plans or initiation of new ones based on subjective data, objective data, and assessment.[7]

Example of a Nutritional Assessment Written from Hospital Admitting Notes

The material on pp. 307–309 are hospital admitting notes and an example of a nutritional assessment. As you read and study this material, pay close attention to the following:

- Separation of the data into objective and subjective categories
- The analysis of the patient's daily diet
- How the plans are related to the subjective, objective, and assessment information

The following questions and comments are based on the information presented on pages 307 and 309. What subjective data indicated to the professional that this patient needed a more thorough nutritional assessment? If you look back at previous information in the chapter, you will see that the data are a loss of 22 lb (10 kg) in the last 2 months, diarrhea, and poorly fitting dentures.

What objective data indicated the need for a more thorough assessment? Again, a review of the previous information shows that the patient's current weight is 16% below his usual body weight and that he has poorly fitting dentures.

What specific anthropometric measurements would be important to verify the assessment of possible PCM? Since the patient's height and weight have already been measured, triceps skinfold thickness and MAMC are important to help assess this problem. If these measurements are well below normal, which laboratory measurements do you think should be ordered in order to reinforce the anthropometric measurements? Serum albumin level, transferrin, hematocrit, and hemoglobin are all good indicators of PCM.

Under plans of the SOAP chart, the suggestion of a high-calorie, high-protein diet is not nearly specific enough (as discussed in the chapter). If the anthropometric and laboratory measurements did verify the assessment of PCM, the attending physician would write specific orders about the diet and treatment.

For further practice and review of assessment and SOAP charts, please consult the review questions at the end of this chapter.

Name: Mr. XY   **Age: 69 years**   **Sex: Male**

1. Height: 5' 11" (177 cm).

2. Present weight: 132 lb (60 kg).
   Normal weight: 154 lb (70 kg), patient statement.

3. Lost 22 lb (10 kg) in the past 2 months, patient statement.

4. Upper and lower dentures fit loosely as a result of weight loss.

5. Likes all foods. "It's been hard to eat with my dentures slipping. I must eat softer foods now with my dentures, and I have diarrhea." Allergic to nuts, shellfish, coconut, chocolate.

6. Breakfast—0600   1 cup oatmeal with 1 tsp sugar, ¼ cup whole milk
                     2 slices white toast with 1 tsp margarine on each
                     2 cups black coffee

   Lunch—1200   ½ cup cottage cheese
                     2 canned peach halves
                     1 glass water

   Dinner—1700   1 cup macaroni and cheese (frozen, heated up)
                     ½ cup applesauce
                     2 cups tea with 1 tsp sugar in each
                     "I know I should be eating better, but I don't have much energy to fix much food. Nothing tastes very good right now when I know I'll be losing it in a few hours."

decubiti Bed sores or skin ulcers that result from interference with blood circulation to the skin.

lethargic Sluggishness, slowness, and sleepiness that often result from drugs.

7. Does not use alcohol or tobacco.

8. Problems with chewing and keeping dentures in place.

9. Thin; bones are prominent, with some **decubiti** forming on the pressure points; pale; **lethargic**; dry skin and hair; numerous bruises.

10. No history of therapeutic diet.

11. Stools—four to five per day for the past 2 months, very loose, black, foul odor; no pain on elimination.

12. Inactive, stays in room; very weak; afraid to go beyond living quarters with diarrhea.

13. Lives in an efficiency retirement apartment partially federally funded; a widower, no children; stove/oven, sink with running water, refrigerator; the building provides a housekeeper to come in once a week to clean; receiving pension and social security.

14. No previous operations or hospitalization.

15. No medications, vitamins, antacids, aspirin.

From the above patient information, the professional prepares the following SOAP chart for the POMR.

SOAP Chart

S: Subjective
Patient states he has lost 10 kg in the past 2 months because of severe diarrhea and no appetite. "Nothing tastes very good right now when I know I'll be losing it in a few hours." He states that the stools are loose, black, and have a foul odor. "It's been hard to eat with my dentures slipping. I know I should be eating better, but I don't have much energy to fix much food."

O: Objective
Very thin—5' 11", 132 lb, therefore 26 lb (16%) below usual body weight.

$$\%UBW = \frac{\text{actual weight (132)}}{\text{usual weight (158)}} \times 100$$
$$= 84\% \text{ or } 16\% \text{ below UBW}$$

Decubiti forming on pressure points, numerous bruises.
Poorly fitting dentures.
Stool specimen is dark, tarry.

1. Cachetic (general ill health and malnutrition), possible PCM.
2. From stated dietary recall, the patient's diet is deficient in all the foods from the Food Guide Pyramid except the bread and cereal group.

P: Plans
1. Request a dietary consultation (an interview of the patient by a dietitian) to do a more thorough nutritional assessment, including anthropometric measurements.

mechanical soft diet
Same as a soft diet.

2. Suggest a high-calorie, high-protein, **mechanical soft diet** with six to seven small feedings a day after diarrhea is under control. Until the diarrhea stops, suggest seven cans of a commercial milk-based nutritional supplement diet (Ensure, Sustacal, Isocal, etc.) every 24 hours, alternating flavors to meet patient's likes.
3. Multivitamin supplement.
4. Ascorbic acid.

etiology Cause.

5. Hold iron medication until the **etiology** of the dark, tarry stools has been determined.

SUMMARY

- The principle of diet therapy: therapeutic nutrition is based on modification of the nutrients in a normal diet; purpose of diet therapy: help to restore homeostasis.
- Four key components of nutritional assessment are physical examinations, anthropometric measurements, laboratory tests, and historical data.
- The triceps skinfold thickness is an indirect measurement of body fat or calorie reserves; the midarm muscle circumference is an indirect measurement of lean body or muscle mass.
- The specific nutrients measured by the following tests are: serum albumin for visceral protein; creatinine height index for skeletal muscle mass; serum transferrin for the amount of iron transported by blood; and hemoglobin-hematocrit for the measurement of iron in RBCs.
- A diet history is important to patients in that it identifies patients who are at high risk of having or developing a nutritional problem, it notes which foods are acceptable to a patient, and it verifies the findings of the clinical examination and lab tests.
- The advantage of using a 24-hour recall diet history is that it is quick and less frustrating to the patient; however, it relies on memory; the previous day's intake may not have been usual; and it does not provide an estimate of quantity of food eaten. The advantage of recording a usual intake pattern is that it is a long-term picture of food intake; the disadvantages are the same as for the 24-hour recall. A food frequency record pinpoints nutrients that are excessive or deficient in the diet; however, it is time consuming and requires a trained interviewer and a computer or hand-calculated analysis. A food diary has advantages in that it may help a subject to understand his or her own food habits; the professional gets a more complete look at a person's lifestyle; and the diary helps identify a person's food allergies.
- Marasmus is characterized by muscle and fat wasting caused by long-term decrease in protein and kcal intake. Indicators are decline in skinfold thickness and MAMC. Marasmus takes months to develop. Kwashiorkor is characterized by acute exhaustion of protein mass in internal organs; a major indicator is a sharp decline in serum albumin and lymphocyte count.

- Four components of a problem-oriented medical record are a defined data base, a problem list, plans, and progress notes.
- SOAP is an acronym that stands for: S—subjective data; O—objective data; A—assessment; P—plans.
- Four possible modifications of normal diets are changes in texture, nutrient level, and frequency of meals, and exclusion of certain foods.
- Hospital diet manuals are important as a guide for physicians in preparing a diet, a reference for nurses, a procedural tool for dietitians, and a teaching tool for new health team members.
- The steps involved in implementing a nutritional care plan are as follows: putting the nutritional care plan into action; providing an adequate normal or modified diet; and providing nutritional education and counseling.
- A nutritional care plan can measure a patient's progress and evaluate the effectiveness of his diet.

REVIEW QUESTIONS

True (A) or False (B)

1. The clinical care process, used in identifying and providing nutritional care to patients, consists of four steps—assessment, planning, implementation, and evaluation. A —true
2. In assessing the nutritional status of a patient, all that is required is to determine his or her dietary background. F
3. When doing a physical examination to detect nutritional deficiencies, an examiner is most interested in examining regions of the body where the turnover of cells is very slow. F
4. Anthropometric measurements are important for determining body size and composition. T
5. Triceps skinfold thickness is an anthropometric measurement of body fat or calorie reserves. F
6. Midarm muscle circumference (MAMC) is an indirect measurement of stored body fat. F
7. Laboratory tests measure changes that have already occurred, whereas anthropometric measurements measure the current nutritional status of the body. F
8. Serum albumin level and creatinine height index are both laboratory indicators of the quantity of iron in the blood. F

9. The serum transferrin laboratory test is a more sensitive indicator of PCM than the serum albumin level. (F)

10. Hemoglobin and hematocrit laboratory values tend to be decreased in PCM. (A)

11. The fourth and final component of nutritional assessment is historical data, which involves medical, diet, and drug histories. (F)

12. A 24-hour recall form, in determining the diet history of a patient, has the disadvantages of taking a long time to fill out and estimates the quantity of food eaten as opposed to the quality. (F)

13. A food frequency record in the diet history of a patient has the advantages of giving a picture of a person's lifestyle and food habits to a professional as well as determining to which foods a person has allergies. (F) diary

14. Iatrogenic malnutrition means physician-induced malnutrition and generally results from overemphasis on medical technology or pharmacologic treatment. (A)

15. The primary underlying cause of marasmus is long-term kilocalorie deficits, and assessment is based primarily on skinfold thickness and MAMC. (T)

16. Kwashiorkor is a malnutrition problem seldom seen in hospitalized patients, since they have an abundance of protein available. (F)

17. There are four basic components of a problem-oriented medical record (POMR)—a defined data base, a problem list, plans, and progress notes. (T)

18. Progress notes in a POMR are written in whatever format the professional chooses. (F)

Multiple Choice

19. The components of a nutritional assessment include:
    1. physical examination
    2. anthropometric measurements
    3. dietary planning
    4. laboratory tests

    A. 1, 2, 3   B. 1, 3   C. 2, 4   D. 4
    E. all of these

20. Which of the following anthropometric measurements and comments is (are) correct:
    1. triceps skinfold thickness: a good indicator of body fat or calorie reserves.

2. height and weight: recent weight loss exceeding 10% of the usual weight is indicative of a need for nutritional assessment.
    3. midarm muscle circumference: indirect indicator of lean body or muscle mass.
    4. anthropometry in children: not important, since they grow so rapidly.

    A. 1, 2, 3   B. 1, 3   C. 2, 4   D. 4
    E. all of these

21. Which of the following laboratory tests and comments is (are) correct:
    1. serum albumin: indicator of prolonged protein depletion
    2. creatinine height index: indicates the status of visceral protein in the body
    3. serum transferrin: protein that transports iron and is a sensitive indicator of PCM
    4. stools: examined for the presence of water and fat-soluble vitamins

    A. 1, 2, 3   B. 1, 3   C. 2, 4   D. 4
    E. all of these

22. Which of the following are ways in which a dietary history is important for a hospitalized person?
    1. identifies the patient who is at high risk of having or developing a nutritional problem.
    2. finds out which foods are acceptable to the patient.
    3. serves as a check on the findings of the clinical examination.
    4. indicates the patient's current dietary deficiencies.

    A. 1, 2, 3   B. 1, 3   C. 2, 4   D. 4
    E. all of these

23. Which of the following is (are) correct concerning methods used to determine food intake?
    1. 24-hour recall: good estimate of the quantity of food eaten
    2. usual intake pattern gives a good picture of short-term food intake
    3. food frequency record: very easy to do and less frustrating for the patient than 24-hour recall
    4. food diary: the person may begin to see and understand his own food habits

    A. 1, 2, 3   B. 1, 3   C. 2, 4   D. 4
    E. all of these

24. PCM can result from _____?
    A. protein deficits
    B. kilocalorie deficits
    C. surviving a long trauma that exhausts the person's nutritional reserves
    D. A, B
    E. A, B, C
25. Which of the following types of PCM and accompanying comments is (are) correct?
    1. marasmus: can develop within 2 weeks, and the underlying cause is very low protein intake
    2. kwashiorkor: can take months or years to develop, and the underlying cause is kilocalorie deficits
    3. marasmic kwashiorkor: characteristic of people who are obese but suddenly are not consuming adequate amounts of protein
       A. 1, 2, 3　　B. 1, 3　　C. 2, 3　　D. 3
       E. None of these
26. The components of a problem-oriented medical record (POMR) are:
    1. progress notes　　3. plans
    2. defined data base　　4. problem list
       A. 1, 2, 3　　B. 1, 3　　C. 2, 4　　D. 4
       E. all of these
27. The format for writing progress notes includes:
    1. subjective data　　3. assessment
    2. objective data　　4. plans
       A. 1, 2, 3　　B. 1, 3　　C. 2, 4　　D. 4
       E. all of these

Matching

28. subjective data
29. objective data

30. assessment

31. plans

A. iron deficiency anemia

B. decrease daily milk intake and increase intake of iron-containing foods

C. 17-month-old girl appears pale to mother recently

D. hemoglobin value low for 17-month-old girl; height and weight for age are only 75% of normal

Completion

32. Name and briefly describe the four key components of nutritional assessment.
33. Name and briefly describe the four possible modifications of normal diets.
34. Discuss what triceps skinfold thickness and midarm muscle circumference measurements measure.

CRITICAL THINKING CHALLENGE

1. A patient has the following values:
   a. triceps skinfold thickness = 2 mm
   b. midarm muscle circumference = 12 cm
   c. very thin appearance
   Determine whether this person has marasmus or kwashiorkor and give the possible underlying cause(s), time course of development, and mortality.
2. Complete the following chart by determining which assessment component each of the tests measure and identifying data that can be obtained by performing the tests.

TEST	ASSESSMENT COMPONENT	ASSESSMENT DATA
a. 24-hour recall		
b. appearance of skin, eyes, and hair		
c. triceps skinfold thickness		
d. serum albumin		
e. usual intake pattern		
f. height and weight measurements		

3. Your client states, "I can't see why I need to have all this lab work done." Your response is based on which of the following statements.
   a. Laboratory tests detect marginal nutritional deficiencies before the onset of overt clinical signs.
   b. The lab work is essential to confirm the subjective data obtained in the nutritional assessment.
   c. Laboratory tests are the only sure way to confirm nutritional deficiencies.
   d. Laboratory tests eliminate the need to complete the other components of the nutritional assessment.

REVIEW QUESTIONS FOR NCLEX

Situation. A 55-year-old male client is hospitalized with the following data: 5 feet 11 inches, actual weight 140 pounds, usual weight 160 pounds. Lost 20 pounds in two months. Dry skin and hair. Very pale. Has had four to five stools per day for the last two months. Very thin.

1. Using the percent usual body weight formula:
   % UBW= actual weight
   _____× 100
   usual weight
   his % UBW is _____ and is indicative of _____ extensive nutritional assessment.
   A. 20.5%; not needing
   B. 15.5% needing
   C. 87.5% needing
   D. 114.5% not needing
2. If you suspected the client might in a state of protein calorie malnutrition (PCM) then which of the following lab tests would be appropriate to verify this assessment?
   A. serum albumin
   B. cholesterol
   C. level of LDLs
   D. triceps skinfold
3. Which anthropometric measurements (remember, height and weight have already been done) could be performed to determine for sure if he is in a state of PCM?
   A. hemoglobin and serum transferrin
   B. triceps skinfold and midarm muscle circumference
   C. head circumference measurements and wrist measurements
   D. creatinine height index and hemoglobin measurements
4. Which of the methods given below is best for pinpointing specific nutrients this client's diet is deficient in but also requires a trained interviewer making calculated analyses.
   A. 24-hour-recall
   B. food diary
   C. food frequency record
   D. hematocrit level

REFERENCES

1. Clay, G., Bouchard, C., & Hemphill, K. (1988). A comprehensive nutrition case management system. *Journal of American Dietetic Association, 88*(2), 196.
2. Morton, G. (1990). *Nurse's clinical guide to health assessment* (pp. 43–50). Springhouse, PA: Springhouse Corporation.
3. Eschleman, M. M. (1992). *Introductory nutrition and diet therapy.* Philadelphia: J. B. Lippincott.
4. Mahan, K. L. (1992). *Krause's food, nutrition and diet therapy* (8th ed.). Philadelphia: W. B. Saunders.
5. Robenoff, R., et al. (1987). Malnutrition among hospitalized patients. *Archives of Internal Medicine, 147,* 1462.
6. Rossouw, J. E. (1989). Kwashiorkor in North America. *American Journal of Clinical Nutrition, 49,* 588.
7. Kozier, B., & Erb, G. L. (1991). *Fundamentals of nursing: Concepts and procedures* (4th ed.). Menlo Park, CA: Addison-Wesley.

14

ENTERAL-PARENTERAL NUTRITION

O B J E C T I V E S

Upon completion of this chapter, you should be able to:

1. Distinguish between enteral and parenteral nutrition.
2. Give four advantages of enteral nutrition.
3. Describe three common types of lique-fied formulas used in tube feedings.
4. Discuss three complications associated with tube feeding.
5. Describe the benefits of parenteral nutrition.
6. Describe the kilocalories, grams of nutrients, and importance of D_5W, crystalline amino acid (3.5%), and 10% fat emulsion solutions.
7. Define total parenteral nutrition (TPN).
8. Distinguish between peripheral TPN and central vein TPN in terms of who can benefit from each and the basic differences in the solutions infused by each method.
9. Describe catheter and metabolic complications of central vein TPN.

INTRODUCTION

enteral nutrition The movement of nutrients through the intestine into the blood.

parenteral nutrition The movement of nutrients that bypass the intestine and are infused directly into the veins.

The majority of hospital patients receive oral diets. In some cases, they may have to receive nutrients through a tube. In either case, they are receiving **enteral nutrition.** Some patients cannot receive nutrients except directly into their veins; these patients are receiving **parenteral nutrition.**

ENTERAL NUTRITION

Enteral feeding has the following advantages:

Intraluminal effect. The presence and absorption of nutrients help to prevent **atrophy** of the intestinal mucosa.

atrophy A decrease in the size of a normally developed organ.

Safety. There is less chance of infection and fluid-electrolyte imbalance if the gastrointestinal tract is used as opposed to direct infusion of the nutrients into the veins.

Normal insulin-glucagon ratio. Absorption of carbohydrates through the intestines helps to keep the blood levels of glucagon and insulin normal.

Reduced cost. Feeding by the enteral route requires less staff and equipment than parenteral nutrition.

Oral feeding is always the first choice in terms of enteral nutrition if the person is able to take food orally. If the person is not able to consume food orally but the gastrointestinal tract is functional, the next choice of enteral nutrition is tube feeding.

Tube Feeding

nasogastric Referring to a tube of soft rubber or plastic that is inserted through a nostril into the stomach. It is used to instill liquid foods or withdraw gastric contents.

esophagotomy Introduction of a tube through the skin into the esophagus.

People who have extreme anorexia, lesions of the mouth, inability to swallow, severe burns, or cancer of the gastrointestinal tract require feeding through a tube. The tube is inserted into the stomach or small intestine through various routes. The most common route is **nasogastric** (see Fig. 14-1), since no incision is required. Over a long period of time, this route can lead to irritation of the mucous membranes of the nose and throat. Therefore, for long-term tube feeding, an **esophagotomy,** a gastrostomy, or jejunostomy is preferred.[1]

The food administered is liquefied so that it can be easily digested and absorbed. Most hospitals use commercially prepared formulas that are composed of purified or synthetically made nutrients and are called

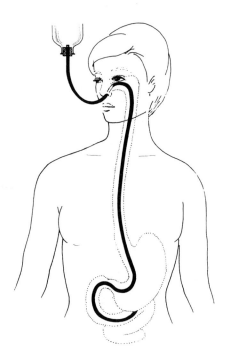

FIGURE 14-1 A nasogastric tube for enteral feeding.

chemically defined (elemental) diets Formulas that are composed of purified or synthetic nutrients.

viscosity The tendency for a fluid to resist flowing.

chemically defined or **elemental diets.** There are three basic types of tube feedings; they differ in osmolality, digestibility, kilocalories, lactose content, **viscosity,** and fat content.

Isotonic formula. This formula contains proteins, fats, and carbohydrates. It has a high molecular weight and an osmolality equal to that of the body (300 mOsm). Normal digestion is required for protein and fat. Isocal and Osmolite are two examples. They supply 1 kcal/ml. These two formulas are lactose free and are therefore appropriate for lactose-intolerant patients.

Elemental formula. This formula contains monosaccharides and amino acids but is almost totally deficient in triglycerides. It requires minimal gastrointestinal function and causes minimal pancreatic stimulation. Vivonex and Vivonex HN are two examples. They supply 1 kcal/ml. Due to the hypertonic concentration, elemental formula should be started at half strength or less and gradually increased to full strength.

Fluid restriction formula. This is a highly concentrated source of kilocalories and is beneficial for patients who have fluid restrictions. Magnacal is an example; it supplies about 2 kcal/ml. Due to the hypertonicity of the formula, it should be started at half strength and gradually increased to full strength.

These formulas may be fed as a **bolus feeding** or continuously by the **gravity-drip method**. The latter method has been found to be better tolerated, with fewer complaints of abdominal discomfort. Generally, about 1,000–1,500 ml (1,000–1,500 kcal) is given daily to maintain nutritional balance. Additional water is needed by most patients in addition to that in the formula.

bolus feeding Intermittent feeding of a formula as meals.

gravity-drip method A method by which liquid formulas flow slowly by gravity through a nasogastric tube.

Complications Associated with Tube Feeding

Patients sometimes experience complications due to tube feeding. Some of the more common complications and the reasons for them are as follows:

Diarrhea. This is the most common complication associated with tube feeding and is generally due to the formula being hypertonic or being administered too rapidly. Hypertonic formulas tend to pull large amounts of water into the intestines (remember that water moves from low-osmotic to high-osmotic fluids). Diarrhea can be reduced by initial dilution of hypertonic formulas followed by a gradual increase in the concentration as the small intestine adapts to the formula. Continuous feeding by the gravity-drip method also allows the intestine to adapt to the formula.

Lactose intolerance is a condition in which the body does not digest and absorb lactose, resulting in a hypertonic condition in the intestines. Lactose intolerance is common in adults and in certain postsurgical patients. In some populations, such as African Americans, Indians, Mexican Americans, Jews, and Orientals, the incidence may be as high as 95%. Some drugs can cause diarrhea. Therefore, drugs that do not cause diarrhea can be considered, or antidiarrheal drugs such as kaolin and pectin (Donnagel) can be administered.

Dehydration. Diarrhea can result in dehydration as well as hyperglycemia. Formulas that are high in carbohydrates can cause hyperglycemia, resulting in "spillage" of sugar into urine and large losses of water. The loss of water is due to the great hypertonicity of the urine as a result of the high sugar content. Diabetics are very susceptible to this problem. Administration of insulin and feeding by the gravity-drip method introduce carbohydrates slowly and lower blood glucose levels, thereby reducing dehydration.

aspiration pneumonia Regurgitation of the stomach contents and inhalation into the lungs.

regurgitation Backup of stomach contents through the esophagus.

Aspiration pneumonia. This problem results from **regurgitation** (backup) of the stomach contents and inhalation into the lungs. Unconscious, comatose, or severely debilitated patients are most likely to experience this problem. Reduction of aspiration is accomplished by elevating the head of the bed by 30 degrees during feeding. Gravity-drip feeding and introduction of the tube by gastrostomy or jejunostomy reduce the chance of developing aspiration pneumonia.

PARENTERAL NUTRITION

As defined previously, parenteral nutrition involves nutrients bypassing the small intestine and entering the blood directly. Parenteral nutrition is used in the following situations:

Unwillingness of the patient to eat. Anorexia nervosa patients frequently have to be fed by parenteral nutrition.

Inability to eat. Patients who are in shock or postoperative generally have to be fed parenterally.

Inadequate oral intake or absorption. Some conditions prevent patients from consuming enough food orally or absorbing the nutrients. Cancer patients undergoing treatment that interferes with gastrointestinal tract functions, people who have been severely burned, and patients who will not receive food for 7–10 days after treatment are examples of people who need parenteral nutrition.

If possible, physicians like to use enteral and parenteral feedings simultaneously in order to prevent atrophy of the intestinal mucosa.

Parenteral nutrition is accomplished by use of a **peripheral** or **central vein.**[2]

peripheral vein A vein near the skin surface in the arm and forearm.

central vein A vein located in the center or midline of the body; an example is the superior vena cava.

dorsum The back or posterior surface of a body or part.

dorsal plexus A network of veins located near the dorsal surface of the foot.

Peripheral Vein

The radial, basilic, and cephalic veins are the peripheral veins most commonly used. The veins on the **dorsum** of the hand and the **dorsal plexus** of the foot are also used if they are large enough (see Fig. 14-2).

FIGURE 14-2 Peripheral veins used in parenteral nutrition. *(a)* Arm and forearm; *(b)* dorsum of the hand; *(c)* dorsal plexus of the foot. (Reprinted with permission from B. Kozier, et al. *Fundamentals of Nursing: Concepts, Process and Practice*, 4th ed. 1991. Redwood City: Addison-Wesley.

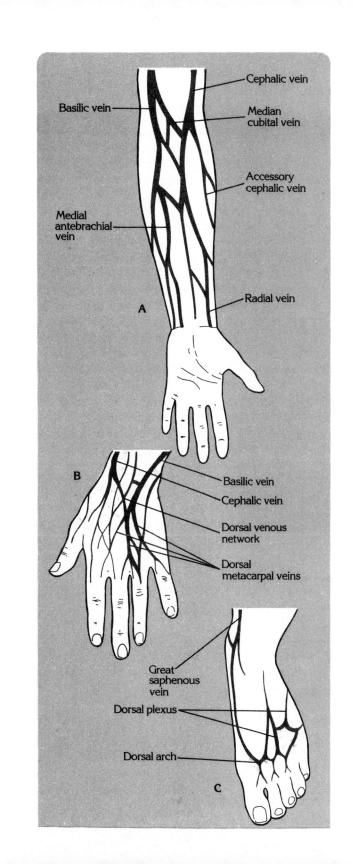

Cephalic vein

Basilic vein

Median cubital vein

Accessory cephalic vein

Medial antebrachial vein

Radial vein

A

B

Basilic vein

Cephalic vein

Dorsal venous network

Dorsal metacarpal veins

Great saphenous vein

Dorsal plexus

Dorsal arch

C

Advantages and Disadvantages

The primary advantage of using peripheral veins is one of safety. It is safer to infuse nutrients into peripheral veins than into a central vein like the superior vena cava or subclavian. The size of the **catheter** inserted into a central vein and entrance into the **thoracic cavity** increases the chances of infection compared to peripheral vein infusion. A disadvantage of using peripheral veins is that hypertonic solutions cannot be infused without causing complications like **phlebitis, thrombosis,** and **sclerosis.** Therefore, peripheral solutions can help most patients meet only their maintenance energy needs, not their repletion needs. Central vein infusion is indicated for patients who need more than 2,500 kcal for tissue repletion, such as those with major burns, trauma, and infection.

Peripheral Vein Solutions

Two common types of solutions infused into peripheral veins are **protein-sparing** and **total parenteral nutrition (TPN).**

Protein-Sparing Solution

A protein-sparing solution is beneficial for patients who have minimal or no protein deficits and are not **hypermetabolic.** Obese people have their protein stores protected but do not receive excess kilocalories. Specific examples of protein-sparing solutions are as follows:

D_5W. This solution contains 5% dextrose (glucose) in water or 50 g dextrose per liter (1,000 ml) water. The dextrose (glucose) used in parenteral solutions is **monohydrous** rather than the **anhydrous** form that is typically found in foods.

Monohydrous dextrose supplies 3.4 kcal/g rather than the usual 4.0 kcal/g. Therefore,

$$\frac{50 \text{ g dextrose}}{\text{liter}} \times \frac{3.4 \text{ kcal}}{\text{g}} = 170 \text{ kcal/liter}$$

As the calculation shows, for every liter of solution infused, a person receives only 170 kcal. Since 3 liters is the maximum amount of fluid that can be infused safely in a 24-hour period, a person would be getting only $3 \times 170 = 510$ kcal. However, 1,600 kcal/day is the basic requirement for an adult on bed rest. This figure is increased by fever and hypermetabolism. This deficit of approximately 1,100 kcal can result in the oxidation of tissue proteins for energy and a negative nitrogen balance. In other words, a kwashiorkor-type malnutrition may result from prolonged use of this type of solution.[3]

The 10 and 20% dextrose solutions, which are hypertonic, are fre-

catheter A slender, flexible tube of rubber or plastic that is inserted into a channel such as a vein.

thoracic cavity Chest cavity.

phlebitis Inflammation of a vein.

thrombosis Blood clot formation.

sclerosis Hardening of a vein.

protein-sparing solution A solution that supplies the needed kilocalories so that proteins can be spared as a source of kilocalories.

Total Parenteral Nutrition (TPN) Infusion of solutions composed of dextrose for energy, amino acids for tissue synthesis, fats for energy, and essential fatty acids plus vitamins and minerals.

hypermetabolic A high metabolic rate following problems like major trauma or burns.

monohydrous Containing one water molecule; an example is monohydrous dextrose, which contains one water molecule connected to a dextrose molecule.

anhydrous Lacking water molecules; an example is anhydrous dextrose, which is found in food.

intralipid A fat emulsion solution that is administered intravenously to supply essential fatty acids and kilocalories.

quently infused along with an **intralipid** solution to increase the kilocalorie intake and reduce the osmolality of the dextrose solution. Dextrose solutions with concentrations higher than 20% should not be infused through a peripheral vein.

Crystalline amino acid solution. This solution supplies a nitrogen source to help achieve a nitrogen balance. Achieving a nitrogen balance is very important in patients stressed by severe trauma, burns, and **sepsis** (pathogenic bacteria in the blood), since more than 75 g of tissue protein and 12 g of nitrogen (6.25 g protein = 1 g nitrogen) are broken down per day for energy.

sepsis Presence of pathogenic bacteria in the blood.

The recommended intake of amino acids for adults varies from 0.8 g/kg/day for nondepleted postoperative patients to 2.0 g/kg/day for hypermetabolic patients (with severe trauma or burns). A 70-kg man would need 56–140 g amino acids, depending upon his condition. *Crystalline amino acid solutions yield 1 g of nitrogen for every 5.9 g of amino acids rather than 1 g of nitrogen for every 6.25 g of protein.*

A 5.5% solution of amino acids supplies the following:

$$\frac{55 \text{ g amino acids}}{\text{liter}} \times \frac{4 \text{ kcal}}{g} = 220 \text{ kcal/liter}$$

$$\frac{55 \text{ g amino acids}}{\text{liter}} \times \frac{1 \text{ g nitrogen}}{5.9 \text{ g amino acids}} = 9.3 \text{ g nitrogen per liter}$$

Amino acid solutions are also supplied in 8.5–15% solutions.

Enough amino acids should be given to help achieve a positive nitrogen balance but not so much that **azotemia** (excess nitrogen in blood) occurs.

azotemia Presence of excess nitrogen in the blood.

Fat emulsion. Fat in parenteral solutions is a mixture of soybean oil (Intralipid) or safflower oil (Liposyn), egg yolk, phospholipid, and glycerol. *A fat emulsion looks like milk and supplies 11 kcal/g, whereas in food 1 g of fat supplies 9 kcal/g.*

A 10% fat emulsion supplies the following:

$$\frac{100 \text{ g fat}}{\text{liter}} \times \frac{11 \text{ kcal}}{\text{g fat}} = 1,100 \text{ kcal/liter}$$

Three reasons for including fat emulsions in parenteral solutions are that they supply concentrated kilocalories in an isotonic solution; they supply linoleic acid and prevent essential fatty acid deficiency; and they enable fat-soluble vitamins to be absorbed.

Fat emulsions are usually infused separately from the rest of the TPN mixture of dextrose and amino acid solutions. If a Y-catheter (Fig. 14-3) is used, both can be infused at the same time, but 2 pumps are required. Mixtures of the different nutrient solutions, called admixtures, are available and widely used because of their convenience. Mixtures with dex-

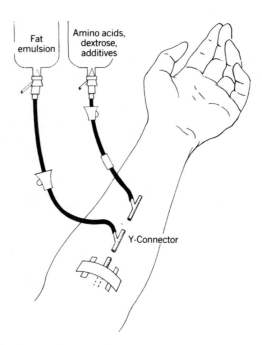

FIGURE 14-3 Tubing from a fat emulsion connected to amino acids, dextrose, and additives solution by a Y connector.

trose and amino acids are referred to as 2-in-1 formulas and mixtures with dextrose, amino acids, and fats are 3-in-1 formulas. As mentioned above, fat emulsions are usually infused separately because questions of stability and compatibility of 3-in-1 formulas still exist. In addition, there is a problem of the larger lipid molecules clogging the filter used for the glucose–amino acid solutions.

Some patients have adverse reactions to intravenous fat solutions such as chills, fever, backache, chest pain, vomiting, headache, and blurred vision. In anticipation and for elimination of these problems, a patient's liver functions, blood count, and plasma lipid levels are evaluated before infusion. Once infusion begins, electrolyte, **blood urea nitrogen (BUN)**, serum triglyceride, and cholesterol levels should be measured regularly.[4]

Blood Urea Nitrogen (BUN) Nitrogenous waste product formed in the liver when amino acids are deaminized (see Chapters 17 and 20).

Peripheral Total Parenteral Nutrition (TPN)

As mentioned above, intralipid and dextrose solutions can be infused simultaneously. In addition, electrolytes and vitamins can be mixed with dextrose and amino acid solutions. These mixtures meet all the body's needs or supply total parenteral nutrition, rather than just supplying kilocalories and sparing proteins.

TPN via a peripheral vein is suitable for patients who require nutritional maintenance for about 7–10 days. An example of a TPN solution infused through peripheral veins for a stable, nonhypermetabolic adult weighing 70 kg is as follows:

Solution	Nutrients	Kilocalories
1 liter crystalline amino acid solution (7%)	70 g amino acids, (11.8 g nitrogen)	280
1 liter dextrose solution (20%)	200 g carbohydrates	680
1 liter fat emulsion (10%)	100 g fats	1,100
Electrolytes and minerals in appropriate amounts[4]		2,060

An analysis of this TPN diet shows that 2,060 kcal is adequate to maintain a nonhypermetabolic 70-kg person. The 70 g of protein is higher than the minimum of 56 g (70 g $\times$ 0.8/kg/day). The fat emulsion supplies essential fatty acids. Appropriate amounts of electrolytes and minerals are also provided.

In essence, the diet should allow for maintenance of the person's tissues. However, if the person were hypermetabolic and needed **repletion,** as a burn patient would, the diet would need to be increased in kilocalories and amino acids and central vein TPN would be required.

repletion Restoration of body composition.

Electrolytes and Vitamins. The major electrolytes (sodium, potassium, calcium, magnesium, chloride, and phosphate) must always be a part of any complete parenteral nutritional support solution, regardless of the duration of therapy. Ideally, they should be added and decreased according to the individual's needs. Additionally, all the essential vitamins, minerals, and trace elements should be added to the solution just before infusion. In severe stress, the requirements for vitamins and minerals may be three times the recommended daily allowances (RDAs). Vitamins and minerals not added to the solution just before infusion are vitamin K, folic acid, vitamin B_{12}, and iron. They are not added because they interact with other vitamins or minerals, causing nutrient imbalances, or they precipitate with other vitamins and minerals and impair availability. They should be administered **intramuscularly.**

intramuscularly Within a muscle.

Central Vein Total Parenteral Nutrition (TPN)

central vein total parenteral nutrition   Infusion of nutrients through a catheter into the subclavian vein and their guidance into the superior vena cava.

subclavian vein   A vein in the shoulder region that is often used for insertion of a TPN catheter.

superior vena cava   A vein that carries blood from the upper part of the body into the heart. A TPN catheter is guided into this vein from the subclavian vein.

hyperalimentation   Feeding by hypertonic solutions (frequently 2,000 mOsm) that are infused through the central vein.

Central vein TPN refers to infusion of nutrients through a catheter into the **subclavian vein** and guided into the **superior vena cava** (see Fig. 14-4). In this chapter, the term *total parenteral nutrition* refers to any intravenous solution that contains dextrose, amino acids, and fats, plus vitamins and minerals, and can be infused into peripheral or central veins. Traditionally, when this term is used alone, it usually refers to central vein TPN. The term **hyperalimentation** is frequently used interchangeably with TPN.

Hypertonic solutions are infused so that a large number of kilocalories in a small volume of fluid can be introduced. A central vein is used for infusion, since it is large in diameter and the large volume of blood flowing through it quickly dilutes hypertonic solutions. Dilution of the solutions is important to reduce the chance of developing phlebitis, thrombosis, and other venous complications.

Who Should Receive Central Vein TPN?

Infusion of hypertonic fluids is important to achieve a positive nitrogen balance. In other words, these high-kilocalorie fluids permit both maintenance of tissues and repletion. Examples of patients who can benefit from central vein TPN are the following:

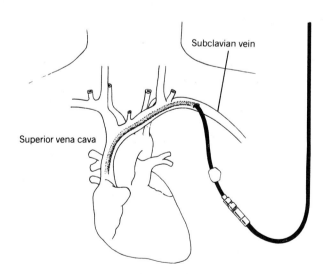

FIGURE 14-4   A central vein TPN catheter inserted into the subclavian vein and guided into the superior vena cava.

- Patients with severe burns
- Patients who require long-term parenteral nutrition
- Patients with protein-kilocalorie malnutrition
- Postoperative patients who cannot receive oral intake for several days
- Patients who have prolonged vomiting
- Patients who have prolonged diarrhea

anabolism A metabolic process whereby large molecules are synthesized from small ones.

The main advantage of central vein TPN, compared to peripheral TPN, is that it can be continued over a longer period of time. It is not usually initiated for periods of less than 2 weeks. In addition, it enables a person to achieve **anabolism** or repletion.

Central Vein TPN Solution and Administration

An example of a solution that may be infused through a central vein is 500 ml $D_{50}W$ plus 500 ml of amino acid solution (8.5%). The kilocalorie content is 850 plus 170, respectively, for a total of 1,020 kcal. The reason for using 500 ml of dextrose and amino acids, as opposed to 1 liter of each, is to dilute the solution. During the first 24 hours, the dilute solution is infused, allowing the person to adapt to the high glucose concentration and osmolality. After the first 24 hours, the kilocalorie intake is increased by 1,000 until, by the third day, the person is getting fat emulsion and full-strength dextrose solutions for a total of approximately 3,000 kcal per 24 hours. The final solution also includes vitamins and minerals, and possibly insulin if hyperglycemia occurs.[5]

aseptic Free from infection or infectious material.

hemothorax Presence of blood in the chest.

superior vena cava thrombosis A blood clot in the superior vena cava.

air embolism Air bubbles in the blood as a result of air leaks through a catheter.

hydrothorax Fluid in the chest.

pneumothorax Air or gas in the chest.

Catheter and Metabolic Complications of Central Vein TPN

The potential for complications with central vein TPN is very great. One major reason is that the catheter must be surgically inserted through the skin into the subclavian vein and then left in place for an extended period of time. A second reason is that the hypertonic, high-kilocalorie, high-fat solutions can cause metabolic imbalances. Sepsis is potentially one of the most serious complications. Septic complications are inversely proportional to careful monitoring and attention to **aseptic** catheter insertion, catheter dressing changes, and changes of IV tubing. Some complications related to catheter insertion and care are **hemothorax, superior vena cava thrombosis, air embolism, hydrothorax,** and **pneumothorax.**

Metabolic complications are also very possible. Examples are as follows:

Hyperglycemia. A temporarily elevated blood glucose level is common the first few days but then clears as the efficiency of glucose removal increases. Persistence of hyperglycemia suggests the possibility of diabetes, sepsis, and stress.

Hypoglycemia. A low blood glucose level usually results from interruption of TPN infusion.

hyperammonemia High blood ammonia levels.

Hyperammonemia. A high blood ammonia level results from impairment of liver functions.

hypophosphatemia Low blood phosphorus levels.

Hypophosphatemia. A low blood phosphorus level usually results from inadequate inorganic phosphate in TPN solutions.

Azotemia. Excess nitrogen in the blood may follow amino acid infusion that is excessive in terms of anabolic needs.

These complications are controlled when central vein TPN is closely monitored by a nutritional support service or team.[6]

TRANSITIONAL FEEDINGS

The interval when a patient changes from one form of feeding to another is termed the *transitional feeding* period. During this period, a patient's nutritional status can usually be maintained by overlapping the two feeding methods. As an example, if a patient has been receiving tube feeding, it should be gradually decreased as the oral intake of food increases.

Patients who have received central vein TPN for an extended period of time may have to proceed first to tube feeding and then to oral feedings. They are gradually weaned from one type of feeding to the other as their tolerance for each increases.[1]

SUMMARY

- Enteral nutrition involves the movement of nutrients through the intestine into the blood. Parenteral nutrition involves nutrients bypassing the intestine and infusing into the blood.
- Four advantages of enteral nutrition are the intraluminal effect, the safety involved, maintenance of the normal insulin-glucagon ratio, and reduction of cost.
- Three types of liquefied formulas are as follows: isotonic, elemental, and fluid restriction.
- Three complications associated with tube feeding are diarrhea, dehydration, and aspiration pneumonia
- People who benefit from parenteral nutrition are people who cannot absorb nutrients through the intestines, cannot ingest food orally, or those who need more calories for repletion of tissues than they can get from tube feeding.
- Total parenteral nutrition contains dextrose, amino acids, fats, vitamins, and minerals.
- Peripheral TPN is infused through the peripheral veins and provides enough nutrients and kcal for nutritional maintenance for 7–10 days. Central vein TPN is infused into a central vein; it provides a more concentrated source of nutrients and kcal and can accomplish repletion.
- Catheter complications from central vein TPN include hemothorax, superior vena cava thrombosis, air embolism, hydrothorax, and pneumothorax. Metabolic complications from central vein TPN include hyperglycemia, hypoglycemia, hyperammonemia, hypophosphatemia, and azotemia.

REVIEW QUESTIONS

True (A) or False (B)

1. Enteral nutrition involves the movement of nutrients through the intestine into the blood. (T)
2. Two advantages of enteral nutrition are increased insulin secretion and decreased thickness of the intestinal mucosa. False, T?
3. An isotonic tube feeding includes proteins and fat, which require normal digestion, whereas an elemental formula contains monosaccharides and amino acids, which require minimal digestion. (T)
4. The advantages of the fluid restriction formula

Magnacal are that it is an isotonic formula and supplies 1 kcal/liter. (F)
5. Constipation is a common complication of tube feeding due to hypotonic formulas pulling water out of the intestines. (F)
6. Tube feedings high in carbohydrates can result in hyperglycemia and dehydration (T)
7. Hyperglycemia and dehydration can be reduced by bolus feeding and decreased administration of insulin. (F)
8. Parenteral nutrition is tube feeding introduced directly into the stomach or jejunum (F)
9. The primary advantage of using peripheral veins for parenteral nutrition is that they are more accessible and fluids can be easily infused (F)
10. A D_5W solution is a protein-sparing solution that contains 50 g dextrose and supplies 170 kcal/liter. (T)
11. A 3.5% amino acid solution supplies 35 g amino acids and 5.9 g nitrogen per liter, which is important for severe trauma, burns, and sepsis patients. (T)
12. A 10% fat emulsion provides 100 g fat per liter and 900 kcal. (F)
13. A 10% fat emulsion cannot be infused simultaneously with dextrose and amino acid solutions because it makes the solution hypertonic and increases the kilocalorie level excessively. (F)
14. A total parenteral nutrition (TPN) solution is always infused through a central vein. (F)
15. The main advantage of central vein TPN over peripheral TPN is that it can be continued over a longer period of time and can help achieve repletion of tissues. (T)

Multiple Choice

16. The advantages of enteral nutrition are
    1. the intracellular effect
    2. a normal insulin-glucagon ratio
    3. infusion of hypertonic solutions
    4. safety

    A. 1, 2, 3   B. 1, 3   C. 2, 4   D. 4
    E. all of these
17. Which of the following is (are) not correctly paired for tube feedings?
    A. elemental formula—contains proteins, fats, and carbohydrates; isotonic and supplies 1 kcal/ml.   Need fat

B. isotonic formula—contains monosaccharides and amino acids that require digestion; hypertonic. *need bat*

C. fluid restriction formula—highly concentrated source of kilocalories; hypertonic and supplies 2 kcal/ml.

D. A, B, C

E. A, B

18. Conditions that can benefit from parenteral nutrition are
   1. anorexia nervosa
   2. shock
   3. cancer of the gastrointestinal tract
   4. malabsorption

   A. 1, 2, 3   B. 1, 3   C. 2, 4   D. 4
   E. all of these

19. A D_5W solution is characterized by:
   1. 50 g dextrose per liter
   2. protein-sparing solution
   3. 170 kcal/liter
   4. 200 kcal/liter

   A. 1, 2, 3   B. 1, 3   C. 2, 4   D. 4
   E. all of these

20. Three important reasons for including fat emulsions in parenteral solutions are:
   A. they provide concentrated kilocalories in a hypertonic solution; they provide essential amino acids; they enable fat-soluble vitamins to be absorbed.
   B. concentrated kilocalories in an isotonic solution; they provide essential fatty acids; they enable absorption of fat-soluble vitamins.
   C. they provide nitrogen for tissue repletion; they provide linoleic acid; they enable absorption of water-soluble vitamins.
   D. none of these

21. A TPN solution is composed of the following nutrients:
   A. dextrose, cholesterol, proteins, vitamins, and minerals.
   B. starch, fatty acids, proteins, minerals, and water
   C. sucrose, linoleic acid, proteins, minerals, and vitamins
   D. dextrose, fatty acids, amino acids, vitamins, and minerals

22. A TPN solution composed of amino acids (5.5%; 55 g/liter), 10% fat emulsion (100 g/liter), and dextrose (20%; 200 g/liter) contains a total of _____ kcal.

A. 1,920
B. 2,305
C. 2,200
D. 2,000

23. TPN solutions infused into peripheral veins differ from those infused into central veins by _____.
   A. containing amino acids, dextrose, fatty acids, vitamins, and minerals.
   B. containing fewer kilocalories and having a lower osmolality.
   C. containing more kilocalories and having a higher osmolality.
   D. containing dextrose only.

24. Two advantages of central vein TPN compared to peripheral TPN are _____ and _____.
   A. continued over a longer period of time—achieve repletion of tissues
   B. use of a less concentrated solution—less chance of hyperglycemia
   C. less chance of infection—easier access to veins
   D. none of these

25. Metabolic complications from the use of central vein TPN are:
   1. hypoglycemia
   2. hyperammonemia
   3. azotemia
   4. hyperglycemia

   A. 1, 2, 3   B. 1, 3   C. 2, 4   D. 4
   E. all of these

Completion

26. Discuss four advantages of enteral nutrition.
27. Distinguish between peripheral TPN and central vein TPN in terms of who can benefit from each and the basic differences between solutions infused by each method.
28. Give four possible catheter complications and four possible metabolic complications of central vein TPN.

CRITICAL THINKING CHALLENGE

1. Using the method shown in the chapter, calculate the following. Show your calculations. (Assume 1 liter of each solution)

% Dextrose/liter	kcal/liter
a. 10	
b. 20	
c. 50	

2. Using the method shown in the chapter, calculate the following. Show your calculations. (Assume 1 liter of each solution)

% Amino Acid Solution	kcal/liter	g of nitrogen/liter
a. 3.5		
b. 7.0		
c. 8.5		
d. 10.0		

3. A TPN solution is composed of the following: (Assume 1 liter of each solution)
   5.5% amino acid solution
   10% fat emulsion
   50% dextrose solution
   Calculate the total g of nutrients for each solution, the total kcal for all three solutions and g of nitrogen for the amino acid solution.

4. Contrast and compare enteral and parenteral nutrition. Address client needs, advantages, disadvantages, and possible complications.

5. Your client questions why he has to have a central line infusion started after the physician orders a hypertonic TPN solution. Which of the following statements will support your response?
   a. TPN should always be administered through a central line.
   b. Hypertonic solutions will always be infused as prolonged therapy.
   c. Vitamins and minerals should be infused in a central line.
   d. The volume of blood flow is important to dilute the hypertonic solution.

REVIEW QUESTIONS FOR NCLEX

Situation. An Oriental male client is hospitalized with mouth cancer and cannot chew or swallow food. His gastrointestinal tract is in a healthy state and functioning normally.

1. The best type of nutrition for this client would be _____.

A. parenteral
B. oral-regular
C. transition
D. enteral

2. A tube feeding formula that might be appropriate for this client is _____.
   A. isotonic
   B. elemental
   C. fluid-restriction
   D. protein-sparing

3. In order to reduce chances of diarrhea, in this Oriental male, his tube feeding formula must be devoid in _____.
   A. glucose
   B. lactose
   C. sucrose
   D. maltose

Situation. A 45-year-old, 120 lb (55 kg) ideal body weight, woman is hospitalized with 2nd and 3rd degree burns over 70% of her body. It was determined that she would need high kcal intake for at least 3 months to achieve repletion. She is placed on central vein TPN with 1 liter of each of the following solutions: 11% amino acid solution, 10% fat emulstion, and 50% dextrose solution.

4. The total kcal for this parenteral solution is _____.
   A. 2100
   B. 2400
   C. 3000
   D. 3240

5. This TPN solution will provide _____ g of protein.
   A. 51
   B. 61
   C. 81
   D. 110

6. Based on her needing 2 g protein/kg of ideal body weight, for repletion, will this solution provide this level?
   A. yes, 240 g
   B. no, 55 g
   C. yes, 110 g
   D. no, 35 g

7. The amount of nitrogen this solution will provide is _____ which is _____ to replace the nitrogen that is lost daily.
   A. 19 g; enough
   B. 9 g; not enough
   C. 29; not enough
   D. 10 g; enough

REFERENCES

1. Ignatiavicus, D. D., & Varnerybayne, M. (1991). *Medical surgical nursing* (pp. 314–324). Philadelphia: W. B. Saunders.
2. Phipps, W. J., et al. (1991). *Medical surgical nursing: Concepts and clinical practice* (4th ed.) (pp. 1257–1264). St. Louis: Mosby Year Book.
3. Kozier, B., et al. (1991). *Fundamentals of nursing: Concepts, process and practice* (4th ed.).
4. Rombeau, J. L., & Caldwell, M. D. (1990). *Clinical nutrition: Enteral and tube feeding* (2nd ed.). Philadelphia: W. B. Saunders.
5. Bennett, K. M., & Roseu, G. H. (1990). Cyclic total parenteral nutrition. *Nutrition in Clinical Practice, 5*, 163.
6. Lenssen, P. (1989). *Monitoring and complications of parenteral nutrition: Dietitians Handbook of Enteral and Parenteral Nutrition*. Rockville, MD: Aspen Publishers.

15   DIABETES MELLITUS

Upon completion of this chapter, you should be able to:

1. Define diabetes mellitus and describe its prevalence.
2. Describe the genesis or cause of insulin-dependent diabetes mellitus (IDDM).
3. Discuss the functions of insulin when there is a normal or increased amount and what happens when there is a deficiency of insulin.
4. Name and give the reasons for the symptoms associated with IDDM.
5. Describe the blood tests and values that are used to diagnose diabetes.
6. Give two advantages of the glycolysated hemoglobin (HbA_{1c}) test for checking diabetes control.
7. Name and give the peak period of activity for the three different types of insulin.
8. Define hypoglycemia, give four causes and five symptoms, and discuss how to correct it.
9. Describe the sequence of steps in diabetic ketoacidosis (DKA) that can ultimately result in death.
10. State what percent of the daily kilocalories should come from carbohydrate, protein, and fat in a diet for a person with IDDM.
11. Discuss the importance of distributing kilocalories and carbohydrate grams throughout the day according to the type of insulin used.
12. Describe the importance of a high-fiber diet to a diabetic.
13. Describe the general characteristics of noninsulin-dependent diabetes mellitus (NIDDM).
14. Discuss the genesis or cause of NIDDM.
15. Describe the sequence of steps that result in hyperglycemic hyperosmolar nonketotic coma (HHNK) and state how it differs from diabetic ketoacidosis.
16. Describe the dietary treatment of IDDM.

INTRODUCTION

Two common metabolic disorders involving altered blood glucose level are diabetes mellitus and hypoglycemia. Diabetes mellitus is the more common disorder; hypoglycemia can occur as a complication. However, hypoglycemia can occur in nondiabetics and will be discussed at the end of the chapter.

DIABETES MELLITUS

Definition and Prevalence

Diabetes mellitus is defined as a group of disorders that have a variety of genetic causes but that have in common hyperglycemia. It is a complex disease involving biochemical and anatomic abnormalities that will be discussed in detail in this chapter.

The term *diabetes* (excessive urine excretion) *mellitus* (honey sweet) literally means excessive excretion of urine with a sweet taste. Another type of diabetes is **diabetes insipidus** (without taste), caused by inadequate secretion of antidiuretic hormone; it is discussed in Chapter 20. The shortened term *diabetes* will be used in this chapter and text to refer to diabetes mellitus only.

diabetes insipidus A type of diabetes that is caused by inadequate secretion of the antidiuretic hormone (ADH).

It is estimated that 10 million Americans, or 5% of the population, may have diabetes. Studies also estimate an approximate 6% growth yearly due to the increased longevity of the population. Due to its complications (heart disease, **stroke,** and kidney failure), diabetes is the third leading cause of death after cardiovascular diseases and cancer. The potential for diabetics to develop severe problems, compared to nondiabetics, is tremendous. Examples show that diabetics have a rate of blindness 25 times higher, kidney disease 17 times higher, gangrene 5 times higher, and heart disease 2 times higher than nondiabetics.[1]

stroke A rupture or blockage of a blood vessel in the brain, resulting in loss of consciousness, paralysis, or other symptoms; it is also called a *cerebrovascular accident.*

TYPE I: INSULIN-DEPENDENT DIABETES MELLITUS (IDDM)

General Characteristics

Approximately 15% or less of diabetics have **insulin-dependent diabetes mellitus (IDDM)** or require injections of insulin to help control their diabetes. Some of the former terms for IDDM are *juvenile diabetes, juvenile-onset diabetes,* and *ketosis-prone diabetes.* The term *juvenile-onset diabetes* was used because it typically has an onset before the age of 20, with the average age being 12. (*See Case Study: Insulin-Dependent Diabe-*

Insulin-dependent diabetes mellitus (IDDM) A type of diabetes in which the person does not secrete enough insulin to control the blood glucose level.

Type I Diabetes—Caused by Milk?

Several correlation studies suggest that the protein in cow's milk might cause type I diabetes. Studies show that the protein in milk possibly triggers an autoimmune reaction resulting in type I diabetes. The studies are correlation studies and some of the findings are[1]:

Country	Cow protein intake	Number of Type I people/100,000
Japan	5 g/day	1
America	19 g/day	15
Finland	30 g/day	28

As the above correlation studies indicate, the greater the amount of cow's milk consumed, the greater the number of people that develop type I diabetes. Mothers in Japan breast-feed infants to a greater extent than those in America and Finland. In countries where a greater percentage of mothers breast-feed, the disease is less prevalent. In Polynesia women breast-feed and then wean infants to fish protein. Only about 2 out of 100,000 persons develop type I. Some animal experiments done with rats that have a genetic tendency toward type I diabetes showed more than half developed the condition when fed cow's milk. The rate of diabetes dropped significantly in the same rats when fed a diet other than cow's milk.[2]

Intervention studies—removal of cow's milk from diets of identified high risk type I infants—has yet to be done. These studies will be able to give a more conclusive answer as to whether cow's milk protein does cause type I diabetes.

REFERENCES

1. Scott, F. W. (1990). Cow's milk and insulin-dependent diabetes mellitus: Is there a relationship? *American Journal of Clinical Nutrition, 51*(3), 489.
2. Scott, F. W., Elliott, R. B., & Kolb, H. (1989). Diet and autoimmunity: Prospects of prevention of Type I diabetes. *Diabetes, Nutrition, and Metabolism, 2*(1), 61.

tes, pp. 356–358, for reinforcement of information on insulin-dependent diabetes.)

The onset of IDDM is sudden and occurs more often in children who have recently had a viral infection such as the mumps or flu. Apparently, the virus results in the destruction of **beta cells** in the pancreas, which secrete insulin. Hyperglycemia is a constant problem and can be controlled only by injection of an **exogenous** source of insulin.

A complication of hyperglycemia is **ketoacidosis,** which can result in a person going into a coma and even dying if the condition is not corrected.

beta cells   Cells in the pancreas that secrete insulin. These cells are often damaged in IDDM, causing an insulin deficiency.

exogenous   Outside of the body.

ketoacidosis   High blood level of ketones (acids).

Genesis or Cause

Much research shows that IDDM results from genetic factors (as mentioned in the definition of diabetes). The genetic factors indicate that some individuals have **genes** on chromosome 6 (a total of 46 **chromosomes** are present in each human cell) that produce certain types of **human lymphocyte antigens (HLA).**

The function of HLAs is, first, to recognize foreign material (e.g., bacteria and protein) and, second, to initiate the formation of antibodies, which attach to and neutralize the bacteria, thereby preventing infection. In other words, the HLAs help to provide immunity.

Certain HLAs, specifically HLA-B8 and HLA-B15, have been found in higher quantities in IDDM patients than in the general population. In addition, high levels of **islet cell antibodies** have been found, which attack the beta cells of the **islets of Langerhans** in the pancreas (see Fig. 15-1). Beta cells secrete insulin; therefore, their destruction and the ensuing insulin reduction result in hyperglycemia and the symptoms of IDDM.

There is much controversy as to what influences the development of islet cell antibodies. Some researchers believe that it may be due to viruses such as coxsackie B-4 (which causes upper respiratory tract infections) and mumps viruses. One possible sequence of events that may ultimately result in IDDM is the following (see Fig. 15-2).

genes   The portion of DNA molecules that contains information necessary to synthesize an enzyme.

chromosomes   Rod-like structures that appear in the nucleus of the cell during mitosis. The chromosomes contain genes.

Human lymphocyte antigens (HLA)   A lymphocyte (a type of white blood cell) that has an antigen attached to its surface.

islet cell antibodies   Antibodies formed in response to islet of Langerhans cell fragments.

islets of Langerhans   Irregular microscopic structures scattered throughout the pancreas. They are composed of alpha cells that secrete glucagon and beta cells that secrete insulin.

1. Coxsackie B-4 or mumps virus invades the beta cells of the islets of Langerhans.
2. Slightly degraded tissue from the beta cells is released into the blood.
3. HLAs recognize the degraded tissue as foreign and initiate the formation of islet cell antibodies.
4. Islet cell antibodies attack and destroy the beta cells.
5. Destruction of the beta cells results in decreased secretion of insulin followed by IDDM.

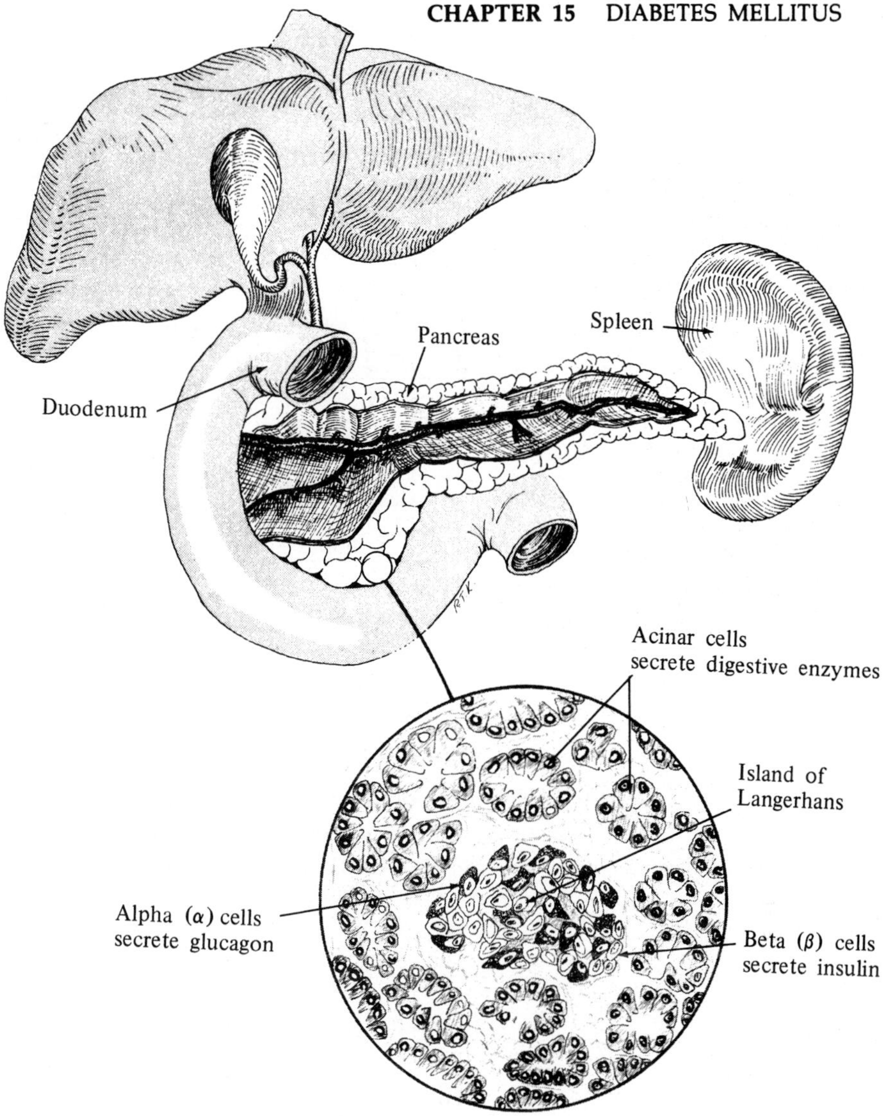

FIGURE 15-1 Pancreas with alpha and beta cells.

It should be emphasized that this is just one possible sequence of events. Some investigators have different theories as to how the HLAs and islet cell antibodies result in decreased insulin secretion.

Most researchers state that IDDM is a result of **autoimmunity**. IDDM persons form islet cell antibodies against their own beta cells, hence the reason for calling it an example of autoimmunity.[2]

autoimmunity A condition in which the body forms antibodies against its own tissues.

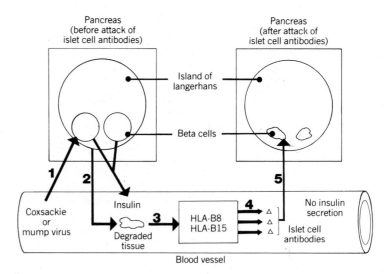

FIGURE 15-2 Five events, in sequence, that may result in IDDM.

Functions of Insulin and Results of Deficiencies

The hyperglycemic problem of IDDM patients is due to inadequate secretion of insulin. To understand the symptoms of IDDM, one needs to know the metabolic functions of insulin and the metabolic changes that result from an insulin deficiency.

The main function of insulin is to promote the transfer of glucose across certain cell membranes so that it can be oxidized for energy. However, insulin is also secreted to facilitate the uptake, use, and storage of fat and amino acids. The action of insulin takes place in three principal tissues: liver, muscle, and fat. These tissues are also the sites of much activity when there is an insulin deficiency. The effects of insulin in normal and deficient amounts on the levels of glucose, fat, and amino acids in liver, muscle, and fat tissues are summarized below.

Normal or increased amounts of insulin:

↓ blood glucose *results from* ↑ uptake of glucose and ↑ synthesis of glycogen in liver and skeletal muscles.

↓ blood fatty acids *result from* ↑ uptake of fatty acids and synthesis of fats by fat cells.

↓ blood amino acids *result from* ↑ uptake of amino acids and synthesis of proteins by muscle cells.

Deficient amounts of insulin:

↑ blood glucose *results from* ↑ breakdown of glycogen and release of glucose by liver; ↓ uptake of glucose and conversion to glycogen by skeletal muscles; ↓ uptake of glucose and conversion to fat in fat cells.

↑ blood fatty acids and ketones *result from* ↑ breakdown of stored fats and release of fatty acids; the liver has ↑ metabolism of fatty acids with ↑ ketones as a by-product. The increased ketones are the reason for the ketacidosis condition that IDDM individuals are prone to develop.

The increased release of fats is partially the reason why IDDM individuals have an increased risk of atherosclerosis.

↑ amino acids *result from* ↑ degradation of proteins in muscles and release of amino acids. This metabolic change is partially the reason why IDDM individuals frequently are underweight when initially diagnosed.[3]

When there is a deficiency of insulin, proteins and fats are degraded to supply energy for the cells. Normally, glucose is used as the energy source, but with an insulin deficiency, not enough glucose can be moved into the cells.

Clinical Symptoms and Complications

The clinical symptoms of IDDM progress from simple complaints at the beginning to potentially very serious complications if the condition is untreated and uncontrolled. The progression through the following symptoms can be very rapid. In fact, the symptoms frequently develop secondary to a viral infection or severe emotional stress; therefore, the parents of an IDDM child may associate the symptoms directly with the infection or stress. It is not uncommon for the initial diagnosis of IDDM to occur when a child is brought to the hospital in a coma due to ketoacidosis.

The symptoms and the underlying cause for each are as follows:

Initial Complaints

polyuria Increased urination.

Polyuria. When the level of glucose in the blood increases above about 170 mg/dl, it begins to spill into the urine. The osmotic pressure of the urine increases due to the high level of glucose, which pulls a great deal of water into the urine and increases urination.

polydipsia Increased thirst.

Polydipsia. Increased urination results in dehydration of the tissues.

polyphagia Increased hunger.

Polyphagia. Glucose is not being properly metabolized; therefore, the cells start metabolizing fat and protein for energy. The result is an increased need for food.

Weight loss. This condition results from the fact that the body does not use glucose properly for energy, but instead starts breaking down fat and protein tissues.

Later Complaints

Blurred vision. One of the complications of IDDM is damage to blood vessels in the retina of the eye.

Skin itching or infection. Skin itching in women is particularly noticeable around the external genitalia (**pruritus vulvae**). This condition results from the excessive excretion of urine that is high in glucose.

Loss of strength (weakness).

pruritis vulvae Itching of the external genitalia of the female.

Life-threatening Symptom

Diabetic ketoacidosis (DKA) A buildup of ketones in the blood that results from uncontrolled IDDM.

Diabetic ketoacidosis (DKA). If IDDM is not properly controlled with insulin and diet, a buildup of ketones in the blood results from the oxidation of fats as the primary source of energy. Ketones are acids, and their increase, combined with hyperglycemia, sets into motion a series of changes shown in Figure 15-3. This sequence of changes can ultimately result in coma and death. Some of the symptoms of ketoacidosis are discussed later in relation to insulin deficiency problems.

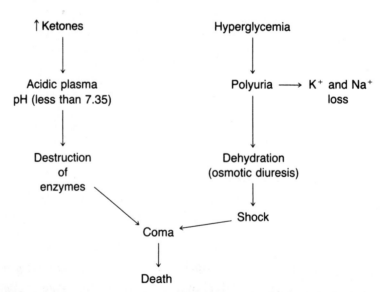

FIGURE 15-3 Sequence of changes that result in diabetic ketoacidosis (DKA).

Chronic Complications

Previously it was mentioned that diabetics often suffer from complications such as blindness, **gangrene,** and cardiovascular disorders. It is because of these complications that diabetes is the third leading cause of death.

The complications can be divided into **large-vessel disease, small-vessel disease,** and susceptibility to infection.

gangrene Death of body tissue due to a loss of the vascular supply, followed by bacterial invasion and putrefaction.

large-vessel disease The development of atherosclerosis in various arteries.

small-vessel disease (microangiopathies) A thickening of small vessels such as arterioles, venules, and capillaries.

Large-Vessel Disease

Large-vessel disease is essentially the development of atherosclerosis in various arteries. Diabetics are more prone to this problem than nondiabetics, since they often have a large amount of fat circulating in the blood. Large vessels supplying blood to the brain, kidneys, heart, and lower extremities are places where atherosclerotic plaques frequently develop.

Atherosclerosis reduces the supply of blood to the above-mentioned organs and regions of the body, leading to the problems of stroke in the brain, kidney failure, heart attack, and gangrene in the lower extremities.

Small-Vessel Disease

Small vessels consist of the microscopic arterioles, venules, and capillaries, and therefore are the source of the term *microangiopathies*. Apparently, the increased glucose and fat circulating through these vessels causes a thickening of the capillary basement membrane.

The capillaries most commonly affected are those supplying the retina of the eye and the kidney, with **diabetic retinopathy** and **diabetic nephropathy,** respectively, being examples of the resultant diseases. As indicated earlier, diabetics have a rate of blindness 25 times higher, kidney disease 17 times higher, gangrene 5 times higher, and heart disease 2 times higher than those of nondiabetics. These statistics show that these diabetic complications are very prevalent; therefore, one of the goals of diabetic therapy (discussed later) is to prevent or delay the onset or progression of the associated complications.

diabetic retinopathy Damage to the retinal blood capillaries as a result of diabetes.

diabetic nephropathy Kidney disease caused by damage to blood vessels that results from diabetes.

Susceptibility to Infection

Diabetics are more susceptible to infections than nondiabetics, since the bacteria multiply and grow in the high-glucose environment.[4] Therefore, all injuries, cuts, and blisters, especially on the lower extremities, should be treated meticulously.

Diagnosis and Monitoring of Diabetes

Two common methods of diagnosing and monitoring diabetes are tests of urine and blood samples.

Urine Testing

reagent A substance that is used to produce a chemical reaction.

Urine is commonly tested for sugar and ketones during a routine physical examination. At home, diabetics monitor their diabetes by checking it sometimes as often as four times daily, before meals and at bedtime. The second-voided specimen is the one that is always tested. The glucose and ketones in urine can be measured by dipping indicator paper strip or **reagent** strips into urine. A color change results that can be compared to a color chart to determine the concentration of glucose in percentages, with 0–0.25% indicating adequate diabetic control. Glucose present in greater quantities in the urine of a person receiving a physical examination suggests the need for blood tests to check for diabetes more thoroughly. Ketones are checked in the same manner.

Blood Testing

If urine tests indicate a high level of glucose, two types of blood tests can be performed to give a definite diagnosis of diabetes.

Fasting blood glucose/sugar (FBG or FBS) A blood glucose test performed on a person's blood after an overnight fast.

Fasting blood glucose/sugar (FBG/FBS). This test is performed on a person's blood after an overnight fast. If the test results show a glucose concentration higher than 140 mg/dl on two separate occasions, the test is positive.

Oral glucose tolerance test (OGTT) A blood glucose test in which a person fasts overnight and is then given a measured amount of glucose in an oral glucose drink.

Oral glucose tolerance test (OGTT). This test is performed on a person's blood after an overnight fast and then the person is given a measured amount of glucose in an oral glucose drink. The amount of glucose for children is calculated as 1.75 g per kilogram of ideal body weight up to a maximum of 75 g, which is the common amount for adults. The person continues to fast and blood samples are taken and analyzed at ½, 1 hour, and 2 hours. If two of the samples show a blood glucose level equal to or greater than 200 mg/dl (see Fig. 15-4), this finding is diagnostic of diabetes. Some physicians may run a second OGTT, since stress, drugs, and inactivity may affect the results. Home monitoring of the blood glucose level by a diabetic is performed by pricking a fingertip, using reagent strips and color changes to determine the amount of glucose present. The tests typically are performed before and 1 hour after meals and at bedtime or when symptoms of hyperglycemia or hypoglycemia occur. Some diabetics may measure their blood glucose level by using a **reflectance photometer** (Glucometer, Glucochex).[4]

reflectance photometer A special device that measures the intensity of light reflected through urine and thereby the amount of glucose that is present.

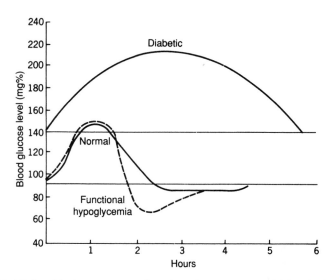

FIGURE 15-4 Glucose curve showing the amount of blood glucose in a diabetic, normal, and functional hypoglycemic person after consumption of a glucose drink. (From S.M. Hunt, J.L. Groff, and J.M. Holbrook, *Nutrition: Principles and Clinical Practice.* New York: John Wiley & Sons, Inc., © 1980. Reprinted by permission.)

Glycated hemoglobin (HbA$_{1c}$)
A test that measures the amount of hemoglobin to which glucose is attached.

Glycated hemoglobin (HbA$_{1c}$). The amount of glycolysated hemoglobin in nondiabetics is about 4–8% of the total hemoglobin. In diabetics, glycolysated hemoglobin may compose 10–28% of the total hemoglobin. Since the amount of HbA$_{1c}$ varies with the blood glucose level, this test can measure blood glucose control.

One advantage of performing this test is that it can be done in a nonfasting state. Also, since the life of glycolysated hemoglobin is about 120 days, a physician can determine how successful diabetes control has been over the past 2–4 months. This factor is important, since some diabetics may have had poor control for a lengthy period but can have a normal urine and blood test by starving or increasing their insulin intake the day before being tested. In addition, the test results are not affected by the time of day, stress, exercise, or food intake.[5]

Treatment of Insulin-Dependent Diabetics

Successful treatment of insulin-dependent diabetics involves coordination of the diet to provide adequate kilocalories for growth and weight gain and to help avoid hypoglycemic or hyperglycemia attacks. The diet must also provide kilocalories for the high activity level of the young diabetic. A key component of successful treatment is injection of the appropriate amounts of exogenous insulin.

Insulin

The primary sources of exogenous insulin are the pancreas of cattle and pigs, commonly called *beef insulin* and *pork insulin*, respectively. New insulins have been recently marketed that are purer than older ones. Even **recombinant DNA** human insulin is now available under the name Humulin.

There are three types of insulin: rapid acting (e.g., regular), intermediate acting (for example, NPH, Lente), and prolonged acting (for example, PZI). Table 15-1 presents information on the three types.

The exact type, amount injected, and time of injection are determined by a physician. These determinations are based on the stage of growth, activity patterns, eating habits, and individual responses of the diabetic. Hyperglycemia and hypoglycemia (the warning signs of each are presented in Table 15-2) are two complications that result if the diabetic gets too little or too much insulin, respectively.

Two basic criteria determine the amount of insulin a diabetic needs: the stage of growth and the activity level. Since these criteria are always changing, so will the amount of insulin a diabetic needs. Basically, a diabetic needs 0.5–1.0 unit of insulin per kilogram of body weight. Insulin is available in the **U100** strength. Interestingly, increased activity increases the glucose needs of the body but decreases the amount of insulin actually required by the diabetic. This relationship results from the

recombinant DNA　DNA in bacteria that has genes spliced into the normal molecule. Frequently, human genes that produce insulin are spliced, thereby forming recombinant DNA insulin; it is also called *artificial human insulin.*

U100　100 units per milliliter of insulin.

TABLE 15-1 TYPES OF INSULIN AND THEIR ACTIVITY

Kind of Insulin	Preparation	Onset of Action (hr)	Maximal Action (hr)	Total Duration of Action (hr)
Short-acting	Regular[a]	0.5–1	2–4[b]	4–6
	Semilente	1–2	3–6	8–12
Intermediate-acting	NPH[c]	3–4	10–16	20–24
	Lente	3–4	10–16	20–24
Long-acting	PZI[d]	6–8	14–20	>32
	Ultralente	6–8	14–20	>32

[a]Also called *crystalline zinc insulin (CZI).*
[b]In some patients, the action of regular insulin may peak later than indicated here (between 4 and 8 hours) and last considerably longer. Therefore, addition of regular insulin to intermediate-acting insulin may cause afternoon hypoglycemia in these patients.
[c]Neutral protamine Hagedorn.
[d]Protamine zinc insulin.

Source: Diabetes Mellitus: Diagnosis and Treatment, by M. B. Davidson, 1981, New York: John Wiley & Sons. © 1981. Reprinted by permission.

fact that exercise increases the number of insulin receptors on muscles, thereby increasing the efficiency of insulin. Exercise tends to lower the blood glucose level; therefore, if the amount of insulin is not lowered during increased exercise, a diabetic will become hypoglycemic.

Injection sites for insulin are surfaces of the arms, thighs, abdomen,

TABLE 15-2 WARNING SIGNS OF HYPOGLYCEMIC AND HYPERGLYCEMIC REACTIONS

Hypoglycemic Reaction (Insulin Reaction)	Warning Signs	Hyperglycemic Reaction (Diabetic Coma)
Sudden	Onset	Gradual
Pale, moist, perspiring	Skin	Flushed, hot, dry
Excited, nervous, trembling, weak, irritable, confused faint, blurred vision	Behavior	Drowsy, weak
Normal	Breath	Fruity odor (acetone)
Normal to rapid shallow	Breathing	Deep, labored
Absent	Vomiting	Present with nausea
Moist, numb, tingling	Tongue	Dry
Present	Hunger	Absent
Absent	Thirst	Present (dehydration)
Headache	Pain	Abdominal
Normal, slight sugar	Urine	Frequent with large amounts of sugar; ketones present
Unconsciousness	Consciousness	Unconsciousness leading to coma
Too much insulin Undereating Vomiting or diarrhea Delayed meal Excessive exercise	Cause	Not enough insulin Overeating Infection Illness Surgery Stress Nausea or vomiting
Orange juice (100 ml) Coke Hard candy (Lifesavers, 4–5) Glucagon if unconscious	Treatment	Check urine Go to bed Keep warm Force fluids Take usual or increased dose of insulin Call doctor

Source: Nutrition in Contemporary Nursing Practice by M. L. Green and J. Harry, 1981, New York: John Wiley & Sons. © 1981. Reprinted by permission.

deltoid muscle Triangular-shaped muscle at the cap of the shoulder. It is frequently used as a site of injections.

and buttocks. Areas that are about to be exercised should be avoided, since the insulin will be absorbed at a faster rate, resulting in hypoglycemia. As an example, a jogger probably would not want to inject himself in the thighs just before jogging. The injection site can also influence when the peak activity of an insulin is achieved. Regular, short-acting insulin peaks fastest when injected into the **deltoid muscle.** Injections into the anterior thigh and the buttocks yield the slowest and lowest peaks, respectively.

A diabetic may have side effects from the use of some types of insulin. Some of the side effects are as follows:

lipoatrophy Loss of fat at the injection site, resulting in indentation.

hypertrophy A buildup of a mound of fat tissue at the injection site.

insulin resistance The deactivation of insulin.

- Allergy: appears as a hivelike rash at the injection site.
- **Lipoatrophy**: loss of fat at the injection site, resulting in indentation.
- **Hypertrophy**: buildup of a mound of fat tissue at the injection site.
- **Insulin resistance**: deactivation of much of the insulin by the body causing the person to take 200 units or more per day.

Most of these problems are eliminated by taking the purified forms of insulin. To avoid lipoatrophy and hypertrophy, a diabetic should be encouraged to rotate injection sites.

Timing of insulin injections needs to be coordinated with meals so that insulin is available when glucose is absorbed into the blood. Some diabetics absorb insulin over a 24-hour period and need only one injection (usually 1 hour before breakfast) of intermediate-acting insulin (NPH or Lente) per day. A few diabetics absorb insulin in less than 24 hours and need two injections of intermediate-acting insulin per day (usually one before breakfast and one 12 hours later). Some diabetics need a mixture of rapidly absorbed insulin (Regular or Semilente) and intermediate-acting insulin before breakfast.

Some diabetics wear an insulin pump. The pump is a small, lightweight machine (about the size of a beeper) that is worn externally. Insulin is contained in a syringe or reservoir in the pump and is delivered into the body through tubing. The tubing is attached to a needle that is inserted under the skin, usually in the abdominal area. Insulin is delivered to the diabetic on a continuous basis, and the amount can be altered in relation to the meals and the blood glucose level of the individual. The main advantage of the pump is elimination of the jolt to the body caused by daily injections of insulin. It may also decrease the damage to the eyes and kidneys that result from daily injections of insulin.

Insulin Shock or Hypoglycemia

insulin shock (insulin reaction) A condition caused by a blood glucose level below 50 mg/dl.

Insulin shock or insulin reaction should be considered synonymous with hypoglycemia (a blood glucose level below 50 mg/dl), since a low blood glucose level precipitates it.

Four basic situations that may cause hypoglycemia are an overdose of insulin, excessive exercise, undereating or skipping meals, and vomiting or diarrhea. The daily activities of a young diabetic may inadvertently increase to the point where he or she forgets to eat. In a nondiabetic, these changes probably would not cause a problem, but a diabetic may start to develop symptoms of an insulin reaction. Diabetics should learn to recognize the symptoms of hypoglycemia, which are summarized in Table 15-2. The onset of the symptoms is sudden, and the diabetic should immediately eat some form of readily absorbed glucose (dextrose). Approximately 15 g of glucose is needed to reverse the symptoms; examples of foods that supply this amount are 4 oz fruit juice, ½ cup of a regular (not sugar-free) soft drink, four to five Life Savers, and two large sugar cubes. After the diabetic has responded to the quick-acting glucose, foods containing either a disaccharide or starch should be eaten. These carbohydrates will be digested and absorbed more slowly, which helps to maintain the blood glucose level, restores liver glycogen, and prevents secondary hypoglycemia.

In severe cases, a diabetic may be so agitated that he spits out food given to him and spills juice. Trying to give food orally in this situation is not advisable. Instead, glucagon should be given subcutaneously, intramuscularly, or intravenously. Glucagon is a hormone whose action is opposite to that of insulin. It stimulates the liver to break down glycogen and release glucose into the blood. The body always releases glucagon from the alpha cells of the pancreas whenever a hypoglycemic condition occurs. Therefore, injection of glucagon enhances the normal response of the body to hypoglycemia. The blood glucose level should rise enough in 5–20 minutes so that food can be given orally until the diabetic is seen by a physician. A diabetic should be encouraged to have glucagon available in the home, and the family should know how to inject it.

Another alternative in emergencies is to use a commercial glucose product (Instant Glucose, Glutol, Glutose) that is gluelike in consistency. This material can be squeezed into the mouth and will be quickly absorbed through the oral tissues into the blood. If neither glucagon nor the commercial products are available, honey placed on the tongue in amounts up to 2 tsp can be used.

Hyperglycemic Reaction

A second potential problem with insulin treatment is hyperglycemia. This problem can result from insufficient injection of insulin or from conditions that require more insulin. Whenever a person is in a stressed state (infection, illness, surgery, injury), the body secretes the stress hormones **cortisone** and epinephrine. These hormones help the body overcome the stress condition by stimulating the liver to break down glycogen and release glucose, thereby, providing more energy to combat

cortisone A hormone secreted from the cortex region of the adrenal glands. It increases the blood glucose level.

stress. If a stress condition occurs in a diabetic, the person must inject more insulin to counter the increased blood glucose level. Table 15-2 compares the symptoms of hyperglycemia and hypoglycemia.

Dietary Treatment of IDDM

The goal of treatment of children with diabetes is to provide a diet that permits normal growth and activity and that controls the disease. The following variables must be considered when planning a diet for these individuals: timing of meals, diet composition, energy content—level of physical activity, and distribution of kcal and carbohydrates.

Timing of Meals

An insulin-dependent diabetic needs to eat regular meals that are evenly spaced. Timing of meals should be planned so that they are 5 hours apart. If a diabetic starts skipping or delaying meals, hypoglycemia or an insulin reaction may result. Tight control of a diabetic's blood glucose level depends on regular eating.

Typically, six meals a day are advised—breakfast, a mid-morning snack, a noon meal, a mid-afternoon snack, an evening meal, and a bed-time snack.

Diet Composition

Carbohydrates should account for 50–60% of the total daily kilocalories. Concentrated sweets or simple carbohydrates should be kept to a minimum. Instead, diabetics should consume complex carbohydrates such as rice, corn, bread, and potatoes, which take longer to metabolize and absorb. This diet will help to supply the blood with glucose in a slow, steady manner. However, recent research has found that some of the traditionally recommended complex carbohydrates, such as bread and potatoes, cause a greater rise in blood glucose level than foods containing simple carbohydrates, such as ice cream.[6] These same studies have found that, in general, carbohydrates from legumes (e.g., beans, peas) and carbohydrates that have been minimally processed (e.g., whole rice as opposed to ground rice) cause a smaller rise in glucose levels when eaten than other carbohydrate sources.

Protein requirements for a diabetic should meet the Recommended Dietary Allowance (RDA) values for the IDDM person's body size and age. The protein allowance should be about 20% of the total kilocalorie intake for young growing diabetics. As IDDM persons complete their growth, their protein requirements decrease, and so should the total percentage of their daily kilocalories from protein. As with a nondiabetic, the protein should be of high quality in order to provide enough essential amino acids.

Fats should compose about 30% of the total kilocalories, with approximately one-third coming from saturated fat and two-thirds from polyunsaturated fats such as soft margarine, corn oil, and safflower oil. Foods high in cholesterol such as eggs, shellfish, and liver should be consumed in small amounts. No more than 300 mg of cholesterol per day should be consumed because of the increased susceptibility of diabetics to cardiovascular disease. See Table 15-3 for an example of a calorie-controlled diet.

Energy Content

The number of kilocalories for young diabetics need to be adequate for their growth and physical activity. The most accurate way to determine this kilocalorie value is to refer to the RDA table for energy intake (Table 9-1) for the child's weight, height, and age. One method for calculating the kilocalorie value is to allow 1,000 kcal for 1 year of age and add 100 kcal for every additional year. According to this method, a 5-year-old child needs 1,600 kcal, whereas a 12-year-old requires 2,200.

The actual kilocalorie requirement will vary from child to child, since their growth rates and physical activity are different. When children know that their physical activity level will be higher than normal, they need to increase their carbohydrate and kilocalorie consumption. A rule

TABLE 15-3 CALORIE-CONTROLLED DIETS

Purpose	Achieve and maintain desirable body weight and near-normal blood glucose levels, and reduce hyperglycemia, glycosuria, and other complications of diabetes mellitus.
Use	Used for people with either insulin-dependent diabetes mellitus, noninsulin-dependent diabetes mellitus, or for weight reduction and maintenance.
Examples of foods	Basically a general diet with calculated amounts of carbohydrates, proteins, and fats and the reduction of concentrated sweets.
Adequacy	Diet is adequate; however, diets with less than 1,200 kcal may be inadequate in some nutrients and therefore a multivitamin supplement is recommended.

Source: From *Manual of Clinical Dietetics* (4th ed.) by the Chicago Dietetic Association, 1992, Chicago, The American Dietetic Association. Reprinted by permission.

of thumb in this respect is to consume an extra 10–15 g (approximately one fruit or bread exchange) of carbohydrate per hour of moderate exercise. For each hour of strenuous activity (running or playing basketball), a person needs an extra 20–30 g of carbohydrate per hour.

Distribution of Kilocalories and Carbohydrates

It is very important that a diabetic's diet be planned so that there is a distribution of carbohydrate and kilocalories to coincide with the type of insulin being used. As an example, if a diabetic injects a mixture of NPH insulin (peak activity of 8–14 hours) and rapid-acting insulin (peak activity of 2–4 hours) at 6:30 A.M., he or she will need to consume more carbohydrate and kilocalories at the noon meal than at the 10 A.M. snack in order to avoid a hypoglycemic reaction. A common distribution of kilocalories and carbohydrate for NPH and rapid-acting insulin is as follows:

Breakfast	4/18 (22%)
Morning snack	2/18 (11%)
Lunch	4/18 (22%)
Afternoon snack	1/18 (5.5%)
Dinner	5/18 (27.5%)
Bedtime snack	2/18 (11%)

Other popular distribution options are in tenths, 2/10ths to 4/10ths of total kilocalories and carbohydrates at each main meal and 1/10th for each snack, 2/7ths for each of the three main meals and 1/7th for a bedtime snack, and 2/5ths for breakfast and evening plus 1/5th for the lunch meal. See the following material on how to calculate a diabetic diet and distribute the kilocalories and carbohydrates using the exchange system.

A young diabetic and his or her parents should be taught how to use the exchange lists. These lists make it possible for diabetics to enjoy eating with their friends and still adhere to their diet. It should be emphasized that diabetics can eat normal foods and do not have to consume expensive dietetic foods for diabetics.[7]

Dietary Fiber and Diabetes

Research shows that increasing the amount of fiber in the diet of some diabetics can help keep blood glucose levels from rising sharply after a meal. Fiber can also reduce the amount of insulin needed by some diabetics who are taking oral drugs or receiving less than 30 units. Insulin-

How to Calculate A Diabetic Diet Using Exchange Lists

The following steps can be used to plan a diabetic diet for both IDDM and NIDDM diabetics.

As an example, let's take a 12-year-old boy who is 59 in. tall and weighs 90 lb.

Step 1. Determine Desirable Body Weight in Pounds

A. Adults
Consult a desirable body weight chart (Table 9-3) for the desirable weight based on height, frame, and sex.

B. Children
Consult a growth pattern on a graph. These growth patterns are readily available at health facilities. The child's growth pattern should be charted every 3–6 months.

Our 12-year-old boy is on about the 50th percentile for his height and weight; therefore, his height and weight are normal for his age.

Step 2. Determine the Total Kilocalorie Needs

A. Adults
1. Kilocalories for basal metabolism:
   desirable body weight (lb) × 10 = _____ kcal
2. Kilocalories for activity level:
   - Sedentary:
   desirable body weight (lb) × 3 = + _____ kcal
   - Moderate:
   desirable body weight (lb) × 5 = + _____ kcal
   - Strenuous:
   desirable body weight (lb) × 10 = + _____ kcal
3. Pregnancy:
   Add 300 kcal/day to gain
   23 lb in 9 months   = + _____ kcal
4. Lactation:
   Add 500 kcal/day   = + _____ kcal
5. Weight loss:
   Subtract 500 kcal/day to
   lost 1 lb/week   = − _____ kcal

   Total kcal needed   = _____ kcal

B. Children

The above steps will not work for estimating total kcal needs for children. Their needs are calculated from Mean Heights and Weights and Recommended Energy Intakes (Table 9-1). When we look up the kcal needs for our 12-year-old, we find he needs 2,700 kcal. Total kcal needed = 2,700 kcal.

Step 3. Divide the Kilocalories into Grams of Protein, Carbohydrate, and Fat

For this example, we will use 20% of total kilocalories from protein, 50% from carbohydrate, and 30% from fat.

Protein:

$$2{,}700 \text{ kcal} \times 20\% = 540 \text{ kcal} \times \frac{\text{g}}{4 \text{ kcal}} = 135 \text{ g}$$

Carbohydrate:

$$2{,}700 \text{ kcal} \times 50\% = 1{,}350 \text{ kcal} \times \frac{\text{g}}{4 \text{ kcal}} = 338 \text{ g}$$

Fat:

$$2{,}700 \text{ kcal} \times 30\% = 810 \text{ kcal} \times \frac{\text{g}}{9 \text{ kcal}} = 90 \text{ g}$$

Step 4. Calculate the Meal Plan in Exchanges

Dietary manuals in health facilities have examples of exchange patterns based on the total number of kilocalories and grams of protein, carbohydrate, and fat. An example of our 2,700-kilocalorie meal plan is as follows:

Exchange group	*Number of Exchanges*	*Carbohydrate (g)*	*Protein (g)*	*Fat (g)*
1. Milk, nonfat	4	48	32	0
2. Vegetables	5	25	10	0
3. Fruit	5	75	0	0
4. Bread	12	180	36	0
5. Meat, low fat	10	0	70	30
6. Fat	9	0	0	45
Total		328	148	75

The actual meal plan for the 12-year-old will depend on his likes and dislikes of certain foods. It is important to stress that the number of kilocalories and grams of protein, carbohydrate, and fat are probably adequate now for this 12-year-old; however, when he becomes a teenager, these values may need to be changed, since this is a period of rapid growth.

Step 5. Determine How Many Kilocalories and Carbohydrate Grams Will Be Consumed at Each Meal

Let us assume that our 12-year-old needs six meals a day, with 4/18ths to 5/18ths of the kilocalories and carbohydrate grams for each major meal and 1/18th to 2/18ths for the three snacks. The distribution might look like this:

$$2700 \text{ kcal} \times 1/18 \ (5.5\%) = 149 \text{ kcal}$$
$$338 \text{ g carbohydrate} \times 1/18 \ (5.5\%) = 19 \text{ g carbohydrate}$$

	Breakfast (4/18)	Mid-morning snack (2/18)	Lunch (4/18)	Mid-afternoon snack (1/18)	Dinner (5/18)	Bedtime snack (2/18)
Energy (kcal)	596	298	596	149	745	298
Carbohydrate (g)	76	38	76	19	95	38

dependent diabetics taking high doses of insulin receive the least benefit from the increased fiber in the diet.[7] How an increase in fiber can reduce the amount of insulin a diabetic needs and lower the blood glucose level is not clear. Some theorize that the increased rate at which food moves through the gastrointestinal tract decreases the amount of glucose absorbed.

A high-fiber diet is one in which the dietary fiber content exceeds 40 g/day. Diabetics should be advised to increase their fiber intake gradually until they are consuming about 45 g/day.

Before a diabetic begins to increase the amount of fiber in the diet, he or she should be cautioned about some of the adverse effects—abdominal fullness, flatulence, and diarrhea. Most of these symptoms, except flatulence, subside with time if the amount of fiber is increased gradually.

TYPE II: NONINSULIN-DEPENDENT DIABETES MELLITUS (NIDDM)

General Characteristics

Noninsulin-dependent diabetes mellitus (NIDDM) A type of diabetes mellitus that is not caused by an insulin deficiency but rather by the ineffectiveness of insulin in moving glucose into the cells.

Maturity-onset diabetes of youth (MODY) NIDDM that occurs in people under 40.

Hyperosmolar hyperglycemic nonketotic coma (HHNK) A complication of type II or noninsulin-dependent diabetes mellitus. Hyperglycemia causes a loss of fluids and electrolytes that can result in coma and death.

Noninsulin-dependent diabetes mellitus (NIDDM) was previously called *adult* or *maturity-onset diabetes*. In a few cases, it occurs in younger people and is called **maturity-onset diabetes of youth (MODY).** This type is much more prevalent, with about 90% of all diabetics being NIDDM. It is usually milder and progresses more slowly than IDDM. NIDDM typically develops later in life, usually after age 40; about 80% of those affected are over age 50.

As the name implies, these diabetics generally do not have an insulin deficiency. Rather, they have a normal amount or even, in some cases, an insulin surplus. However, their insulin is ineffective in moving glucose into cells. From 60 to 90% of NIDDM people are obese, which may be part of the reason why their insulin is ineffective, as described below. Most NIDDM patients can be controlled by a weight loss diet, increased exercise, and decreased stress.

NIDDM patients are not ketoacidosis prone, but they are prone to **hyperosmolar hyperglycemic nonketotic coma (HHNK).** They usually have less vascular damage to small vessels but more atherosclerosis, possibly due to age. (*See Case Study: Noninsulin-Dependent Diabetes, pp. 359–360, for application, and reinforcement of information on noninsulin-dependent diabetes mellitus.*)

Genesis or Cause

There are two basic theories concerning the cause of NIDDM. One theory is that the number of insulin receptors is decreased in obese people (see Fig. 15-5). When they lose weight, the number of insulin receptors returns to normal. Insulin must combine with a receptor before its functions can begin. As a result of the decreased number of receptors, the cells are less responsive to insulin and hence less capable of using glucose.

A second theory is that the problem is within the target cells after insulin binds to the receptors. The biochemical changes within the cell, normally initiated by attachment of insulin to receptors, do not occur. The consequence is less use of glucose.[1]

No relation to the HLA antigens exists in NIDDM people, and they rarely show an elevated level of islet cell antibodies.

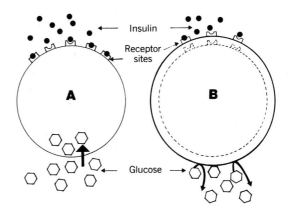

FIGURE 15-5 Cause of NIDDM. (*a*) The number of insulin receptors and the permeability of the cell to glucose are shown in the non-obese condition. (*b*) A reduced number of insulin receptors and a decreased permeability to glucose are shown in the obese condition.

Symptoms and Complications

The symptoms of NIDDM are the same as those of IDDM: polyuria, polydipsia, and hyperglycemia. Diagnosis is based on glucose tolerance test results.

As described earlier, NIDDM people do not have as many of the chronic cardiovascular complications as IDDM people, except for atherosclerosis. One very serious complication of NIDDM is HHNK. This problem is very similar to diabetic ketoacidosis (DKA) in that it is initiated by a hyperglycemic condition and the sequence of changes shown in Figure 15-6 occur. If you compare this sequence of changes with that of DKA, you will see that there is no increase in ketones; therefore, the blood does not become acid. No ketones are formed because the body secretes enough insulin to avoid the breakdown of fats but not enough to prevent hyperglycemia. The coma is the result of both dehydration and hyperosmolarity.

HHNK is diagnosed by a high blood glucose value, a high level of glucose in urine, and the lack of a corresponding increase in ketones (e.g., acetone) in urine. While insulin is the key to treating DKA together with fluid and electrolyte replacement, only the latter is important in treating HHNK. In fact, giving ample amounts of water may be the key to preventing this syndrome. The mortality of HHNK (60–70%) is higher than that of DKA (as low as 0%) because the patients are older and often have serious complications (pneumonia, **pancreatitis,** thrombosis, and **cerebrovascular accidents**).[8]

pancreatitis Inflammation of the pancreas.

cerebrovascular accidents Same as stroke.

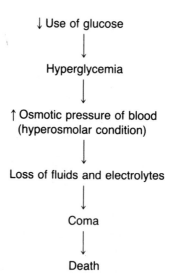

↓ Use of glucose

Hyperglycemia

↑ Osmotic pressure of blood
(hyperosmolar condition)

Loss of fluids and electrolytes

Coma

Death

FIGURE 15-6 Sequence of changes that result in hyperosmolar hyperglycemic nonketotic coma (HHNK).

Treatment

The goal of treatment for NIDDM patients is the same as that of IDDM patients. The main difference between the two is that NIDDM people can usually control their blood glucose level with diet alone, since they have insulin that is circulating but not being used. Since 60–90% of NIDDM diabetics are obese, they need to be on a weight loss diet to achieve and maintain a desirable body weight. This diet requires a reduction of total daily kilocalories to below their normal needs. Some NIDDM diabetics may have to use drugs in addition to diet.

Dietary Treatment

As mentioned above, the diet for most NIDDM diabetics is a low-kilocalorie weight loss diet. At first, their intake per day may be as low as 600 kcal in order to lower their blood glucose to an acceptable level. A weight loss of 5–10 lb should provide considerable improvement in their blood glucose level. The basic reason is that as they lose weight, the number of insulin receptors increases greatly, thereby improving the effectiveness of their insulin. Once their blood glucose level has been lowered, the number of kilocalories they should be consuming daily to lose weight at a rate of 1–2 lb/week needs to be determined. A procedure for doing this is shown in the box titled "How to Calculate a Diabetic Diet

Using Exchange Lists." A reduction of 500 kcal/day from the diabetic's normal intake will result in a deficit of 3,500 kcal/week and a loss of 1 lb. Frequently, though, diabetics are placed on a 1,000–1,200 kcal/day diet.

NIDDM diabetics need to be taught how to use the exchange lists. Usually, only three meals a day are recommended. The timing and distribution of the kilocalories are not critical.

Exercise

Exercise is one of the most important aspects of treatment for NIDDM diabetics. Increasing exercise lowers the blood glucose and fatty acid levels. Exercise has also been found to raise the levels of high-density lipoproteins (HDL), which benefit the diabetic by lowering cholesterol and triglyceride levels.

Exercise can be risky for some diabetics who have cardiac disease or other diabetic complications. Diabetics whose blood glucose level is uncontrolled (over 300 mg/dl) or who have ketones in their urine should not begin to exercise until control has been established.

A diabetic should exercise when the blood sugar level is at its peak (after a meal) rather than when the insulin or oral hypoglycemic dose is having its peak effect.

Oral Hypoglycemic Drugs

Some NIDDM diabetics cannot control their blood glucose level by diet and exercise alone. These people may be required to take oral hypoglycemic drugs or insulin. The effects of insulin were discussed earlier in the chapter.

Oral hypoglycemics are not a form of oral insulin. Insulin is a protein that, if taken orally, would be digested or broken down into individual amino acids by the stomach. Oral hypoglycemics stimulate the beta cells of the pancreas to secrete more insulin and to increase the affinity of insulin receptors in peripheral tissues.[2]

The oral hypoglycemics currently approved by the Food and Drug Administration are known as *sulfonylurea drugs.* Common examples are tolazamide (Tolinase), tolbutamide (Orinase), and chlorpropamide (Diabinese). The possible side effects of these drugs are as follows:

Hypoglycemia. Reduction of the blood glucose level is what these drugs are designed to accomplish. However, a combination of these drugs and certain conditions (reduction in kidney or liver functions, infection, surgery, or other stress conditions) can cause the blood glucose level to drop into the hypoglycemic range (below 50 mg/dl).

Gastrointestinal irritation. The symptoms are usually mild and may involve only nausea and occasional vomiting or diarrhea.

Allergic skin reactions

Alcohol sensitivity. Some diabetics who consume alcohol and oral drugs may have a reaction that makes them appear drunk—stumbling and slurring of words. They may also experience facial flushing and a pounding headache.[4]

The most likely candidates for oral therapy are diabetics who are ketoacidosis resistant or who have NIDDM, cannot control their blood glucose level by diet and exercise alone, and generally need fewer than 40 units of insulin per day. The biggest advantages of oral therapy are ease of administration and acceptance. Use of oral drugs, as opposed to insulin, has allowed some diabetics to keep jobs whose working hours are highly irregular (construction workers, railroad workers, etc.).

CRITICAL THINKING—CASE STUDY: INSULIN-DEPENDENT DIABETES

Billy, an 11-year-old boy, has recently been diagnosed as an insulin-dependent diabetic. He is 5 ft 5 in. tall and weighs 78 lb (his ideal weight should be 105–114 lb). His condition was diagnosed after he was brought to the hospital unconscious. The symptoms he exhibited at the time of admission included deep, labored breathing, polyuria, and flushed, hot, dry skin. His laboratory data and medications are as follows:

Laboratory Findings		Normal values
Serum glucose	325 mg/100 ml	70–110 mg/dl
Urine ketones (acetone)	4+	none
Blood pH	7.1	7.35–7.45
Serum sodium	130 mEq/liter	136–145 mEq/liter
Blood urea nitrogen (BUN)	74 mg/dl	10–20 mg/dl

$$\% \text{ ideal body weight (IBW)} = \frac{\text{actual weight (78 lb)}}{\text{ideal weight (105 lb)}} \times 100 = 68\%$$

Medications
Insulin-NPH   32 units/day

1. Billy's symptoms at the time of admission indicated that he was unconscious due to a _____ reaction.
   A. hypoglycemic
   B. hyperglycemic
2. According to Billy's ketone and pH values, his condition could also be described as _____.
   A. ketoacidosis
   B. HHNK
3. The elevated BUN level and UBW only 68% of normal indicate that glucose is not being properly used for energy; therefore,

   _____.

   A. protein digestion and absorption are being decreased.
   B. increased metabolism of tissue proteins and formation of urea.
   C. there is decreased fat digestion and metabolism.
   D. none of these

Billy's diet includes the following number of exchanges:

1. milk (skim)   4
2. vegetable   3
3. fruit   5
4. bread   9
5. meat   8
      3 lean
      5 medium
6. fat   6

Using the information in Table 2-5, calculate the answers to questions 4–8.

4. The number of grams of carbohydrate in the diet is _____.
   A. 153
   B. 273
   C. 248
   D. 303
5. The number of grams of protein in the diet is _____.
   A. 121
   B. 92
   C. 83
   D. 164
6. The number of grams of fat in the diet is _____.
   A. 34
   B. 55
   C. 48
   D. 77

7. The total number of kilocalories in the diet is _____.
   A. 1,816
   B. 1,978
   C. 2,152
   D. 2,269

8. The percentages of kilocalories due to carbohydrate (C), protein (P), and fat (F) are _____.
   A. C—40%
      P—30%
      F—30%
   B. C—60%
      P—30%
      F—10%
   C. C—48%
      P—21%
      F—31%

Billy's diet plan includes between-meal snacks, with 30 g of carbohydrate in the morning and 30 g before bedtime. Which of the following exchanges and foods can he consume and achieve the 30 g of carbohydrate? Use the information in Table 2-5 to answer questions 9–13.

   Key: a = food and exchange can be consumed
        b = food and exchange cannot be consumed

9. _____ 1 bread + 1 fruit; example: 2 graham crackers + 1 apple
10. _____ 2 fruits; example: 1 whole banana
11. _____ ½ milk + 1 bread; example: ½ cup milk and ¾ cup unsweetened cereal
12. _____ 1 meat + 1 bread; example: 1 slice cheese + 6 crackers
13. _____ 2 meats: example: 2 boiled eggs

14. Billy plays soccer and basketball and runs track at his school. Would the snacks given above provide Billy with enough extra carbohydrate for 1 hour of these strenuous activities?
    A. Yes, all of them would.
    B. No, none of them would, since he would need more than a minimum of 30 g of extra carbohydrate per hour of increased activity.
    C. Yes, examples 9, 10, and 11 would, since the extra carbohydrate should be adequate per hour of increased activity.
    D. none of these

CRITICAL THINKING—CASE STUDY:
NONINSULIN-DEPENDENT DIABETES

Mr. N is a 34-year-old man with NIDDM. He is 6 ft 3 in. tall, with a medium frame, and weighs 245 lb (recommended weight, 167–182 lb). He works in an office and recently began having spells of extreme thirst, headache, dizziness, blurred vision, abdominal pain, labored breathing, and rapid pulse. Mr. N. admitted that he had not been following his diet or taking his medications properly, and frequently had been drinking excessive amounts of beer.

His laboratory data and medications are as follows:

Laboratory Findings		Normal Values
Serum glucose	310 mg/dl	70–110 mg/dl
Serum triglycerides	525 mg/dl	10–200 mg/dl
Blood pressure	152/97	90–140/50–90
% ideal body weight (IBW) =	$\dfrac{\text{actual weight (245 lb)}}{\text{ideal weight (182 lb)}}$ = 135% over ideal weight	

Medications		
tolbutamide (Orinase)	500 mg tablets	four times a day

1. Is Mr. N. obese, since 115–120% of IBW is indicative of obesity?
   A. No
   B. Yes
2. How many kilocalories should Mr. N be required to consume in order to allow weight loss but still be adequate?
   A. 2,000 kcal
   B. 1,800 kcal
   C. 900 kcal
   D. 1,500 kcal
3. What other steps besides dietary restriction should be taken to control Mr. N's diabetes?
   A. diet alone should be adequate
   B. he should begin a moderate, regular exercise program
   C. he should check his blood sugar 4 times daily
   D. adequate rest is essential for normal glucose metabolism

Occasionally, when stressful events occur at work, Mr. N. experiences episodes of hypoglycemia. Which of the following would supply approximately 15 g of glucose and therefore be most suitable to correct his hypoglycemia?

Use the following key to answer questions 4–8.

Key: a = suitable
     b = unsuitable

4. _____ 1 cup milk

5. _____ ½ cup pineapple juice

6. _____ ½ cup diet cola

7. _____ 4 or 5 Life Savers

8. _____ go for a brief walk

9. How many meals should Mr. N consume per day?
   A. any number would be suitable
   B. three, with a snack when hypoglycemia occurs
   C. six are essential to control his diabetes
   D. only one in order to facilitate weight loss

10. What nutrient distribution is recommended for Mr. N.?
   A. 20% protein, 30% carbohydrate, 50% fat
   B. 10% protein, 50% carbohydrate, 40% fat
   C. 20% protein, 50% carbohydrate, 30% fat
   D. none of these

11. If Mr. N. consumes beer while taking his tolbutamide (Orinase) tablets, which of the following possible side effects might he experience?
   A. stumbling
   B. blurred vision
   C. confusion
   D. shortness of breath

SUMMARY

- Diabetes is a group of disorders with a variety of genetic causes but which have hyperglycemia in common.
- The genesis or cause of diabetes is the presence of HLAs that are stimulated to produce antibodies by certain viruses.
- Insulin increases the uptake of glucose, fatty acids, and amino acids from the blood. Therefore, the blood glucose level of these nutrients decreases.

  Deficiency of insulin is evidenced by a decreased uptake of glucose, fatty acids, and amino acids from the blood. Therefore, the blood glucose level of these nutrients increases.
- Blood tests to diagnose diabetes are the fasting blood glucose/sugar (FBG/FBS) and oral glucose tolerance test (OGTT).
- Advantages of glycolysated hemoglobin (HbA$_{1c}$) are that it can measure control over a period of 2–4 months and can be performed on a diabetic in a nonfasting state.
- Peak period of activity for insulins are as follows: short-acting, 2–4 hours; intermediate, 10–16 hours; long-acting, 14–20 hours.
- Hypoglycemia is defined by a blood glucose level below 50 mg/dl.

  Four causes of hypoglycemia are an overdose of insulin, excessive exercise, undereating or skipping of meals, or vomiting or diarrhea.
- Steps involved in causing diabetic ketoacidosis are as follows:

  increased ketones → acidic plasma → destruction of enzymes → coma → death

  hyperglycemia → polyuria → dehydration → shock → coma → death
- Percentage of daily kcal from nutrients for IDDM are as follows: carbohydrates—50–60%; proteins—20%; and fats—30%.
- It is important to distribute kcal and carbohydrates throughout day to have adequate carbohydrates available to cells when insulin has peak activity.
- A high-fiber diet is important to a diabetic in that it decreases the amount of insulin required.
- General characteristics of noninsulin-dependent diabetes mellitus (NIDDM), the most common type of diabetes, include the fact that 90% of diabetics have this type; NIDDM develops usually after age 40; 80% of people diagnosed with NIDDM are over age 50; and generally they do not have insulin deficiency.
- The genesis or cause of NIDDM is a decreased number of insulin receptors. In obese people, target cells do not bring about proper biochemical changes in glucose after it is absorbed.
- The sequence of steps leading to HHNK is as follows:

  decreased use of glucose → hyperglycemia → increased osmotic pressure of blood → loss of fluids and electrolytes → coma → death
- NIDDM can be treated by diet alone; most NIDDM are obese and should be on a weight-loss diet.

REVIEW QUESTIONS

True (A) or False (B)

1. Diabetes is not a genetic but rather a biochemical problem.
2. Diabetes, although a serious problem, is not a leading cause of death.
3. Insulin-dependent diabetes mellitus (IDDM) is the most common type of diabetes and is caused by early-onset obesity in children.
4. IDDM people almost always have a higher level of human lymphocyte antigens HLA-B8 and HLA-B15, plus islet cell antibodies.
5. Many researchers believe that IDDM is an example of autoimmunity, since the body forms islet cell antibodies against its own pancreas tissue.
6. Normal or increased amounts of insulin result in increased amounts of blood glucose, blood fatty acids, and blood amino acids.
7. The symptoms of IDDM develop very rapidly, usually secondary to a viral infection or severe emotional stress.
8. The symptoms of IDDM are polyuria, polydipsia, polyphagia, skin itching, and diabetic ketoacidosis (DKA).
9. DKA is characterized by a high plasma pH, hypoglycemia, edema, shock, and coma.
10. Retinopathy and nephropathy result from too much fat damaging the walls of the microscopic vessels supplying the retina and kidney, respectively.
11. A fasting blood glucose (FBG) test result of 120 mg/dl and two oral glucose tolerance test values of 140 mg/dl are indicative of diabetes.

12. The advantages of glycolysated hemoglobin (HbA_{1c}) tests are that it allows a physician to check how successful diabetes control has been over the past 2–4 months and can be performed on a person in a nonfasting state.

13. As the exercise level of a diabetic increases, the need for insulin decreases.

14. Insulin should not be injected into areas of the body that are about to be exercised, since it will be absorbed faster and result in hypoglycemia.

15. Situations that may cause a hypoglycemic or insulin shock reaction are lack of exercise, overeating, and stress.

16. Symptoms of a hypoglycemic reaction are drowsiness, weak, deep, labored breathing, and vomiting.

17. In a severe insulin shock reaction, glucagon may be given to increase glucose by breaking down glycogen.

18. In a stress condition, the diabetic should increase the amount of insulin injected to counter the increased blood glucose level.

19. An IDDM diet should be low in carbohydrates and high in protein, with a medium amount of fat.

20. The diet mentioned in question 19 is high in protein so that the excess can be converted to carbohydrates without stimulating the release of insulin.

21. Recent research has shown that complex carbohydrates such as bread and potatoes cause a greater rise in blood glucose level than foods containing simple carbohydrates such as ice cream.

22. Carbohydrates from legumes (e.g., beans, peas) and carbohydrates that have been minimally processed cause less of a rise in glucose level than other carbohydrate sources.

23. The kilocalorie level of IDDM diabetics should be low, since these persons are usually obese.

24. It is very important that the distribution of kilocalories and grams of carbohydrates for IDDM diabetics coincide with the type of insulin being used.

25. All diabetics can keep their blood glucose levels from rising sharply by increasing their dietary fiber intake up to 45 g/day.

26. A high-fiber diet supposedly reduces that rapid rise in blood glucose level following a meal because fiber prevents the digestion of carbohydrates to glucose.

27. NIDDM diabetics have hyperglycemia because obesity reduces the number of insulin receptors.

28. One very serious possible complication of NIDDM diabetes is hyperglycemic hyperosmolar nonketotic coma (HHNK).

29. The major difference between DKA and HHNK is that the latter does not result in an increase in ketone levels.

30. A weight loss diet for an NIDDM diabetic should be low enough in kilocalories that the person loses weight at a rate of 5 lb/week until the recommended weight is achieved.

31. Some NIDDM diabetics must take oral insulin such as tolazamide (Tolinase), tolbutamide (Orinase), and chlorpropamide (Diabinese) to control their blood glucose level.

32. A pregnant diabetic needs an extra 300 g of protein and 30 kcal/day for her increased needs and those of the fetus.

33. During the first trimester of an IDDM pregnancy, the insulin requirements generally decrease, since a large amount of glucose shifts from the mother into the fetus.

34. Oral hypoglycemics generally are not recommended during pregnancy, since they may cause prolonged hypoglycemia and possibly death of the fetus.

Multiple Choice

35. A possible sequence of events that could lead to the development of IDDM is:
    1. recognition of degraded pancreas tissue by HLA cells
    2. islet cell antibodies attack and destroy beta cells
    3. virus invades and causes the release of degraded pancreas beta cell tissue
    4. decreased secretion of insulin followed by IDDM

    A. 1, 2, 3   B. 3, 2, 1, 4   C. 3, 1, 2, 4
    D. 2, 3, 1, 4

36. Which of the following is (are) correctly paired when a person has an increased secretion of insulin?

A. decreased blood glucose—increased uptake of glucose and synthesis of glycogen in the liver
B. increased blood fatty acids—increased breakdown of stored fats
C. decreased blood amino acids—increased uptake of amino acids and synthesis of proteins by muscle cells
D. A, C
E. A, B

37. The following changes can occur when an IDDM diabetics has DKA. Select the one answer that presents the changes in the correct order.
1. destruction of enzymes
2. acidic plasma
3. coma
4. increase in ketone level
   A. 2, 4, 1, 3   B. 4, 1, 2, 3   C. 4, 2, 1, 3
   D. 2, 1, 4, 3

38. Which of the following tests are indicative of diabetes or inadequate diabetic control?
1. fasting blood glucose level of 130 mg/dl on two separate occasions
2. 1% glucose level in urine
3. oral glucose tolerance test (OGTT) values of 150 mg/dl at 1 hour and 130 mg/dl at 2 hours
   A. 1, 2, 3   B. 2   C. 2, 3   D. 1, 3
   E. 3

39. Two basic criteria determine the amount of insulin an IDDM diabetic needs: _____ and _____ .
A. stage of growth—activity level
B. age—weight
C. basal metabolic rate—age
D. time of meals—total kilocalorie intake

40. Four situations that might cause hypoglycemia or an insulin reaction are:
1. overdose of insulin   3. undereating
2. lack of exercise   4. edema
   A. 1, 2, 3   B. 1, 3   C. 2, 4   D. 4
   E. all of these

41. Symptoms of hypoglycemia are:
1. agitation, nervousness, trembling   3. normal to rapid shallow breathing
2. vomiting   4. lack of hunger
   A. 1, 2, 3   B. 1, 3   C. 2, 4   D. 4
   E. all of these

42. A diet composition for an IDDM might be _____ percent of the total daily kilocalories.

A. carbohydrates 50–60; proteins, 20; fats 30
B. carbohydrates, 30–40; proteins, 30; fats 30
C. carbohydrates, 10–15; proteins, 50; fats 40
D. none of these

43. The benefit to a diabetic from a high-fiber diet is to _____ and a high-fiber diet is defined as dietary fiber that exceeds _____ g/day.
A. help prevent hypoglycemia—20
B. prevent a rapid rise in the glucose level after a meal—40
C. prevent hyperglycemia—30
D. prevent colon cancer—50

44. One theory as to why obesity can result in NIDDM is that _____ .
A. fat infiltration into the pancreas destroys beta cells.
B. fat prevents the liver from synthesizing glycogen.
C. the number of insulin receptors attached to cells is reduced.
D. none of these

45. The treatment of NIDDM consists of the following:
1. low-kilocalorie weight-loss diet   3. oral hypoglycemic drugs for some NIDDM people
2. increased exercise   4. eating large amount of dietetic foods
   A. 1, 2, 3   B. 1, 3   C. 2, 4   D. 4
   E. all of these

Completion

46. Discuss the effects of a deficient amount of insulin on the levels of blood glucose, blood fatty acids and ketones, and amino acids.
47. Discuss the importance of distributing kilocalories and carbohydrate grams throughout the day according to the type of insulin used.
48. Name and give the peak period of activity for the three different types of insulin.

CRITICAL THINKING CHALLENGE

1. A diabetic patient's diet prescription is protein 90 g, fat 50 g, carbohydrate 250 g. Carbohydrate 2/7, 2/7, 1/7, 2/7.

a. What is the percentage of carbohydrate, fat, and protein? Show calculations.

b. Calculate how many grams of carbohydrate are to be provided at each of the four meals (use the carbohydrate fractions for each of the four meals given above).

c. Give specific names and number of exchanges that can be prescribed for each meal to provide the grams of carbohydrate that you calculated in b. Show all calculations.

2. An IDDM patient's diet contains the following exchanges for lunch and dinner:

    4 lean meat
    1 vegetable
    1 fruit
    3 bread
    4 fat
    1 skim milk

He tells you that he has a favorite food, a frozen entree, that he would like to include in his diet today. The information on the label of the food states that there is 36 g of carbohydrate, 14 g of protein, and 15 g of fat. Which of the above exchanges will have to be removed when he consumes this entree? Show all calculations.

3. A 54-year-old noninsulin-dependent diabetic female office worker is 5 ft 3 in tall and weights 165 lb. Her fasting blood glucose has been between 150 and 170 mg/dl.

a. Using Table 9-3, Suggested Weights for Adults, determine whether she is overweight. If so, how much?

b. Using the Resting Energy Expenditure (REE) formula in Chapter 9, calculate the total caloric consumption for her assuming a sedentary level of physical activity. Show all calculations.

c. Calculate how many kcal she should consume to lose two pounds per week? Show all calculations.

4. Prepare a dietary teaching plan for an insulin-dependent diabetic. Include aspects of:

a. diet composition
b. energy content
c. distribution of kcal and carbohydrates
d. timing of meals
e. physical activity

REVIEW QUESTIONS FOR NCLEX

Situation. John is a 10 year old newly diagnosed insulin dependent diabetic (IDDM). His height and weight place him on about the 30 percentile, therefore, he is placed on a 2700 kcal per day diet. You are asked to prepare a nursing care plan for John and his parents concerning the following aspects of his diabetes condition.

1. John's type of diabetes is found in about _____% of diabetics.
   A. 45
   B. 35
   C. 25
   D. 15

2. John's condition is one that is _____.
   A. curable, with proper surgery
   B. treatable, with proper diet and exercise
   C. uncurable and untreatable
   D. curable, but only with a pancreas transplant

3. The excess glucose (hyperglycemia) in John's blood is the result of _____.
   A. him consuming too much sugar
   B. the pancreas not secreting enough insulin
   C. all body cells being insensitive to insulin
   D. his liver excessively breaking down glycogen

4. What is the most important reason for instructing John to rotate insulin injection sites?
   A. to avoid lipoatrophy (loss of fat at injection site)
   B. to avoid insulin resistance
   C. to avoid decreased effectiveness of insulin
   D. to avoid excess pain when inserting the needle

5. John's weight and height being below the average (50 th percentile) for his age is due _____.
   A. to his body utilizing excess glucose for energy
   B. his body not utilizing glucose for energy but instead broke down fat and protein tissue
   C. inadequate secretion of growth hormone during the first nine years of his life
   D. inadequate secretion of metabolic hormones and therefore his metabolic rate being too low for adequate growth

6. What percent of John's daily total kcal should come from carbohydrate?

A. 20–30 percent
B. 30–40 percent
C. 40–50 percent
D. 50–60 percent

7. After instructing John and his family on how to use the exchange system for determining daily food intake, which of the following combinations will achieve a 2700 kcal diet? (Use kcal value for exchanges to make calculations.)
   A. 4 skim milk, 5 vegetable, 5 fruit, 12 bread, 10 lean meat, 9 fat
   B. 5 skim milk, 6 vegetable, 7 fruit, 10 bread, 10 lean meat, 7 fat
   C. 3 skim milk, 8 vegetable, 5 fruit, 14 bread, 11 lean meat, 6 fat
   D. 5 skim milk, 7 vegetable, 8 fruit, 13 bread, 12 lean meat, 10 fat

8. Regular (short-acting) insulin is ordered for John. The first dose is administered at 7:00 a.m. What time should John and his family be taught that maximal action and therefore hypoglycemia might occur?
   A. 5–7 pm
   B. 4–6 pm
   C. 10–12 midnight
   D. 9–11 am

9. Which of the following are symptoms of hypoglycemia that John and his family need to be taught?
   A. flushed, hot dry skin
   B. fruity odor to breath
   C. vomiting with nausea
   D. normal to rapid breathing

10. John plays youth basketball, therefore, he is instructed that to avoid hypoglycemia, when playing, he needs to _____.

A. reduce his intake of carbohydrates by 10–15 g per hour
B. consume an extra 20–30 g carbohydrates per hour
C. consume an extra 20–30 g protein per hour
D. reduce his intake of fat by 10–15 g per hour

REFERENCES

1. Nerup, J., Mondrup-Paulsen, T., & Hokfelt, B. (Eds.). (1989). *Genes and gene products in the development of diabetes* (pp. 7–69). Amsterdam: Elsevier Science Publications.
2. Sakomoto, N., Alberti, K.G.M.M., & Hotta, N. (Eds.). (1990). *Current status of prevention and treatment of diabetic complications* (pp. 195–210). Amsterdam Elsevier Science Publications.
3. Robinson, C. H., Lawler, M. R., Chenoweth, W. L., & Garwick, A. E. (1990). *Normal and therapeutic nutrition* (17th ed.). New York. Macmillan.
4. Davidson, B. M. (1991). *Diabetes mellitus, diagnosis and treatment* (3rd ed.). New York: Churchill Livingstone.
5. Larsen, M. L., Harder, M., & Magensen, E. F. (1990). Effect of long-term monitoring of glycosylated hemoglobin levels in IDDM. *New England Journal of Medicine, 323,* 1021.
6. Jenkins, D.J.A., & Wolener, T.M.S. (1988). Dietary fiber in management of diabetes. *Diabetes Care, 11,* 160.
7. Ninik, A. I., & Jenkins, D.J.A. (1988). Dietary fiber in management of diabetes. *Diabetes Care, 11,* 160.
8. Alberti, K.G.M.M., & Kroll, L. P. (Eds.). (1991). Hyperglycemic emergencies: A further look. *The Diabetes Annual, 6,* 403–404.

16 DISEASES OF THE GASTROINTESTINAL TRACT

Upon completion of this chapter, you should be able to:

1. Describe the structure and function of the esophagus.
2. Give the cause, symptoms, and diet therapy for hiatal hernia.
3. List four functions of the stomach.
4. Recognize the cause, symptoms, and diet therapy for acute gastritis.
5. Give the cause, symptoms, and diet therapy for a peptic ulcer.
6. Describe the symptoms of and reasons for the dumping syndrome.
7. Give the dietary treatment of dumping syndrome.
8. Describe the long-range nutritional problems after a subtotal gastrectomy.
9. Give three functions of the small intestine.
10. Recognize the cause, symptoms, and diet therapy for nontropical sprue (celiac disease).
11. Describe the cause, symptoms, and diet therapy for lactose intolerance.
12. Give the cause, symptoms, and diet therapy for Crohn's disease.
13. Recognize three functions of the large intestine.
14. Give the cause, symptoms, and diet therapy for diverticulosis and diverticulitis.
15. Give the cause, symptoms, and diet therapy for ulcerative colitis.

INTRODUCTION

alimentary canal A muscular tube that extends from the mouth to the anus.

The **alimentary canal** is the muscular tube (see Fig. 16-1) into which one ingests food, digests it, and absorbs it and from which feces are excreted. The canal is specialized in certain regions for particular functions. In this chapter, we will study the esophagus, stomach, and small and large intestinal regions in terms of their functions and therapeutic nutrition for disorders of these areas.

ESOPHAGUS

bolus A round mass of food.

peristaltic contractions Rhythmic waves of smooth muscle contractions.

The esophagus (Fig. 16-1) begins at the base of the pharynx, extends through the thorax, posterior to the trachea, continues through the diaphragm, and finally joins the stomach. It functions as the passageway for food from the pharynx to the stomach. It moves a **bolus** into the stomach by **peristaltic contractions** of the muscular wall (Fig. 16-2). A sphincter-type valve is present at the entrance of the stomach. It opens to allow food into the stomach and closes to prevent regurgitation.

Disorders

Hiatal Hernia

The most common form of a hiatal hernia is one in which the esophagus–stomach junction slides through the diaphragm when the person lies down (see Fig. 16-3).

Cause. Hiatal hernia can result from a congenital weakness of the diaphragm muscle as well as from aging, obesity, pregnancy, and tight-fitting clothes.

pyrosis Heartburn.

reflux Regurgitation.

dysphagia Difficulty in swallowing.

Symptoms. The most common complaint is **pyrosis,** which results from a **reflux** of stomach contents. Other complaints are **dysphagia,** substernal pain, and vomiting.

Diet Therapy. The primary goal of the diet is to prevent reflux. The diet is bland, with small, frequent feedings. Antacids are frequently taken to help neutralize the acidity in the stomach. Foods should not be eaten for 3–4 hours before bedtime. It is important that the patient avoid physical activity that requires stooping forward after eating. The head of the bed should be elevated to avoid reflux.[1] A weight-reduction diet may be appropriate for hiatal hernia, since many people with this condition are obese. The principles of a restricted bland diet are provided in Table 16-1. Table 16-2 gives a summary of the above information.

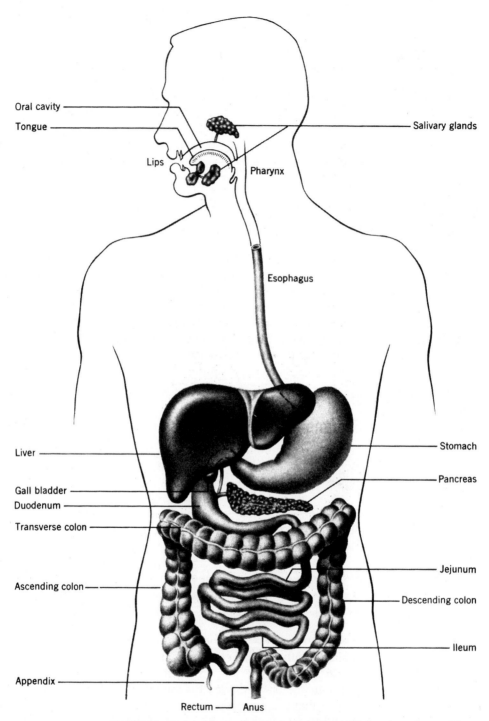

Oral cavity

Tongue

Lips

Pharynx

Salivary glands

Esophagus

Liver

Gall bladder

Duodenum

Transverse colon

Ascending colon

Appendix

Rectum

Anus

Stomach

Pancreas

Jejunum

Descending colon

Ileum

FIGURE 16-1 Alimentary canal and specialized regions. (From S.R. Burke, *Human Anatomy and Physiology for the Health Sciences*, 3rd ed. Albany: Delmar Publishers, Inc. © 1992. Reprinted by permission.)

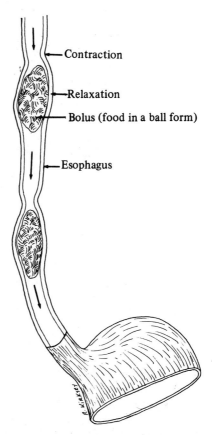

- Contraction
- Relaxation
- Bolus (food in a ball form)
- Esophagus

FIGURE 16-2 Peristaltic contractions of the esophagus that move a bolus of food from the pharynx to the stomach.

STOMACH

The stomach (see Fig. 16-4) has four basic functions:

chyme Semifluid mass of food that is formed in the stomach and released into the duodenum.

Storage. It temporarily stores **chyme,** which is released to the duodenum for further digestion.

Mixing. Peristaltic contractions mix food thoroughly with gastric juices to form chyme.

pyloric sphincter valve A circular muscle that controls the movement of food from the pyloric region of the stomach into the duodenum.

Regulation of the flow of chyme. Chyme is released in small quantities into the duodenum through opening and closing of the **pyloric sphincter valve** (Fig. 16-4).

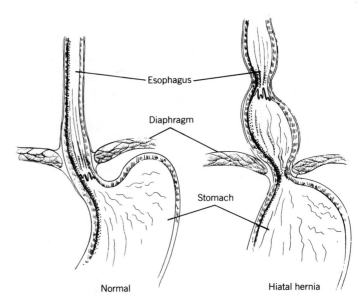

FIGURE 16-3   A hiatal hernia.

Facilitates absorption of vitamin B₁₂, iron, and calcium. The stomach secretes an intrinsic factor that aids the absorption of vitamin B_{12} in the small intestine. Also, the hydrochloric acid (HCl) in the stomach helps to convert iron from a +3 charge to a +2 charge, which is more readily absorbed. HCl increases the solubility and thereby the absorption of calcium.

Any stomach disorder interferes with one or more of these functions.

Disorders
Gastritis

gastritis A condition in which the gastric mucosa is inflamed.

Gastritis involves inflammation of the gastric mucosa, which is the mucous membrane lining the stomach. The most common form, acute gastritis, will be discussed.

Acute Gastritis

edematous Refers to a condition of edema.

Acute gastritis is a common disorder characterized by a reddened, **edematous** mucosa, with small erosions and hemorrhages.

TABLE 16-1 RESTRICTED BLAND DIET

Purpose	Designed to decrease peristalsis and avoid irritation of the gastrointestinal tract.
Use	Used in treatment of hiatal hernia. Also used as a transitional diet in treatment of various diseases of the gastrointestinal tract in which inflammation or spasms are present.
Examples of foods	Foods that are chemically, mechanically, or thermally irritating are removed from the diet. Some examples of foods that are eliminated are fried foods, most raw fruits and vegetables, caffeine, alcohol, coarse breads and cereals, and highly seasoned foods.
Adequacy	Diet is adequate.

Source: From *Manual of Clinical Dietetics* (4th ed.) by the Chicago Dietetic Association, 1992, Chicago, The American Dietetic Association. Reprinted by permission.

Cause. Probably the most common cause is alcohol, especially when consumed in combination with aspirin. Spicy foods composed of pepper, vinegar, and mustard are also known to cause gastritis.

epigastric pain Same as epigastric distress.

Symptoms. An affected person may complain of anorexia, **epigastric pain,** and in some cases severe vomiting.

Diet Therapy. The inflammation subsides when the offending foods are withheld; therefore, if vomiting persists, no foods can be given by mouth and parenteral nutrition should be instituted. Once the vomiting stops, a bland diet and antacids should be given.

peptic ulcer A deterioration or lesion in the mucosal lining of the stomach or duodenum.

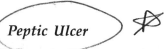

Peptic Ulcer

There are two types of **peptic ulcers.**

TABLE 16-2 SUMMARY OF HIATAL HERNIA

Pathophysiology	Causes	Symptoms	Diet Therapy
Protrusion of part of stomach through esophagus opening in diaphragm	Congenital weakness of diaphragm Aging process Obesity Pregnancy Tight-fitting clothes	Pyrosis Reflux Dysphagia	Bland diet Small, frequent feedings No foods eaten 3–4 hours before bedtime Elevation of head of bed

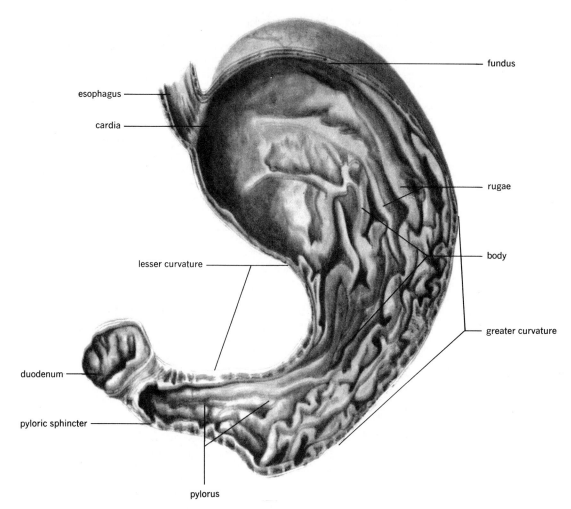

esophagus

cardia

fundus

rugae

lesser curvature

body

greater curvature

duodenum

pyloric sphincter

pylorus

FIGURE 16-4 Anatomy of the stomach. (From J.R. McClintic, *Basic Anatomy and Physiology of the Human Body.* New York: John Wiley & Sons, Inc., © 1980. Reprinted by permission.)

gastric ulcer A deterioration of the gastric mucosa generally located along the lesser curvature of the stomach.

duodenal ulcer A deterioration of the mucosal lining of the duodenum.

Gastric. Deterioration of the gastric mucosa (see Fig. 16-5) along the lesser curvature of the stomach causes most **gastric ulcers** (see Fig. 16-6). This type occurs most frequently in people 40–55 years of age and about two and a half times more often in men than in women.

Duodenal. Duodenal ulcer occur in the mucosal lining of the duodenum (see Fig. 16-6). They are the most common type of ulcers accounting for about 80% of all peptic ulcers. A younger group of people, 25–50 years old, tend to develop this type.

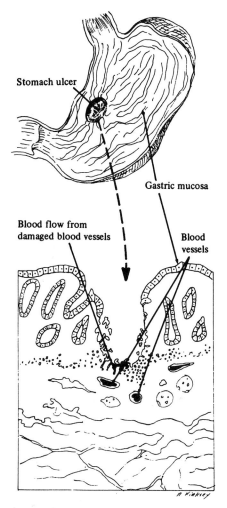

FIGURE 16-5   A gastric ulcer.

Cause. The exact cause of ulcers is not known. However, ulcers seem to occur when there is an imbalance between the amount of hydrochloric acid (HCl), pepsin enzyme, and mucosal resistance. Normally, the gastric and duodenal mucosae are very effective in preventing deterioration of the stomach and duodenal walls. An imbalance can result from a variety of factors. Most often it occurs in people who are tense, hard-driving, and anxious. Research has also shown that alcohol, caffeine, and nicotine tend to predispose a person to the development of ulcers.

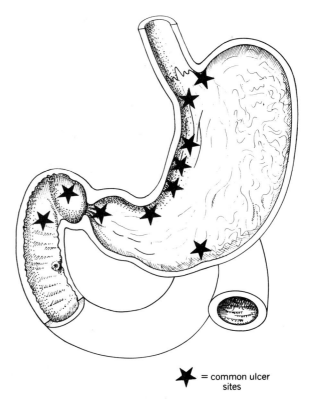

FIGURE 16-6 Sites of gastric and duodenal ulcers.

Symptoms. Epigastric pain, occurring 1–3 hours after eating or at night, is a common symptom. Apparently the pain results from HCl coming in contact with exposed nerve endings in the lesion. Eating a meal relieves the pain, since chyme coats the nerve endings and blocks the HCl. Other symptoms tend to vary depending upon whether the ulcer is duodenal or gastric. These symptoms are as follows:

Gastric Ulcer	Duodenal Ulcer
Nausea	Heartburn
Anorexia	Good appetite
Vomiting	Weight gain
Weight loss	Constipation

Apparently the weight gain in duodenal ulcers results from the fact that the patient has a good appetite and consumes food to reduce pain.[2]

Diet Therapy. The primary goal of dietary management is to buffer or inhibit acid secretions. This goal is accomplished by eating small, frequent meals and avoiding alcohol and caffeine, which stimulate secretion of HCl.

Antacid drugs are prescribed to neutralize activity up to about pH 5 (from a normal pH of 1–3), which significantly reduces pepsin enzyme activity.

Rest is prescribed, since it reduces vagus nerve activity. The **vagus nerve** stimulates the release of HCl from glands in the stomach.

vagus nerve The tenth cranial nerve. It stimulates gastric glands in the stomach to secrete hydrochloric acid and pepsin enzyme.

Current Dietary Treatment

The current dietary treatment for ulcers is a more liberal individualized diet than the traditional bland diet. The objectives of the diet are as follows:

- To decrease gastric acid secretion
- To neutralize gastric acidity
- To promote healing of the ulcer

Most nutritionists and research studies indicate that a strict bland diet is not necessary when the ulcer patient shows no symptoms. General guidelines for an ulcer diet for a symptom-free person are as follows:

Three meals should be eaten rather than six small feedings per day. Three meals per day cause less stimulation of gastric acid secretion than six small meals. In addition, the extra meals interfere with antacid therapy to reduce gastric acidity, and thus are more harmful than three meals.

Bedtime snacks should be eliminated. The traditional approach was to include bedtime snacks in order to coat the ulcer while the person was sleeping. However, this practice is not now recommended, since the snacks actually stimulate gastric acid secretion.

Milk and cream feedings should not be used to reduce acidity. While milk should be included, it should not be used as a way to lower gastric acidity. Milk protein does initially neutralize HCl, but it also stimulates secretion of the acid. Cream is high in saturated fat, which can promote weight gain and increase the risk of atherosclerosis.

Completely eliminating certain foods is unwarranted. Research does not indicate that totally eliminating certain foods is beneficial. If a food causes repeated discomfort, it should be eliminated. Caffeine-containing beverages (coffee, tea, cola drinks) typically do increase gastric acid secretion but may be taken in moderation.

Omission of foods containing fiber has not been found to be beneficial to ulcer patients. Omission of gas-forming foods such as baked beans, cabbage, milk, nuts, and onions has not been found to aid the healing of ulcers. However, black pepper, chili powder, and nicotine may cause distress and need to be limited.[3]

Excessive alcohol intake should be avoided. Alcohol can damage the gastric mucosa; therefore, excessive intake should be avoided in order to increase the healing of ulcers.

In reference to specific details, the diet should contain an adequate level of protein for healing. In addition, it should contain a moderate amount of fat for suppression of gastric secretions and peristaltic contractions. The principles of a chronic peptic ulcer diet are provided in Table 16-3. Table 16-4 provides a summary of the pathophysiology, causes, symptoms, and diet therapy for a gastric ulcer. See the sample menu for a liberal peptic ulcer diet.

Complications. Complications of peptic ulcers are as follows:

Hemorrhage. Approximately 25% of peptic ulcer patients lose blood at some time. Duodenal ulcers tend to bleed more often than gastric ulcers.

Perforation. This is an opening through the gastric or duodenal wall.

Pyloric obstruction. Sometimes the pyloric sphincter becomes scarred and stenosed (the opening becomes narrowed).

Patients who develop these complications generally are treated surgically, with a subtotal gastrectomy (see Fig. 16-7) being one example. This procedure removes the distal 50–75% of the stomach.

perforation An opening through the gastric or duodenal wall.

pyloric obstruction A condition in which the pyloric sphincter becomes scarred and stenosed (the opening is narrowed).

TABLE 16-3 CHRONIC PEPTIC ULCER DIET

Purpose	Decrease gastric irritation and excessive gastric acid irritation.
Use	Treatment of chronic peptic ulcer disease.
Examples of modifications	Three regular meals are recommended. Eliminate between meal and bedtime snacks, as they interfere with antacid therapy. Alcohol should be eliminated. Anatacids should be given 1 hour and 3 hours after meals and prior to bedtime in order to keep the acidity of the stomach within tolerable limits.
Adequacy	Diet is adequate in all nutrients.

Source: From *Manual of Clinical Dietetics* (4th ed.) by the Chicago Dietetic Association, 1992, Chicago, The American Dietetic Association. Reprinted by permission.

TABLE 16-4 SUMMARY OF GASTRIC ULCER

Pathophysiology	Causes	Symptoms	Diet Therapy
Lesion in mucosal lining of stomach or duodenum	Not known, but results from imbalance of HCl, pepsin, and mucosal resistance	Epigastric pain 1–3 hours after eating Nausea Anorexia Heartburn Weight loss	Avoidance of alcohol, caffeine, and other mucosal irritants Liberal diet or one that allows wide variety of foods

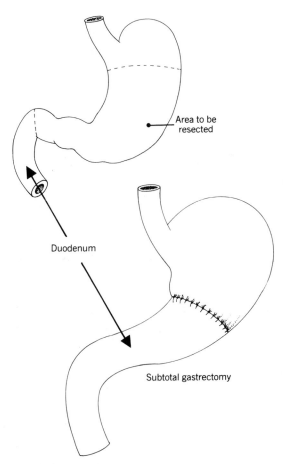

Area to be resected

Duodenum

Subtotal gastrectomy

FIGURE 16-7 A subtotal gastrectomy surgical procedure.

Sample Menu for a Liberal Peptic Ulcer Diet

Exchange	
	Breakfast
1 fruit	½ cup orange juice
1 bread	½ cup oatmeal
½ milk	4 oz milk (whole or lowfat)
1 medium-fat meat	1 poached egg or egg substitute
2 fat	2 slices broiled bacon or bacon substitute
1 bread	1 slice toast
1 fat	1 tsp butter or margarine
	1 tbsp jelly
	2 tsp sugar
	1 cup coffee, if tolerated
	Lunch
1½ vegetable	6 oz vegetable soup
2 medium-fat meat	2 oz beef patty on bun
1 vegetable	Sliced tomato and lettuce
1 fat	1 tbsp french dressing
1 fruit	4 apricot halves
	2 sugar cookies
1 milk	8 oz milk (whole or lowfat)
	Dinner
1 vegetable	½ cup tomato juice
3 lean meat	3 oz broiled chicken
1 bread	½ cup mashed potatoes
1 vegetable	½ cup peas
1 fruit	½ cup fruited jello salad
	½ cup orange sherbet
1 bread	1 slice bread
1 fat	1 tsp butter or margarine
½ milk	4 oz milk (whole or lowfat)

Analysis and Comments

- An analysis of this diet shows 2 milk, 4½ vegetable, 3 fruit, 4 bread, 6 meat, and 5 fat exchanges. This menu reinforces the point that a liberal diet should not exclude certain foods but rather should be an optimum diet with foods from all exchange groups.
- The number of milk exchanges is 2, which reinforces the point that a great deal of milk should not be used for antacid therapy.
- The 5 fat exchanges provide a moderate amount of fat for suppression of gastric secretions and peristaltic contractions.

Source: Adapted from *Manual of Clinical Dietetics* (4th ed.) by the Chicago Dietetic Association, 1992, Chicago, The American Dietetic Association. Reprinted by permission.

Dumping Syndrome (Postgastrectomy Syndrome)

tachycardia An abnormally rapid heartbeat.

After a gastrectomy, a person may experience a combination of symptoms: weakness, a desire to lie down, nausea, profound sweating, **tachycardia,** and dizziness. The changes in blood vessels and the small intestine related to the dumping syndrome are shown in Figure 16-8 and are as follows:

Rapid entrance of food into the duodenum. Chyme enters the duodenum rapidly as a result of the removal of the majority of the stomach and pyloric sphincter. Normally, the stomach and pyloric sphincter store and gradually release food into the duodenum.

Increased osmotic pressure in the intestines. Osmotic pressure increases considerably in the duodenum and small intestine as a result of the rapid entrance of a large amount of food.

Movement of a large volume of water into the intestines. A higher osmotic pressure in the intestines compared to the blood results in the movement of a large volume of water into the intestines. This movement of water by osmosis results from the fact that water moves through all membranes from a low osmotic to a high osmotic pressure.

Decreased blood pressure. The movement of water out of the blood into the intestines results in a drop in blood pressure and is the cause of weakness, sweating, tachycardia, and dizziness.

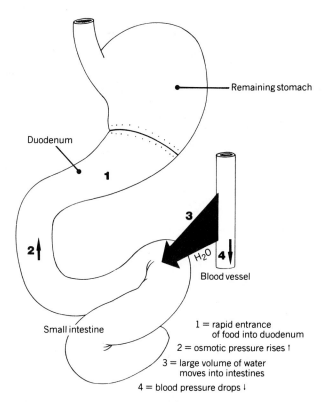

Remaining stomach

Duodenum

1

2

3

H₂O **4**

Blood vessel

Small intestine

1 = rapid entrance
of food into duodenum

2 = osmotic pressure rises ↑

3 = large volume of water
moves into intestines

4 = blood pressure drops ↓

FIGURE 16-8 Dumping syndrome and changes in blood vessels and the small intestine.

Dietary Treatment. Dumping syndrome can be best controlled by diet. Objectives of diet therapy and explanation of the dumping syndrome are discussed below. The principles of a postgastrectomy diet are provided in Table 16-5.

Minimize the quantity of food eaten at meals and increase the number of meals. Eating small meals means that smaller amounts of food are released into the duodenum. Therefore, the osmotic pressure in the intestine will be lower. The number of meals should be increased to six per day.

Avoid simple sugars. Simple sugars in the intestines increase osmotic pressure more than fats and proteins, causing great movement of water out of blood into the intestines. Simple sugars that move into the blood also cause temporary hyperglycemia, with increased insulin secretion. This action is followed by hypoglycemia, with symptoms of weakness and dizziness, about 2–3 hours after rapid entrance of sugar into blood.

TABLE 16-5 POSTGASTRECTOMY DIET

Purpose	Designed to retard the rapid passage of food into the intestine and decrease the formation of a concentrated hyperosmolar solution. Adequate kilocalories are provided for tissue building and for prevention of weight loss.
Use	Used for persons who have undergone surgical procedures that accelerate the normal emptying time of the stomach; total gastrectomy and Billroth I and II anastomoses are examples.
Examples of foods	Simple sugars are kept to a minimum. Proteins and fats are increased. Meals are small and frequent. Liquids are generally served between meals rather than with meals, thus slowing the passage of food from stomach into the intestines.
Adequacy	Adequacy of the diet depends upon the extent of surgery; vitamin B_{12} absorption is inadequate due to loss of intrinsic factor when the stomach is removed; therefore, vitamin B_{12} injections are required.

Source: From *Manual of Clinical Dietetics* (4th ed.) by the Chicago Dietetic Association, 1992, Chicago, The American Dietetic Association. Reprinted by permission.

Avoid liquids 30 minutes before and 1 hour after meals. Liquid ingested during these times will move large amounts of food (chyme) out of the stomach and into the intestines faster than the food would move without liquid consumption.

Increase the ratio of calories from polyunsaturated fat and proteins. Since carbohydrates are reduced, calories come primarily from polyunsaturated fat and proteins. Fat also delays emptying of the stomach, thereby reducing the chance of rapid movement of food into the duodenum and initiating dumping syndrome symptoms.

Increase caloric intake to 2,000–3,500 kcal.[4]

See the sample menu for the dumping syndrome diet.

Long-Range Nutritional Problems After a Subtotal Gastrectomy. The nurse, as well as all members of the health team, needs to be aware of and plan for possible long-term nutritional problems in a patient who has undergone a subtotal gastrectomy. Some of the more common problems are discussed below (see Fig. 16-9).

Hypocalcemia. The previous discussion of stomach functions mentioned that the HCl in the stomach increases the absorption of calcium by increasing its solubility. With the removal of a large portion of the stomach, the ability to absorb calcium is reduced. This reduction can result in the following problems:

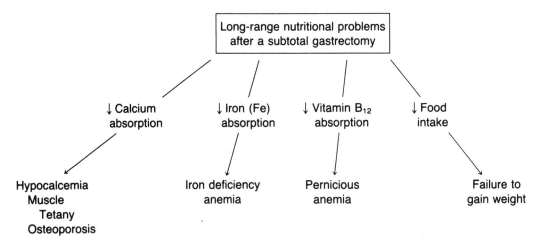

FIGURE 16-9   Long-range nutritional problems after a subtotal gastrectomy.

Muscle tetany: abnormal skeletal muscle contraction.

Osteoporosis: a decline in bone mass. The reduction in calcium absorption results in the removal of calcium from bones, causing their mass to decline.

Anemia. A patient may suffer from iron-deficiency anemia as a result of decreased iron absorption. The stomach aids in the absorption of iron, as discussed at the beginning of this chapter, and this function is decreased as a result of a subtotal gastrectomy. Since iron is essential to red blood cell (RBC) production, this surgery results in a decreased production of RBCs or anemia.

The stomach aids the absorption of vitamin B_{12} by secreting an intrinsic factor. Vitamin B_{12} is also important to the synthesis of RBCs, and its absorption is reduced by subtotal gastrectomy. This reduction results in another anemia called *pernicious anemia.*

Reduced Food Intake and Absorption. A person who has undergone a subtotal gastrectomy may develop a fear of eating, since the dumping syndrome is brought on by consumption of food. Failure to gain weight *ultimately will* result from this fear.

Dietary Counseling. A nurse, doctor, or nutritionist will probably counsel a subtotal gastrectomy patient regarding diet and ways to prevent symptoms of dumping once he or she is discharged from the hospital. Recommendations include the following:

Sample Menu for the Dumping Syndrome (Postgastrectomy Syndrome)

Exchange	
	Breakfast
2 medium-fat meat	2 fried eggs
2 bread	2 slice toast
2 fat	2 tsp butter
	1 cup coffee
	(take 30–60 minutes after eating)
	Mid-Morning Snack
1 low-fat meat	$\frac{1}{4}$ cup cottage cheese
1 bread	2 graham crackers
	Lunch
3 medium-fat meat	3 oz hamburger patty
2 bread	1 cup mashed potatoes
1 fat	1 tsp margarine
1 fruit	$\frac{1}{4}$ cantaloupe
	iced tea with lemon and sugar substitute
	(take 30–60 minutes after eating)
	Mid-Afternoon Snack
1 medium-fat meat	2 tbsp peanut butter
1 bread	6 saltine crackers
	Supper
4 medium-fat meat	4 oz boiled ham
2 bread	1 cup rice
1 vegetable	$\frac{1}{2}$ cup carrots
2 fat	2 tsp butter
1 fruit	$\frac{1}{4}$ cup unsweetened peach slices
	iced tea with lemon and sugar substitute
	(take 30–60 minutes after eating)
	Evening Snack
1 high-fat meat	1 oz cheddar cheese
1 fat	1 strip bacon
1 bread	1 slice bread

Analysis and Comments

- An analysis of this diet indicates the following exchanges:
  1 vegetable
  2 fruit
  9 bread
  12 meat
    1 low-fat
    10 medium-fat
    1 high-fat
    6 fat
- The totals of the three nutrients are as follows:
  Fat—91 g
  Carbohydrate—160 g
  Protein—104 g
- Of the 160 g of carbohydrate, 140 g are starch from the bread and vegetable exchanges and only 20 g are disaccharides from the fruit group. This breakdown is important since, as discussed previously, the major cause of the dumping syndrome is the large amount of simple and double sugars entering the duodenum in a short period of time. The large amount of starch in this diet is important, since it decreases the osmotic pressure of fluid entering the duodenum and decreases the rate at which glucose enters the blood. The slow absorption rate is important in decreasing the chance of developing hypoglycemia.
- The amount of fat being almost equal to the amount of protein is important because it delays the rate of gastric emptying, thereby decreasing the chance of developing the dumping syndrome. In addition, the high fat content supplies needed kilocalories.
- Notice that milk is missing from this diet. The reason is that the carbohydrate in milk is lactose, which increases the osmotic pressure of fluid in the duodenum.

1. *Small frequent feedings.* Advise the patient to eat about six meals a day.
2. *Emphasis on protein, fat, and limited carbohydrate.* Using the person's cultural background as a basis, a list of foods high in protein and fat should be stressed in the everyday diet. Foods in the culture that are high in sugar content should be pinpointed as foods to be avoided.
3. *Gradual addition of foods.* It should be stressed that foods that are not on these lists can be added gradually; however, the person needs to add them slowly in order to determine if he or she can tolerate them.

This is best done by introducing only one new food at a time, such as a low-sugar vegetable or fruit. Next should be a starchy food. However, high-fiber foods should be avoided, since they tend to pull large volumes of water into the intestines.

4. *No fluids at meals.* People from cultures that traditionally consume wines, beer, coffee, and other beverages with their meals may be quite concerned when told not to consume fluids at meals. It should be stressed that they can have their favorite beverage or fluid 45 minutes before or after the meal.

5. *The necessity of taking vitamin and mineral supplements.* It should be stressed that the patient should be very conscientious in taking calcium, iron, and vitamin B_{12} and D supplements, if prescribed.

SMALL INTESTINE

As we move distally from the stomach, the small intestine is the next region of the alimentary canal. It winds and coils around for about 6–7 m (19–23 ft) from the stomach to the large intestine. The three regions of the small intestine are the duodenum, jejunum, and ileum (see Fig. 16-10).

Three important functions occur in the small intestine:

Complete digestion of food. Enzymes are secreted here that complete the digestion of food.

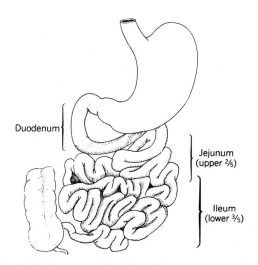

FIGURE 16-10 The regions of the small intestine.

Absorption of nutrients. The end products of carbohydrate, fat, and protein digestion are absorbed across the intestinal wall at specific sites (see Fig. 16-11) into blood and lymph. In addition, water, electrolytes, and vitamins are absorbed at specific sites. Knowledge of these absorption sites is necessary in order to understand how disease of the intestine may cause specific nutritional deficiencies.

Secretion of hormones. Various hormones (ex-gastrin and cholecystokinin) are secreted that affect the activity of stomach, pancreas, and gallbladder.

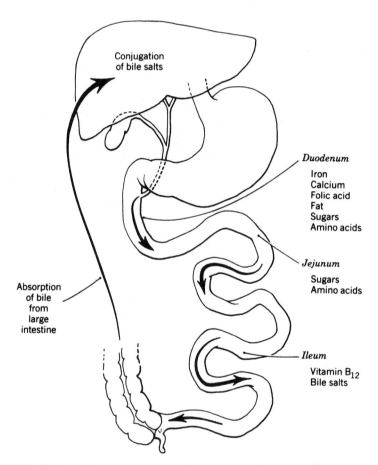

FIGURE 16-11 Specific sites along the small intestine where nutrients are absorbed. (Reproduced with permission from S.A. Price and L.M. Wilson, *Pathophysiology: Clinical Concept of Disease Processes,* 2nd ed. New York: McGraw-Hill Book Company, 1982.)

Malabsorption Disorders

Nontropical Sprue (Celiac Disease, Gluten-Sensitive Enteropathy)

Nontropical sprue affects both children and adults. It appears in children primarily between the ages of 1 and 5 years and in adults primarily between 30 to 40.

Celiac disease is characterized by degeneration and atropy of intestinal villi induced by the ingestion of foods containing **gluten** (a water-insoluble protein found in wheat, rye, barley, and oats).

Cause. The exact cause is unknown, but two theories suggest an inborn error of metabolism and an immune reaction. The inborn error of metabolism is an inherited inability to produce a **peptidase** enzyme. Lack of the enzyme allows a buildup of a harmful peptide, resulting in damage to the villi. The immune reaction theory proposes that gluten causes a hypersensitive reaction to the intestinal mucosa.

Pathophysiology. The intestinal mucosa reacts to gluten in ways that cause the intestinal villi to atrophy, shorten, become club-shaped, or fuse. The end result is that the absorption surface area is decreased; therefore, the afflicted individual does not absorb nutrients very efficiently.

Symptoms. Diarrhea is a common symptom, with the stools being fatty (steatorrhea), foul-smelling, greasy, and bulky. This symptom is common in both children and adults. Other symptoms in children are more subtle, such as irritability, failure to gain weight, and muscle wasting. A child may go into a **celiac crisis.** These problems can cause dehydration, acidosis, and even death.

Diet Therapy. Diet therapy involves a low-gluten diet. The principles of a gluten-restricted diet are provided in Table 16-6. Ideally, the diet should exclude all foods that contain gluten. However, this plan is impossible to implement, so the best one can hope for is to reduce dietary gluten to a minimum. Table 16-7 lists foods containing gluten, as well as the by-products of gluten-containing foods. See the sample menu for a gluten-restricted diet.

Other aspects of diet therapy for celiac sprue are given in Table 16-8. The diet has to be supplemented with vitamins, minerals, and electrolytes, since they are not absorbed adequately. The diet should also be high in kilocalories, since food is not adequately absorbed.[5]

Celiac disease   A disease characterized by the degeneration and atrophy of the intestinal villi, induced by the ingestion of foods containing gluten.

gluten   A water-soluble protein found in wheat, rye, barley, and oats.

peptidase enzyme   An enzyme that catalyzes the degradation of a harmful peptide.

celiac crisis   An attack of watery diarrhea and vomiting.

TABLE 16-6 GLUTEN-RESTRICTED DIET

Purpose	Diet is designed to avoid foods that contain the protein gluten.
Use	Used for patients who have nontropical sprue (celiac disease or gluten-induced enteropathy).
Examples of foods	General diet with elimination of all foods containing the grains wheat, rye, oats, barley, and buckwheat.
Adequacy	Diet is adequate.

Source: From *Manual of Clinical Dietetics* (4th ed.) by the Chicago Dietetic Association, 1992, Chicago, The American Dietetic Association. Reprinted by permission.

Lactose Intolerance (Lactase Deficiency)

Lactose (disaccharide) is hydrolyzed, or broken down, into glucose and galactose by the enzyme lactase. This enzyme normally is located in the brush border of the intestinal mucosa. Some people have a deficiency of lactase; therefore, the quantity of lactose builds up, resulting in increased osmotic pressure in the small intestine (see Fig. 16-12). This increased osmotic pressure causes a large amount of water to shift into the intestine, resulting in increased motility and diarrhea. Malabsorption of nutrients occurs due to the motility.

congenital lactase deficiency
A rare inherited intolerance of lactase throughout life.

Cause. There are three causes of lactase deficiency. **Congenital lactase deficiency** is a rare inherited condition. Persons who have it are intoler-

TABLE 16-7 GLUTEN-CONTAINING FOODS

Foods	
Wheat	Barley
Oats	Rye
By-Products	
Flours	Malted milk
Cereals	Beer and ale
Many commercial soups	Bread and crackers
Puddings (except cornstarch and tapioca ones)	Breaded meats
	Wheat germ
Macaroni, spaghetti, noodles, oatmeal, and granola	

TABLE 16-8 SUMMARY OF CELIAC DISEASE

Pathophysiology	Causes	Symptoms	Diet Therapy
Atrophy, shortening, and decrease in size of intestinal villi	Inborn error of metabolism Immune reaction	Diarrhea Irritability Muscle wasting	Eliminate gluten-containing foods Diet prescription: high protein, high carbohydrate, low to moderate fat, and high calories Vitamin, mineral, and electrolyte supplementation

secondary lactase deficiency A condition that may develop as a secondary problem in a person who has a disease of the small intestine such as celiac disease, Crohn's disease, or protein-calorie malnutrition.

developmental lactase deficiency A condition that results from a gradual decrease in lactase during childhood and adolescence.

ant of lactose throughout their lives. **Secondary lactase deficiency** may develop as a secondary problem in a person who has a small intestine disease such as celiac disease, Crohn's disease, or protein-calorie malnutrition (PCM). **Developmental lactase deficiency** results from a gradual decrease in the lactase level during childhood and adolescence, until it is quite low in the adult. Approximately 70% of African Americans have this condition, along with significant percentages of Orientals and American Indians.

The tolerance of milk by these groups varies considerably, and many are able to tolerate and benefit from inclusion of moderate amounts of milk and other dairy foods in their diet.

Symptoms. The increased osmotic pressure in the small intestine from ingestion of milk results in a bloated feeling, flatulence, belching, cramps, or diarrhea.

Diet Therapy. An infant who has a congenital lactase deficiency can obtain the necessary nutrients from soybean formulas that contain low levels of lactose. Adults with secondary and developmental deficiencies can frequently tolerate partially fermented dairy products (which have reduced or absent lactose) such as cottage cheese, buttermilk, sour cream, yogurt, and hard cheese. The principles of a lactose-restricted diet are provided in Table 16-9.

A lactase enzyme powder (Lact-Acid) can be added to milk, thereby hydrolyzing lactose to galactose and glucose. This makes it possible for lactase-deficient individuals to drink milk without experiencing the previously mentioned symptoms. Table 16-10 summarizes important information about lactase deficiency.[6]

Sample Menu for a Gluten-restricted Diet

Exchange

	Breakfast
1 fruit	½ cup orange juice
1 bread	¾ cup corn flakes
2 fat	2 strips bacon
1 bread	1 slice low-gluten bread
1 fat	margarine
1 milk	1 cup skim milk
	1 cup coffee with sugar
	Lunch
3 lean meat	3 oz baked fresh fish (halibut, trout, red snapper, etc.)
1 bread	1 small baked potato
1 vegetable	½ cup sliced tomatoes plus lettuce
1 bread + 1 fat	1 piece corn bread (2 × 2 × 1 in.) (made without flour)
1 fat	1 tsp margarine
1 fruit	4 apricot halves
	iced tea with lemon and sugar
	Dinner
	7 oz beef bouillon
3 lean meat	3 oz broiled chicken
1 vegetable	½ cup green beans
1 bread	1 slice low-gluten bread
1 fat	1 tsp margarine
	cherry gelatin (1 envelope)
1 milk	1 cup skim milk
	iced tea with lemon and sugar

Analysis and Comments

- An analysis of this menu shows that it contains 2 milk, 2 vegetable, 2 fruit, 5 bread, 6 meat, and 6 fat exchanges.

- In reference to the exchanges, the following foods should be eliminated:

  Milk: commercial chocolate milk and malted milk.

  Vegetables: creamed or breaded.

  Fruit: none.

  Bread: all breads made with wheat, rye, oats, barley, and buckwheat should be eliminated. Notice that this menu includes low-gluten bread and cornbread. Any breads or cereals that contain corn (cornbread, corn tortillas) or rice (rice wafers, Rice Krispies, and puffed rice) are allowed and should definitely be included, since they are the only grain sources that can be tolerated.

  Meat: meats excluded are prepared meats such as sausage, frankfurters, bologna, luncheon meat, and commercial hamburger, meat loaf, croquettes, gravy, cream sauce and processed cheese.

  Fat: cream substitutes, whipped toppings, and commercial salad dressings (typically contain gluten stabilizers) must be eliminated.

  Miscellaneous: puddings (except cornstarch and tapioca) must be eliminated. All beverages that contain wheat, rye, oats, or barley, such as beer and ale, must be eliminated. In addition, chili sauce, soy sauce, and bottled meat sauces contain these grains and must be eliminated.

- Sometimes the gluten-restricted menu initially decreases the number of fat exchanges and fiber to decrease diarrhea and steatorrhea.
- Between meals, bedtime snacks are given to achieve a high kilocalorie intake.
- This menu and similar ones are typically deficient in thiamin and iron, since wheat, barley, oats, and rye must be eliminated. Therefore, it is recommended that the diet be supplemented with daily vitamins and minerals.

Source: Adapted from *Diet Manual* (5th ed.) by the Texas Dietetic Association, 1988, Austin: The Texas Dietetic Association. Reprinted by permission.

Crohn's disease An inflammatory disease that is located primarily in the ileum region of the small intestine and may extend into the large intestine.

granuloma A tumor-like mass of granulation tissue.

serosa The outer layer of the intestine.

Crohn's Disease (Inflammatory Bowel Disease)

Crohn's disease is an inflammatory disease that is located primarily in the ileum region of the small intestine but may extend into the large intestine. The intestinal wall may also have **granulomas** extending through all layers, including the **serosa** (see Fig. 16-13). The disease occurs frequently in young adults and is seen in mild, moderate, and severe forms.

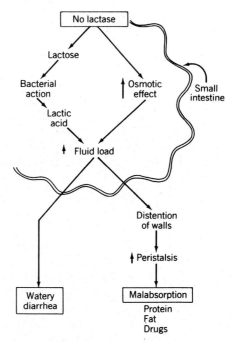

FIGURE 16-12 The effects on the small intestine caused by lactase deficiency. (Reproduced with permission from R.B. Howard and N.H. Herbold, *Nutrition in Clinical Care.* New York: McGraw-Hill Book Company, 1978.)

Cause. The exact cause is unknown. Some theories focus on infectious agents, autoimmune disease, and possibly a genetic link.

Symptoms. The symptoms tend to vary depending on the severity of the condition and the area of the gastrointestinal tract affected. Mild intermittent bloody diarrhea, two to five stools per day, and pain in the lower abdomen are common symptoms. Some patients also develop steatorrhea, weight loss, and anemia. Other malabsorption symptoms may be present. Young children may experience growth retardation.[7]

Diet Therapy. The general dietary goals are to rest the small intestine so that healing can occur and to avoid nutritional deficiency states. These goals are best achieved by excluding foods that are high in fiber (raw fruits and vegetables) and residue. See the sample menu for a minimum-residue diet. Table 16-11 provides the pathophysiology, cause, symptoms, and diet therapy for Crohn's disease.

Medium chain triglycerides (MCTs) should be used to replace the fats that are not being absorbed.

cecum The first portion of the large intestine to which the small intestine attaches and from which the appendix extends.

ileocecal valve A valve that is located between the ileum and the cecum.

To promote healing of the intestinal wall, the diet should be high in protein and carbohydrate and low in fat. Supplementation with vitamin B_{12} may be necessary due to malabsorption (see Fig. 16-11 for site of vitamin B_{12} absorption). Supplementation with iron and folic acid may be necessary due to blood loss from tissue destruction. Patients with severe Crohn's disease respond very favorably to total parenteral nutrition (hyperalimentation), especially when they are to undergo surgery.[8]

LARGE INTESTINE (COLON)

ascending colon The portion of the large intestine that ascends upward on the right side of the body from the cecum to the liver.

transverse colon The portion of the large intestine that extends across the abdomen from the right to the left.

descending colon The portion of the large intestine that extends downward along the left side of the abdomen.

The large intestine is a continuation of the alimentary canal from the small intestine. It is a muscular tube about 5 ft in length and is noticeably larger in diameter than the small intestine. It extends from the **cecum** to the anal canal and is divided into the cecum, colon, and rectum (see Fig. 16-14). The **ileocecal** valve guards the entrance into the cecum. The colon is subdivided into the **ascending, transverse, descending,** and **sigmoid** colons. The last major region of the large intestine is the rectum. The final inch of the rectum is called the *anal canal* and is guarded by internal and external sphincter muscles.

The functions of the large intestine are related to the final processing of materials that enter from the small intestine:

TABLE 16-9 LACTOSE-RESTRICTED DIET

Purpose	Provide foods that contain a minimum of lactose.
Use	Used to reduce symptoms in people who do not tolerate lactose well due to a deficiency of the enzyme lactase.
Examples of foods	General diet, with a reduction of milk and milk products that contain lactose. Most people can tolerate about 4 to 8 oz of milk if consumed with meals. Yogurt and other fermented foods are generally tolerated, since lactose is altered by fermentation. Breast milk contains more lactose than cow's milk, so breast feeding is not recommended for infants born with congenital lactose intolerance.
Adequacy	Diet will lack calcium but will be adequate in all other nutrients; calcium supplements or the use of milk substitute is recommended.

Source: From *Manual of Clinical Dietetics* (4th ed.) by the Chicago Dietetic Association, 1992, The American Dietetic Association. Reprinted by permission.

TABLE 16-10 SUMMARY OF LACTOSE INTOLERANCE

Pathophysiology	Causes	Symptoms	Dietary Treatment
Lack of lactase enzyme activity	Congenital Secondary Developmental	Bloated feeling Flatulence Belching Cramps Diarrhea	Lactose-free formula for infants Partially fermented dairy products—cottage cheese, buttermilk, sour cream yogurt—generally can be pretty well tolerated.

sigmoid colon The S-shaped portion of the large intestine between the descending colon and the rectum.

Reabsorption of water and electrolytes. About 600 ml of water with electrolytes are absorbed through the colon wall into the blood, compared with about 8,000 ml absorbed by the small intestine.

Elimination of wastes (feces). Nonabsorbed residue, bacteria, nonabsorbed water, and electrolytes are excreted as feces by the anal canal.

intestinal flora Bacteria in the large intestine.

Synthesis of vitamins. **Intestinal flora** synthesize several vitamins, including vitamin K and some of the B complex group.

Disorders

Colonic Diverticulosis and Diverticulitis

colonic diverticulosis A condition characterized by small, saclike herniations of the colon mucosa called *diverticula*.

Colonic diverticulosis is a condition characterized by small, saclike herniations of the colon mucosa (see Fig. 16-15) called *divertculae*. The most common initial site of diverticula formation is the sigmoid colon.

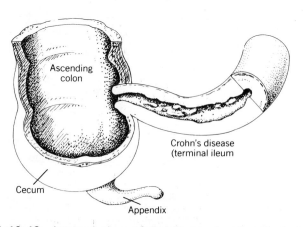

FIGURE 16-13 Internal view of the ileum showing Crohn's disease.

TABLE 16-11 SUMMARY OF CROHN'S DISEASE (INFLAMMATORY BOWEL DISEASE)

Pathophysiology	Etiology	Symptoms	Diet Therapy
Inflammation of intestinal mucosa in ileum region Granulomas extending through wall of intestine	Exact cause unknown Possibly due to infectious agents, autoimmune, or genetic component	Mild diarrhea Lower abdominal pain Steatorrhea Weight loss Anemia	Rest the small intestine Low-fiber, low-residue diet High protein and carbohydrate levels Supplementation with iron, folate, and vitamin B_{12}

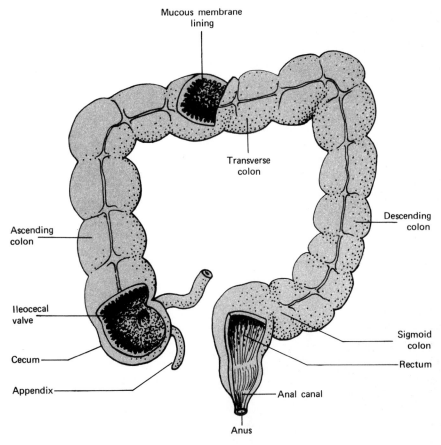

FIGURE 16-14 The large intestine and its subdivisions. (From S.R. Burke, *Human Anatomy and Physiology in Health & Disease*. Albany. Delmar Publishers, 1992. Reprinted by permission.)

Sample Menu for a Minimum-residue Diet

Exchange	
	Breakfast
1 fruit	½ cup strained orange juice
1 bread	½ cup cream of wheat
2 medium-fat meat	2 poached eggs
2 bread	2 slices of white toast
2 fat	2 tsp margarine
	Lunch
2 low-fat meat	2 oz tender, lean roast beef
1 vegetable	½ cup buttered rice
1 vegetable	½ cup tomato juice
1 bread	1 slice white bread
1 fat	1 tsp margarine
	angel food cake
	iced tea
	Dinner
	1 cup beef broth
1 bread	½ cup macaroni
1 fruit	¼ cup grape juice
1 bread	slice white bread
1 fat	1 tsp margarine
	plain orange gelatin
	iced tea

Analysis and Comments

- An analysis of this menu shows 0 milk, 2 vegetable, 2 fruit, 6 bread, 4 meat, and 4 fat exchanges.
- Notice that the fruits and vegetables are either juices or soft vegetables as opposed to fresh whole fruits and fibrous vegetables. These adaptations reduce the level of residue.
- Foods from the meat exchange list are either soft foods (eggs) or tender beef, which are low in fiber and will form little residue.
- Notice that there are no milk exchanges. The reason is that milk

can be fermented by bacteria in the large intestine, thereby forming a large amount of residue.

▪ Due to its adaptations and exclusions, this menu is deficient in the
RDA levels of calcium, iron, vitamin A, riboflavin, and vitamin D.
If it is to be followed for a long period, these vitamins and miner-
als should be supplemented.

Source: Adapted from *Diet Manual* (5th ed.) by the Texas Dietetic Association, 1988, Austin:
The Texas Dietetic Association. Reprinted by permission.

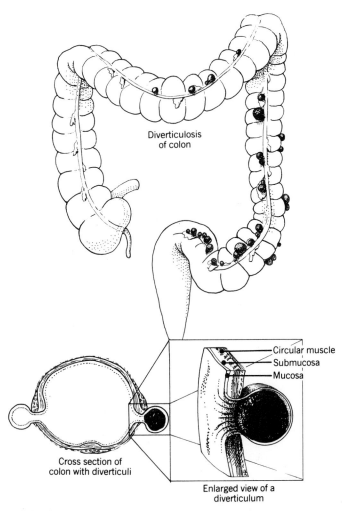

FIGURE 16-15   Diverticulosis of the large intestine.

diverticulitis Inflammatory condition of diverticula caused by bacterial growth and action arising from food residues and fecal matter.

The incidence of diverticulosis is higher in people over 40 years of age than in younger people. Between 15 and 30% of diverticulosis cases develop into the inflammatory condition called **diverticulitis.**

Cause. One basic cause of this disease is a low-fiber diet. The mechanism by which a low-fiber diet results in the formation of diverticula is as follows:

Low-fiber→ foods	increased segmenta- → tion of colon to move residue along	increased → intraluminal pressure within intestine	protrusion of intestinal mucosa through intestinal wall

A high-fiber diet basically prevents diverticulosis, since the feces occupy a greater volume and are heavier. This condition results in less segmentation of the colon in moving the feces along, thereby generating less intraluminal pressure.

Symptoms of Colonic Diverticulosis. Symptoms are minimal, with occasional abdominal discomfort. Constipation is not a symptom of diverticulosis but rather an indication that conditions are right for its development.

Diet Therapy of Colonic Diverticulosis. The treatment consists of prevention, which is accomplished by increasing the amount of fiber and bulk in the diet. This diet decreases intraluminal pressure and reduces the possible development of diverticula. If diverticula are already present, they may revert to a normal state if a high-fiber diet is consumed and intraluminal pressure remains lowered over a period of time. The principles of a high-fiber diet are provided in Table 16-12.

Symptoms of Diverticulitis. If diverticulosis develops into diverticulitis, the symptoms are an increase in the total white blood cell count, fever, left lower quadrant abdominal pain, abdominal distention, flatulence, slight nausea, and constipation. Occasionally, bloody stools and/or intestinal obstructions may occur.

fistulas Abnormal tubelike passages within the body tissue, usually between two internal organs.

abscesses Localized collections of pus in cavities formed by the disintegration of tissues.

Diet Therapy for Diverticulitis. The initial treatment of an acute attack of diverticulitis is bed rest, antibiotics, stool softeners, and a liquid diet. If there is no evidence of obstruction, **fistulas, abscesses,** or perforation, the diet may progress to normal. Bulk agents such as Metamucil or bran may be gradually included, but large quantities should be avoided. After the inflammation has subsided, a high-fiber diet may be followed.

TABLE 16-12 HIGH-FIBER DIET

Purpose	Promotes regular elimination and increases fecal excretion.
Use	Used in treatment of diverticular disease, atonic constipation, and irritable bowel syndrome.
Examples of foods	Almost all foods on a general diet are included; includes three to four servings of food high in indigestible carbohydrates (fiber).
Adequacy	The diet is adequate.

Source: From *Manual of Clinical Dietetics* (4th ed.) by the Chicago Dietetic Association, 1992, Chicago, The American Dietetic Association. Reprinted by permission.

Ulcerative Colitis (Inflammatory Bowel Disease)

Ulcerative colitis is similar to Crohn's disease in that it is also an inflammatory disease and has other features common to Crohn's disease. It mostly occurs in adults between the ages of 20 and 40 years. Ulcerative colitis is about five times more common than Crohn's disease.

The ulcers are located in the mucosa (see Fig. 16-16) and submucosa of the large intestine, as opposed to the granulomas in Crohn's disease extending through all layers of the small intestine wall. The initial ulcers are located in the rectum and sigmoid colon regions, from which they tend to spread upward.

Cause. As with Crohn's disease, the exact cause is unknown. Some theories are as follows:

- Genetic. There is a strong familial relationship in colitis.
- Autoimmunity. Antibodies from the colon and the diseased region have been found in the serum of ulcerative colitis patients.
- Psychological stress. Much controversy has been generated over this theory. It is now considered to play a secondary role.

Symptoms. The symptoms vary depending on whether the patient has **acute fulminating, chronic intermittent (recurrent),** or **chronic continuous** colitis. Most ulcerative colitis patients have the chronic intermittent (recurrent) type. The attacks are short and may occur at intervals ranging from months to years. There may be little or no fever. It is common for the patient to suffer frequent **exacerbations** and repeated hospitalizations.

The chronic loss of blood and mucus may result in anemia, dehydration, and hypoproteinemia. Chronic poor protein intake may also contribute to hypoproteinemia. Crampy abdominal pain and weight loss are

acute fulminating A condition that occurs suddenly with great intensity.

chronic intermittent (recurrent) A type of ulcerative colitis that is characterized by mild diarrhea and intermittent, slight bleeding.

chronic continuous A condition that persists for a long time and shows either little change or an extremely slow progression over a long period.

exacerbations Increased severity and complications.

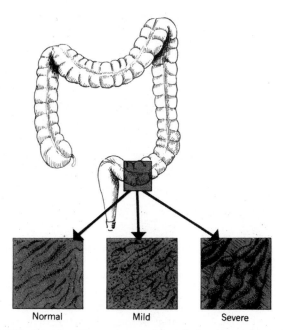

FIGURE 16-16 Ulcerative colitis of the large intestine.

common symptoms. Patients may be deficient in vitamin B$_{12}$ if the ileum region of the small intestine is affected.

Ulcerative colitis patients frequently exhibit an intolerance to milk, since lactase depletion is secondary to the disease.

Diet Therapy. The principal goals of diet therapy are to control inflammation, maintain the patient's nutritional status, give symptomatic relief, and prevent infection.

A bland, low-residue diet may be helpful during attacks but is not believed to help prevent the symptoms. A new and quite successful approach to treating acute attacks of this chronic disease is 4–6 weeks of total parenteral nutritional therapy with simultaneous drug therapy.

The protein in the diet should be high, 1.5 g per kilogram of desired body weight per day. The caloric level should be 2,400–3,600 kcal/day. If eggs or milk are not well tolerated, manufactured (packaged) nutritional supplement formulas are excellent for providing kilocalories and protein, provided they do not present the intestine with an **osmotic overload.**

Any foods that may irritate the mucosa, such as raw fruits and vegetables, are eliminated.

Iron should be supplemented, due to loss of blood, but because of diarrhea and malabsorption it should be administered parenterally or intramuscularly. Vitamin B$_{12}$ should also be administered parenterally.[9]

osmotic overload A condition that results in the movement of large amounts of water into the intestines from the blood.

anticholinergic drugs Drugs that block the passage of impulses through the parasympathetic nerves.

total colectomy   Removal of the colon.

ileostomy   An opening into the ileum for drainage of fecal matter.

Anticholinergic drugs help to relieve cramps and diarrhea. Emotional support from the health team is very important to successful treatment.

If dietary, drug, and emotional help fail, surgical intervention is indicated. The most common procedure is a **total colectomy** and the creation of a permanent **ileostomy.**[10]

Table 16-13 summarizes information about ulcerative colitis.

CASE STUDY: PEPTIC ULCER AND THE DUMPING SYNDROME

John is a 45-year-old Spanish-American who is admitted to a hospital with complaints of epigastric fullness, nausea, dizziness, tachycardia, and generalized malaise 2–3 hours after eating.

Family History. Father died of a heart attack last year. Mother, age 63, alive and well. Five brothers and three sisters.

Personal History. Frequent alcohol but no tobacco use. No medications. Subtotal gastrectomy 6 years ago. Has not been taking vitamin and mineral supplements or following the prescribed diet.

Laboratory Findings		Normal Values
Serum iron	40 μg/dl	65–150 μg/dl
Serum calcium	7.3 mg/dl	9–11 mg/dl
Serum glucose	40 mg/dl	70–120 mg/dl
	at 2 hours of oral glucose tolerance test	
Bone biopsy indicated Osteoporosis		
Hemoglobin	8 g/dl	13–16 g/dl
Hematocrit	33%	42–50%

TABLE 16-13 SUMMARY OF ULCERATIVE COLITIS

Pathophysiology	Etiology	Symptoms	Diet Therapy
Ulcers in mucosa and submucosa of large intestine	Exact cause unknown Theories Genetic Autoimmunity Stress	Diarrhea Crampy abdominal pain Anemia Hyproteinemia	Low-residue diet Bland diet Total parenteral nutrition High protein level High calorie level Eliminate milk if patient is intolerant Supplement iron and vitamin B$_{12}$

Present illness. A diagnosis of early postprandial (after-meal) dumping syndrome, anemia, and osteoporosis.

Using the above information plus material in this chapter, answer the following questions.

1. John's subtotal gastrectomy probably was for a _____ ulcer.
   A. gastric
   B. duodenal
2. The basis for the low serum iron and calcium values is _____.
   A. partial stomach removal.
   B. decreased amount of mucus.
   C. decreased amount of HCl
   D. decreased pepsin enzyme
3. John's laboratory values indicate that he is probably suffering from _____ anemia.
   A. pernicious
   B. iron deficiency
   C. folic acid
   D. none of these
4. The following dumping syndrome diet has been planned for John. Using the exchange lists (Appendix A), calculate the protein, fat, and carbohydrate values in grams; then choose from the answers below:

	Exchanges	Protein (g)	Fat (g)	Carbohydrate (g)
Meat (all medium fat)	15			
Fat	18			
Fruit	2			
Vegetables	2			
Bread	3			
Total				

   A. protein, 118 g; fat, 165 g; carbohydrate, 85 g
   B. protein, 105 g; fat, 90 g; carbohydrate, 185 g
   C. protein, 185 g; fat, 75 g; carbohydrate, 150 g
   D. protein, 110 g; fat, 150 g; carbohydrate, 100 g
5. The total kilocalories for this diet are:
   A. 3,510
   B. 1,985
   C. 2,297
   D. 3,247

6. The caloric ratio is protein, 1.5; fat, 5; and carbohydrate, 1. The reason(s) why the fat and protein ratios are high and the carbohydrate ratio low is (are):
   A. fat and protein supply needed calories
   B. fat delays gastric emptying
   C. simple carbohydrates increase osmotic pressure in intestines more than fats and proteins
   D. A, B, C

7. Food from one exchange list is intentionally omitted from the diet, which is _____ and the reason is due to its _____ content.
   A. cereal—carbohydrate
   B. milk—fat
   C. liquid—water
   D. milk—carbohydrate (lactose)

8. In reference to question 7, which important mineral (contained in an omitted food) is lacking and therefore must be given as an oral supplement?
   A. sodium
   B. cobalt
   C. potassium
   D. calcium

9. The basis for some of John's dumping syndrome symptoms is rapid movement of water from the blood into the intestines, thereby lowering blood pressure.
   A. true   B. false

10. John has not been following his prescribed diet, and an increased intake of simple sugars is probably a major reason for the symptoms and activity mentioned in question 9.
    A. true   B. false

SUMMARY

- Hiatal hernia is caused by a congenital weakness of the diaphragm, aging, obesity, pregnancy, or tight-fitting clothes. Symptoms include heartburn, dysphagia, substernal pain, and vomiting. Diet therapy involves a bland diet, small frequent feedings, and no foods 3–4 hours before bedtime.
- Acute gastritis is caused by alcohol consumed with aspirin, and spicy foods. Symptoms include anorexia, epigastric pain, and vomiting. Diet therapy involves removing offending foods.
- A peptic ulcer is caused by an imbalance between the amount of HCl and pepsin enzyme, and mucosal resistance. Symptoms include epigastric pain 1–3 hours after eating, heartburn, anorexia, vomiting, weight loss, and constipation. Diet therapy involves a liberal diet, adequate protein, and a moderate amount of fat.
- Symptoms of dumping syndrome include weakness, nausea, sweating, tachycardia, and dizziness, due to rapid entrance of food into the duodenum and subsequent increased osmotic pressure in the intestines. Dietary treatment involves minimizing the quantity of food and increasing the number of meals, avoiding simple sugars, and avoiding liquids 30 minutes before and 1 hour after eating meals.
- Long-range nutritional problems after a subtotal gastrectomy include hypercalcemia, anemia, and reduced food intake and absorption.
- Celiac disease is caused by an inborn error of metabolism or an immune reaction to gluten. Symptoms include diarrhea and stetorrhea in adults, irritability and failure to gain weight in children. Diet therapy involves a low-gluten diet and vitamin, mineral, and electrolyte supplements.
- Lactose intolerance causes are congenital, secondary, and developmental. Symptoms include a bloated feeling, flatulence, belching, cramps, and diarrhea. Diet therapy involves a lactose-free formula for infants and partially fermented dairy products for adults.
- Crohn's disease is caused by infectious agents, autoimmune disease, or a genetic factor. Symptoms include diarrhea, pain in the lower abdomen, steatorrhea, weight loss, and anemia. Diet therapy involves a low-fiber diet, with high protein and carbohydrate and low fat levels; the diet is supplemented with iron, folate, and vitamin B_{12}.
- Diverticulosis and diverticulitis occur when low-fiber foods cause increased intraluminal pressure in the large intestine. Symptoms of diverticulosis include minimal constipation; diet therapy involves high fiber and bulk in diet. Symptoms of diverticulitis include increased total white blood cell count, fever, left lower quadrant pain, flatulence, slight nausea, and constipation; diet therapy involves antibiotics, stool softeners, and a liquid diet initially, with a gradual progression to a normal diet. After inflammation subsides, a high-fiber diet may be followed.
- Ulcerative colitis is caused by a genetic component, autoimmunity, or psychological stress. Symptoms include chronic intermittent colitis and diarrhea, slight bleeding, anemia, dehydration, hypoproteinemia, and vitamin B_{12} deficiency. Diet therapy involves a bland, low-residue diet during attacks, with a high-calorie diet and iron supplements when there is no attack.

REVIEW QUESTIONS

True (A) or False (B)

1. The primary goal of the diet in hiatal hernia is to prevent reflux by a bland diet and small frequent feedings.
2. A person who is receiving a hiatal hernia diet should not eat food 3–4 hours before bedtime.
3. A gastric ulcer is the most common type of peptic ulcer.
4. The exact cause of peptic ulcers is known to be the result of being tense, hard-driving, and anxious.
5. A constant state of epigastric pain is a common symptom of a gastric or duodenal ulcer.
6. The primary goal of peptic ulcer dietary management is to buffer or inhibit acid secretions in the stomach.
7. General guidelines for an ulcer diet for a symptom-free person are three meals rather than six small meals per day, elimination of bedtime snacks, avoidance of milk and cream feedings to reduce acidity, and avoidance of excessive alcohol.
8. The dumping syndrome is a combination of symptoms—weakness, a desire to lie down,

nausea, profound sweating, tachycardia, and dizziness—that often develop after a subtotal gastrectomy.

9. Dietary treatment of the dumping syndrome includes increased consumption of simple sugars and decreased consumption of fats.

10. Some of the long-term problems related to a subtotal gastrectomy are hypercalcemia and constipation.

11. One theory about the cause of nontropical sprue is that the protein gluten, found in wheat, causes an immune reaction to the intestinal mucosa.

12. Some of the common symptoms of nontropical sprue are diarrhea, fatty stools (steatorrhea), and muscle wasting.

13. All products that may contain wheat, and thus gluten, must be eliminated from the diet, with breaded vegetables, chicken fried steak, and gravy being examples.

14. All breads and cereals that contain wheat, corn, and rice must be eliminated from a gluten-restricted diet. (For the answer, consult the analysis and comments on the sample menu for the gluten-restricted diet.)

15. A gluten-restricted diet involves merely increasing the amount of food consumed to achieve adequacy in the intake of certain nutrients such as thiamine and iron. (The comments for question 15 are applicable here.)

16. Congenital lactase deficiency is the most common type of lactase deficiency and is very prevalent in African Americans and Orientals.

17. Lactase deficiency can result in malabsorption of nutrients due to increased motility and diarrhea.

18. A lactose-intolerant individual must avoid all dairy products, including cottage cheese, buttermilk, sour cream, yogurt, and hard cheese.

19. Symptoms of Crohn's disease include bloody diarrhea, pain in the lower abdomen, and possibly steatorrhea.

20. The dietary goal of Crohn's disease is to rest the small intestine, which is best accomplished by excluding foods high in fiber and residue.

21. A person who has diverticulitis has herniations of the small intestine mucosa, constipation, and few other minimal symptoms.

22. The treatment of diverticulosis is a liquid diet, bed rest, antibiotics, and stool softeners.

23. A high-fiber diet is recommended for diverticu-

litis after inflammation has subsided, since it decreases intraluminal pressure, thereby decreasing the chance of diverticuli formation.

24. Ulcerative colitis is characterized by ulcers in the mucosa of the rectum and sigmoid colon, with diarrhea, crampy abdominal pain, and weight loss being common symptoms.

25. The principal goals of diet therapy for ulcerative colitis are to control inflammation, maintain the patient's nutritional status, give symptomatic relief, and prevent infection.

26. An ulcerative colitis diet should consist of high levels of protein and decreased amounts of raw fruits and vegetables, plus iron and vitamin B_{12} supplements.

Multiple Choice

27. Hiatal hernia is characterized by:
    1. possibly being caused by aging and obesity
    2. complaints of heartburn, reflux, and difficulty in swallowing
    3. diet therapy consisting of a bland diet and small, frequent feedings
    4. no food being eaten 3–4 hours before bedtime
       A. 1, 2, 3   B. 1, 3   C. 2, 4   D. 4
       E. all of these

28. The exact cause of peptic ulcers is not known; however, the condition can result from:
    1. an imbalance in the amount of HCl
    2. an imbalance in the amount of pepsin enzyme
    3. an imbalance in mucosal resistance of the gastric mucosa
    4. eating a chronic low-fiber diet
       A. 1, 2, 3   B. 1, 3   C. 2, 4   D. 4
       E. all of these

29. Current dietary therapy for peptic ulcer includes
    1. six small meals per day
    2. inclusion of a bedtime snack
    3. consumption of whole milk as opposed to skim milk
    4. limitation of black pepper, chili powder, and nicotine
       A. 1, 2, 3   B. 1, 3   C. 2, 4   D. 4
       E. all of these

30. The symptoms or changes in blood vessels and the small intestine that may result from a subto-

tal gastrectomy are _____ and the reason(s) is (are) _____.

1. increased osmotic pressure in the intestines—rapid entrance of food into the duodenum
2. increase in blood pressure—large volume of water moving out of the intestines
3. weakness, sweating, and tachycardia—drop in blood pressure due to movement of water out of the blood
4. slow entrance of food into the duodenum—removal of the majority of the stomach and pyloric sphincter
   A. 1, 2, 3   B. 1, 3   C. 2, 4   D. 4
   E. all of these

31. The dietary treatment for control of dumping syndrome is (are)
    1. an increased quantity of food at three meals
    2. avoidance of simple sugars
    3. drinking liquids with meals
    4. increasing the number of kilocalories from polyunsaturated fat and proteins
       A. 1, 2, 3   B. 1, 3   C. 2, 4   D. 4

32. Long-range nutritional problems that are possible following a subtotal gastrectomy are
    1. hypocalcemia and osteoporosis
    2. iron deficiency and pernicious anemia
    3. fear of eating
    4. high blood cholesterol level
       A. 1, 2, 3   B. 1, 3   C. 2, 4   D. 4
       E. all of these

33. The immune theory of the cause of celiac disease is that _____ causes the intestinal villi to _____, thereby decreasing absorption.
    A. simple sugars—be destroyed
    B. corn and rice—enlarge and become distorted in shape
    C. gluten—atrophy, shorten, and fuse
    D. fats—become ulcerated

34. Infants who have congenital lactose intolerance can obtain necessary nutrients from _____ and adults with secondary lactose intolerance can tolerate partially fermented dairy products such as _____.
    A. fat formulas—skim milk and skim cheese
    B. soybean—cottage cheese and buttermilk formulas
    C. sucrose—low-fat butter and ice cream formulas
    D. none of these

35. A menu for a minimum-residue diet, such as for Crohn's disease, has the following characteristics and adaptions:
    1. numerous servings of fresh fruits and fibrous vegetables
    2. two servings of skim milk
    3. six servings of high-fiber bread
    4. supplements of calcium, iron, vitamin A, riboflavin, and vitamin D
       A. 1, 2, 3   B. 1, 3   C. 2, 4   D. 4
       E. all of these

36. A chronic low-fiber diet may cause diverticulosis, and the mechanism that results in the formation of diverticula is
    A. low-fiber foods → increased segmentation → of colon

    → increased intra-luminal pressure within intestine   → protrusion of intestinal mucosa through intestinal wall

    B. high-fiber foods → decreased segmentation → of colon

    → decreased intra-luminal pressure within intestine   → protrusion of intestinal mucosa through intestinal wall

37. Initial treatment of an acute attack of diverticulitis consists of:
    1. a high-fiber diet   2. stool softeners
    3. a high-residue diet   4. a liquid diet
       A. 1, 2, 3   B. 1, 3   C. 2, 4   D. 4
       E. all of these

38. Chronic intermittent ulcerative colitis typically occurs in the mucosa and submucosa layers of the _____ regions of the large intestine and is characterized by _____.
    A. ascending and transverse—severe diarrhea and bleeding
    B. cecum and ascending—steatorrhea and constipation
    C. rectum and sigmoid—mild diarrhea and slight bleeding
    D. none of these

39. Dietary and drug therapy for ulcerative colitis includes

1. total parenteral nutrition
2. decreased amounts of raw fruit and vegetables
3. iron and vitamin B_{12} supplements
4. administration of anticholinergic drugs
   A. 1, 2, 3   B. 1, 3   C. 2, 4   D. 4
   E. all of these

Completion

40. Discuss the general guidelines for a liberal, individualized diet for peptic ulcer.
41. Describe the mechanism by which a low-fiber diet may cause diverticulosis.
42. Discuss the causes, symptoms, and diet therapy for ulcerative colitis.

CRITICAL THINKING CHALLENGE

1. Determine which of the lunches below would be part of a
   a. minimum-residue diet
   b. gluten-restricted diet
   c. liberal peptic ulcer diet

Lunch 1

1½ vegetable	6 oz vegetable soup
2 medium-fat meats	2 oz beef patty
1 vegetable	½ sliced tomato
1 fat	1 tbsp French dressing
1 fruit	4 apricots
1 milk	8 oz milk (whole or lowfat)

Lunch 2

2 low-fat meats	2 oz tender, lean roast beef
1 vegetable	½ cup buttered rice
1 vegetable	½ cup tomato juice
1 bread	1 slice white bread
1 fat	1 tsp margarine

Lunch 3

3 lean meats	3 oz baked fresh fish
1 bread	1 small baked potato
1 vegetable	½ cup sliced tomatoes
1 bread + 1 fat	1 pc corn bread
1 fat	1 tsp margarine
1 fruit	4 apricots

2. State and explain why which of the lunches from question 1 would be appropriate for: Crohn's disease, nontropical sprue, and gastric ulcer.
3. Your client is diagnosed with ulcerative colitis. You have identified the nursing diagnosis Altered Nutrition: Less Than Body Requirements related to diarrhea, dietary restrictions, and pain. Which of the following would *not* be dietary goals for the client?
   a. Maintaining nutritional status
   b. Reducing inflammation
   c. Preventing infection
   d. Stimulating peristalsis

REVIEW QUESTIONS FOR NCLEX

Situation. Mr. C is admitted to the hospital with a diagnosis of possible duodenal ulcer. His job is one that requires him to work long hours under a lot of stress. He drinks approximately 6–8 cups of coffee per day. In addition he smokes two packs of cigarettes per day.

1. Mr. C probably did not exhibit which symptom at the time of admission?
   A. weight loss
   B. heartburn
   C. constipation
   D. good appetite
2. Mr. C asks why his diet does not allow coffee and an explanation might be that caffeine _____.
   A. hinders absorption of food
   B. aggravates the nerve endings in stomach wall resulting in pain
   C. causes constipation and decreases digestion of food
   D. stimulates secretion of HCl
3. In discussing Mr. C's diet with him it would be explained that the primary goal of his dietary management is to _____.
   A. buffer or inhibit acid secretions
   B. aid him in gaining weight
   C. reduce vomiting
   D. reduce nausea and anorexia
4. Mr. C is symptom free therefore, which of the following do not characterize a liberal ulcer diet?

A. three meals per day rather than six
B. meals that are high in cream and fat
C. bedtime snacks
D. complete elimination of foods such as baked beans and cabbage

5. Mr. C's duodenal ulcer does not respond to medical treatment and he is advised to have surgery. He undergoes a pyloric antrectomy (removal of the pyloric region of the stomach), truncal vagotomy (severing of the vagus nerve at the stomach) with a Billroth II reconstruction (joining of the gastric stump to the jejunum). Postoperatively, after bowel sounds have returned, how would you describe his diet to prevent dumping syndrome?
A. high carbohydrate, low fat, low protein, and three meals per day
B. low carbohydrate, low fat, low protein, and 6 meals per day
C. low carbohydrate, high fat, high protein, and 6 meals per day
D. high carbohydrates, high fat, high protein, and 6 meals per day

REFERENCES

1. Williams, S. R. (1991). Nutrition and diet therapy (6th ed.) (pp. 732–733). St. Louis: Times Mirror/Mosby College Publishing.
2. Mulholland, M. W., & Debas, H. T. (1987). Chronic duodenal and gastric ulcer. *Surg. Clin. North America, 67,* 489.
3. Hollander, D. (1988). Diet therapy of peptic ulcer disease. *Nutrition and the M.D., 14*(2), 1.
4. Mahan, K. L., & Arlin, M. (1992). *Food, nutrition, and diet therapy* (8th ed.) (pp. 446–448). Philadelphia: W. B. Saunders.
5. Holmes, G.K.T., et al. (1989). Malignancy in coeliac disease—Effect of a gluten free diet. *Gut 30,* 333.
6. Rosado, J. L., Allen, L. H., & Solomons, N. W. (1987). Milk consumption symptom response and lactose digestion in milk intolerance. *American Journal of Clinical Nutrition, 45,* 1457.
7. Jayanthi, V., Probert, C.S.V., Sher, K. S., & Mayberry, J. F. (1991). Current concepts of the etiopathogenesis of inflammatory bowel disease. *Gastroenterology, 86,* 1566–1572.
8. Christie, P. M., & Hill, G. L. (1990). Effect of intravenous nutrition on nutrition and function in acute attacks of inflammatory bowel disease. *Gastroenterology, 99,* 730–736.
9. Farraye, F. A., & Peppercorn, M. A. (1988). Advances in the management of ulcerative colitis and Crohn's disease. *Consultant, 28*(10), 39.
10. Peppercorn, M. (1989). Advances in drug therapy for inflammatory bowel disease. *Annals of Internal Medicine, 112*(1), 50.

17 DISORDERS OF THE LIVER, GALLBLADDER, AND PANCREAS

OBJECTIVES

Upon completion of this chapter, you should be able to:

1. Name and give examples of the four liver functions.
2. Give the cause and symptoms of hepatitis.
3. Name the most common cause of cirrhosis and describe the underlying causes of portal hypertension, esophageal varices, and ascites.
4. Describe the dietary treatment of hepatitis and cirrhosis in terms of the amounts of kilocalories, protein, carbohydrate, fat, vitamin supplements, and sodium.
5. Discuss the drug treatments of hepatitis and cirrhosis and their possible side effects.
6. Name the precipating factor that results in hepatic coma, as well as the symptoms.
7. Discuss how the dietary treatment of

hepatic coma is different from that of hepatitis and cirrhosis.
8. Discuss the roles of antibiotics and lactulose in the treatment of hepatic coma.
9. Discuss the theories of what causes formation of gallstones.
10. Describe the dietary treatment of gallstones.
11. Describe the location and functions of the pancreas.
12. Name the symptoms of pancreatitis.
13. Discuss the dietary and drug treatments of pancreatitis.
14. Explain how mucus produced in cystic fibrosis affects the pancreas and lungs.
15. Describe the dietary and drug treatments of cystic fibrosis.

INTRODUCTION

The gallbladder, pancreas, and liver attach to the intestinal portion of the gastrointestinal tract (see Fig. 17-1). These accessory digestive organs contribute important chemical compounds to the small intestine. In addition, the pancreas and liver play important roles in metabolic reactions.

LIVER

Functions

The liver (see Fig. 17-1) is the largest organ in the body and carries on many metabolic reactions. These functions can be grouped into four areas: synthesis, decomposition, storage, and detoxification.

bile   A fluid secreted by the liver that emulsifies fat molecules in the small intestine.

fibrinogen   A blood protein that contributes to blood clotting.

albumin   A blood protein that regulates the osmotic pressure of the blood.

Synthesis

Production of bile. The liver produces approximately 600–800 ml bile per day.

Production of blood proteins. **Fibrinogen** and prothrombin proteins are vital to blood clotting. A third protein is **albumin,** which is the primary contributor to the osmotic pressure of the blood.

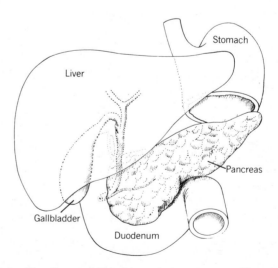

FIGURE 17-1 The liver, gallbladder, and pancreas. (Courtesy of the National Institute of Public Health.)

Glycogenesis. Insulin promotes the synthesis of glycogen by combining many glucose molecules.

Cholesterol. Liver cells synthesize cholesterol, some of which become a component of bile.

Synthesis of lipoproteins. Very low density lipoproteins (VLDL) and low-density lipoproteins (LDL) are synthesized and transport cholesterol and other lipids to the tissues.

Urea. Urea is synthesized from ammonia molecules, which result from deamination of amino acids.

Decomposition

phagocytic cells Cells that carry on phagocytosis, such as some white blood cells.

Destruction of red blood cells (RBCs). **Phagocytic cells** decompose wornout RBCs. **Bilirubin** is a product of this decomposition and is incorporated into bile.

bilirubin A pigment produced by the breakdown of heme and secreted into bile.

Glycogenolysis. Decomposition of glycogen and release of glucose is stimulated by glucagon when the blood glucose level drops below 70 mg/dl.

Hydrolysis of lipids. The liver hydrolyzes cholesterol, phospholipids, and lipoproteins to fatty acids and glycerol.

Steroid hormone inactivation. Several steroid hormones (aldosterone, glucocorticoids, estrogen, progesterone, and estrogen) are inactivated.

Storage

Vitamin and mineral storage. Fat-soluble vitamins, vitamin B_{12}, copper, and iron are stored in the liver.

Detoxification

Drug and alcohol detoxification. Liver cells can decompose, thereby detoxifying most drugs and alcohol. This function is one reason why chronic alcoholism can result in cirrhosis (discussed later).

hepatic coma A coma that results from the buildup of ammonia, which increases as a result of the liver's inability to convert ammonia to urea.

Detoxification of ammonia to urea. As mentioned above, the liver synthesizes urea; however, another way of describing this function is detoxification of ammonia. When this function fails, ammonia can build up to a toxic level, resulting in **hepatic coma.**

hepatitis A viral infection that results in inflammation of the liver tissue.

Diseases

Three common liver diseases are **hepatitis,** cirrhosis, and hepatic coma. These conditions are discussed in an increasing order of severity.

Hepatitis

Hepatitis A and B are the two most common forms. A comparison of the two is as follows:

	Hepatitis A	Hepatitis B
Synonyms	Infectious hepatitis	Serum hepatitis
Groups with highest incidence	Young children, especially in institutions	All age groups; common in drug addicts and hemodialysis patients
Transmission	Fecal-oral route; shellfish	Blood transfusion is most common
Symptoms	Fatigue, anorexia, jaundice, light stools, dark urine, elevated enzyme levels (**SGOT and SGPT**), enlargement of the liver, and abnormal liver function test	

SGOT Serum glutamic oxaloacetic transaminase, an enzyme found especially in the heart and liver. An elevated level in the blood is indicative of liver damage.

SGPT Serum glutamic pyruvic transaminase, an enzyme found in several tissues including the liver. An elevated level in the blood is indicative of liver disease.

chronic persistent hepatitis An inflammation of the liver that may last for 4–8 months.

interstitial Between parts. Interstitial fluid, which is located between cells, is an example.

Laennec's cirrhosis Cirrhosis caused by chronic alcoholism.

biliary atresia Congenital destruction or closure of one or more bile ducts in the liver.

hemochromatosis An inherited disease in which a person absorbs and deposits excessive amounts of iron in the liver.

The majority of hepatitis A and B infections are mild, with complete recovery. In hepatitis A, the symptoms are sometimes so mild that the person may think he or she simply has the flu.

Treatment of viral hepatitis is nonspecific, but bed rest and a nutritious diet (discussed below) are essential. Most hepatitis cases show signs of recovery 1–2 weeks after the onset of jaundice. Stools regaining their abnormal color, jaundice lessening, and lightening of the urine color are examples of normal recovery signs.

From 5 to 10% of hepatitis patients experience **chronic persistent hepatitis,** which lasts for 4–8 months. Approximately the same percentage experience a relapse as a result of alcohol ingestion or excessive physical activity. A small number of hepatitis patients experience destruction of liver tissue and cirrhosis.[1]

Cirrhosis of the Liver

The term *cirrhosis* means inflammation and scarring of **interstitial** (between parts) tissue. Cirrhosis of the liver results in destruction of liver cells, which are replaced by scar tissue. Destruction of liver cells and replacement by scar tissue result in decreased functioning of the liver. (See Case Study: Liver Disease, pp. 428–430, for reinforcement and application of information about cirrhosis of the liver.)

Causes. In the United States, chronic alcoholism is the most common cause and is called **Laennec's cirrhosis.** Chronic severe hepatitis can also cause cirrhosis. Other causes of cirrhosis include obstruction and absence of or injury to bile ducts. For example, **biliary atresia** and **hemochromatosis** can also result in cirrhosis.

palmar erythema Bright red palms.

spider angioma Spider-shaped blood vessels.

inferior vena cava The vein that drains the blood from the lower part of the body to the right atrium of the heart.

hepatic veins Veins that drain the blood from the liver into the inferior vena cava.

portal hypertension Abnormally increased pressure in the portal circulation.

collateral channels Veins that are used as detour routes from the liver connecting to veins from the lower esophagus.

esophageal varices Dilation of esophageal veins.

ascites The accumulation of fluids in the abdominal cavity.

hyperaldosteronism An increased level of the hormone aldosterone.

Symptoms. The early onset of cirrhosis is subtle, including symptoms such as anorexia, weight loss, and fatigue. Other examples of early symptoms are **palmar erythema** and **spider angioma.** Decreased inactivation of the steroid hormone estrogen results in the formation of spider-shaped blood vessels. These are seen in the skin, especially in the neck, shoulder, and chest regions. Intense itching is often reported; it results from deposits of bile in the skin. This condition and jaundice occur because pigments are not being processed normally by the liver. A later symptom is the accumulation of triglycerides or the development of fatty liver. These problems result from the inability to synthesize enough lipoproteins to transport fats out of the liver. All of these symptoms result from the loss of various liver functions.

A second group of symptoms results from scar tissues altering the normal flow of blood through the liver. Normally, the liver receives about one-third of the blood the heart pumps each minute. The major blood supply is from the portal vein (see Fig. 17-2), through which the liver receives products of digestion from the gastrointestinal tract. After the blood flows through the liver, it empties into the **inferior vena cava** through the **hepatic veins.** Scar tissue decreases blood flow into the liver through the portal vein. This decreased flow results in **portal hypertension** and the development of detour routes around the liver. These detour routes are called **collateral channels** and involve veins from the liver connecting to veins from the lower esophagus (see Fig. 17-3). Portal hypertension often results in **esophageal varices.** About 70% of advanced cirrhosis patients experience these varices, and bleeding from them is a common cause of death.

A major symptom or complication of scar tissue in the liver is **ascites.** Many of the dietary modifications for cirrhotic patients are based on preventing or reducing ascites; therefore, it is important to understand the three major changes that lead to ascites:

Decreased albumin. The development of scar tissue results in gradual loss of liver functions such as synthesis of albumin. Decreased albumin in the blood results in a lowering of blood osmotic pressure. This low osmotic pressure in the veins of the gastrointestinal tract prevents the normal pulling of fluids into veins. Instead, the fluid is pulled into the abdominal cavity, where the osmotic pressure is higher.

Portal hypertension. Increased pressure in the portal vein helps to force fluids out of the blood into the abdominal cavity.

Hyperaldosteronism. This hormone stimulates the absorption of sodium by the kidneys and normally is degraded by the liver. Hyperaldosteronism causes increased retention of sodium, which further aggravates the ascites.

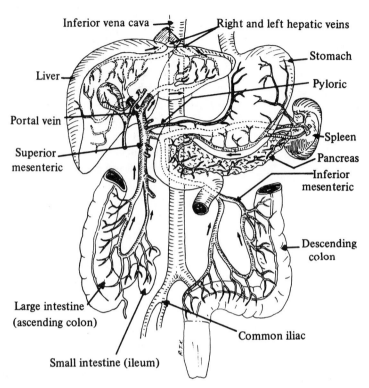

FIGURE 17-2 The portal vein, which supplies most of the blood to the liver, and the hepatic veins, which drain blood from the liver into the inferior vena cava.

Dietary Treatment of Hepatitis and Cirrhosis

The two goals of diet therapy in hepatitis and cirrhosis are:

- To maintain homeostasis by providing kilocalories and nutrients
- To enhance the functions of the liver and allow for healing and cellular renewal

Nausea, vomiting, and anorexia are the most difficult symptoms to deal with, since they directly affect food intake and malnutrition complicates liver disease. When the symptoms are severe, intravenous solutions or parenteral fluids of 5–10% glucose and 3.5% protein hydrolysates should be given until the symptoms subside.

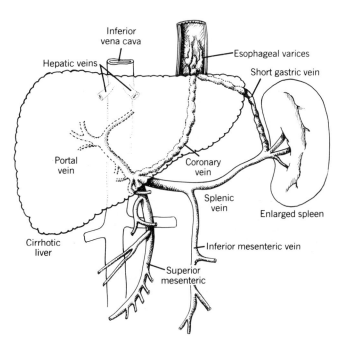

FIGURE 17-3 Collateral venous channels that drain blood around the liver in cirrhosis. (Courtesy of the National Institute of Public Health.)

Diet Treatment. The diet prescription for hepatitis and cirrhosis is the same: high kilocalories, high protein, high carbohydrate, and moderate fat.

The caloric content should be 35–50 kcal per kilogram of recommended body weight, or approximately 2,000–3,000 kcal for an adult. The increase in kilocalories over the normal amount a sedentary person needs (about 30 kcal/kg) is important for regeneration of liver tissue. See the sample menu for a high-protein, moderate-fat, high-carbohydrate diet.

A high protein intake should provide 1.5–2.0 g of protein per kilogram of desired body weight. This protein intake is two to almost three times the Recommended Dietary Allowance (RDA) for protein for adults with 0.8 g per kilogram of body weight. The increased protein is important for several reasons:

- To protect the liver from further degeneration
- To repair and restore liver tissue
- To form bile acids

- To replenish plasma proteins
- To provide lipotropic factors

lipotropic factors Compounds that contribute to the formation of lipoproteins that transport fats out of the liver.

Protein sources should be of high biological value and especially high in foods that contain **lipotropic factors.** Foods especially rich in lipotropic factors are egg yolks, meat, fish, and cereals. If the condition progresses to hepatic coma, protein must be restricted.

Carbohydrate intake should be 300–400 g/day, or approximately 60% of the total kilocalories. Carbohydrate intake is important so that protein can be spared from being used as an energy source.

Sample Menu for a High-protein, Moderate-fat, High-carbohydrate Diet

Exchange	
	Breakfast
1 fruit	½ grapefruit
1 bread	½ cup bran flakes
1 medium-fat meat	1 scrambled egg
2 bread	2 slices whole wheat toast
2 fat	2 tsp margarine
	1 tbsp jelly* (3 tsp)
	1 cup coffee
	Lunch
4 lean meat	4 oz broiled fish
1 bread	1 small baked potato
1 fat	1 tsp margarine
1 vegetable	½ cup asparagus
2 bread	2 slices whole wheat bread
2 fat	2 tsp margarine
	1 tbsp jelly* (3 tsp)
2 fruit	1 banana
1 milk	1 cup skim milk
	Mid-Afternoon Snack
1 milk	1 cup skim milk
1 bread	2 graham crackers

	Dinner
4 lean meat	4 oz broiled chicken (skin removed)
1 bread	1 small baked potato
2 fat	2 tsp margarine
1 vegetable	½ cup string beans
2 bread	2 plain rolls
1 fat	1 tsp margarine
	1 tbsp apple jelly* (3 tsp)
1 milk	1 cup skim milk
	Evening Snack
1 milk	1 cup skim milk
2 bread	2 slices whole wheat bread
	2 tbsp jelly* (6 tsp)
	Totals

Analysis of Menu and Calculations

- An analysis of this menu shows that there are 4 milk, 2 vegetable, 3 fruit, 12 bread, 9 meat, and 8 fat exchanges.
- In order to achieve a high-protein diet while achieving a moderate-fat diet, there are eight servings of lean meat, one serving of medium-fat meat, and no servings of high-fat meat.
- Notice that much of the carbohydrate in the menu is from the sugar group, which is not one of the exchanges. The amount of carbohydrate in each tablespoon and teaspoon is given.
- Fat is kept to a moderate level by including skim milk rather than whole milk. The 8 fat exchanges should be polyunsaturated rather than saturated fat. This is especially important, since the fat in the 9 meat exchanges is all saturated.

*The asterisk (*) in the menu indicates foods that are not part of an exchange list. Rather, these foods are members of the sugar group. The amount of carbohydrate in a tablespoon (3 tsp) of jelly is 5 g/tsp or 15 g/tbsp.

Moderate fat consumption of 25–40% of the kilocalories is recommended. Whole dairy products and eggs should be the main source of fat, as opposed to greasy foods. Medium chain triglyceride (MCT) oils may help to reduce fat infiltration in the liver, since they do not use the chylomicron transport system. However, since MCTs are metabolized in the liver, some authorities recommend that they not be given to cirrhosis patients. Fat is important for absorption of fat-soluble vitamins and energy, and to increase the palatibility of the meals. The principles of a low-fat diet are provided in Table 17-1.

Vitamin supplements include thiamin, which is important for the metabolism of carbohydrates, proteins, fats, and vitamin B_{12}. Vitamin K is given to counteract the bleeding tendency that results from decreased synthesis of prothrombin. Vitamin C helps to provide collagen, which is important for tissue regeneration.

If a person has ascites, this condition can be helped by restricting sodium in the diet, with 22–40 mEq/day (500–920 mg/day) being a common amount. A major problem with this restriction is that protein may also be restricted, since many foods high in protein are also high in sodium (see Appendix E for the sodium content of foods). Powdered protein supplements can be used to help offset this problem. In addition, low-sodium milk (Lonalac) is a good source of protein and allows the use of other foods with a higher sodium content. Water intake often has to be limited to 1,000–1,500 ml/day.[2]

Hepatic Coma

Hepatic coma occurs when cirrhosis progresses to the point where the liver cannot adequately detoxify ammonia to urea. A person experiencing this condition usually is not in a comatose state but rather exhibits mental disturbances such as disorientation and behavioral changes. Sleep patterns may be altered and a flapping tremor of the hands may occur when the arms are extended.

Ammonia results from the deamination of amino acids, with the gastrointestinal tract being the main source. Intestinal bacteria produce ammonia by interacting with cells from the intestinal mucosa and blood cells that result from esophageal varices. Ammonia levels increase in the blood to the point where they cause malfunction of the brain tissue;

TABLE 17-1 LOW-FAT DIET (40–45 g)

Purpose	The diet is designed to limit the total amount of fat to 40–45 g.
Use	Used in diseases of the liver, gallbladder, or pancreas in which there is an impairment of fat digestion and absorption.
Examples of foods	Foods with a high fat content are omitted and those that cause gaseous distention may be omitted.
Adequacy	Diet is adequate.

Source: From *Manual of Clinical Dietetics* (4th ed.) by the Chicago Dietetic Association, 1992, Chicago, The American Dietetic Association. Reprinted by permission.

hepatic encephalopathy A condition caused by increased levels of ammonia in the blood, which leads to a malfunction of brain tissue.

therefore, the name **hepatic encephalopathy** is often used to describe this condition.

Dietary Treatment. Regulating protein intake is the key to treating hepatic coma. Since ammonia can also be formed by bacterial action, antibiotic therapy is used to destroy intestinal bacteria.

Low protein, low fat, high carbohydrate levels and high kilocalories are the diet prescription for hepatic coma. Elimination of foods that contain preformed ammonia (certain cheeses, chicken, salami, peanut butter, and potatoes) is essential.

Dietary protein intake should be decreased to 0.5 g per kilogram of body weight, or 20–40 g of protein per day. See the sample menu for a 20-g protein diet. A diet containing less than 40 g of protein is deficient in many nutrients, such as protein, niacin, riboflavin, thiamin, calcium, phosphorus, and iron. If a person is in a coma, he or she must be placed on a zero protein diet for a few days until the ammonia decreases to a safe level. This diet involves complete elimination of some exchanges, such as milk, vegetables, and meat. Other exchanges, such as bread, allow some foods, such as low-protein bread and pasta only. Also, only certain fruits are allowed, such as cranberry juice and apple juice. The diet is high in carbohydrates and fat and should supply 1,500–2,000 kcal to prevent breakdown of tissue proteins.[3]

As the person's condition improves, protein intake can be increased gradually by 10–15 g/week to 40–50 g/day.

Sample Menu for a 20-g Protein Diet

Exchange	
	Breakfast
1 fruit	½ cup orange juice
1 bread	½ cup oatmeal
1 milk	1 cup skim milk
3 fat	3 strips of bacon
1 bread	1 slice low-protein bread
2 fat	2 tsp margarine
	1 tbsp jelly
	1 cup coffee
	4 tsp sugar

Mid-Morning Snack

8 oz Kool-Aid with ¼ cup high-calorie, low-protein powder (e.g., Contralyte) added

Lunch

1 vegetable	½ cup sliced tomatoes
1 fat	1 tbsp French dressing
1 fruit	½ cup peaches
1 fruit	½ cup applesauce
	½ cup fruit cocktail
1 bread	1 slice low-protein bread
3 fat	3 tsp margarine
	1 tbsp jelly
	8 oz ginger ale

Mid-Afternoon Snack

8 pieces candy
8 oz Seven-Up

Dinner

1 medium-fat meat	1 poached egg
1 bread	1 slice low-protein bread
1 vegetable	½ cup spinach
1 vegetable	½ cup asparagus
1 fat	1 tbsp French dressing
	1 cup Italian water ice
3 fat	3 tsp margarine
	1 cup tea
	2 tsp sugar

Bedtime Snack

8 oz Kool-Aid with ¼ cup high-calorie, low-protein powder (e.g., Controlyte) added

Analysis and Comments

- An analysis of this diet shows that it contains 1 milk, 3 vegetable, 3 fruit, 4 bread, 1 meat, and 13 fat exchanges.
- In order to keep the protein level at 20 g, the menu includes only 1 meat and 1 milk exchange. The four bread exchanges are low-protein bread, which contains 0.5 g protein or less, compared to 2 g per slice in normal bread.
- The high number of fat exchanges is important to provide kilocalories. In addition, kilocalories are provided by the foods from the sugar group (e.g., jelly, Kool-Aid) and the high-kilocalories, low-protein powder.
- Due to the restriction in protein, the menu is deficient in protein, niacin, riboflavin, thiamin, and calcium.

Source: Adapted from *Manual of Clinical Dietetics* (4th ed.) by the Chicago Dietetic Association, 1992, Chicago, The American Dietetic Association. Reprinted by permission.

GALLBLADDER

Function

cholecystokinin A hormone that stimulates the gallbladder to contract and release bile.

The gallbladder is a sac whose walls consist of smooth muscle and have a mucosal lining. It is located on the inferior surface of the liver (see Fig. 17-1). Storage and concentration of bile from the liver are the functions of the gallbladder. Concentrated bile is released into the duodenum through the common bile duct when the gallbladder is stimulated to contract. The hormone **cholecystokinin** stimulates the gallbladder to contract when it is secreted from the duodenum on the entrance of fat from the stomach.

Bile is composed of bile salts, cholesterol, bilirubin, and lecithin. The liver secretes about 700 ml of bile per day, which is important in emulsification and digestion of fats (see Chapter 4 for details).

cholecystitis An inflammation of the gallbladder that results from bacterial infection or gallstones.

gallstones Stonelike masses that form in the gallbladder.

cholelithiasis The formation of stones in the gallbladder.

Disorders

Cholecystitis is inflammation of the gallbladder and frequently results from bacterial infection or **gallstones**. **Cholelithiasis** is the formation of stones in the gallbladder. About 80% of all gallstones are composed chiefly of cholesterol.

Gallstone Formation and Symptoms

It is believed that gallstones develop when cholesterol in bile becomes too concentrated. Two reasons for the increased cholesterol level are increased cholesterol synthesis and a decrease in the amount of bile. Cholesterol gradually precipitates out of solution, with the end result being the formation of gallstones (see Fig. 17-4).

Many persons have gallstones but no symptoms, that is, they have "silent gallstones." Others may experience severe, steady pain in the epigastric area that lasts for at least 20 minutes and usually up to 2–4 hours. There may be pain between the shoulder blades or in the right shoulder. There may be nausea or vomiting. Frequently, gallstones move into the **cystic duct** (see Fig. 17-4), which causes cholecystitis. The symptoms appear after a person eats fatty foods. When fat enters the duodenum, it causes secretion of the hormone cholecystokinin, which stimulates the gallbladder to contract and release bile into the duodenum.

cystic duct A duct that drains bile from the gallbladder to the common bile duct.

Women are three times more likely than men to develop gallstones. Both men and women who are obese and eat many dairy products plus animal fats are likely to form gallstones.[4]

Dietary Treatment

The goal of diet therapy is to avoid foods that produce painful symptoms or cause the gallbladder to contract. Persons with cholecystitis or cholelithiasis may experience bloating and belching after eating greasy or rich

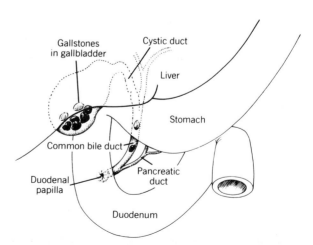

FIGURE 17-4 Gallstones in the gallbladder and common bile duct. (Courtesy of the National Institute of Public Health.)

foods or specific foods such as garlic, onions, bell peppers, apples, or other gas formers. Individual food intolerances should be avoided, and a low-fat diet of about 40 g/day will bring relief. See Table 17-2 for foods on each exchange list that are allowed and disallowed.

Protein intake should be normal, but carbohydrate and total kilocalorie intake generally should be decreased, since most people who have gallbladder problems are obese. Restriction of dietary cholesterol has not been shown to reduce the amount of cholesterol synthesized by the liver. The reason is that the liver synthesizes about 60% of the total cholesterol in the body, despite the amount in the diet.

cholecystectomy Surgical removal of the gallbladder.

If a **cholecystectomy** is performed, a low-fat diet should be continued for a few months. Since bile is synthesized by the liver, after a few months fat can be gradually increased to the amount tolerated by the person.

PANCREAS

Functions

The pancreas, a rather large gland, extends from the duodenum behind the stomach to the spleen (see Fig. 17-1). Its functions are to secrete digestive enzymes and sodium bicarbonate into the duodenum. See chapters 3, 4, and 5 for the specific roles of the enzymes. The sodium bicarbonate neutralizes the acidic chyme that enters the duodenum from the stomach. In addition, the pancreas secretes insulin and glucagon, as described in Chapter 15.

Disorders

Pancreatitis

autodigestion Self-digestion

Pancreatitis is inflammation of the pancreas and may be acute or chronic. This inflammation is an example of **autodigestion.** Normally, the pancreatic enzymes are secreted in an inactive form into the duodenum, where they are activated. Autodigestion is initiated when these inactive enzymes accumulate in the pancreas and become activated. The protein-digesting enzyme trypsin is especially responsible for degradation of the pancreas tissue. The normal endocrine functions (secretion of insulin and glucagon) and exocrine functions (secretion of enzymes) are lost as the pancreatic tissue is degraded and replaced by fibrous tissue.

Causes and Symptoms. Exactly how the enzymes become activated is not understood. Their blockage and accumulation have been found to result from blockage of the pancreatic duct by gallstones, alcohol abuse,

TABLE 17-2 40-g FAT DIET

Food Group	Foods Allowed	Foods Not Allowed
Milk group (2 cups daily):		
Milk	Skim milk, nonfat dry milk, buttermilk made from skim milk, condensed skim milk, cocoa made from skim milk, yogurt made from skim milk.	All other milk, including whole milk and lowfat milk (2%), low-fat yogurt.
Meat group (two servings daily)		
Meat poultry, and fish	Limited to 5 oz daily: lean beef, lamb, ham, veal, or poultry; lean fish such as cod, flounder, haddock, bluefish, perch, bass, whitefish; water-packed salmon and tuna. All meats prepared without fat and served without sauces or gravies.	Fatty meats, bacon, sausage, luncheon meats, frankfurters, corned beef; processed meats, fish, or poultry; fatty fish or fish canned in oil; fried meats; poultry skin.
Eggs	Egg whites as desired; one egg yolk per day may be substituted for 1 oz of meat, if tolerated.	Egg yolks in excess of one per day.
Meat substitutes	Low-fat cheese and uncreamed cottage cheese; dried beans and peas if they do not cause gaseous distress.	All cheese other than those allowed, peanut butter, nuts.
Vegetable and fruit group		
Potato and substitute	White and sweet potatoes; macaroni, noodles, spaghetti and rice.	Fried potatoes, potato chips, potatoes prepared with cream sauce or butter.
Vegetables	All fresh, frozen, or canned vegetables except those on the avoid list.	All buttered, creamed, or fried vegetables. Omit the following if they cause distress: broccoli, brussel sprouts, cabbage, cauliflower, chives, corn, cucumber, garlic, onion, green pepper, radishes, rutabagas, turnips, sauerkraut.
Fruit	All except those on the avoid list.	Avocado, olives, coconut. If the following cause gaseous distress, they should be omitted: raw apple, melon, and banana.
Bread and cereal group (four servings daily)		
Bread and crackers	Whole grain and enriched breads except those on the avoid list; graham crackers, soda or saltine crackers.	Hot breads such as muffins, biscuits, pastries, sweet rolls, doughnuts, pancakes, waffles, french toast; high-fat snack crackers.

TABLE 17-2 *(Continued)*

Food Group	Foods Allowed	Foods Not Allowed
Cereals	All except those on the avoid list.	Cereals prepared with chocolate, fat, coconut, or nuts.
Miscellaneous foods Fats	3 level tsp daily: butter, margarine, or oil, which may be used on bread or in cooking. One strip of crisp bacon may be substituted for 1 tsp of fat if well tolerated.	Any fat in excess of the amount allowed; all fried foods, cream, salt pork, lard, visible fat on meat, gravies, and salad dressings.
Soups	Fat-free broth and bouillon, homemade soup made with skim milk and allowed vegetables.	Commercial soups, cream soups prepared with whole milk.
Desserts and sweets	Gelatin desserts, sherbet, fruit ices, angel food cake, meringue cookies, pudding made with skim milk; sugar, syrup, honey, jam, jelly, gum drops, plain sugar candy.	Ice cream, rich pastries, pie, cake, cookies. Any prepared with chocolate, coconut, or nuts.
Beverages	Coffee, tea, carbonated beverages	None.
Miscellaneous	Salt, pepper, herbs and spices in moderation, catsup, mustard, vinegar, cocoa, lemon juice, flavoring extracts, nonstick cooking pan spray.	Garlic, barbeque sauce, chili sauce, steak sauce, cream sauce, gravy, nuts, olives, pickles, chocolate, popcorn.

Source: Menu adapted from *Diet Manual* (5th ed.) by the Texas Dietetic Association, 1988, Austin: The Texas Dietetic Association. Reprinted by permission.

Cystic fibrosis A genetic disorder characterized by the production of very thick mucus by mucus-producing glands and increased concentration of sodium in sweat.

Pleurisy Inflammation of the pleura membrane that lines and covers the lungs in the thoracic cavity.

certain drugs (corticosteroids and thiazide diuretics), and **cystic fibrosis.** It is not understood how these factors produce the attacks.[5]

The symptoms usually begin with a mild, steady pain in the upper abdomen, which usually increases in severity and may last for several days. Other symptoms include nausea, vomiting, low-grade fever, increased pulse rate, jaundice, **pleurisy,** and shortness of breath. In the most severe cases, bleeding can occur in the pancreas, leading to shock and often death.

Frequently, acute pancreatitis can result in elevated blood glucose levels due to decreased secretion of insulin and elevated blood lipid levels. Characteristically, amylase (a carbohydrate-splitting enzyme) is found in elevated amounts in the blood

Dietary Treatment. The goal of treatment is to relieve pain by reducing the stimulation of the pancreas and to prevent additional damage to the pancreas.

To reduce stimulation of the pancreas, no food is given by mouth for 24–48 hours. Intravenous fluids or tube feedings of elemental formulas are administered during this time. Also, to help relieve pain, a nasogastric tube may be inserted and the stomach contents suctioned out.

Once the pain subsides, the diet should consist of clear liquids followed by progression to a low-fat, high-carbohydrate, high-protein diet. The low-fat diet basically is the same as the one prescribed for gallbladder problems—a 40-g low-fat diet (see Table 17-2).

The low-fat diet is important because pancreatitis is almost always accompanied by steatorrhea as a result of a decreased level of pancreatic lipase. In addition to low-fat foods, the diet should include MCT oils (which are readily absorbed without requiring digestion), MCT margarines, or preparations that combine sugar, vitamins, essential fatty acids, and minerals with MCT oils such as Portagen or Pregestimil. Approximately 3 tbsp of MCT oil can be added each day to foods such as skim milk, homemade salad dressing, and milkshakes made of whole milk, sugar, and vanilla. The MCTs should reduce the steatorrhea as well as enhance the absorption of fat-soluble vitamins, which should be increased.[6]

Alcohol, as well as any other gastric irritants, must be totally eliminated. Gradually the person progresses to six small, bland meals. As mentioned above, it is not uncommon for pancreatitis to result in decreased insulin secretion; therefore, if the blood glucose level begins to rise, the amount of carbohydrates should be lowered and complex carbohydrates should be generally used.

Cystic Fibrosis

Cystic fibrosis is a genetic disorder that is usually evident in early infancy, with the diagnosis being often made before 6 months of age. This disorder is characterized by production of very thick mucus by the mucus-producing glands and an increased concentration of sodium in sweat. Cystic fibrosis can affect many organs, but the lungs and pancreas are affected most severely, as described:

Pancreas. The thick mucus blocks the entrance of pancreatic enzymes into the duodenum. As a result, the digestion of carbohydrates, proteins, and especially fats is impaired. The buildup of enzymes gradually results in destruction, atrophy, and replacement of pancreatic tissue with fibrous tissue.

Lungs. Mucus clogs the bronchi and bronchioles (cartilaginous air tubes in the lungs), which can result in overinflation, emphysema, and **atelectasis.** In addition, the mucus leads to recurrent pulmonary infections such as pneumonia and even respiratory failure. Management of pulmo-

atelectasis A collapsed state of the lungs, which may involve all or part of the lungs.

nary complications is critical in determining the survival of a cystic fibrosis patient.

The impairment of digestion and absorption in cystic fibrosis often causes the child to be malnourished or fail to gain weight. As a result, many young patients experience growth failure, and are short and very thin for their age. Fat malabsorption in cystic fibrosis is especially serious, with steatorrhea, osteoporosis, and low levels of fat-soluble vitamins being the result.

Dietary Treatment. The goals of dietary treatment of cystic fibrosis are as follows:

- To provide adequate protein for growth and immunity
- To provide adequate kilocalories for growth and development
- To prevent or control pulmonary infections
- To maintain electrolyte balance (especially sodium)

In reality, providing adequate nutrients and kilocalories requires increases in most of them, since a cystic fibrosis patient does not absorb nutrients very efficiently.

Protein intake should be 6–8 g per kilogram of ideal body weight, or about twice the normal amount for growth, to compensate for the amount that is not absorbed. Infants with cystic fibrosis are usually given high-protein formulas (e.g., Pregestimil and Albumaid) with protein **hydrolysates** that do not require digestion. For noninfant CF patients, the best protein foods are those that provide the most protein, vitamins, and minerals while keeping dietary fats to a minimum. Broiled, stewed, or roasted lean meats, fish, and fowl are best.

hydrolysates Solutions with amino acids.

Kilocalorie intake should be increased by 50–100% over the child's RDA, or to about 150 kcal/kg of ideal body weight per day. This increased amount is required to offset malabsorption and to help fight the frequent infections that occur. In addition, the increased kilocalories are required for the patient's laborious breathing.

Simple carbohydrate intake should be high in order to help supply the increased level of kilocalories. However, complex carbohydrates should be decreased, since they require the enzyme amylase to be digested.

If the person experiences steatorrhea and abdominal pain, fat intake may have to be reduced to 25–30 g/day. If there is no steatorrhea, the level of fat tolerated can be individualized. MCT oils are recommended especially for those who do not tolerate fat well.

An increase in salt to 2–4 g/day may be needed to offset that lost through perspiration, especially during periods of fever, diarrhea, and increased sweating. Iron must also be increased, since pancreatic enzymes decrease its absorption.

Water- and fat-soluble vitamin supplements are usually given, with riboflavin being especially important due to the high level of kilocalories. Vitamin A is very important since it maintains the integrity of the respiratory and digestive mucosae. Another fat-soluble vitamin that must be increased is vitamin K, since antibiotic therapy destroy many intestinal bacteria. Fat-soluble vitamins should be given in a water-miscible form, since they can be absorbed in water or in the absence of fat.[7]

CASE STUDY: LIVER DISEASE

Mr. E. is an alcoholic who has been drinking heavily for the past 8 years. Recently, he has been experiencing abdominal pain, fatigue, and anorexia and has noticed jaundice in his eyes. In addition, he complains of frequent itching of his skin. The physical and laboratory findings are as follows:

Physical Findings:

2+ peripheral edema	Palmar erythema
Jaundice	Weight loss (156 lb), with
Spider angiomas	usual weight being 166 lb

Laboratory Findings:		*Normal Values*
Serum albumin	2.8 g/dl	3.5–5.0 g/dl
Serum potassium	3.0 mEq/liter	3.2–4.6 mEq/liter
Total bilirubin	1.6 mg/dl	0.15–1.0 mg/dl
Prothrombin time	14 seconds	12 seconds
Hemoglobin	9.7 g/dl	13–16 g/dl
Hematocrit	27.6%	42–50%
Serum triglycerides	453 mg/dl	10–200 mg/dl

An upper gastrointestinal tract series reveals esophageal varices.

Diet Prescription:	*Medications:*
High protein	Aldactone
High carbohydrate	Folic acid
Moderate fat	Iron
Low sodium	Cholestyramine
Fluid restriction 1,000 ml/day	
Smooth diet	

1. Which of the following statements made by Mr. E. indicate a need for teaching?
   A. "My skin really itches. It's hard to believe the liver can cause itching."
   B. "I keep coughing up blood. I guess I've really got some damage in my throat."
   *C. "The doctor said my triglycerides are up. Guess I won't be getting to eat any fat."
   D. "Guess I'll be eating some sweets. The dietitian told me sugar was important for me."

2. Which of the following nutrient values ordered for Mr. E. should the nurse question?
   *A. 10–15 g protein
   B. 400 g carbohydrate
   C. 100 g fat
   D. 3,000 kcal

3. Mr. E. states, "Low sodium! That means I can't have salt!" Which of the following should the nurse explain to Mr. E. to help him accept the sodium restriction?
   A. Sodium is deposited in the liver.
   *B. Sodium restriction helps to reduce ascites and peripheral edema.
   C. Rest for the kidney is important in his treatment plan.
   D. Sodium restriction is important for better utilization of protein.

4. Based on Mr. E's weight (156 lb or 71 kg) and the normal allowance of protein on a high-protein intake, Mr. E's protein intake should be _____ g.
   A. 100–142
   B. 55–85
   C. 23–32
   D. none of these

5. If Mr. E's condition worsened to prehepatic coma, which of the protein values in question 4 would be appropriate for this condition?
   A. 100–142 g
   B. 55–85 g
   C. 23–32 g
   D. none of these

6. Which of the following foods are the best sources of protein and lipotropic factors?
   A. sardines, liver, egg yolks, cereals
   B. milk, pinto beans, peanuts, soybeans
   C. hard cheese, legumes, peanut butter
   D. none of these

7. A moderate amount of fat is prescribed to _____
   A. absorb fat-soluble vitamins
   B. increase the palatibility of meals

C. provide kilocalories

D. all of these

8. The smooth diet will help relieve which of Mr. E's problems?

A. portal hypertension

B. low albumin levels

C. esophageal varices

D. none of these

9. To facilitate the metabolism of carbohydrates, help correct the decreased prothrombin level, and provide collagen for tissue regeneration, his diet should include which of the following vitamin supplements?

A. thiamin, vitamin A, vitamin E, and vitamin B_{12}

B. thiamin, vitamin K, vitamin C

C. vitamin A, vitamin D, vitamin E

D. none of these

SUMMARY

- The liver functions in the following ways: synthesis—production of bile; decomposition—destruction of wornout RBCs; storage of vitamins and minerals; and drug and alcohol detoxification.
- Cirrhosis can be caused by chronic alcoholism or chronic severe hepatitis and causes portal hypertension, esophageal varices, and ascites.
- The dietary treatment of hepatitis and cirrhosis is as follows: high kcal—35–50 kcal/kg of ideal body weight or 2,000–3,000 kcal/day; high protein—1.5–2.0 g/kg of ideal body weight; carbohydrate—300–400 g/day; moderate fat—25–40% of total kcal per day; and vitamin and mineral supplements.
- Hepatic coma is caused by the liver's inability to detoxify ammonia to urea; dietary treatment involves decreasing protein to 20–40 g/day.
- It is theorized that gallstones are formed when cholesterol in bile becomes too concentrated and the amount of bile formed is decreased; dietary treatment involves a low-fat, 40 g/day diet, with proteins normal and carbohydrates low.
- Pancreatitis is caused by a blockage of enzymes from the pancreas entering the duodenum; symptoms include pain in the upper abdomen, nausea, vomiting, and low-grade fever. Dietary treatment involves reducing stimulation to pancreas (that is, no food for 24–48 hours), followed by a progression to clear liquid diet, then to low-fat, high-carbohydrate, high-protein diet.
- In cystic fibrosis, mucus blocks the enzymes from the pancreas entering the duodenum. Dietary treatment is as follows: high protein—6–8 g/kg of body weight; high kcal—increase by about 50–100% or about 150 kcal/kg of ideal body weight; high carbohydrate—simple carbohydrates increased but complex carbohydrates reduced; low-fat—25–30 g/day; increased salt—2–4 g/day to offset that lost through perspiration.

REVIEW QUESTIONS

True (A) or False (B)

1. The metabolic functions of the liver can be grouped into synthesis, decomposition, storage, and detoxification.
2. The most common cause of cirrhosis is hepatitis.
3. Development of fatty liver in cirrhosis results from the inability of the liver to synthesize enough lipoproteins to transport fats out of the liver.
4. Portal hypertension followed by the development of collateral blood channels and esophageal varices results from the inability of the liver to detoxify urea.
5. Many of the dietary modifications for cirrhotic patients are based on preventing or reducing ascites.
6. Three major changes that lead to the development of ascites are decreases in the following—hydrolysis of lipids, vitamin and mineral storage, and synthesis of cholesterol.
7. The diet prescription for hepatitis and cirrhosis is high kilocalories (30 kcal/kg), high protein (0.8 g/kg), high carbohydrate (150 g/day), and moderate fat.
8. Three important roles of protein in hepatitis and cirrhosis are to repair and restore liver tissue, to form bile acids, and to provide lipotropic factors.
9. Restricting sodium in cases of ascites is common but may also restrict sources of protein, since foods high in sodium frequently are also high in protein.
10. A person showing signs of hepatic coma (disorientation and behavioral changes) should be on a diet that includes 60–80 g protein per day.
11. Two possible reasons for the formation of gallstones are increased cholesterol synthesis and a decreased amount of bile synthesized by the liver.
12. The persons most likely to develop gallstones are men and women who are obese and eat many dairy products and animal fats.
13. The diet for patients with cholecystitis or cholelithiasis is very low in fat (20 g or less), high in protein (1.5 g/kg), and high in carbohydrates (300–400 g).
14. A person who has had the gallbladder surgically removed (cholecystectomy) has to be on a low-fat diet, due to decreased bile production, for the rest of his or her life.
15. Pancreatitis is an example of autodigestion, in which pancreatic enzymes are not secreted and their accumulation results in digestion of pancreatic tissues.
16. The dietary goals of treatment of pancreatitis are

to relieve pain by reducing stimulation of and prevent additional damage to the pancreas.

17. Steatorrhea may be a problem with cirrhosis but not with pancreatitis.

18. MCTs are important in a pancreatic diet because they enhance the absorption of proteins.

19. Cystic fibrosis is a genetic disorder that severely affects the liver and intestines.

20. Cystic fibrosis results in little digestion of nutrients, especially fats, since mucous blocks the secretion of pancreatic enzymes.

21. A cystic fibrosis diet might include 6–8 g of protein per kilogram of body weight for growth and to compensate for the amount that is not absorbed.

22. Vitamins A and K are increased in cystic fibrosis diets, with K being important to maintain the integrity of respiratory and digestive mucosa.

Multiple Choice

23. Hepatic coma can result from which liver malfunction?
    A. hydrolysis of lipids
    B. synthesis of cholesterol
    C. detoxification of ammonia to urea
    D. production of bile

24. Major changes in a cirrhosis patient that lead to the development of ascites are:
    1. decreased albumin
    2. portal hypertension
    3. hyperaldosteronism
    4. decreased bile production
    A. 1, 2, 3   B. 1, 3   C. 2, 4   D. 4
    E. all of these

25. Which of the following are a correct diet prescription for hepatitis and cirrhosis?
    1. high kilocalories (35–60 kcal/kg)
    2. high fat (60–80 g)
    3. high protein (1.5–2.0 g/kg)
    4. high sodium (2–4 g/day)
    A. 1, 2, 3   B. 1, 3   C. 2, 4   D. 4
    E. all of these

26. Two sources of ammonia that can result in hepatic coma are _____ and _____.
    A. deamination of amino acids—intestinal bacteria from the gastrointestinal tract
    B. conversion of urea in the liver—preformed ammonia in foods

C. portal vein—liver
D. none of these

27. Cholelithiasis and cholecystitis patients may receive relief from a diet that consists of:
    A. low fat (60–80 g/day)
       high protein (1.5 g/kg/day)
       high carbohydrate (300–400 g/day)
    B. low fat (40 g/day)
       normal protein (0.8 g/kg)
       decreased kilocalories for weight loss
    C. moderate fat (90–120 g/day)
       low protein (0.4 g/kg)
       normal carbohydrate (50% of total kilocalories)
    D. none of these

28. Symptoms of gallstones are:
    1. epigastric pain   2. nausea and vomiting
    3. pain in the right   4. appearance of
       shoulder   symptoms after
                             eating fatty foods
    A. 1, 2, 3   B. 1, 3   C. 2, 4   D. 4
    E. all of these

29. Pancreatitis can result in loss of _____ and _____, which are the normal pancreatic functions.
    A. insulin and glucagon secretion—secretion of cholecystokinin
    B. bile secretion—cholesterol synthesis
    C. insulin and glucagon secretion—enzymes secretion
    D. none of these

30. Cystic fibrosis patients experience great difficulty in digesting and absorbing nutrients, especially fats; the reason is _____.
    A. damage to the liver
    B. thick mucus blocks the secretion of enzymes from the pancreas
    C. there is no bile from the gallbladder
    D. an acidic condition in the stomach destroys enzymes

31. Dietary treatment for cystic fibrosis includes:
    1. high protein (6–8 g/kg) for growth
    2. low kilocalories for weight loss
    3. high carbohydrate intake but a decrease in complex carbohydrates, since they require the enzyme amylase for digestion
    4. low salt level due to the presence of edema
    A. 1, 2, 3   B. 1, 3   C. 2, 4   D. 4
    E. all of these

Completion

32. Describe the dietary treatment of hepatitis and cirrhosis in relation to the amounts of kilocalories, protein, carbohydrate, fat, vitamin supplements, and sodium.
33. Discuss the dietary and drug treatments of pancreatitis.
34. Discuss how the dietary treatment of hepatic coma is different from that of hepatitis and cirrhosis.

CRITICAL THINKING CHALLENGE

1. Jimmy is a 10-year-old cystic fibrosis patient. Information and data about Jimmy are:
   - weight = 60 lb
   - steatorrhea is present
   a. Calculate the approximate amount of protein that should be included in his daily diet. Show calculations.
   b. Give the approximate amount of fat that should be included in his daily diet. Explain why.
   c. Give the amount of kcal that should be included in his daily diet. Explain why.
   d. Give which vitamin supplements are important for him and why.

REVIEW QUESTIONS FOR NCLEX

Situation. Mr. E is admitted to the hospital with severe left midepigastric pain and nausea and vomiting. He is diagnosed as having pancreatitis.

1. Which of the following would you rule out as possible causes of Mr. E's pancreatitis?
   A. blockage of pancreatic duct by gallstones
   B. alcohol abuse
   C. cystic fibrosis
   D. gastric ulcer
2. In answering Mr. E's question, as to why he can't have any food orally for 24-48 hours and must instead receive intravenous fluids, you would tell him that this will _____ than if he was fed orally.
   A. provide more nutrients for healing of the pancreas

   B. prevent stimulation of the pancreas and reduce pain
   C. allow more rapid digestion of food
   D. provide more milk and other good sources of protein
3. Once Mr. E's pain subsides the diet should consist of _____.
   A. high protein, high carbohydrate, and moderate fat
   B. high protein, moderate carbohydrate, and high B-complex vitamins
   C. clear liquids, low fat, high carbohydrate, and high protein
   D. low fat, low carbohydrate, low protein, and clear liquids
4. As a result of malfunctioning of the pancreas, Mr. E's blood needs to be monitored for a possible increase in _____.
   A. glycogen
   B. triglycerides
   C. protein
   D. glucose

REFERENCES

1. Diehl, A. M. (1988). Alcoholic liver disease. In S. J. Chobanian and M. M. Van Ness (Eds.), *Manual of clinical problems in gastroenterology.* Boston, Little, Brown.
2. Mezitis, N.H.E. (1988). Nutritional management in liver disease. *Nutrition in clinical practice, 3*(3), 108.
3. Hiyama, D. T., & Fischer, J. E. Nutritional support in hepatic failure: Current thought in practice. *Nutrition in Clinical Practice, 3*(3), 96.
4. Maclure, K. M. et al. (1989). Weight, diet, and the risk of symptomatic gallstones in middle aged women. *New England Journal of Medicine, 321,* 563.
5. Hyder, S. A., & Borkin, J. S. (1990). A new look at acute pancreatitis. *Contemporary Gastenterology, 3*(6), 34.
6. Frey, C. F., Gerzof, S. G., et al. (1989). Progress in acute pancreatitis. *Patient Care, 23*(5), 38.
7. Drurie, P. R., & Pencharz, P. B. (1989). A rational approach to the nutritional care of patients with cystic fibrosis. *Journal of Royal Society of Medicine, 82,* 11.

18

DISEASES OF THE CARDIOVASCULAR SYSTEM

OBJECTIVES

Upon completion of this chapter, you should be able to:

1. Describe atherosclerosis in terms of the modifications of blood vessels.
2. Name the nonmodifiable and modifiable risk factors of atherosclerosis.
3. Discuss how dietary modifications of cholesterol, polyunsaturated versus saturated fats, and fiber can influence the development of atherosclerosis.
4. Distinguish between type II and type IV hyperlipoproteinemia in terms of lipid elevation, age range and frequency, and characteristics.
5. Distinguish between dietary and drug treatment of type II and type IV hyperlipidemia.
6. Discuss the role of kilocalories, sodium intake, calcium and magnesium, and potassium on essential hypertension.
7. Name the components of a stepped care approach in the treatment of hypertension.
8. Discuss specific details of a moderate sodium-restricted diet in treating hypertension.
9. Describe three nutritional ways in which the workload on the heart can be reduced in a myocardial infarct patient.

INTRODUCTION

Cardiovascular diseases are diseases of the blood vessels and the heart. Cardiovascular diseases have declined during the past decade but are still the leading cause of death in the United States. It is responsible for about 650,000 deaths a year, 150,000 of which occur in people over 65 years of age. In addition to the high number of deaths, the total economic cost of cardiovascular disorders is estimated to be $60 billion annually, more than 20% of the total cost of illness in the United States.[1]

ATHEROSCLEROSIS

atherosclerosis The thickening and loss of elasticity of the walls of arteries.

atheroma An abnormal mass of fatty or lipid material with a fibrous covering often found in the inner lining of arteries.

lumen Inner open space in a tube such as blood vessel or the intestine.

coronary arteries Arteries that supply blood to the myocardium (heart tissue).

ischemia The lack of blood flow and oxygen to a body part that is often due to an obstruction of an artery, as in atherosclerosis.

A major cardiovascular disease is **atherosclerosis.** "Hardening of the arteries," the lay term for atherosclerosis, occurs in the walls of medium- and large-sized arteries. There are several causes of atherosclerosis, but the only one that is treatable by nutrition is the accumulation of fatty plaques. The thickening of the arterial walls results from **atheroma** (see Fig. 18-1). The plaques initially are composed primarily of cholesterol and later may become encapsulated by fibrous tissue. As the plaques enlarge, they decrease the **lumen** and elasticity of the arteries. These changes decrease the amount of blood flowing through the arteries, as well as their ability to dilate and contract. The amount of blood reaching the tissues decreases and the heart has to work harder to pump blood through the narrowed arteries.

Atherosclerosis of the **coronary arteries** initially results in **ischemia,** which is indicated by **angina pectoris** pain. Prolonged ischemia heart disease can result in **necrosis.** The lay term for this condition is *heart attack* and the medical term is **myocardial infarction.**

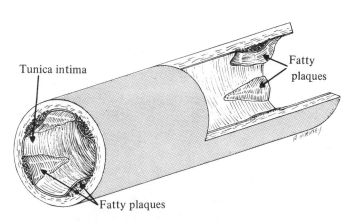

Tunica intima

Fatty plaques

Fatty plaques

FIGURE 18-1   Fatty plaques inside arteries.

angina pectoris Acute pain in the chest resulting from ischemia of the heart muscle.

necrosis Death of tissue.

myocardial infarction A condition in which a portion of the heart tissue becomes necrotic. Commonly referred to as a *heart attack.*

Causative Factors

It is believed that many factors interact to cause atherosclerosis. They are referred to as *risk factors* and are classified as nonmodifiable and modifiable factors.

Nonmodifiable Biologic Risk Factors

Age, sex, and family history are examples of nonmodifiable factors.

Age. Research and statistics show that cases of coronary atherosclerosis increase with age, especially after age 40.

Sex. Women before menopause are less susceptible to atherosclerosis than men. After menopause, women are equally susceptible. Estrogen has been theorized as the possible reason why women have greater immunity than men.

Family history. The chances of developing atherosclerosis appear to be higher if it has been detected in close relatives (parents, brothers, and sisters). It is not known how genetic inheritance predisposes a person to atherosclerosis; however, it is theorized that it may be linked to familial disorders (type III and type V hyperlipidemia) or obesity.

Modifiable Risk Factors

Major risk factors in the development of atherosclerosis are elevated blood lipid level, hypertension, cigarette smoking, diabetes mellitus, and a high-fat diet. All these factors can be altered, decreasing the chances of developing atherosclerosis.

Elevated blood lipids levels. An elevation of the level of blood lipids (cholesterol, triglycerides, and phospholipids) is called *hyperlipidemia* and is a potent indicator of the severity and prematurity of the disease. The blood cholesterol level relates most directly to the risk of developing atherosclerosis. The American Heart Association states that a person whose blood cholesterol level is consistently above 250 mg/dl has a threefold increased risk of developing atherosclerosis. The optimal cholesterol level is under 200 mg/dl.

Hypertension. High blood pressure, or hypertension, exists when the systolic pressure is over 140 mm Hg and the diastolic pressure is 90 mm Hg. Increased blood pressure pushes lipids into the arterial wall with great force; therefore, a greater risk of plaque development exists. A person with a systolic blood pressure above 150 mm Hg has twice as great a risk of developing atherosclerosis as a person with a systolic pressure under 120 mm Hg.

Cigarette smoking. Smoking is apparently related to atherosclerosis in that the nicotine in cigarettes is a vasoconstrictor, which decreases blood flow through arteries.

Diabetes mellitus. Research has shown that diabetics experience a greater number and more severe cases of atherosclerosis than nondiabetics. The exact reason is unknown, but it may result from their high level of blood lipids.

High-fat diet. A diet that has a high concentration of cholesterol and saturated fat contributes to hyperlipidemia and obesity. Both of these conditions increase the stress or workload on the heart.[2]

Three other risks that contribute to coronary heart disease are sedentary lifestyle, psychological stress, and personality type. Stress always results in the release of large amounts of epinephrine and norepinephrine, which can result in an increase in blood pressure and pumping by the heart. Research shows that psychological stress is handled by some people in such a way as to increase their risk of developing atherosclerosis. These people have a personality characterized by intense competitiveness, ambition, aggressiveness, and a sense of time urgency.

As mentioned at the beginning of the discussion of atherosclerosis, various factors interact to cause the disease. This statement is reinforced by the fact that in the presence of two or more factors the risk of developing atherosclerosis is not additive but rather **synergistic.** As an example, if a person has a high blood cholesterol level and elevated diastolic blood pressure and smokes, his or her chances of having a coronary heart attack are eight times greater than those of someone who does not have any of these risk factors. However, if an individual has only two of these risk factors, his or her chances of having an attack are four times greater than someone who does not have any of them.

synergistic The combined effect is greater than the sum of the parts.

Diet as a Modifiable Risk Factor

Nutritional experts do not all agree that diet alone can lower the risk of atherosclerosis. However, groups such as the American Heart Association do believe that certain modifications in the diet can reduce the level of cholesterol and triglycerides.

Cholesterol. Chapter 4 discussed the chemical structure, functions, and endogenous and exogenous sources of cholesterol. It was indicated that cholesterol is definitely important in the body. However, an excessive level of cholesterol in the blood is one of the major risk factors in atherosclerosis.

Cholesterol absorption is directly proportional to cholesterol intake. About 40% of dietary cholesterol is absorbed. Therefore, lowering the intake of cholesterol should lower the amount absorbed into the blood. Cholesterol from dietary sources does not have as powerful an effect on serum cholesterol as saturated fat does. Consuming a diet that is low in saturated fat, high in polyunsaturated fat, and low in cholesterol will decrease serum cholesterol levels from 8 to 18%. If cholesterol intakes are reduced to less than 300 mg/day, serum cholesterol levels will decrease regardless of endogenous cholesterol production. Appendix B lists the cholesterol and saturated fat content of some common foods. The principles of a fat-controlled diet are provided in Table 18-1.

It was noted in Chapter 4 that cholesterol and other lipids are transported in the blood as lipoproteins [chylomicrons, very low density lipoprotein (VLDL), low-density lipoprotein (LDL), and high-density lipoprotein (HDL)], with VLDL and LDL transporting the majority of cholesterol from the liver to the tissues. HDL transports cholesterol from the tissues or plaques to the liver, where it is decomposed into bile. Research shows that the higher the level of LDL, the greater the risk of atherosclerosis. However, the higher the level of HDL, the lower the risk of atherosclerosis, since this lipoprotein actually lowers the level of serum cholesterol. Dietary LDL is lowered when the saturated fat intake is reduced. Serum HDL levels apparently cannot be increased by diet but rather by increasing exercise. Sustained aerobic exercise for 20 minutes at least four times a week is necessary to raise the serum HDL level.[3]

Polyunsaturated versus Saturated Fats. Research shows that an increase in polyunsaturated fats (review the discussion of saturated and unsaturated fats in Chapter 4) can reduce the serum cholesterol level. The desirable ratio of polyunsaturated to saturated fats (P : S) is 1 : 1 and

TABLE 18-1 FAT-CONTROLLED DIET

Purpose:	To reduce serum lipid levels.
Use:	Used for persons with elevated serum cholesterol levels or people who are high-risk candidates for atherosclerosis and coronary heart disease.
Examples of foods:	Based on a general diet with the following adjustments: • Fat is limited to 30% of total kilocalories. • Dietary cholesterol should be limited to 250–300 mg. • Simple sugars and alcohol may be limited, since they can cause elevation of serum triglyceride levels, which is a causative factor in atherosclerosis.
Adequacy:	Diet is adequate.

Source: Chicago Dietetic Association, *Manual of Clinical Dietetics,* 4th edition. Philadelphia, W.B. Saunders Company, 1981. Reprinted by permission.

may be achieved in three ways. One way is to add polyunsaturated fat to the diet. The second way is to consume less saturated fat. Table 4-1 presents some suggestions on how to decrease the amount of saturated fat in the diet. The third way is to decrease saturated fat and increase unsaturated fat until a ratio of 1 : 1 is achieved.

Fiber. The soluble fiber has been shown to help lower LDL cholesterol levels by approximately 15%. It is suggested that the dietary fiber reduces the absorption of bile acids from the intestinal tract. This reduction causes more cholesterol from the liver to be degraded to bile acids, thereby reducing the serum cholesterol level.

Elevated Blood Lipid Levels

hyperlipoproteinemia Elevated blood lipoprotein level.

Persons who have atherosclerosis often have elevated levels of blood lipids, with chylomicrons, triglycerides, and cholesterol being the most common. Hyperlipidemia refers to elevated blood lipid levels and **hyperlipoproteinemia** refers to elevated blood lipoprotein levels. It is not unusual for these two terms to be used interchangeably.

Types of Hyperlipoproteinemia

There are six basic types of hyperlipoproteinemia: types I, IIa, IIb, III, IV, and V. Types II and IV are the most common, and types I and V are not associated with an increased incidence of atherosclerotic disease. The types of hyperlipoproteinemia are based on which of the classes of lipoproteins (see Chapter 4 for details of the five classes of lipoproteins) are elevated; LDL and VLDL are the ones most commonly elevated.

LDL transport more cholesterol than any other lipoproteins, and VLDL transport primarily triglycerides. Therefore, the two lipids that are primarily elevated are cholesterol and triglycerides. Table 18-2 presents information on which lipids are elevated, as well as the age range, frequency, and characteristics of the four types of hyperlipoproteinemia that are associated with atherosclerosis.

autosomal dominant trait A dominant gene that is present on one of the 22 pairs of genes known as *autosomes.*

nephrosis Kidney disease that is characterized by a large loss of proteins in the urine and edema (see Chapter 20).

Type IIa is a relatively common type of hyperlipoproteinemia, since it can be inherited as an **autosomal dominant trait.** It is not unusual for the problem to be detected in infants by 1 year of age. Premature atherosclerosis occurs rapidly, often resulting in death by age 30. This type of lipoproteinemia, as well as the others, can result from either primary causes (inherited disorders) or secondary causes (conditions such as diabetes, **nephrosis,** or obesity). Secondary causes of type IIa include nephrosis, hypothyroidism, and biliary obstruction. Once elevated blood lipid levels are detected, secondary causes must be ruled out before the appropriate treatment can be determined.

TABLE 18-2 SUMMARY OF HYPERLIPOPROTEINEMIAS

Hyperlipoproteinemia Type	Cholesterol (Normal, 120–220 mg/dl)	Triglycerides (Normal 10–200 mg/dl)	Age Range and Frequency	Characteristics
IIa (autosomal dominant)	300–600	Normal	All ages; severe cases occur in early childhood	Xanthoma (yellowish lesion) in tendons; corneal arcus (whitish line around edge of cornea); premature atherosclerosis
IIb	300–600	150–400	Usually adult; common	Xanthoma (palmar) premature atherosclerosis
III	350–800	400–800	Adult	Xanthoma (palmar) premature atherosclerosis
IV (familial)	Normal or slightly elevated	200–1,000	Adult; very common	Obesity; often develops as a secondary problem with diabetes mellitus

Type IV is probably the most common form of hyperlipoproteinemia. While it can be genetically inherited, most causes result from the diet. Secondary causes include uncontrolled diabetes, alcohol abuse, renal dialysis, pregnancy, and pancreatitis. It is very common to find type IV hyperlipoproteinemia associated with diabetes and obesity.[3]

Goals and Principles of Diet Therapy

The goals of the therapy are to reduce cholesterol and triglycerides to desirable levels. Its achievement requires permanent changes in eating habits that must be followed for life. Generally, drugs are not used to treat hyperlipoproteinemia unless diet therapy has been unsuccessful for at least 3 months.

Lowering the cholesterol level with diet therapy generally can be achieved by:

- Restricting cholesterol intake to less than 300 mg/day
- Reducing saturated fat intake
- Increasing polyunsaturated fat intake

An elevated level of cholesterol is the basic problem with type II hyperlipoproteinemia; therefore, the following comments are applicable to lowering cholesterol levels. (See Case Study: Hyperlipoproteinemia, pp.

457–459, for reinforcement and application of hyperlipoproteinemia information.)

The P : S ratio is more important than the amount of fat in the diet. A P : S ratio of 2 : 1 is most beneficial in reducing blood cholesterol level. In order to restrict cholesterol, the diet must exclude egg yolks and liver. In addition, beef and pork intakes should be limited. (See Appendix B for cholesterol values of specific foods.)

The P : S ratio can be accomplished by increasing the intake of poly-unsaturated foods such as tub margarines and liquid oils and increasing the intake of vegetables. Saturated fats can be reduced by restricting the consumption of butter, whole milk, coconut oil (used in popping corn commercially), palm oil (found in nondairy creamers), and animal fat as on steaks, chops, and bacon. See the sample menu for type IIa hyperlipoproteinemia.

Persons who follow this diet and increase their physical activity should be able to lower their LDL level and thereby their cholesterol. Increased physical activity will also increase their HDL level, which will lower their cholesterol level.

Lowering triglyceride levels by diet therapy generally can be achieved by:

- Weight reduction
- Carbohydrate restriction
- Elimination of concentrated sweets
- Reduction of alcohol intake

Elevated triglyceride levels is the common lipid disorder in type IV hyperlipoproteinemia. As mentioned above, this disorder is frequently a complication of obesity and diabetes. Therefore, a reduction in daily kilocalories to lose weight will reduce triglyceride levels as well as help reduce obesity and diabetes.

Carbohydrate intake should be almost exclusively from complex carbohydrate sources. Concentrated sweets should be restricted. A major difference in the type IV diet compared to the type II diet is the recommended reduction in alcohol. Alcohol has been found to increase triglyceride levels, whereas it does not affect cholesterol levels. See the sample menu for type IV hyperlipoproteinemia.

Treatment and Prevention

In 1987 the National Cholesterol Education Program (NCEP) was initiated to reduce coronary heart disease (CHD) by producing blood cholesterol to less than 200 mg/dl and LDL to less than 130 mg/dl.

Sample Menu for Type IIa Hyperlipoproteinemia

Exchange	
	Breakfast
1 fruit	½ cup orange juice
1 bread	¾ cup corn flakes
2 bread	2 slices whole wheat toast
1 fat	1 tsp margarine
	1 tsp jelly
1 milk	1 cup skim milk
	1 cup coffee
	Lunch
2 lean meat	2 oz slices chicken sandwich
2 bread	2 slices bread
1 vegetable	½ cup sliced tomatoes
	½ cup shredded lettuce
1 fat	1 tsp mayonnaise
	iced tea with lemon and sugar
	Dinner
	1 cup beef bouillon
4 lean meat	4 oz broiled fish
1 vegetable	½ cup green beans
1 bread	1 slice whole-wheat bread
1 fat	1 tsp low-fat margarine
1 fruit	1 medium peach
1 milk	1 cup skim milk

Analysis and Comments

- An analysis of the menu shows that it contains 2 milk, 2 vegetable, 2 fruit, 6 bread, 6 meat, and 3 fat exchanges.
- The cholesterol level is kept to less than 300 mg/day by modifications in certain exchanges:

Milk: skim milk is used as opposed to whole milk, thereby reducing the saturated fat intake.

Meat: three modifications are used to reduce fat and cholesterol intake. First, all 6 meat exchanges are from the lean group. Second, there are no eggs. Third, the number of ounces of meat exchanges is 6. In order to reduce cholesterol intake, it is best to keep the total number of meat exchanges to 9 or fewer.

Bread: no sweet rolls or other breads with added fat should be used.

Vegetables: vegetables should not be prepared with butter or cream sauces and should not be fried.

Fat: margarines should be low in fat.

Miscellaneous: beef bouillon helps to provide some nutrients without adding much cholesterol. Some examples of desserts that are high in cholesterol and should be excluded are commercial cakes, pies, cookies, ice cream, and desserts, which contain whole milk or egg yolks.

Source: Menu adapted from Texas Dietetic Association, *Diet Manual*, 5rd ed. Austin: Texas Dietetic Association, 1988. Reprinted by permission.

Dietary Modifications

The dietary modifications are recommended in a stepwise fashion with Step 1 and Step 2 diets.

	Step 1 Diet	*Step 2 Diet*
Saturated fatty acids	less than 10%	less than 7%
Monounsaturated fatty acids	10–15%	10–15%
Polyunsaturated fatty acids	up to 10%	up to 10%
Carbohydrate	50–60%	50–60%
Protein	up to 20%	up to 20%
Cholesterol	less than 300 mg/day	less than 200 mg/day
Total calories	to achieve and maintain weight	

An average reduction in cholesterol levels from the Step 1 diet of 30 to 40 mg/dl can be expected. The Step 2 diet may lower these levels another 15 mg/dl and reduce LDL to varying degrees.

Step 1 and Step 2 diets can help in accomplishing one of two goals:

1. Food choices to assist individuals in accomplishing the Step 1 Diet are listed in Table 18-3 (page 446). This diet is appropriate for people who do not need to lose weight.
2. To help people accomplish the goals of this diet, and lose weight, Table 18-4 (page 448) gives the suggested number of servings of foods grouped by similar nutrient, especially fat content, for diets containing 30% of their calories from fat.

Sample Menu for Type IV Hyperlipoproteinemia (1,200 kcal)

Exchange	
Breakfast	
1 fruit	½ cup orange juice
1 bread	¾ cup corn flakes
1 fat	1 tsp margarine
1 milk	1 cup skim milk
	coffee with sugar substitute
Lunch	
3 lean meat	3 oz broiled chicken (no skin)
1 bread	½ cup rice
1 vegetable	½ cup green beans
1 vegetable	½ cup sliced tomatoes
1 fruit	1 small apple
2 fat	2 tsp margarine
1 milk	1 cup skim milk
	iced tea with sugar substitute
Dinner	
3 lean meat	3 oz baked fish (e.g., halibut, trout, red snapper)
1 bread	½ cup mashed potatoes
1 vegetable	½ cup cooked cabbage
1 fruit	12 fresh grapes
1 fat	1 tsp margarine
	iced tea with sugar substitute

Analysis and Comments

- An analysis of this menu shows that it contains 2 milk, 3 vegetable, 3 fruit, 3 bread, 6 meat, and 4 fat exchanges.
- The bread and fruit exchanges are few in order to reduce the amount of carbohydrates.
- Foods from the miscellaneous and other group are limited to those that are low in carbohydrate.
- The intake of saturated fat is reduced, while the total fat intake is not limited.

Source: Menu adapted from *Diet Manual* (5th ed.) by the Texas Dietetic Association, 1988, Austin: The Texas Dietetic Association. Reprinted by permission.

HYPERTENSION

Hypertension is a symptom that is manifested as an elevated systolic and/or diastolic blood pressure. The major effect of hypertension is on the blood vessels. The increased tension and pressure cause the lining of the blood vessels to become thickened and the lumen narrowed. This thickening and narrowing change the flow of blood to the heart and kidneys and can eventually cause damage to these organs. Hypertension is a major risk factor for heart disease, stroke, and renal disease and affects approximately 18% of adult Americans.

Diagnosis

The diagnosis of hypertension is based on three consecutive readings that are elevated by two or more standard deviations above the norm for the age group. The upper limit of normal blood pressure for the 18- to 44-year-old age group is:

$$\frac{140 \text{ mm Hg (systolic)}}{90 \text{ mm Hg (diastolic)}}$$

Hypertension and degrees of severity are as follows:

Mild hypertension: diastolic pressure 90–104 mm Hg

Moderate hypertension: diastolic pressure 105–114 mm Hg

Severe hypertension: diastolic pressure 115–129 mm Hg

Malignant hypertension: diastolic pressure greater than 130 mm Hg

TABLE 18-3 RECOMMENDED DIET MODIFICATIONS TO LOWER BLOOD CHOLESTEROL: THE STEP 1 DIET

Food Group	Choose	Decrease
Fish, chicken, turkey, and lean meats	Fish, poultry without skin, lean cuts of beef, lamb, pork or veal, shellfish	Fatty cuts of beef, lamb, or pork, spare ribs, organ meats, regular cold cuts, sausage, hot dogs, bacon, sardines, roe
Skim and lowfat milk, cheese, yogurt, and dairy substitutes	Skim or 1% fat milk (liquid, powdered, evaporated), buttermilk	Whole milk (4% fat): regular, evaporated, condensed; cream, half and half, 2% milk, imitation milk products, most nondairy creamers, whipped toppings
	Nonfat (0% fat) or lowfat yogurt	Whole-milk yogurt
	Lowfat cottage cheese (1% or 2% fat)	Whole-milk cottage cheese (4% fat)
	Lowfat cheeses, farmer or pot cheeses (all of these should be labeled no more than 2–6 g fat/oz)	All natural cheeses (e.g., blue, Roquefort, Camembert, cheddar, Swiss)
	Lowfat or "light" cream cheese Lowfat or "light" sour cream	Cream cheeses, sour cream
	Sherbert Sorbet	Ice cream

(continued)

Types and Causes

essential hypertension A type of hypertension for which there is no known cause.

Essential Hypertension

About 90% of all cases of hypertension are essential. While there is no known cause of essential hypertension, factors that can influence it are genetic predisposition (approximately 20% of the population is so predisposed), race (approximately twice as many African Americans as whites), body weight, level of exercise, cigarette smoking, psychological stress, and diet. The following discussion concerns the role of various dietary factors on blood pressure.

Kilocalorie intake. Research shows that weight reduction in overweight hypertensives can reduce their blood pressure.

Sodium intake. Many researchers believe that some of the genetically predisposed individuals are sensitive enough to their current levels of sodium intake to cause hypertension. However, other researchers disagree. Currently, scientific and medical research has not shown that there is a

TABLE 18-3 *(Continued)*

Food Group	Choose	Decrease
Eggs	Egg whites (2 whites = 1 whole egg in recipes), cholesterol-free egg substitutes	Egg yolks
Fruits and vegetables	Fresh, frozen, canned, or dried fruits and vegetables	Vegetables prepared in butter, cream, cheese, or other sauces
Breads and cereals	Homemade baked goods using unsaturated oils sparingly, angel food cake, lowfat crackers, lowfat cookies	Commercial baked goods: pies, cakes, doughnuts, croissants, pastries, muffins, biscuits, high-fat crackers, high-fat cookies
	Rice, pasta	Egg noodles
	Whole-grain breads and cereals (oatmeal, whole wheat, rye, bran, multigrain, etc.)	Breads in which eggs are a major ingredient
Fats and oils	Baking cocoa	Chocolate
	Unsaturated vegetable oils: corn, olive, canola oil, safflower, sesame, soybean, sunflower	Butter, coconut oil, palm oil, palm kernel oil, lard, bacon fat, cocoa butter
	Margarine or shortening made from one of the unsaturated oils listed above	
	Diet margarine	
	Mayonnaise, salad dressings made with unsaturated oils listed above	Mayonnaise, dressings made with egg yolk
	Lowfat dressings and mayonnaise Seeds and nuts	Coconut

Source: Adapted from Expert Panel on Detection, Evaluation and Treatment of High Blood Cholesterol in Adults: High Blood Cholesterol in Adults. National Cholesterol Education Program (*NIH Publ No 89-2925*), Washington, DC, NHLBI, USDHHS, NIH, 1989.

causal relationship between hypertension and sodium consumption at the present levels.[4]

Calcium and magnesium. Calcium and magnesium are closely interrelated, and some studies have shown that when they are reduced, an increase in blood pressure can occur.[5]

Potassium. The ratio of sodium to potassium may be more important in causing hypertension than the level of sodium alone. The relationship between sodium and potassium is normally inverse. In other words, when there is a high level of potassium there is a low level of sodium. Research indicates that this is the best relationship for preventing hypertension. Current diets tend to be high in sodium and low in potassium; this may be the reason for hypertension in genetically predisposed individuals.[6]

TABLE 18-4 EATING PLANS FOR STEP 1 AND STEP 2 DIETS

Food Group	Daily Portions—Step 1 Diet			
	1,200 kcal	1,600 kcal	2,000 kcal	2,500 kcal
Fats and oils	3	4	6	8
Fish, poultry, meat	6 oz	6 oz	6 oz	6 oz
Egg yolks	3/wk	3/wk	3/wk	3/wk
Dairy foods	2	3	3	4
Bread, beans, grains, and starches	3	4	7	10
Fruit	3	3	3	5
Vegetables	4	4	4	4
Sugars, sweets, alcohol	0	2	2	2

Food Group	Daily Portions—Step 2 Diet			
	1,200 kcal	1,600 kcal	2,000 kcal	2,500 kcal
Fats and oils	3	5	7	8
Fish, poultry, meat	6 oz	6 oz	6 oz	6 oz
Egg yolks	1/wk	1/wk	1/wk	1/wk
Dairy foods	2	2	2	3
Bread, beans, cereals, and starches	4	5	8	10
Fruit	3	3	4	7
Vegetables	4	4	4	5
Sugars, sweets, alcohol	0	2	2	2

Secondary Hypertension

primary aldosteronism An excessive secretion of the hormone aldosterone from the adrenal gland. It is characterized by hypertension, hypokalemia, muscular weakness, and polydipsia.

Secondary hypertension can be traced to a specific disease or disorder such as kidney disease, **primary aldosteronism,** and **Cushing's disease.**

Stepped Care Treatment Program for Hypertension

Cushing's disease A condition caused by an excessive secretion of hormones from the cortex region of the adrenal glands.

People who have at least mild, essential hypertension (basically those with a diastolic pressure between 90 and 104 mm Hg) have recently been helped by a stepped care approach. This approach involves the following:

- Dietary sodium restriction
- Weight-control measures
- Moderate exercise
- Drug therapy

Essentially, in this approach the mild hypertensive implements the first three steps (weight control only if necessary) simultaneously. If these steps are not successful in lowering blood pressure to 90 mm Hg or below, drug therapy is also implemented. Only dietary sodium restriction and drug therapy will be discussed at this point, since weight control and exercise have been adequately covered in previous chapters.[7]

Dietary Sodium Restriction

Sodium Level in the Normal Diet. It is estimated that Americans consume about 3 g (1 tsp) to 12 g (5 tsp) of salt (NaCl) per day. However, the amount of sodium (Na) in these same diets varies from 1.2 to 4.8 g. The reason for the difference in the amount of salt (NaCl) and sodium (Na) is that salt is composed of 40% Na and 60% chloride (Cl).

As mentioned in Chapter 7, animal foods generally contain more sodium than plant foods. Therefore, exchange lists that, on the average, contain more sodium are list 1 (milk) and list 5 (meat), but only cured meats such as ham and bacon and some cheeses such as cheddar. One exception to the statement that list 2 (vegetables) is lower in sodium is canned vegetables that do not state "no salt added," since canning normally involves addition of salt. Table 18-5 lists the sodium values for each exchange list.

Sodium Measurement. Sodium may be measured in grams (g), milligrams (mg), and milliequivalents (mEq). The relationships between the three are as follows:

1 g sodium = 1000 mg sodium

1 tsp salt = 2,300 mg sodium = 100 mEq

1 mEq sodium = 23 mg sodium

Levels of Sodium-Restricted Diets. Physicians often use a variety of terms for ordering a sodium-restricted diet. Diet orders should specify the level of sodium in either milligrams or milliequivalents. The following terms are nonspecific, open to a wide range of interpretation, and should not be used without specific *sodium* levels being given: *low salt, no salt, salt free, salt poor, sodium restricted,* and *low sodium*.

The following are standard sodium levels for sodium-restricted diets:

Mild (2,000–3,000 mg, 87–130 mEq sodium) (Approximately 1 to 1¼ tsp of salt)
- No more than ½ tsp (1,150 mg salt) of salt added in cooking.
- No salt added to food at the table.
- No salty foods (crackers, pretzels, potato chips, corn chips, etc.).
  This diet is frequently used as a maintenance diet for hypertension, renal, and heart patients at home. See sample menu for 2,000- to 3,000-mg diet.

TABLE 18-5 SODIUM VALUES FOR FOODS ON THE SIX EXCHANGE LISTS

Exchange List	Food Group	Amount	Na+ (mg)	Na+ (mEq)
1	Milk			
	Whole	1 cup	120	5
	Skim	1 cup	120	5
	Milk, low sodium	1 cup	7	—
	Buttermilk, salted	1 cup	280	13
2	Vegetables			
	Cooked, raw, fresh, frozen	½ cup	9	—
	Canned	½ cup	230	10
3	Fruits	1 serving	2	—
4	Bread or cereal			
	Low sodium or made without salt	1 slice	5	—
	Salted yeast bread	1 slice	150	7
5	Meat, poultry, fresh fish cooked without salt	1 oz	25	1
	Cheese, cottage (dry)	¼ cup	5	—
	cheddar	1 oz	207	9
	Egg	1	70	3
6	Fat			
	Unsalted	1 tsp	—	—
	Salted		50	2

Moderate (1,000 mg, 44 mEq sodium) (Slightly less than ½ tsp of salt)
- No salt used in cooking.
- No salt added to food at the table.
- No salty foods.
- Some natural-sodium foods replaced with foods processed without salt (e.g., salt-free canned vegetables, bread).
- Foods containing moderate amounts of sodium may be limited, such as milk, eggs, and desserts.
This level is very difficult to achieve as a maintenance diet at home. See sample menu for 1,000 mg/44 mEg salt diet.

Strict (500 mg, 22 mEq sodium) (Approximately ¼ tsp of salt)
- First three comments for the above restriction applicable here.
- Meat limited to 5–6 oz total per day
- All natural-sodium foods replaced with foods processed without salt.
- Milk limited to 2 cups or servings per day.
- Unsalted margarine is used.
This level of restriction is extremely difficult to achieve and should be used for only short term or tests in a hospital.

Severe (250 mg, 11 mEq sodium) (Approximately 1/10 tsp of salt)
- Identical to the 500-mg sodium diet except that 2 cups of regular milk must be replaced by low-sodium milk.

Sample Menu for a 2,000- to 3,000-mg Diet

Exchange	
	Breakfast
1 fruit	½ cup orange juice
1 bread	½ cup oatmeal
1 milk	1 cup skim milk
1 medium-fat meat	1 poached egg
1 bread	1 slice toast
1 fat	1 tsp margarine
	1 tsp jelly
	1 cup coffee
	4 tsp sugar
	Lunch
2 vegetable	1 cup unsalted vegetable soup
2 medium-fat meat	2 oz beef patty
1 vegetable	½ cup sliced tomatoes
	1 tbsp oil and vinegar dressing
1 fruit	4 halves of dried apricots
	2 sugar cookies
1 milk	1 cup skim milk
	Dinner
1 vegetable	½ cup low-sodium tomato juice
3 lean meat	3 oz broiled chicken
1 bread	½ cup mashed potatoes
1 vegetable	½ cup peas (frozen)
1 fruit	½ cup fruited gelatin salad
1 bread	1 slice bread
1 fat	1 tsp margarine
	½ cup orange sherbert
	1 cup coffee

Analysis and Comments

- An analysis of this menu shows that it consists of 2 milk, 5 vegetable, 3 fruit, 4 bread, 6 meat, and 2 fat exchanges.
- The menu does not limit any exchanges. The main restrictions are in foods from the miscellaneous or other group. Notice that the soups are unsalted and that an oil and vinegar dressing is used as opposed to other dressings that are higher in sodium. Also notice that no salty foods (crackers, pretzels, potato chips, or corn chips) are included.

Source: Menu adapted from Chicago Dietetic Association, *Manual of Clinical Dietetics*, 4th ed. Philadelphia: W.B. Saunders Company, 1981. Reprinted by permission.

This diet should be used only in cases of extreme edema or for hospital tests. The principles of sodium-controlled diets are provided in Table 18-6.

Another source of sodium that needs to be considered is the public water supply. The sodium standard for public water should be about 20 mg/liter, as recommended by the American Heart Association, to help protect heart and kidney patients. However, public water supplies may contain more or less sodium, depending on the geographic location. Water containing over 100 mg/liter of sodium probably should be avoided by hypertensives, who instead should use bottled, distilled water for drinking and cooking.

Specific Details of Dietary Restriction. Moderate sodium restriction (to approximately 1,000 mg sodium) in two recent controlled trials has been found to be successful in lowering blood pressure.

In addition to lowering sodium, increasing potassium in the diet is important. These two dietary changes help to achieve a low-sodium, high-potassium diet, which, as discussed earlier, is beneficial in lowering blood pressure. Foods naturally high in potassium are those on the fruit exchange, 4, list with oranges, bananas, and dried fruits. Foods from the meat exchange list, 5, and the vegetable exchange list, 2, contain smaller amounts.

Mechanism of the Low-Sodium Diet in Lowering Blood Pressure. Essentially, a low-sodium diet functions as a natural diuretic to reduce the volume of extracellular fluid. As a result, the work on the heart is reduced, as is **peripheral resistance** in the arterioles and capillaries. Reduction in peripheral resistance is apparently the main factor responsible for the long-term effect of salt restriction on blood pressure. It may take

peripheral resistance
Resistance to the passage of blood through small blood vessels, especially the arterioles.

Sample Menu for a 1,000-mg Diet

Exchange

	Breakfast
1 fruit	½ cup orange juice
1 bread	½ cup unsalted oatmeal
1 milk	1 cup skim milk
1 medium-fat meat	1 unsalted poached egg
1 bread	1 slice regular toast
1 fat	1 tsp unsalted margarine
	1 tbsp jelly
	1 cup coffee
	4 tsp sugar

	Lunch
2 vegetable	1 cup unsalted vegetable soup
3 medium-fat meat	3 oz unsalted beef patty
1 vegetable	½ cup sliced tomatoes
	1 tbsp vinegar and oil dressing
1 fruit	4 dried apricot halves
1 milk	1 cup skim milk

	Dinner
1 vegetable	½ cup low-sodium tomato juice
3 lean meat	3 oz unsalted broiled chicken
1 bread	½ cup unsalted mashed potatoes
1 vegetable	½ cup low-sodium canned peas
	½ cup fruited gelatin salad
1 bread	1 slice regular bread
1 fat	1 tsp unsalted margarine
	½ cup orange sherbert
	1 cup coffee
	2 tsp sugar

Analysis and Comments

- An analysis of this menu shows that it contains 2 milk, 5 vegetable, 3 fruit, 4 bread, 7 meat, and 2 fat exchanges.
- Notice that the only major difference between this menu and the 2,000- to 3,000-mg menu is the use of salt-free or low-salt foods.

Source: Menu adapted from Chicago Dietetic Association, *Manual of Clinical Dietetics*, 4th ed. Philadelphia: W.B. Saunders Company, 1981. Reprinted by permission.

a few weeks to a couple of months for a hypertensive person to benefit from a low-sodium diet. The more successful the person is in restricting the sodium intake, the less likely will be the need for drug therapy.

Suggestions to Help Reduce Sodium Intake. Hypertensives often find it difficult to reduce their sodium intake drastically, primarily because the food tastes unpalatable. One way to increase compliance with the diet is to introduce the person to spices that add flavor to food but do not contain sodium. Some sodium-free spices are the following:

Allspice	Paprika
Bay leaves	Pepper
Curry powder	Sage
Lemon juice	Thyme
Nutmeg	Vanilla extract

Learning to read labels for sources of sodium is important. Some substances in foods that contain sodium are the following:

Baking powder	Monosodium glutamate
Baking soda	Sodium alginate
Disodium phosphate	Sodium benzoate
Sodium propionate	

In general, processed foods, milk, and dairy products are high in sodium. Some medications, such as antacids, antibiotics, cough medicines, laxatives, pain relievers, and sedatives, may contain sodium. Even some toothpastes and mouthwashes contain sodium.

TABLE 18-6 SODIUM-CONTROLLED DIETS

Purpose:	Sodium-controlled diets are designed to avoid excessive retention of sodium.
Use:	Used for persons with fluid retention caused by cardiovascular, renal, or hepatic diseases.
Sodium restriction:	Examples of specific sodium-controlled diets:

No added salt (approximately 4 g sodium or 174 mEq)

  All foods on the general diet are used, but salt is not used at the table.

2,000–3,000 mg sodium (87–130 mEq)

  $\frac{1}{2}$ tsp regular table salt may be used, either in the preparation of food or at the table.

  Foods with high salt content are omitted but can be calculated into the diet in place of the $\frac{1}{2}$ tsp table salt.

1000 mg (43 mEq). *This level is not recommended for home use.*

  No salt is used in the preparation of food or at the table. Canned or processed foods containing sodium are omitted. Four servings of regular bread are allowed daily.

500 mg sodium (22 mEq). *This level should be used for the short term or tests only.*

  No salt is used in the preparation of food or at the table. Canned or processed foods containing sodium are omitted. Certain vegetables containing high levels of natural sodium are omitted.

250 mg sodium (11 mEq). *This diet is not recommended, but could be used for the short term or tests only.*

  No salt is used in the preparation of food or at the table. Canned or processed foods containing sodium are omitted. Certain vegetables containing high natural sodium are omitted. Low-sodium milk is used instead of regular milk.

Adequacy:	All the sodium modifications are adequate, with the possible exceptions of the 250-mg and 500-mg sodium diets. Unless carefully planned, these two diets can be inadequate in some nutrients.

Source: Chicago Dietetic Association, *Manual of Clinical Dietetics*, 4th ed. Philadelphia, W.B. Saunders Company, 1981. Reprinted by permission.

MYOCARDIAL INFARCTION

A myocardial infarction (also known as *heart attack, coronary occlusion,* or *coronary*) is a condition in which a portion of the heart tissue is necrotic. As discussed earlier in the chapter, the main contributor is atherosclerosis of the coronary arteries.

Diet Therapy

The basic dietary principle for a heart attack patient is to reduce the workload on the heart and improve cardiac output. This can be accomplished nutritionally in three ways:

- Keep the size of the meals small
- Reduce to ideal body weight if necessary
- Eliminate excess body fluid

In addition, the following foods are avoided, since they can cause stress on the heart: foods that cause gaseous discomfort or distention, very hot or cold foods, and foods containing stimulants.

A diet progression for a myocardial infarct patient may be as follows:

First 24–48 hours

- Nothing is given by mouth; an intravenous line is established for intravenous fluids and drugs.

After 1–2 days

- Usually the first oral meals are clear liquids and skim milk (the possibility of distention due to lactose intolerance should be monitored).
- No caffeine is given.
- Fluids are usually limited to 1,000–1,500 ml.
- Sodium restriction is necessary if edema is present.

After about 3 or 4 days

- A soft, low-kilocalorie, mildly restricted sodium diet (2,000 kcal) is given.
- Fat and cholesterol are restricted.
- Six small meals are given to avoid distention.

Rehabilitation phase

- A moderate-fat and cholesterol-controlled diet (depending on blood lipid levels) is given.
- There is mild sodium restriction (2,000–3,000 mg).
- Caffeine is restricted.

CONGESTIVE HEART FAILURE

congestive heart failure
A condition in which the heart is damaged to the point where it is unable to pump blood adequately to the tissues.

decompensation Inability of the heart to maintain adequate circulation of blood.

Congestive heart failure is a condition in which the heart is damaged to the point where it is unable to pump blood adequately to the tissues. This condition is often called **decompensation**. The term *congestion* comes from the fact that this condition often results in pulmonary edema. Since the kidneys, like all body tissues, do not receive enough blood, they set into motion a mechanism to conserve sodium and water throughout the body. The end result is peripheral edema and ascites. The excess fluid increases the load on the heart and can further weaken it.

Diet Therapy

The diet principle in congestive heart failure is basically like that of a myocardial infarction patient: to reduce the workload of the heart. Therefore, a low-kilocalorie (if the patient is overweight or obese), sodium-restricted, and sometimes fluid-restricted diet is common for congestive heart failure. Also, a soft diet with avoidance of gaseous food and foods containing stimulants is common in diet therapy.[8]

CASE STUDY: HYPERLIPOPROTEINEMIA

Mr. T is a 52-year-old ex–vice president of a bank. He has come into a clinic for a yearly health checkup. Below are the assessment findings for this person.

Physical Findings	*Normal Values*
Height: 5 ft 9 in. (69 in.)	
Weight: 191 lb.	148–160 lb
Blood pressure: $\dfrac{145 \text{ mm Hg}}{95 \text{ mm Hg}}$	Upper limit $\dfrac{140 \text{ mm Hg}}{90 \text{ mm Hg}}$
Laboratory Findings	
Serum cholesterol: 480 mg/dl	Upper limit for age 50+ is 330 mg/dl
Serum triglycerides: 100 mg/dl	10–190 mg/dl
LDL: 200 mg/dl	60–120 mg/dl
HDL: 56 mg/dl	57–80 mg/dl
Other Information	
Occupation: retired early because of disability	

Activity: minimal physical activity; spends days reading and watching TV.

Nutrition: eats three meals per day and an evening snack; three or four beers per day.

Other: no known present or previous disorders; smokes two packs of cigarettes per day.

Using the above information and material in this chapter answer the following questions.

1. What type of hyperlipoproteinemia does Mr. T have?
   A. type IIa   C. type III
   B. type IIb   D. type IV
2. The modifiable risk factor(s) that Mr. T has for the development of heart disease is (are):
   A. overweight   D. age
   B. sex   E. A, C
   C. elevated cholesterol level
3. The basic diet for Mr. T should be one of _____.
   A. low saturated fat, restricted carbohydrates, no alcohol consumption
   B. weight reduction, restricted carbohydrate, salt restriction
   C. decreased saturated fat and increased polyunsaturated fat, increased HDL, weight loss, exercise
   D. none of these

For the fats listed below, choices 4 through 12, mark an A or a B based on the following key:
   A = polyunsaturated fat and should be increased in Mr. T's diet
   B = saturated fat and should be decreased in Mr. T's diet

__ 4. coconut oil   __ 9. Crisco

__ 5. safflower oil   __ 10. soybean oil

__ 6. corn oil   __ 11. bacon drippings

__ 7. butter   __ 12. skim milk

__ 8. tub margarines

13. The following meal represents a typical breakfast for Mr. T before being put on a low-cholesterol diet. Use information in Appendix B to calculate the total amount of cholesterol in this meal.

    2 scrambled eggs, 4 slices bacon
    Swiss cheese (1 cu in.) on an English muffin
    6 oz orange juice
    coffee with nondairy creamer, 2 tsp sugar

The total amount of cholesterol for this meal is _____ mg.
   A. 330
   B. 540
   C. 780
   D. 920

14. The major source of cholesterol in Mr. T's breakfast is _____ and a suggestion for decreasing the cholesterol from this source but still retaining some of its nutrients is _____.
   A. bacon—to substitute beef bacon for pork
   B. cheese on muffin—to substitute low-kilocalorie bread and cheese
   C. eggs—to eat the egg whites only or egg substitute.
   D. nondairy creamer—to eliminate cream from his coffee

15. For his other meals, Mr. T can increase his P : S ratio by increasing his consumption of _____ and decreasing his consumption of _____.
   A. tub margarines, liquid oils, and vegetables—butter, whole milk, coconut oil, and animal fat
   B. skim milk, butter, and animal fat—liquid oils, vegetables, and animal fats
   C. egg whites, whole milk, and animal fat—skim milk, sweets, and low-kilocalorie bread
   D. none of these

16. Part of Mr. T's dietary advice is to increase his intake of fiber, like the kind he might get naturally from fruits and oat bran, and to increase his exercise level. The increase in fiber is to _____ and the increase in exercise is designed to _____.
   A. increase HDL—decrease Mr. T's weight
   B. decrease LDL—increased HDL
   C. decreased synthesis of cholesterol—increase degradation of cholesterol in the liver
   D. decrease HDL—increase LDL

SUMMARY

- Atherosclerosis is the thickening and loss of elasticity of arterial walls.
- Modifiable risk factors of atherosclerosis are elevated blood lipid levels, hypertension, cigarette smoking, diabetes mellitus, and high fat intake; nonmodifiable risk factors are age, sex, and family history.
- The cholesterol level in the blood can be reduced by decreasing cholesterol and saturated fat in the diet, plus increasing polyunsaturated fat; increasing fiber will decrease cholesterol absorption.
- Type II hyperlipoproteinemia is caused by elevated LDL and cholesterol levels, is an autosomal dominant trait, and causes premature atherosclerosis. Type IV hyperlipoproteinemia is the most common type, where elevated triglycerides is the basic problem. Most cases result from diet, but secondary causes include diabetes, alcohol abuse, renal dialysis, pregnancy, and pancreatitis; type IV hyperlipidemia is commonly associated with diabetes and obesity.
- Certain dietary factors can have an effect on essential hypertension: 1) a decrease in kcal and weight can reduce blood pressure; 2) research is inconclusive as to whether reduced sodium alone reduces blood pressure; 3) reduction of calcium and magnesium can increase blood pressure; 4) a low sodium, high potassium diet is beneficial in reducing blood pressure.
- Components of a stepped care program are sodium restriction, weight control, moderate exercise, and drug therapy.
- Moderate sodium-restricted diet includes 1,000 mg (approximately ½ tsp of salt), with no salt in cooking, no salt added to food at table, no salty foods, and replacement of some natural-sodium foods with foods processed without salt. Foods containing moderate amounts of sodium may be limited (for example, milk, eggs, and desserts).
- Three nutritional ways for a myocardial infarct patient to reduce the workload on the heart are to eat small meals, reduce body weight to ideal body weight, and eliminate excess body fluid.

REVIEW QUESTIONS

True (A) or False (B)

1. Atherosclerosis is a weakening of arterial walls with the formation of outer extending sacs.
2. Atherosclerosis can decrease the lumen of coronary arteries, resulting in angina pectoris.
3. The risk of developing atherosclerosis, for anyone who has two or more modifiable risk factors, is not additive but rather synergistic.
4. Cholesterol from dietary sources has a more powerful effect on serum cholesterol levels than does saturated fat.
5. If cholesterol intake is reduced to less than 300 mg/day, serum cholesterol level will decrease regardless of endogenous cholesterol production.
6. Increasing the blood level of high-density lipoproteins (HDL) will lower the level of blood cholesterol.
7. Increasing the blood level of low-density lipoproteins (LDL) will lower the level of blood cholesterol
8. Blood LDL levels will increase when the intake of saturated fats is reduced.
9. Type IIa hyperlipoproteinemia can occur at any age, since it is inherited and is characterized by a high level of cholesterol.
10. Type IV hyperlipoproteinemia is characterized by a high level of triglycerides and is often associated with diabetes and obesity.
11. The diet for a person with type IIa hyperlipoproteinemia is one in which P : S level is 1 : 2.
12. The amount of polyunsaturated fat in the diet could be increased by increasing the consumption of butter, whole milk, coconut oil (popping corn oil), and palm oil (found in nondairy creamers).
13. Scientific and medical research has proven that there is a definite causal relationship between sodium consumption and hypertension.
14. A decrease in both sodium and potassium levels in the diet is beneficial in reducing hypertension.
15. Low dietary calcium intake can cause an increase in blood pressure.
16. In general, animal foods contain more sodium than plant foods; therefore, the milk and meat exchange lists contain more sodium than the other lists.

17. A strict sodium (500 mg, 22 mEq) diet has been found easy to achieve for people who have mild essential hypertension.
18. A person on a moderate (1,000 mg, 44 mEq) sodium-restricted diet cannot add salt to food and needs to limit the intake of milk and eggs.
19. Reduction in peripheral resistance is apparently the main factor responsible for the long-term effect of salt restriction.
20. The basic dietary principle for a heart attack patient is to increase foods and drugs that will increase the strength of heart muscle contractions.
21. A person who has suffered a myocardial infarct should be kept on total parenteral nutrition for a lengthy period of time to allow maximum relaxation and healing of the heart.
22. A heart attack patient who is receiving the drug quinidine should also have a diet that is low in alkaline ash foods (milk, vegetables, and fruits except cranberries, prunes, and plums).

Multiple Choice

23. Modifiable risk factors in developing atherosclerosis include:
    1. elevated blood lipid levels
    2. cigarette smoking
    3. diabetes mellitus
    4. age
    A. 1, 2, 3,   B. 1, 3   C. 2, 4   D. 4
    E. all of these
24. Which of the following comments about cholesterol and atherosclerosis is not true?
    A. Cholesterol absorption is inversely proportional to intake
    B. Cholesterol from dietary sources has a more powerful effect on blood cholesterol levels than saturated fat
    C. Consuming a diet that is high in saturated fat and low in polyunsaturated fat will decrease serum cholesterol levels
    D. A, B
    E. A, B, C
25. Type IIa hyperlipoproteinemia can be described as:
    1. an elevated level of triglycerides
    2. an elevated level of cholesterol
    3. a problem that can be helped by weight loss
    4. a problem that can be helped by increasing the P:S ratio
    A. 1, 2, 3   B. 1, 3   C. 2, 4   D. 4
    E. all of these
26. Type IV hyperlipoproteinemia is characterized as:
    1. an elevated level of triglycerides
    2. a frequent complication of obesity and diabetes
    3. being helped by reducing the consumption of alcohol
    4. a problem that is helped more by restricting total kilocalories than fat intake
    A. 1, 2, 3   B. 1, 3   C. 2, 4   D. 4
    E. all of these

Choose either A, B, or C

A = reduction in this factor can reduce blood pressure
B = increase in this factor can reduce blood pressure
C = this factor cannot be altered but can influence blood pressure

___ 27. kilocalorie intake
___ 28. genetic predisposition to hypertension
___ 29. calcium and magnesium
___ 30. potassium
___ 31. sodium

32. Which of the following presents the steps, in the proper sequence, for a stepped care treatment program for hypertension?
    A. dietary sodium restriction, drug therapy, weight-control measures, and moderate exercise
    B. drug therapy, moderate exercise, weight-control measures, and dietary sodium restriction
    C. dietary sodium restriction, weight-control measures, moderate exercise, and drug therapy
    D. none of these
33. The mechanism of a low-sodium diet in lowering blood pressure is initial reduction of _____, which is followed by reduction of _____.
    A. blood cholesterol—body weight and blood pressure

B. the volume of extracellular fluid—work on the heart and peripheral resistance
C. edema—sodium and calcium
D. none of these

34. After a heart attack, which of the following help to reduce the workload of the heart?

1. keep size of meals small
2. increase fiber in diet
3. eliminate excess body fluid
4. increase foods like ice cream, which contain many kilocalories in small portions

A. 1, 2, 3   B. 1, 3   C. 2, 4   D. 4
E. all of these

CRITICAL THINKING CHALLENGE

1. Analyze the menu below and compare to Table 18-4 Step 1 Diet as to the number of kcal in the diet and the number of daily portions in each food group.

Breakfast	Food Group Portions
	1 dairy
margarine, (1 tsp)	1 fat
bagel (½)	1 breads
½ grapefruit	1 fruit

Lunch	
broiled chicken (2 oz)	2 meats
milk, 1% (1 cup)	1 milk
tossed salad	
carrot (1 cup raw)	1 vegetable
lettuce (1 cup)	free vegetable
tomato (1 tomato)	1 vegetable
mushrooms (4)	free vegetable
oil and vinegar dressing	
olive oil (1 tsp)	1 fat
vinegar (2 tsp)	free
saltine crackers (6)	1 bread
nectarine (1)	1 fruit

Dinner	
broccoli (½ cup)	1 vegetable
carrot-raisin salad	
shredded carrot	
(½ cup)	1 vegetable
raisins (2 T)	1 fruit
mayonnaise (1 tsp)	1 fat

broiled fish (4 oz)	4 lean meats
roll (1)	1 bread
margarine (1 tsp)	1 fat
milk, 1% (1 cup)	1 milk

2. Your client has been following a 2,000–3,000 mg sodium-restricted diet but the doctor has changed the diet prescription to 1,000 mg. Contrast and compare the two diet prescriptions as you prepare a teaching plan to simplify your client's adjustment to the new diet prescription.

3. Your client has received lab results indicating elevated cholesterol and triglycerides. He tells you he just cannot imagine meals with no fat or flavor. Prepare a simple plan to implement the modifications necessary for the client to reduce his serum cholesterol and triglyceride levels.

REVIEW QUESTIONS FOR NCLEX

Situation. Mr. G is a black hypertensive male. His history indicates his father died from a heart attack at 57 years of age. Physical findings: obesity for his height; blood pressure = 152/104 mmHg; no edema in the extremities.

1. The factors, described above, that might be influencing Mr. G's essential hypertension are _____.
   A. race, genetic predisposition, and body weight
   B. blood pressure, exercise, and edema
   C. body weight, blood pressure, and exercise
   D. smoking, diet, and exercise

2. Which choice below gives all the dietary factors that might influence Mr. G's hypertension?
   A. kcal intake, sodium intake, protein intake and carbohydrate intake
   B. protein intake, sodium intake, potassium intake, and weight
   C. kcal intake, sodium intake, calcium and magnesium, potassium
   D. B complex vitamins, water soluble vitamins, sodium and potassium

3. Mr. G. is prescribed a 2,000-3,000 mg mild sodium restricted diet. Two exchanges that will have to be limited, in order to achieve the above levels of sodium are _____.
   A. fruit and vegetables
   B. bread and fat
   C. fruits and meat
   D. milk and meat

4. In preparing a teaching care plan for Mr. G, which three restrictions characterize the 2,000-3,000 mg sodium restricted diet?
    A. no more than 1/2 tsp of salt added in cooking, no salt added to food at table, and no salty foods
    B. no salt used in cooking, no salt added to food at table, no salty foods
    C. milk is limited to 2 cups per day, meat limited to 5-6 oz per day, and salt free foods
    D. unsalted margarine, no salt added to food, and use all unsalted foods
5. Mr. G should be cautioned to read food labels for the presence of sodium. Which of the following substances, that might appear on a label, do not contain sodium?
    A. baking soda
    B. sodium benzoate
    C. baking powder
    D. vanilla extract

REFERENCES

1. Williams, S. R. (1989). *Nutrition and diet therapy* (6th ed.) (p. 778). St. Louis: Mosby College Publishing.
2. Committee on Diet and Health, Food and Nutrition Board. National Research Council: Diet and Health. (1989) Implications for reducing chronic Disease Risk. Washington, DC: National Academy Press, 1989.
3. Expert Panel on Detection, Evaluation, and Treatment of High Blood Cholesterol in Adults: National Cholesterol Education Program, (1989) NHLBI, USDHHS, NIH Publication, no. 89-2925. Washington, DC, NIH, 1989.
4. Intersalt: An International Study of Electrolyte Excretion and Blood Pressure. (1988). Results of 24 hour urinary sodium and potassium excretion. *British Medical Journal, 297*, 319.
5. Chockalingham, A., Abbott, D. et al. (1990). Recommendation of the Canadian Consensus Conference on non-pharmacological approaches to the management of high blood pressure. *Canadian Medical Association Journal, 142*, 397.
6. Potassium supplements for hypertension. (1990). *New England Journal of Medicine, 322*, 623.
7. Stamler, R. et al. (1987). Nutritional therapy for high blood pressure, final report of a four-year randomized controlled trial—the hypertension control program. *Journal of the American Medical Association, 257*, 1484.
8. Kaufman, A. M., & Kahn, T. (1986). Congestive heart failure with hyponatremia. *Archives of Internal Medicine, 146*, 402.

19

DISEASES OF THE RESPIRATORY SYSTEM

OBJECTIVES

Upon completion of this chapter, you should be able to:

1. Describe bronchitis in terms of tissue changes, characteristic problems exhibited by bronchitis patients, and underlying causes.
2. Describe emphysema in terms of tissue changes, characteristic problems exhibited by emphysema patients, and underlying causes.
3. Discuss diet therapy for bronchitis and emphysema.
4. Discuss two reasons why malnutrition is common in respiratory insufficiency and respiratory failure.
5. Give the formula for calculating basal energy expenditure (BEE) for men and women.
6. Discuss lung cancer (bronchiogenic cancer) in terms of symptoms, nutritionally related side effects of therapy, and dietary treatment.

INTRODUCTION

Nutrition is important in regard to respiratory diseases. Poor nutrition in children has been associated with increased frequency of respiratory infections. In some studies, starving children and adults have been found to have emphysema-like changes. Recovery from pulmonary diseases can be affected by the type of nutritional care the person receives.

This chapter discusses some of the more common respiratory disorders and the role that nutrition may play in recovering from them.

CHRONIC OBSTRUCTIVE PULMONARY DISEASE

Chronic obstructive pulmonary disease (COPD) A group of disorders that obstruct the air flow into and out of the lungs.

Chronic obstructive pulmonary disease (COPD) refers to a group of disorders that obstruct air flow into and out of the lungs. COPD includes bronchitis, emphysema, and asthma.

The severity of COPD is significant. The death rate is more than 40,000 per year, making it the sixth leading cause of death. In addition, more than 13 million Americans suffer from emphysema and chronic bronchitis. COPD is found primarily in men over 45 years of age; however, the incidence in women is now steadily increasing.

Bronchitis

Bronchitis is a chronic infection of the lower respiratory tract or the bronchial tree (see Fig. 19-1). The condition is characterized by a regularly returning cough due to excessive mucus secretion and an inability to expel it. In addition, the bronchioles become constricted, resulting in decreased **ventilation** and **dyspnea.** Decreased ventilation often results in a **cyanotic** condition. The body build of chronic bronchitis sufferers often tends toward obesity, and because of their persistent bluish color, clinicians often refer to them as "blue boaters."

ventilation The ability to move air into and out of the lungs.

dyspnea Labored breathing.

cyanotic Bluish color of the skin due to reduced level of oxygen.

emphysema A disease characterized by the gradual destruction of alveoli, enlargement of distal air spaces, and trapping of air.

cor pulmonale Hypertrophy of the right side of the heart.

The underlying cause of bronchitis is frequent respiratory infections. The condition can progress to **emphysema** and can result in **cor pulmonale.** Cor pulmonale results from increased difficulty of the right side of the heart in pumping blood to the lungs. As the bronchioles become constricted, thereby decreasing blood flow to them, the right side of the heart has to work harder to pump blood to the lungs.

Pulmonary Emphysema

Emphysema is characterized by gradual destruction of alveoli, enlargement of distal air spaces, and trapping of air (see Fig. 19-2). Loss of elas-

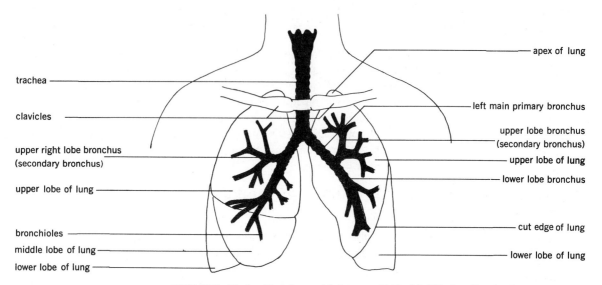

FIGURE 19-1   The bronchial tree. (J.R. McClintic, *Basic Anatomy and Physiology of the Human Body.* New York: John Wiley & Sons, Inc., copyright 1980. Reprinted by permission.)

barrel chest   An appearance of the chest often seen in people who suffer from chronic asthma attacks.

pulmonary therapy   Treatment of lung diseases.

intermittent positive-pressure breathing   The use of a ventilator for treatment of patients with inadequate breathing.

ticity allows the bronchi to collapse during expiration, making it very difficult for them to expire. There is progressive loss of lung tissue and destruction of alveolar blood capillaries. Mucus secretions are increased and accumulate due to ineffectual coughing. As more and more alveoli are hyperextended, the lungs become overdistended, causing the diaphragm to flatten. As a result, it becomes more and more difficult to breathe with the diaphragm. Instead, the person becomes more of a chest breather, relying on the intercostal muscles. These changes result in the formation of a **barrel chest.**

Unlike bronchitis, there is adequate oxygenation of tissues and no cyanosis develops; therefore, clinicians frequently refer to these patients as "pink puffers." People suffering from emphysema characteristically are thin, with muscle wasting and recent weight loss. There are three basic reasons for these changes:

- Extra energy is required to eat
- Increased physical effort is required to eat
- The full stomach presses on the diaphragm and causes dyspnea

The basic cause of emphysema is chronic irritation of the lungs. Cigarette smoking and inhaled irritants are the two most common sources.

Drugs are used to liquefy secretions, dilate the bronchi, and treat infections. In addition, **pulmonary therapy, intermittent positive-**

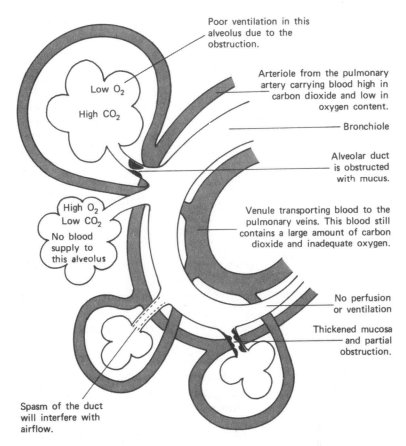

Poor ventilation in this alveolus due to the obstruction.

Low O$_2$

High CO$_2$

Arteriole from the pulmonary artery carrying blood high in carbon dioxide and low in oxygen content.

Bronchiole

Alveolar duct is obstructed with mucus.

High O$_2$
Low CO$_2$
No blood supply to this alveolus

Venule transporting blood to the pulmonary veins. This blood still contains a large amount of carbon dioxide and inadequate oxygen.

No perfusion or ventilation

Thickened mucosa and partial obstruction.

Spasm of the duct will interfere with airflow.

FIGURE 19-2 Emphysema is characterized by gradual destruction of alveoli, enlargement of distal air spaces, and trapping of air. (Reproduced by permission from S.R. Burke, *The Composition and Function of Body Fluids*, 3rd ed. St. Louis, 1980, The C.V. Mosby Co.)

pressure breathing, aerosol treatments, and oxygen in low concentrations are used in treating emphysema.

Diet Therapy

Eating is often very difficult for chronic bronchitis and emphysema patients. Dyspnea accompanied by air swallowing, coughing, persistent mucus production, and side effects of medications often result in anorexia and weight loss. In addition, when they do eat a large meal, the resulting full stomach pushes up on the diaphragm, decreasing the ability of the lungs to inflate.

The general diet plan is a high-kilocalorie diet with five to six small meals per day. Small meals require less energy to consume and decrease the fear that eating will bring on coughing spells and increase breathing difficulties.

In addition to high kilocalories, high protein and especially high levels of vitamins A and C are important in a COPD diet. The possibility of protein-calorie malnutrition (PCM) of the marasmic type should be assessed in patients with COPD, especially those with emphysema. It is important to include enough protein in the diet to prevent a negative nitrogen balance. A negative nitrogen balance will result in the catabolism of the intercostal and diaphragm muscles, predisposing the person to **acute respiratory failure.**

Vitamin A is important for maintenance and restoration of respiratory epithelial tissues. Without maintenance and restoration of this tissue, the person is strongly predisposed to respiratory infection and **bronchial pneumonia,** which could be fatal. Vitamin C is important for synthesis of collagen for the respiratory mucosa and blood vessels. Liquid blenderized or commercial formulas may be beneficial. Administering oxygen while the person is eating may be helpful. High-kilocalorie between-meal snacks should be offered to help achieve a high kilocalorie intake.

A COPD patient should be encouraged to consume an adequate level of fluids for hydration and **liquefaction** of mucus secretions. Gas-producing foods should be avoided, since they can cause upward pressure on the diaphragm, increasing dyspnea. (See Case Study: COPD in a 45-Year-Old Man, pp. 470–472, for reinforcement and application of COPD information.)[1]

Nutrition in Respiratory Insufficiency and Respiratory Failure

COPD can worsen into **respiratory insufficiency** failure. **Respiratory failure** can develop if the blood pH becomes too acidic, the pCO_2 increases, and the pO_2 decreases. Patients who go into acute respiratory failure (ARF), including **adult respiratory distress syndrome (ARDS),** require special mechanical ventilatory techniques and are very susceptible to malnutrition. There are two reasons why malnutrition may develop. First, an **endotracheal tube,** required for mechanical ventilation, decreases oral intake of food. Second, it is more difficult for the patient to communicate a feeling of hunger.

As discussed previously, a negative nitrogen balance can result in catabolism of the diaphragm and intercostal muscles, as well as decreasing the ability to produce the **alveolar surfactant.**

The patient's fat stores can be assessed by measuring skinfold thickness and muscle mass by measuring midarm muscle circumference. It is important to make sure that the total kilocalorie intake is adequate for

Acute respiratory failure (ARF) Inadequacy of the respiratory function in maintaining the body's need for an oxygen supply and for carbon dioxide removal while at rest.

bronchial pneumonia Inflammation of the bronchi in the lungs.

liquefaction Conversion into a liquid form.

respiratory insufficiency A condition that results when the exchange of oxygen and carbon dioxide is insufficient for the body's needs during normal activities.

respiratory failure A condition that develops when the blood pH becomes too acidic, the pCO_2 increases, and the PO_2 decreases.

Adult respiratory distress syndrome (ARDS) A variety of acute lung lesions that cause deficient oxygenation of the blood.

endotracheal tube An airway catheter inserted into the trachea that removes secretions and maintains an adequate air passageway.

alveolar surfactant A protein compound that is important in inflating the lungs.

Basal Energy Expenditure (BEE) The amount of energy expended by a person is at rest.

the patient's metabolic needs. One formula that can be used to estimate the **Basal Energy Expenditure** (BEE) of resting individuals who are not under stress is given in Chapter 9.

If possible, the enteral route is best for providing nutrients. However, aspiration is a complication of feeding by the enteral route, especially with the already-compromised respiratory system (see Chapter 14 for other complications of enteral nutrition). Total parental nutrition (TPN) by a central vein is the best alternative after enteral nutrition (see Chapter 14 for details of TPN).

LUNG CANCER (Bronchiogenic Cancer)

bronchiogenic cancer A malignant tumor of the lung that originates in the epithelial lining of the bronchi.

Bronchiogenic cancer is a malignant tumor of the lung that originates in the epithelial lining of the bronchi. Lung cancer is the most common type found in men, and the incidence in women has been increasing in the last several years. The most common cause is cigarette smoking, with persons who smoke one pack per day or more being at greatest risk. Another possible cause of lung cancer is preexisting pulmonary diseases such as tuberculosis and COPD.

metastasis The transfer of a cancerous tumor.

Metastasis frequently occurs from the lungs to other regions of the body by the blood and lymph. Some of the symptoms are a persistent cough that may be productive of sputum, dyspnea, wheezing, chest pain, and repeated infections of the upper respiratory tract. Later symptoms are weight loss, fatigue, anorexia, nausea, and vomiting.

Medical management involves surgical therapy, radiation therapy, chemotherapy, and immunotherapy. Surgical therapy offers the only type of cure and is usually successful only in the early stages of the disease. Radiation therapy and chemotherapy may be helpful in slowing the metastasis of cancer and providing symptomatic relief.

dysphagia Difficulty in swallowing.

When the lungs and chest are treated by radiation therapy, the esophagus may be irritated, resulting in **dysphagia.** As a result, tube feedings may be necessary. The drugs used in chemotherapy are among the most powerful and destructive of tissues that are available. They often cause nausea, vomiting, and anorexia, as well as tissue destruction and diarrhea. Some drugs prevent absorption of folic acid and cause iron deficiency through blood loss. As a result of these problems, hyperalimentation is the only alternative.

Diet Therapy

Patients suffering from lung cancer, as well as other cancers, often experience PCM. This results from many factors such as internal metabolic changes, anorexia, vomiting, nausea, and malabsorption of nutrients.

To avoid or correct PCM, a cancer patient needs approximately 1.2–1.5 g protein per kilogram of body weight daily. To be sure that the protein is used properly, 2,000 kcal/day are required for patients who are not malnourished. A malnourished patient may need as many as 4,000 kcal/day.

In addition to having protein deficits, cancer patients frequently are low in vitamins and minerals, requiring therapeutic doses.

Due to anorexia, an altered sense of taste, and vomiting, oral feeding will not meet the nutritional needs of the cancer patient. As a result, tube feeding and TPN are required. TPN is especially important if the patient has lost 7% of his or her body weight within 2 months or has been unable to eat for 5 days and is unlikely to eat for another week. Some practical dietary suggestions for lung cancer and other cancer patients are as follows[3]:

- Encourage small, high-calorie, high-protein snacks such as yogurt, peanut butter, cream soups, eggs, and fresh fruits.
- Additional kilocalories at meals or snacks can be provided by milkshakes, eggnog, pudding, custard, ice cream, butter, and gravy.
- Pain and nausea interfere with eating; therefore, pain and antinausea medications could be timed to be given 30 minutes before meals.
- For dry mouth problems, foods can be moistened with butter, gravy, cheese sauce, and cream.
- Nausea can be helped by giving the patient dry crackers, toast, and carbonated drinks.

CASE STUDY: COPD IN A 45-YEAR-OLD MAN

Mr. L is a 45-year-old man who has a long history of COPD. He has had many previous hospitalizations for congestive heart failure.

Four days before his admission, he noticed increasing shortness of breath and generally felt ill. On admission, he was described as a thin, middle-aged man who was experiencing adult respiratory distress syndrome (ARDS) and appeared chronically ill. It was decided to place Mr. L on a respirator.

Physical Findings	*Normal Values*
Height: 5 ft 11 in. (71 in.)	
Weight: 142 lb	154–166 lb (medium frame)
Blood pressure: $\dfrac{160 \text{ mm Hg}}{90 \text{ mm Hg}}$	Upper limits: $\dfrac{140 \text{ mm Hg}}{90 \text{ mm Hg}}$

Laboratory Findings

Blood gases

PaO_2 = 40 mm Hg	75–100 mm Hg
$PaCO_2$ = 62 mm Hg	35–45 mm Hg
pH = 7.28	7.35–7.45
Bicarbonate = 21 mEq/liter (HCO_3^-)	20–30 mEq/liter
Protein in urine	Negative

Using the information above and the material in this chapter, answer the following questions.

1. A major nutritional factor that health professionals need to monitor in Mr. L's case is _____.
   A. weight gain
   B. dehydration
   C. malnutrition
   D. metabolic alkalosis
2. Mr. L's diet should prevent a negative nitrogen balance, since this condition can result in catabolism of which respiratory muscles?
   A. triceps and biceps
   B. diaphragm and intercostals
   C. pectoralis major and rectus abdominis
   D. sternocleidomastoid and deltoid
3. The metabolic needs of Mr. L using the BEE formula (see Chapter 9) multiplied by 1.5 are
   A. 2,060 kcal
   B. 2,360 kcal
   C. 3,158 kcal
   D. 3,090 kcal
4. If possible, the best route to administer the kilocalories to Mr. L is _____ but a complication is _____.
   A. parenteral—edema
   B. enteral—osmotic overload
   C. parenteral—hyperglycemia
   D. enteral—aspiration
5. Since Mr. L, when admitted, was experiencing retention of CO_2, which was contributing to his acidotic condition, which nutrient should contribute the majority of kilocalories to his diet?
   A. carbohydrate   B. protein   C. fat

6. The diet for Mr. L, in addition to the previous comments, should contain adequate to increased amounts of
    A. vitamin A
    B. liquids
    C. vitamin C
    D. A, B, C

SUMMARY

- Bronchitis is characterized by chronic coughing due to excess mucus, dyspnea, and cyanosis, and is caused by frequent respiratory infections.
- Emphysema is characterized by destruction of alveoli, enlargement of distal air spaces and trapping of air. People with emphysema experience hyperextension of the lungs and difficulty in expiration; they breathe with the intercostal muscles instead of the diaphragm. Emphysema is caused by chronic irritation of lungs from smoking and inhaled irritants.
- Diet therapy for bronchitis and emphysema includes a high level of kcal, 5–6 small meals per day, a high-protein diet, and high levels of vitamins A and C.
- Malnutrition in a patient with respiratory insufficiency or respiratory failure may develop due to an endotracheal tube decreasing oral food intake, or the fact that it is more difficult for patient to communicate feeling of hunger.
- Symptoms of lung cancer include a persistent cough, dyspnea, wheezing, and chest pain; the most common cause is smoking. Diet therapy involves 1.2–1.5 g protein per kg of ideal body weight; 2,000 kcal/day for nonmalnourished and 4,000 kcal/day for malnourished patients; TPN for a patient who cannot consume food orally or if patient has lost 7% of body weight within 2 months or has been unable to eat for 5 days and is unlikely to eat for another week.

REVIEW QUESTIONS

True (A) or False (B)

1. Chronic obstructive pulmonary disease (COPD) includes problems like tuberculosis, pneumonia, and lung cancer.
2. Bronchitis involves collapse of alveoli and trapping of air.
3. People suffering from emphysema frequently are thin, with muscle wasting and recent weight loss.
4. Emphysema patients are thin and wasted because extra energy is required to eat, increased physical effort is required to eat, and a full stomach presses on the diaphragm and causes dyspnea.
5. The general diet plan for COPD is low kilocalories, high protein, and high levels of vitamins D and K.
6. Adequate to high levels of fluids are important in COPD to lower temperature and aid dysphagia (difficult swallowing).
7. It is common for people who are in respiratory insufficiency or respiratory failure to be susceptible to malnutrition.
8. The energy needs of a patient in respiratory insufficiency or respiratory failure are less than those when the patient is not in this condition.
9. TPN is always the best method for feeding respiratory patients.
10. The general diet plan for pneumonia is a low-fluid, low-protein, high-carbohydrate diet.
11. Exchange of gases in tuberculosis is hampered by tubercles (lesions) that destroy epithelial and blood tissues.
12. Radiation therapy and chemotherapy for cancer often alter the patient's metabolism such that less kilocalories, protein, and vitamins are needed.
13. Management of respiratory problems related to cystic fibrosis involves optimal nutrition, intermittent aerosol therapy, mist tent, postural drainage, expectorants, and antibiotics.
14. Tetracyclines should be administered with milk to reduce irritation to the gastrointestinal tract.
15. One reason for increasing the vitamin content in the diet of cystic fibrosis patients is to compensate for losses caused by some tetracycline antibiotics.

Multiple Choice

16. Common characteristics of emphysema patients are:

    1. overweight
    2. thinness
    3. recent weight gain
    4. muscle wasting

    A. 1, 2, 3   B. 1, 3   C. 2, 4   D. 4   E. all of these

17. Some of the common nutritional problems of COPD patients are:

    1. increased metabolism and voracious appetite
    3. decreased absorption of nutrients

473

2. negative nitrogen   4. large meals
   balance   causing dyspnea
   A. 1, 2, 3   B. 1, 3   C. 2, 4   D. 4
   E. all of these

18. A negative nitrogen balance or malnutrition in a COPD patient can result in:
    1. catabolism of intercostal muscles
    2. catabolism of the diaphragm
    3. decreased synthesis of epithelial tissue in the respiratory mucosa
    4. increased predisposition to acute respiratory failure
       A. 1, 2, 3   B. 1, 3   C. 2, 4   D. 4
       E. all of these

19. Which of the following two meals is appropriate for a COPD patient who needs high kilocalories, high protein, and high levels of vitamins A and C?
    A. cheeseburger on a bun with mayonnaise, ½ tomato with lettuce, french fries, and 1 cup whole milk
    B. ½ cup cream of wheat, lettuce salad, ½ cup peas, 1 cup skim milk, 1 banana

20. An adequate to high level of fluid intake in COPD patients is important for:
    A. reducing temperature
    B. replacing fluids lost due to diarrhea
    C. replacing fluids lost because of increased perspiration
    D. liquefaction of mucus secretions

21. The basal energy expenditure (BEE) for patients who are in acute respiratory failure (ARF) or adult respiratory distress syndrome (ARDS) is _____.
    A. lower than when patients are not in this condition.
    B. 1.2–1.5 times the BEE if the patients are stressed.
    C. 0.5–1.0 times the BEE if the patients are stressed.
    D. none of these

22. Dietary treatment for lung cancer includes:
    A. a low-kilocalorie, low-fat, low-protein diet to reduce the work of the lungs
    B. 0.8 g of protein per kilogram of ideal body weight, 1,200 kcal, and low fat
    C. high calcium, high levels of vitamins D, E, and K, and normal protein intake

    D. 1.2–1.5 g protein per kilogram of body weight per day, 4,000 kcal, and high vitamins plus minerals

CRITICAL THINKING CHALLENGE

1. Identify the diet therapy measures you would discuss with a client with chronic bronchitis and/or emphysema. Include measures you could implement to overcome the fatigue associated with the physical effort and energy required to eat.

2. You have been asked to speak with the local cancer support group about the nutritional needs of patients with cancer. Prepare a list of dietary suggestions to increase food acceptance and tolerance while increasing caloric intake. Identify resources available in your community where family members can obtain further assistance in meeting dietary needs of the client.

REVIEW QUESTIONS FOR NCLEX

Situation. Mr. R is diagnosed as having acute respiratory failure. He is intubated (insertion of tube for respiratory purposes) and placed on mechanical ventilation. Mr. R is 47 years old, 5 ft. 9 in. and weighs 145 lb.

1. Enteral feeding products that produce the most kcal from fat, versus carbohydrates, will produce the least amount of CO_2, therefore, stress to the respiratory system. Which of these products will be best for this patient.
   A. Ensure—31.5% kcal from fat
   B. Traumacal—38% kcal from fat
   C. Osmolite—31.4% kcal from fat
   D. Pulmocare—55.2% kcal from fat

2. Mr. R will need to be assessed regularly for malnutrition and two reasons why he might become malnourished are _____ and _____.
   A. lack of interest in eating; cannot swallow very well
   B. malfunction of the digestive tract; difficult to communicate feelings of hunger.
   C. decreased oral food intake due to tube; difficult to communicate hunger

D. increased REE (resting energy expenditure) or BEE; malfunction of the digestive tract

3. Assessment of Mr. R's fat stores to prevent negative nitrogen balance can be done by measuring _____ and _____.
   A. skinfold thickness; midarm muscle circumference
   B. body weight; resting energy expenditure
   C. waist size; and wrist measurements
   D. body weight; and wrist size

4. In Mr. R's diet it is very important for him to get vitamin _____ for maintenance and restoration of respiratory tissues.
   A. E
   B. D
   C. B complex
   D. A

5. Using the REE formula $66 + (13.7 \times wt) + (5 \times ht) - (6.8 \times age)$ and information about Mr. R's age, height and weight from above, calculate his REE $\times$ 1.5 for the stress condition he is in. His total kcal requirement for REE $\times$ 1.5 for stress is _____ kcal.
   A. 1,667
   B. 2,567
   C. 2,867
   D. 3,117

REFERENCES

1. Efthimiou, J. et al. (1988). Effect of supplementary oral nutrition in poorly nourished patients with chronic obstructive pulmonary disease. *American Review of Respiratory Diseases*, 137, 1075.

2. Keim, N. L. et al. (1986). Dietary evaluation of outpatients with chronic obstructive pulmonary disease. *Journal of the American Dietetic Association*, 86, 902.

3. Lindmark, L. et al. (1986). Thermic effect and substrate oxidation in response to intravenous nutrition in cancer patients who lose weight. *Annals of Surgery*, 204, 628.

20 DISEASES OF THE KIDNEYS

O B J E C T I V E S

Upon completion of this chapter, you should be able to:

1. Name and give four examples of each of the main functions of the kidneys.
2. Give and describe the three major functions of the nephrons.
3. Describe the symptoms of acute glomerulonephritis.
4. Discuss the dietary treatment of acute glomerulonephritis.
5. Give the characteristic symptoms of nephrotic syndrome.
6. Describe the dietary modifications necessary to alleviate edema, protein malnutrition, and hyperlipidemia associated with nephrotic syndrome.
7. Describe the causes of acute renal failure and the dietary treatment to correct this problem.
8. Describe the causes of chronic renal failure and the dietary treatment to alleviate the symptoms.
9. Distinguish between peritoneal dialysis and hemodialysis in terms of the method of operation and the disadvantages of each.
10. Discuss the dietary treatment of calcium phosphate and calcium oxalate.

INTRODUCTION

dialysis The separation of small molecules from large ones by passage through a semipermeable membrane.

Renal disease is found in about 8 million people, with deaths related to kidney disease being estimated at about 55,000 annually. However, with new treatment methods including **dialysis** and transplants, the outlook for kidney disease is now brighter.

Dietary modifications of people with renal disease depend on the specific disease. In general, these modifications do not result in a cure, but they do prevent further degeneration of the kidneys or help improve their functions.

FUNCTIONS OF THE KIDNEYS

The functions of the kidneys can be grouped into two main categories: excretory and endocrine.

Excretory Function

The excretory function is clearly the more important of the two, since the kidneys are responsible for maintaining the volume and composition of body fluids. Examples of substances that the kidneys excrete are as follows:

creatinine A nitrogenous waste that is formed from protein, muscle, and purine metabolism.

Urea, uric acid, and creatinine. These compounds are nitrogenous wastes and are formed from protein, muscle, and purine metabolism.

Excess water. The water level of the body in general, especially of the blood, is regulated by the kidneys in excreting excess water or retaining water if a deficit exists.

Electrolytes and acid-base composition. The kidneys regulate the amounts of the electrolytes sodium, potassium, chloride, bicarbonate, phosphorus, calcium, and others. The pH of the blood is partially regulated by the kidneys in excreting acids or bases whenever they occur in excess.

Excretion of foreign substances. Some medications are excreted, along with other foreign substances, by the kidneys.

Endocrine Function

The kidneys secrete hormones that affect every organ and system of the body. Hormones secreted by the kidneys and their functions are as follows:

erythropoietin   A hormone, secreted by the kidneys, that stimulates erythropoiesis.

Erythropoietin. Stimulation of erythropoiesis (maturation of red blood cells in the red bone marrow) is the role of this hormone.

Renin. This hormone causes formation of the compound angiotensin, which ultimately raises blood pressure by vasoconstriction.

renin   A hormone that causes the formation of the compound angiotensin.

Active form of vitamin D. Vitamin D enters the kidneys in an inactive form and is secreted in the active form 1,25-dihydroxycholecaciferol (calcitriol), which increases the absorption of calcium and phosphorus from the intestine, from the bones, and in the kidneys.

nephron   The structural and functional unit of the kidney.

These functions show that the kidneys play a major role in regulating the internal environment of the body.

NEPHRON: FUNCTIONAL UNIT OF THE KIDNEY

glomerulus   A capillary tuft within the Bowman's capsule of a nephron.

The functional unit of the kidney is the **nephron** (see Fig. 20-1). Since renal diseases affect different regions and functions of the nephron, it is important to have some knowledge of them. The nephron has three major functions: filtration, reabsorption, and secretion. These functions and the locations where they occur in the nephron will be discussed next.

Bowman's capsule   A proximal portion of a renal tubule that encloses the glomerulus of a nephron.

Glomerular Filtration

filtrate   A fluid present in Bowman's capsule. It is formed by filtration of blood in the glomeruli.

Blood enters the **glomerulus** of each **Bowman's capsule** under high pressure, which causes large amounts of **filtrate** to be filtered from the blood. The filtration process is not selective; therefore, both nutrients and wastes are filtered from the blood.

Glomerular filtration rate (GFR)   The amount of filtrate formed.

The **glomerular filtration rate (GFR)** averages about 125 ml/min, or about 180 liters/day. **Creatinine clearance** (normal values = 95–135 ml/min) is used as a measure of the GFR. Kidney disease frequently decreases the creatinine clearance rate, resulting in decreased filtration of the wastes out of the blood. When the filtration decreases to a certain level, dialysis is required. This topic will be discussed later.

creatinine clearance   The rate at which the nitrogen compound creatinine is filtered out of the blood by the kidneys.

threshold level   The amount of nutrients that will be reabsorbed into the blood of the nephrons. When this level is reached, no more reabsorption of the nutrients will occur.

Reabsorption

The tubular system of the kidney reabsorbs the important nutrients that were filtered out according to the **threshold level** of each substance. In other words, most of the nutrients are found in the blood at a certain threshold level, and when the absorption of each nutrient has been reached, the excess will be excreted in the urine.

proximal tubule   The portion of the renal tubule attached to Bowman's capsule. Most reabsorption of nutrients occurs here.

About 80% of the reabsorption occurs in the **proximal tubule** (see Fig. 20-1). The hormone aldosterone (secreted by the adrenal gland)

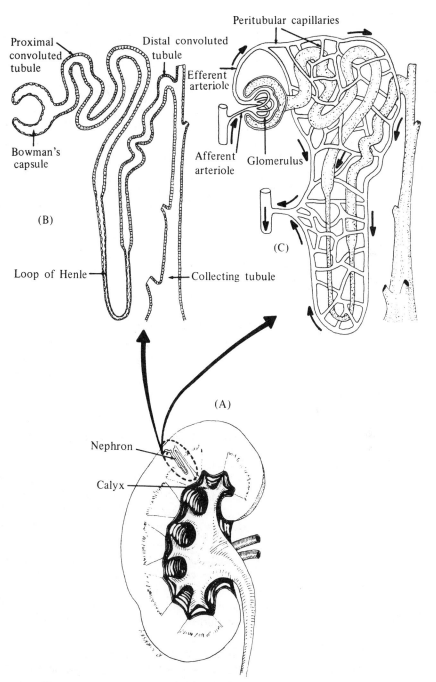

FIGURE 20-1 Parts of the kidney. (*a*) The sagittal section of a kidney shows a nephron. (*b*) The sagittal section of a nephron shows the regions. (*c*) A glomerulus within a Bowman's capsule and peritubular capillaries surrounding the regions of a nephron.

distal convoluted tubule
The portion of the renal tubule that is farthest from Bowman's tubule. Some water reabsorption and secretion occur here.

collecting duct   A duct that carries urine from the distal convoluted tubule of the nephron to the pelvic region.

stimulates the absorption of sodium and the excretion of potassium from the **distal convoluted tubule** and the **collecting duct.**

Secretion and Blood pH

The kidneys help to regulate the pH of the blood by secreting hydrogen ions and reabsorbing basic bicarbonate ions. Metabolic reactions produce an excess of hydrogen ions; therefore, to keep the pH of the blood within the normal range (7.35–7.45), the kidneys secrete the hydrogen ions from the blood in the distal convoluted tubule into the urine. In addition, basic bicarbonate ions are reabsorbed into the blood.

In addition, many different medications are secreted from the blood into the urine.

KIDNEY DISEASES

Acute renal disease   Sudden onset of kidney disease.

Chronic renal disease
Gradual onset of kidney disease.

Kidney diseases may result from temporary or permanent damage to the nephrons and may occur as either **acute renal disease** or **chronic renal disease.** In acute renal disease, there is usually recovery; however, with chronic disease, there is usually little if any recovery, and dialysis or transplantation is generally the only way to avoid death.

Acute Glomerulonephritis

acute glomerulonephritis   A form of kidney disease that involves inflammation of the glomeruli.

porosity   The state of being porous.

septic abortion   An abortion in which a uterine infection is spread to the general circulation.

hematuria   Blood in the urine.

proteinuria   Protein in the urine.

albuminuria   Albumin in the urine.

Acute glomerulonephritis involves inflammation of the glomeruli, frequently as a result of streptococci infections. The inflammation increases the **porosity** of the glomerular membrane to the point where large molecules (proteins and red blood cells) are filtered out of the blood. However, other substances such as urea and creatinine are not filtered out adequately, since the glomeruli are damaged from the infection.

Besides streptococcal infections other possible causes of acute glomerulonephritis include shock, **septic abortion,** surgery in other areas of the body, and drugs.

Symptoms and their causes associated with acute glomerulonephritis are as follows:

Hematuria. Blood in the urine results from the increased porosity of the glomeruli, as well as from damage to them.

Proteinuria. Protein in the urine also results from the increased porosity of the glomerular membranes. Frequently the protein is albumin; therefore, the symptom is often called **albuminuria.**

Edema. Loss of protein causes a reduction in the osmotic pressure of the blood therefore, an imbalance occurs in the exchange of fluids in the capillaries (see Chapter 7 for details on this fluid exchange).

oliguria   Diminished urine output.

Oliguria. This is diminished urine output to about 500 ml/day, or about a 50% drop from a normal of about 1,000–1,500 ml/day. This decrease results from increased damage to the nephrons.

The following symptoms may occur with acute glomerulonephritis but are not always present.

Increase in blood urea nitrogen (BUN). Diminished urine output frequently results in an increase in the waste compound urea.

Hypertension. Damage to the glomeruli results in reduced blood flow through the nephrons. This activates the renin-angiotensin mechanism in a compensatory step to increase blood flow to the kidneys. The end result is an increase in blood pressure.

In addition, frequently the person with acute glomerulonephritis exhibits nausea and anorexia.[1]

Dietary Treatment

The basic dietary treatment for acute glomerulonephritis is as follows:

- During oliguria, fluid intake needs to be limited to the amount lost during the previous day.
- Fruit juices are given orally to supply carbohydrates and to help maintain energy needs and spare protein breakdown, but the total amount should be within the prescribed fluid limits. The person needs to be monitored for hyperkalemia, which is a potential problem with oliguria and consumption of fruit juices. See Table 20-1 for approximate amounts of potassium per exchange list.
- Protein needs to be limited to about 40 g/day during a period of oliguria. Once oliguria has ended, protein intake is increased to compensate for urinary losses and to restore lost serum protein.
- Sodium restriction is necessary with edema. See Table 20-1 for approximate amounts of sodium per exchange list.[1]

Chronic Glomerulonephritis

Repeated episodes of glomerulonephritis lead to loss of nephrons and of kidney function, especially filtration. The problem is characterized by increased loss of protein and by accumulation of urea and creatinine.

TABLE 20-1 SODIUM AND POTASSIUM VALUES OF EXCHANGE LISTS

Exchange	Serving Size	Sodium (mg)	Potassium (mg)
Milk			
Whole or skim	1 cup	120	335
Low sodium	1 cup	7	600
Vegetables	½ cup	9	110–245
Starchy vegetables	Varies	2–10	110–190
Fruits	Varies	2	135–200
Bread			
Regular	1 slice	60	30
Low sodium	1 slice	5	30
Meat	1 oz or equivalent	25	100
Fat	1 tsp or equivalent	—	—

Comments

The values above are average values for each exchange list.
Specific comments about each exchange list

- Milk. Foods to be avoided due to their high sodium and potassium levels are chocolate milk, condensed milk, ice cream, malted milk, milkshake, milk mixes, and sherbet.

- Vegetable. Vegetables to be avoided due to their high potassium levels are baked beans, dried beans, lima beans, fresh broccoli, brussels sprouts, raw carrots, raw celery, peas, spinach (fresh or frozen), and potatoes (in skin or frozen). Vegetables to be avoided due to their high sodium levels are carrots, spinach, canned beets, turnips, dandelion greens, collards, and mixed vegetables.

- Fruit. For potassium- and sodium-restricted diets, the following fruits should be avoided: all dried and frozen fruits with sodium sulfite added, fresh apricots, avocado, bananas, glazed fruits, maraschino cherries, nectarines, prunes, and raisins.

- Bread. The following foods on the bread exchange list should be avoided on sodium- and potassium-restricted diets: yeast breads or rolls made from commercial mixes, quick breads made with baking powder, commercial baked products, graham crackers (except low-sodium dietetic ones), self-rising flour, salted popcorn, potato chips, pretzels, and waffles.

- Meat. Meats to avoid are all canned, salted, or smoked meats (e.g., bacon, bologna, corned beef, ham, sausage, kosher meats, and luncheon meats); all canned, salted, or smoked fish (e.g., anchovies, caviar, cod, herring, halibut, sardines, salmon, and tuna); cheddar, cottage, American, and Swiss cheeses should be avoided on sodium-restricted diets.

Source: Reprinted with permission of Macmillan Publishing Company from *Normal and Therapeutic Nutrition,* 16th edition, by Corinne H. Robinson and Marilyn R. Lawler. Copyright © 1982 by Macmillan Publishing Co.

nephrotic syndrome   A stage of kidney disease that is characterized by large losses of protein in the urine, severe edema, low serum protein levels, elevated levels of cholesterol and other serum lipids, and anemia.

Dietary treatment of chronic glomerulonephritis is identical to that of acute glomerulonephritis unless the condition worsens to a stage termed **nephrotic syndrome.**

Nephrotic Syndrome

Nephrotic syndrome is characterized by large losses of protein in the urine, severe edema, low serum protein levels, elevated levels of cholesterol and other serum lipids, and anemia. The massive losses of protein can result in tissue wasting, which is often masked by edema. The elevated cholesterol level is a result of increased lipoprotein production (especially low-density lipoproteins) by the liver. Anemia results from decreased secretion of erythropoietin.

The goal of dietary and drug treatment of nephrotic syndrome is to alleviate the symptoms of edema, protein malnutrition, and hyperlipidemia. The most effective means of preventing edema and initiating **diuresis** is severe sodium restriction. Nephrotic syndrome results in very little sodium excretion or about 230 mg/day (10 mEq/day). Therefore, dietary sodium intake must be equally low and must not exceed 10 mEq/day.

diuresis   Increased urine flow.

Protein malnutrition can be helped by high protein intake (65–200 g/day or, more accurately, 1.5 g per kilogram of ideal body weight). As with any high-protein diet, it needs to be accompanied by a high kilocalorie intake (35–50 kcal per kilogram of ideal body weight). When necessary, high-protein supplements and tube feeding may be used.

The hyperlipidemia problem that accompanies nephrotic syndrome is often type IIa and IIb, with type V being the most common. The diet should be appropriate for the type of hyperlipoproteinemia.

Losses of calcium, potassium, and vitamin D may occur with nephrotic syndrome. The symptom of bone pain may indicate calcium deficiency and muscular pain indicates potassium deficiency. Diets should contain adequate amounts of these minerals and iron in order to prevent deficiency symptoms.

renal failure   A condition in which kidney damage is severe enough that the kidneys no longer excrete the nitrogenous wastes or maintain the electrolytes in the blood.

Renal Failure

Renal failure results when enough damage to the kidneys has occurred so that they no longer adequately excrete nitrogenous wastes (urea, uric acid, and creatinine) and maintain the composition of the various electrolytes in the blood. Diagnosis is generally based on azotemia. The volume of urine decreases to the point of oliguria and even to **anuria.** If renal failure progresses to a severe stage, the person may develop **uremic syndrome,** which is a complex of symptoms caused by azotemia. The symptoms and their sources are discussed later.

anuria   Execretion of less than 50 ml of urine per day.

uremic syndrome   A complex of symptoms that result from an extremely high level of nitrogenous wastes in the blood.

acute renal failure Sudden onset of renal failure.

chronic renal failure Gradual onset of renal failure.

Like the other renal diseases, renal failure can be sudden or **acute renal failure** and the person can regain normal function of the kidney tissue. Alternatively, the failure may occur gradually and is referred to as **chronic renal failure.**

Acute Renal Failure

A rapid drop in the urine volume to about 500 ml can result from dehydration, fever, allergic reactions, immunologic reactions, shock, and glomerulonephritis. When the urine volume drops below 600 ml/day, the excretion of urea, uric acid, and creatinine is not adequate and these waste products may increase to toxic levels.

Dietary Treatment. Dietary treatment of acute renal failure is as follows:

Discover and treat the cause. Since acute renal failure is an abrupt problem that results from a cause other than damage to the kidneys, it is important to determine the cause and treat it before permanent damage to the kidneys occurs.

insensible water loss Fluid lost through the skin, vomiting, diarrhea, and fever (averages about 400–600 ml per day).

Maintain fluid homeostasis. Fluid intakes should replace urine output plus **insensible water loss,** with about 400 ml/day allowed for this loss. During the oliguric phase, fluid intake will be low, but during the diuretic phase, it must be increased in order to prevent **hypovolemic shock** and dehydration. Diuretics may be necessary during the oliguric phase to prevent uremic syndrome and edema.

hypovolemic shock Shock caused by low blood volume.

Maintain mineral homeostasis. Potassium is not excreted in acute renal failure and may build up in the blood, since it is a by-product of tissue destruction. Potassium intake should be restricted to 30–50 mEq/day (1,200–2,000 mg/day). Dialysis may be used when there is an urgent need to reduce serum potassium levels. It is possible to lose large amounts of potassium during the diuretic phase, which may result in hypokalemia. When this occurs, potassium chloride may be added to the diet.

peritoneal dialysis Infusion of dialysate fluid through a tube into the abdominal cavity. Nitrogenous wastes, excess fluids, and electrolytes are exchanged from the blood through the peritoneum into the dialysate fluid. The fluid is then drained out.

Prevent malnutrition. Prevention of possible malnutrition may hasten recovery and improve survival. Protein catabolism in cases of vomiting and diarrhea is prevented by administering amino acids and glucose in parenteral solutions. The majority of the kilocalorie intake should come from carbohydrates and fat, since their waste products are not excreted through the impaired kidneys. Kilocalorie intake should be high (50 kcal per kilogram of ideal body weight) to prevent tissue breakdown and promote synthesis of new tissue.

hemodialysis Circulation of arterial blood from the body into a machine called a *dialyzer.* Through diffusion and osmosis, nitrogenous wastes, excess fluid, and electrolytes are exchanged from the blood into the dialysate. The cleansed blood is then returned to the body.

Prevent uremic syndrome. If the levels of urea and other wastes are high, **peritoneal dialysis** or **hemodialysis** may have to be used to diminish their toxic effects.[2]

Chronic Renal Failure

Chronic renal failure occurs over a long period of time and is usually secondary to other diseases such as diabetes mellitus, chronic glomerulonephritis, atherosclerosis, and malignant hypertension.

Chronic renal failure can progress through four stages. Stage 1 is characterized by loss of 50 to almost 70% of the kidney tissue. This stage is frequently not distinguishable, since the kidneys can continue to function normally even with this amount of damage. Stage 2 is characterized by damage to more than 75% of the kidney tissue. At this stage, the ability of the kidneys to filter out nitrogenous wastes is decreased to the point where mild azotemia occurs. Stage 3 is characterized by moderate to severe azotemia. Stage 4 occurs when 90% of the kidney tissue is damaged. This stage is often called **end-stage renal disease (ESRD).** At this point, the GFR has decreased to about 10–12 ml/min (normal, 95–135 ml/min), with the end result being **uremia (uremic syndrome).**

Some of the symptoms of uremic syndrome are fatigue, weakness, decreased mental alertness, hyperglycemia, hyperlipidemia, hypertension, anorexia, nausea, and vomiting. In later stages, pH and metabolic imbalances result in gastrointestinal ulcers and bleeding. A major complication of ESRD is **renal osteodystrophy.** Renal failure results in retention of phosphorus and loss of calcium (refer to Chapter 7 for information on the reciprocal relationship of calcium and phosphorus).

Dietary Treatment. The basic goals of nutritional care in chronic renal failure include the following:

Regulation of protein intake. As renal function and the GFR decrease, so does dietary protein intake. Table 20-2 presents the amount of protein intake in relation to creatinine clearance. The **Giordano-Giovannetti (G-G) diet** is frequently used to supply protein, kilocalories, sugar, and fats. The diet (Table 20-3) provides about 20 g of high-quality protein with almost all the essential amino acids. The low level of protein intake causes the body to use some of the urea to make the nonessential amino

End-stage renal disease (ESRD) The stage of chronic renal failure in which 90% of the kidney tissue is damaged.

uremia (uremic syndrome) A complex of symptoms that result from an extremely high level of nitrogenous wastes in the blood.

renal osteodystrophy A complication of end-stage renal disease that is characterized by the loss of calcium from the bones and bone mass.

Giordano-Giovannetti (G-G) diet A diet used to treat chronic renal failure.

TABLE 20-2 PROTEIN INTAKE IN RELATION TO CREATININE CLEARANCE

Creatinine Clearance (ml/min)	Protein Allowance (g/day)
30–20	50
20–15	40
15–10	30
10–5	25

TABLE 20-3 GIORDANO-GIOVANNETTI DIET

20 g protein per day	Amount of protein per exchange
1 egg	(7 g)
¾ cup milk or 1 oz meat	(7 g)
½ lb low-protein bread or 1 piece of regular bread	(1.5 g)
2–4 vegetable exchanges	(2 g per exchange)
Fats and sweets as desired to supply adequate kilocalorie intake	

acids. The end result is a positive nitrogen balance and a reduction in urea levels.

Fluid intake to balance urinary output and insensible losses. Fluid intake should not exceed urinary output and the amount from the insensible losses. Allowing about 400–600 ml for insensible losses, plus the amount excreted in the urine, is usually adequate.

Regulation of sodium intake to balance output. Sodium intake is dependent on urinary sodium excretion, the presence of edema, the serum sodium level, and blood pressure. When hypertension, edema, and oliguria are present, sodium intake must be restricted to equal urinary sodium output. When vomiting and diarrhea are present, sodium intake needs to be increased.[3]

Determination of potassium balance. Hyperkalemia may occur when the volume of urine formed is very low or anuric. Potassium restriction depends on serum potassium levels and urinary potassium loss.

Control phosphorus intake. As mentioned earlier, ESRD results in retention of phosphorus; therefore, the amount in the diet depends on the degree of renal function. Generally, a low-protein diet is low in phosphorus. However, foods that are high in phosphorus and therefore may need to be restricted are dried beans and peas, dried fruit, milk, nuts, whole-grain breads, whole-grain cereals, and peanut butter. Another method used to control the phosphorus level is to administer aluminum hydroxide medications such as Amphojel, Basaljel, and Alu-Caps. These compounds bind with phosphorus in the intestines and prevent its absorption. The advantage of these compounds is that they do not require restriction of foods that are high in phosphorus. However, some people find them unpalatable, and they can cause constipation.[4]

Control energy requirements. Kilocalorie requirements range from 1,800 to 3,500 per day, based on the individual's height, age, weight, sex, and activity level. Since individuals suffering from ESRD frequently do not have much desire to eat, it is difficult to get them to consume this level of kilocalories. Therefore, their diet frequently must include concentrated caloric sources such as honey, heavy cream, sugar, hard candy, butter, jam, and jelly. This high-kilocalorie intake is very important to avoid protein degradation and, therefore, an elevation of the urea level.

Provide vitamin and mineral supplementation. A diet that is low in protein is also low in various vitamins such as thiamin, riboflavin, niacin, pyridoxine, ascorbic acid, and vitamin D. It is also deficient in iron and calcium. Ironically, renal failure results in iron and calcium deficiencies, with iron deficiency resulting from gastrointestinal tract ulcers. Calcium deficiency results from the inability of the kidneys to activate vitamin D or secrete calcitriol (dihydroxycholecalciferol). Calcium should be supplied from supplements, with 1,200–1,600 mg/day being necessary to prevent loss of bone mass. A multivitamin preparation can provide iron and the above-mentioned vitamins. The principles of a protein-sodium-potassium controlled diet for renal disease are provided in Table 20-4. (See Case Study: Chronic Renal Failure, pp. 491–492, for reinforcement and application of chronic renal failure information.)

DIALYSIS TREATMENT

Diet alone is not always successful in preventing uremia. At this point, the nitrogenous wastes have to be removed by dialysis, or else the per-

TABLE 20-4 PROTEIN-SODIUM-POTASSIUM-CONTROLLED DIET FOR RENAL DISEASE

Purpose:	Designed to minimize complications frequently associated with acute and chronic renal failure and to maintain ideal body weight (IBW).
Use:	A guide for planning diets for persons with acute or chronic renal failure.
Examples of foods:	Diet provides specific amounts of protein, electrolytes, and fluid, depending on the individual's needs.
Adequacy:	Diets containing less than 40 g protein are deficient in the following nutrients: protein, niacin, riboflavin, thiamin, calcium, phosphorus, and iron for both men and women. Levels of protein between 40 and 60 g are deficient in niacin, riboflavin, thiamin, and calcium for men and calcium and iron for women.

Source: Chicago Dietetic Association, *Manual of Clinical Dietetics,* 4th ed. Philadelphia, W.B. Saunders Company, 1981. Reprinted by permission.

son will die from complications of ESRD. The determination of when dialysis is required is based on the GFR. A commonly used figure is a GFR of 5–10 ml/min compared to a normal level of 125 ml/min. There are two types of dialysis: hemodialysis and peritoneal dialysis.

Hemodialysis

In hemodialysis (see Fig. 20-2), the person's arterial blood, rich in nitrogenous wastes, is circulated from the body into a machine called a *dialyzer*. The blood circulates through semipermeable dialysis membranes that are bathed by a **dialysate** fluid. This fluid is similar in composition to normal plasma. By diffusion and osmosis, the nitrogenous wastes, excess fluid, and electrolytes are exchanged from the person's blood into the dialysate. The cleansed blood is returned to the patient by a vein. The entire process takes about 4–6 hours and is repeated about three times per week.

One disadvantage of hemodialysis is loss of about 9–12 g of amino acids per 6-hour treatment. Hepatitis is a potential complication with nutritional implications. Another disadvantage is the cost; hospital-based hemodialysis is estimated to cost about $25,000 per year and home hemodialysis about $18,000 per year.

dialysate A fluid that bathes semipermeable dialysis membranes in dialyzer.

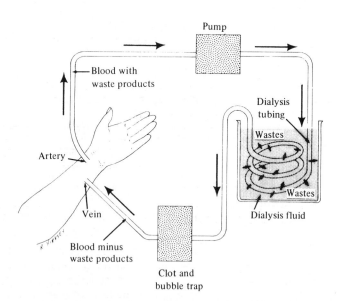

FIGURE 20-2 A dialysis kidney machine removes wastes from blood through dialysis tubing. (From T. Randall Lankford, *Integrated Science for Health Students*, 3rd ed., 1984.)

Peritoneal Dialysis

peritoneum membrane A membrane that covers most of the abdominal pelvic organs and through which exchange of nutrients and wastes occurs in peritoneal dialysis.

Peritoneal dialysis utilizes the **peritoneum membrane.** Dialysate fluid is infused through a tube into the person's abdominal cavity (see Fig. 20-3). The nitrogenous wastes, excess fluids, and electrolytes are exchanged from the person's blood through the peritoneum into the dialysate fluid. After about 20–40 minutes, the dialysate fluid with the wastes is drained out. For chronic but not acute cases, the procedure is repeated over 8–12 hours, three to five times a week. For acute conditions, the procedure is repeated over 36–72 hours.

Intact proteins can be lost (about 6–8 g/day) with peritoneal dialysis. Another disadvantage of peritoneal dialysis is the potential for hyperglycemia due to the diffusion of large amounts of glucose into the blood.

Diet Therapy for Dialysis Treatments

The diet therapy for hemodialysis and peritoneal dialysis is basically the same as for predialysis for most nutrients, with the exception of proteins and fluids.[5]

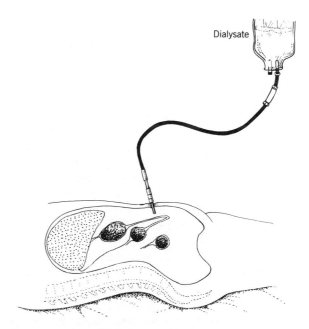

Dialysate

FIGURE 20-3 Peritoneal dialysis.

	Hemodialysis	Peritoneal Dialysis	Comments
Proteins	Higher than for predialysis	Higher than for predialysis	Increased protein is required for both, due to loss of amino acids by hemodialysis and loss of intact proteins by peritoneal dialysis.
Fluids (ml/day)	Lower than for predialysis	Lower than for predialysis	With 90% of the nephrons destroyed and a GFR of 5–10 ml/min, the amount of fluid removed is very low compared to that of a predialysis person; if fluid intake is not restricted, the person experiences edema and weight gain.

RENAL CALCULI (KIDNEY STONES)

kidney stones (renal calculi) Material that is composed of calcium phosphate, calcium oxalate, or a mixture of both.

hyperparathyroidism An excessive secretion of the parathyroid hormone from the gland.

Kidney stones (renal calculi) are composed primarily of calcium phosphate, calcium oxalate, or a mixture of both. Various problems can cause these salts to precipitate out of urine, such as **hyperparathyroidism,** bone disease, and ingestion of excessive amounts of antacids (as is common in peptic ulcer treatment). Kidney stones may develop either in the kidney or the bladder, where they can obstruct the urinary system, resulting in infection and pain.

Dietary Treatment

Many physicians do not consider diet to be important in treating kidney stones. Others use diet along with medications.

A high fluid intake of about 2,400–4,000 ml (at least 10–12 glasses) per day is very important to dilute the concentration of calcium in the urine. A reduction in the calcium level to about 400–600 mg/day is commonly recommended. This restriction is usually achieved by the removal of milk and dairy products. (See the sample menu for a calcium-restricted diet.) Increasing the acidity of urine helps to prevent the formation of calcium stones; this is accomplished by giving medications

acid ash diet A diet that includes foods that will form an acid urine.

along with an acid ash diet. An **acid ash diet** includes foods that form an acid urine, such as cereals, meat, bread, fish, and eggs; foods high in protein tend to be good acid formers.[6]

If tests indicate that a person is forming calcium oxalate stones, foods high in oxalic acid should be restricted. Foods high in oxalic acid include asparagus, spinach, cranberries, plums, tea, cocoa, coffee, green beans, tomatoes, almonds, and cashews.

CASE STUDY: CHRONIC RENAL FAILURE

Ms. White, age 78, is admitted to the emergency room in a semicomatose state with severe nausea, vomiting, lack of coordination, and a complaint of weakness. She has been a diabetic for several years.

Sample Menu of a Calcium-restricted Diet

Exchange	
	Breakfast
1 fruit	$\frac{1}{2}$ cup raspberries
1 bread	$\frac{3}{4}$ cup corn flakes
1 milk	1 cup skim milk
1 medium-fat meat	1 soft-cooked egg
1 bread	1 slice Italian bread
1 fat	1 tsp margarine
	1 tsp jelly
	1 cup coffee
	Lunch
3 lean meat	3 oz cold sliced turkey
2 bread	2 slices Italian bread
1 bread	1 small potato
2 fat	2 tsp margarine
	4 oz angel food cake
1 fruit	$\frac{3}{4}$ cup strawberries
	Dinner
3 medium-fat meat	3 oz pork loin
1 bread	$\frac{1}{2}$ cup noodles
1 fat	1 tsp margarine
1 vegetable	$\frac{1}{2}$ cup zucchini squash
1 bread	1 hard roll made without milk
1 fat	1 tsp margarine
	$\frac{1}{2}$ cup fruit salad
	iced tea with lemon

Analysis and Comments

- An analysis of this menu shows the following exchanges, with the approximate amount of calcium in parentheses: 1 milk (290 mg), 1 vegetable (25 mg), 2 fruit (25 mg), 7 bread (35 mg), 7 meat (25 mg), and 5 fat (0 mg). The total amount of calcium is 400 mg.
- In order to achieve a calcium-restricted diet of 400–600 mg, the following exchanges and comments are important:

Milk. This is the most important exchange group that has to be limited, since 1 cup contains 290 mg. In addition, since it is important that an acid ash diet be followed for the treatment of calcium stones, it is important to restrict milk, since it causes an alkaline ash diet.

Vegetables. This exchange group does not provide much calcium; however, there are some vegetables that should be avoided due to their higher calcium levels: dried beans, broccoli, green cabbage, greens, and okra. In addition to avoiding these vegetables, this exchange group in general does not help provide an acid ash diet, but rather an alkaline ash.

Fruit. Fresh, canned, or cooked fruits are low in calcium. Cranberries and plums are also good acid formers. Dried fruits should be avoided.

Bread. Many breads have to be avoided, since they are prepared with milk. Examples of breads that can be readily consumed are French or Italian breads (without added milk), pretzels, saltines, matzoh, and water rolls.

Meat. Beef, lamb, veal, pork, and poultry all contain little calcium. However, seafood such as crabs, lobster, oysters, salmon, and sardines should be avoided.

Fat. All fats are low in calcium, except for mayonnaise, sweet cream, and sour cream.

Source: Menu adapted from C.H. Robinson and M.R. Lawler, *Normal and Therapeutic Nutrition*, 16th ed. New York: Macmillan, 1982. Reprinted by permission.

Laboratory Values	Normal Values
Hemoglobin 8.6 g and hematocrit 27.0%	12–14 g/dl 40–48%
Serum potassium 6.3 mEq/liter	3.5–5.0 mEq/liter

Physical Findings	Normal Values
Height 62 in.	
Weight 150 lb	118–132 lb
Blood pressure 220/98 mm Hg	Upper limit, 140/90 mm Hg
Edema in lower extremities	
Laboratory Values	
Blood urea nitrogen (BUN) 52 mg/dl	10–20 mg/dl
Creatinine clearance 15 ml/min	95–135 ml/min
Serum phosphorus 5.9 mg/dl	3–6 mg/dl
Serum calcium 7.1 mg/dl	8.5–10.5 mg/dl

Ms. White is diagnosed as having ESRD with severe chronic renal failure, severe fluid overload, hypertension, uremia, and anemia.

1. Ms. White's diagnosis of severe chronic renal failure and uremia are based primarily on which laboratory values?
   A. hemoglobin and hematocrit
   B. blood pressure values
   C. BUN, creatinine, and phosphorus
   D. calcium and blood pressure values
2. Ms. White's high BUN values indicate
   A. she has been eating too much protein
   B. a significant decrease in filtration by nephrons
   C. her kcal intake has been high
   D. increased insensible fluid loss
3. Ms. White could suffer cardiac arrhythmias as a result of which substance that is present in an abnormal amount, according to the laboratory values?
   A. calcium
   B. iron
   C. phosphorus
   D. potassium

In order to reduce Ms. White's BUN level but still provide an adequate amount of proteins to avoid tissue breakdown, she is placed on the G-G (Giordano-Giovannetti) diet.

Using the key below and information in Table 20-3, determine which meals would provide 20 g of high-quality protein, and kilocalorie from sugars and fats.

Key:

a = meal allowed

b = meal not allowed

4. 2 eggs

6 oz meat

½ lb normal bread (approximately 8 slices)

1 cup green beans

2 tbsp of jelly

2 tsp of butter

5. 1 egg

1 oz meat

½ cup asparagus

½ cup carrots

1 slice of bread + 1 teaspoon of butter + 2 tbsp jelly

6. Ms. White's fluid intake: per 24 hours, 3,500 ml; urine output per 24 hours, 900 ml. This record indicates that Ms. White is experiencing

A. normal fluid output with intake

B. fluid retention

C. edema

D. A, C

E. B, C

7. In reference to the fluid figures given in question 6, what could be done to improve this condition?

A. limit fluid intake to 3,500 ml

B. limit fluid intake to 900 + 400 to 600 ml

C. place Ms. White on dialysis

D. A, C

E. B, C

8. If Ms. White is placed on periodic peritoneal dialysis, her diet should be higher in _____ than a nondialysis diet.

A. kilocalories

B. carbohydrates

C. fats

D. proteins

E. none of these

9. Ms. White is taking Basaljel tablets, which help her condition by

_____.

A. decreasing her edema

B. increasing her serum calcium level

C. decreasing her serum phosphorus level

D. decreasing her urea level

10. Ms. White is also taking the medication ferrous gluconate, which will help her _____ condition.
    A. potassium
    B. phosphorus
    C. anemic
    D. creatinine

SUMMARY

- The kidneys function in two ways, excretory and endocrine: 1) urea, uric acid, creatinine, excess water, electrolytes, and foreign substances are all excreted by the kidneys; 2) the hormones secreted are erythropoietin, renin, and an active form of vitamin D.
- Symptoms of acute glomerulonephritis are hematuria, proteinuria, edema, oliguria, an increase in BUN, and hypertension; dietary treatment involves limiting fluid intake to the amount lost the previous day during oliguria, increasing carbohydrate intake, limiting protein, and, during edema, restricting sodium.
- Nephrotic syndrome symptoms include large losses of protein in urine, severe edema, low serum protein level, elevated blood cholesterol level, and anemia; dietary treatment involves a severe sodium restriction to about 230 mg/day; a high protein intake, to 1.5 g/kg of ideal body weight; a high kcal intake, to 35–50 kcal/kg of ideal body weight, a diet appropriate for the type of hyperlipidemia, and an increased intake of calcium, potassium, and vitamin D.
- The causes of acute renal failure include dehydration, fever, allergic reactions, immulogic reactions, shock, and glomerulonephritis; dietary treatment involves treating the cause, maintaining fluid and mineral homeostasis, and preventing malnutrition and uremic syndrome.
- Chronic renal failure is usually secondary to diseases such as diabetes, chronic glomerulonephritis, atherosclerosis, and malignant hypertension; dietary treatment involves regulating protein intake, regulating fluid intake to balance output and insensible losses, regulating sodium intake, restricting potassium intake, controlling phosphorus intake, increasing concentrated carbohydrates and fats to increase the energy level, and vitamin and mineral supplementing the diet with vitamins and minerals.
- Hemodialysis involves removing wastes from a person's blood by exchanging wastes for nutrients in a dialysate fluid; a disadvantage to this process is the loss of 9–12 g of amino acids per 6-hour treatment.
- Peritoneal dialysis involves using the peritoneum membrane to remove wastes from the blood and exchange nutrients from dialysate fluid in the abdominal cavity; a disadvantage to this process is the loss of 6–8 g of intact proteins per day of treatment.

REVIEW QUESTIONS

True (A) or False (B)

1. A major function of the kidneys is excretion of aldosterone, renin, and erythropoietin.
2. A person who has damaged kidneys may have anemia due to decreased secretion of erythropoietin.
3. Filtration is a major function of the kidneys and can be determined by measuring the creatinine clearance.
4. Reabsorption of sodium and potassium occurs in the proximal tubule of the nephron.
5. Nephrons help regulate the normal pH of the blood by typically secreting bicarbonate and absorbing hydrogen ions.
6. Dietary treatment of acute glomerulonephritis includes high fluid intake to flush out the wastes plus high protein intake during oliguria to restore damaged tissues.
7. The diet for nephrotic syndrome is high protein (1.5 g per kilogram of ideal body weight) and high kilocalories (35–50 kcal per kilogram of ideal body weight).
8. Renal failure occurs when the kidneys no longer adequately excrete the nitrogenous wastes (urea, uric acid, and creatinine) and the volume of urine produced drops to 50% of normal.
9. Two components of dietary treatment of acute renal failure are restriction of potassium and intake and provision of kilocalories primarily from carbohydrates and fat.
10. Stage 4 of chronic renal failure is called *end-stage renal failure*, and the GFR is decreased to about 10–12 ml/min.
11. As renal function and GFR decrease in chronic renal failure, protein intake is increased to restore damaged tissue.
12. The Giordano-Giovannetti (G-G) diet supplies only about 20 g of protein, with almost all the essential amino acids and urea used to synthesize nonessential amino acids.
13. A major complication of ESRD is renal osteodystrophy, which is retention of too much calcium.
14. ESRD diets frequently have a restriction on foods high in phosphorus, such as dried beans and peas, dried fruit, milk, nuts, and whole grain cereals.
15. Hemodialysis has the disadvantage of causing

amino acids to be lost (about 9–12 g per 6-hour treatment).

16. Peritoneal dialysis does not involve any nutrient losses and can be completed in a shorter period of time than hemodialysis.

17. Dietary treatment of calcium phosphate or calcium oxalate renal stones is an alkaline ash diet and reduction of foods high in protein.

Multiple Choice

18. Substances that the kidneys excrete are:
    1. urea, uric acid, and creatinine
    2. renin
    3. excess amounts of sodium, potassium, and hydrogen ions
    4. active form of vitamin D

    A. 1, 2, 3   B. 1, 3   C. 2, 4   D. 4
    E. all of these

19. Kidney diseases can affect the functions of the nephrons, which are:
    1. filtration
    2. reabsorption
    3. secretion
    4. synthesis of fats

    A. 1, 2, 3   B. 1, 3   C. 2, 4   D. 4
    E. all of these

20. Symptoms associated with glomerulonephritis and the reasons for them are:
    1. hematuria—protein in the urine results from decreased porosity of the glomeruli.
    2. edema—retention of protein results in increased osmotic pressure
    3. proteinuria—blood in the urine results from damage to glomeruli.
    4. oliguria—diminished urine output to about 500 ml/day results from increased damage to nephrons

    A. 1, 2, 3   B. 1, 3   C. 2, 4   D. 4
    E. all of these

21. The anemia of ESRD results from
    A. decreased synthesis of renin
    B. decreased synthesis of erythropoietin
    C. bleeding from gastrointestinal ulcers
    D. A, B
    E. B, C

22. Uremia and uremic syndrome associated with ESRD results from a buildup of _____ due to decreased _____ in the nephrons.

A. hydrogen ions—secretion
B. nitrogenous wastes—reabsorption
C. sodium and potassium—filtration
D. nitrogenous wastes—filtration

23. Increased intake of calcium in renal failure is necessary to reduce _____.
    A. loss of bone mass, or renal osteodystrophy
    B. potential for cardiac arrhythmias
    C. edema
    D. anemia

24. A renal failure diet may include the restriction of milk, nuts, whole-grain breads, and peanut butter and the administration of Amphojel, Basaljel, or Alu-Caps to control the level of _____.
    A. potassium
    B. phosphorus
    C. sodium
    D. calcium

25. Concentrated sugars and fats such as honey, sugar, heavy cream, butter, and jam are included in a renal failure diet is to achieve a _____ without producing nitrogenous wastes.
    A. high level of protein
    B. low level of calcium
    C. high energy intake
    D. none of these

CRITICAL THINKING CHALLENGE

1. A chronic renal failure patient has the following lab values and assessment:
   - creatinine clearance 5–10 ml/min
   - urine output 500 ml/day
   - potassium output in urine is low
   - high level of phosphorus in blood
   - edema is present

   Based on the above data and information, calculate and prepare a teaching plan for the following for this patient.
   a. protein intake
   b. sodium intake
   c. potassium intake
   d. phosphorus intake
   e. level of kcal

2. Your patient with acute glomerulonephritis has developed hyperkalemia. Which of the following foods would be most responsible for the elevated serum level?

a. whole milk
b. rare beef
c. potatoes
d. fruit juices

3. Your client has been diagnosed with nephrotic syndrome. Which of the following orders should the nurse question?
   a. Give multivitamin supplement
   b. Restrict protein intake
   c. Restrict sodium intake
   d. Limit saturated fats

REVIEW QUESTIONS FOR NCLEX

Situation. Ms. E is admitted to the hospital in acute renal failure. Her symptoms include oliguria, hypertension, edema and elevated blood urea nitrogen (BUN).

1. The elevated level of Ms. E's blood urea nitrogen (BUN) is due to _____.
   A. increased intake of protein and thereby formation of urea
   B. decreased ability of kidneys to filter and remove urea from blood
   C. increased retention of urea by the bladder
   D. increased BEE (basal energy expenditure) and decreased excretion by the kidneys

2. During oliguria Ms E's fluid intake should be _____.
   A. limited to 2,500 ml per day
   B. restricted to 1,000 ml per day
   C. limited to what she gets from the foods she eats
   D. limited to the amount lost during the previous day

3. Ms. E's protein intake is probably _____ for the purpose of _____.
   A. limited to about 40 g/day; decreasing her urea level

B. increased to about 2g/kg per day; improving chances of healing kidneys
   C. limited to the amount lost the previous day; decreasing her edema
   D. high, 0.8 g/kg; healing her damaged nephrons

4. Which mineral, in Ms. E's diet and blood, should be monitored for the purposes of reducing her edema and hypertension?
   A. calcium
   B. potassium
   C. iron
   D. sodium

5. Ms. E's diet includes giving fruit juices for the purpose of providing _____ but she should be monitored for _____ which can occur from consumption of fruit juices and having oliguria.
   A. proteins; azotemia
   B. fluids; hypertension
   C. carbohydrates; hyperkalemia
   D. sodium and potassium; hypernatremia

REFERENCES

1. Ahmed, F. E. (1991). Effect of diet on progression of chronic renal disease. *Journal of the American Dietetic Association, 91,* 1266–1269.
2. Kahr, S. (1989). The modification of diet in renal disease study. *New England Journal of Medicine, 320,* 864.
3. Wilkens, K. (Ed.). (1986). *Suggested guidelines for nutrition care of renal patients.* Chicago: American Dietetic Association.
4. Coburn, J. W., & Salusky, I. B. (1989). Control of serum phosphorus in uremia. *New England Journal of Medicine, 320,* 1140.
5. Foulkes, C. (1988). Nutritional evaluation of patients on maintenance dialysis therapy. *American Nephrology Nurses Association Journal, 15*(1), 13.
6. Goldfarb, S. (1988). Dietary factors in the pathogenesis and prophylaxis of calcium nephrolithasis. *Kidney International, 34,* 544.

21

NUTRITION AND CANCER

Upon completion of this chapter, you should be able to:

1. Define cancer and compare its rate of occurrence in younger and older people.
2. Give six dietary recommendations that may prevent cancer.
3. List four possible reasons for anorexia in cancer patients.
4. Describe cachexia in terms of its characteristics, major problems resulting from it, and two complications.
5. Describe diet therapy for cancer patients in terms of protein, kilocalories, and vitamin intake.
6. Give three ways in which diet can be modified to alleviate nausea and vomiting.
7. Discuss the advantages of tube feeding and parenteral nutrition in treating cancer.

INTRODUCTION

neoplasm Tumor.

Cancer is an abnormal growth or **neoplasm** of the body cells. It tends to grow without control and can spread to secondary sites. It is the second leading cause of death in the United States.

The majority of cancers are now thought to be preventable. Diet is responsible for 35 percent of all cancers, as estimated by the National Cancer Institute.[1]

DIET AND CANCER PREVENTION

As mentioned above, the National Cancer Institute (NCI) believes that the majority of cancers are preventable; therefore, this organization plus the American Cancer Society and others offer some broad public recommendations to help prevent cancer.

1. *Avoid obesity.* The risk of breast, colon, prostate, gallbladder, ovary, and uterine cancers increase in individuals who are 40 percent or more overweight. Men have a 33 percent and women 55 percent greater chance of cancer than those of normal weight.[2]
2. *Increase intake of high-fiber foods such as whole-grain cereals, fruits, and vegetables.* Population studies show that consuming 20–30 g of fiber per day per person reduces the incidence of colon and rectum cancers. This would mean each American would need to double their intake of fiber per day since they consume on average 10–15 g per day.[3]
3. *Reduce total fat intake.* Diets high in total fat may be linked to the development of breast, colon, and prostate cancers. Another benefit of reducing total fat intake is reduction of the chance that a person will become obese.[4]
4. *Include foods rich in vitamins A and C in daily diet.* Studies have shown that people who consume foods high in vitamins A and C may lower their risk of developing cancer of the larynx, esophagus, and lung. Dark green and orange vegetables plus citrus fruits will provide these nutrients.[5,6]
5. *Moderate consumption of salt-cured, smoked, and nitrite-cured foods.* Smoked hams, sausages, fish, bacon, and so on, are high in tars that may cause stomach and esophageal cancers. Nitrites are preservatives that are commonly added to foods to protect against food poisoning and to improve food and color. While nitrites are beneficial, they also have been found to lead to the formation of nitrosamines, powerful cancer-causing chemicals.[7]

6. *Include cruciferous vegetables in the diet.* Cauliflower, broccoli, cabbage, and Brussels sprouts all are examples of cruciferous vegetables. Some studies have shown that consumption of these vegetables may reduce risk of respiratory and gastrointestinal tract cancers.
7. *Moderate consumption of alcohol.* Heavy consumption of alcoholic beverages may increase risk of oral cavity, larynx, and esophagus cancers. This is especially true with people who both smoke and drink heavily.[8]

NUTRITIONAL PROBLEMS AND DIET THERAPY FOR CANCER PATIENTS

cachexia A problem characterized by extreme weight loss, weakness, and severe wasting of tissues.

Two common nutritional problems associated with common cancers are anorexia and **cachexia.**

Anorexia

Anorexia, or decreased appetite, is the primary nutritional problem in cancer and is a major cause of cachexia. No one knows exactly what causes anorexia, but some of the possible reasons are altered tastes, a feeling of fullness, altered metabolism, and nausea or vomiting. The side effects of cancer therapy often result in anorexia.

Cachexia

Cachexia and malnutrition are synonymous. Loss of tissue protein is the major problem in cachexia, and one reason for the loss is that cancer results in increased metabolism. This is coupled with anorexia (decreased appetite and reduced protein intake) and the fact that tumors have a tendency to retain nitrogen. In addition, serum albumin tends to leak out of the blood into the tissue fluids. The end result of anorexia, retention of nitrogen in tumors and loss of albumin is less synthesis of proteins in the tissues.

In addition to protein deficiencies, cachexia typically results in anemia and vitamin A and vitamin C deficiencies (see Table 21-1). Anemia typically results from decreased availability of iron. The reasons for the vitamin A and C deficiencies are not known.

The major complications of cachexia are increased susceptibility to infections (due to decreased synthesis of protein antibodies) and decreased tolerance of cancer therapies (surgery, chemotherapy, and radiation therapy).[9]

TABLE 21-1 HOW THE CANCER PATIENT WASTES AWAY

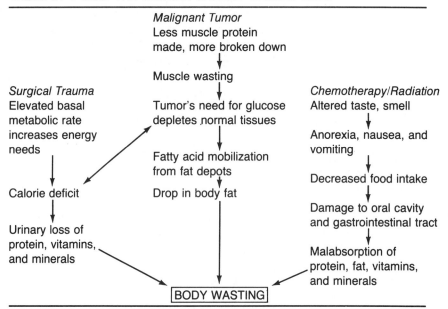

Source: Published in *RN,* a full-service nursing journal. Copyright © 1985 Medical Economics Company Inc., Oradell, N.J. March 1985, vol. 48. pp. 22–27. Reprinted by permission.

Diet Therapy

Two objectives of diet therapy for cancer patients are to meet the increased metabolic needs of the body and to alleviate the symptoms of the disease or the side effects of the treatment. Specific details of diet therapy are as follows:

High protein. Increased protein intake is important to replace the tissue losses and increase the body's resistance to infection. Approximately 1 g protein per kilogram of ideal body weight is often adequate for a well-nourished patient and 2–3 g/kg for a malnourished patient.

High kilocalories. Due to the hypermetabolic condition that accompanies cancer, the diet should contain 2,000–4,000 kcal. Most of these kilocalories should be from nonprotein sources so that proteins can be spared for tissue synthesis. Since most cancer patients exhibit anorexia, getting them to increase their intake of kilocalories and proteins is not always easy. Some examples of how to accomplish this goal are as follows:

- Add milk powder to milk, cereals, soups, gravies, and ground meat.
- Add ground meat and cheese to dishes like soups and sauces.
- Increase the consumption of foods like eggs and peanut butter by adding them to other dishes.

Vitamin intake. Vitamins A and C typically need to be increased for most cancer patients, since they are usually deficient in these nutrients. Thiamin is usually increased to metabolize the high kilocalorie intake. Increased amounts of vitamin B_{12} and folacin help to alleviate anemia.

Nausea and vomiting are common side effects of chemotherapy. Anti-nausea medications can be given 30 minutes before meals to help alleviate this problem. However, they are frequently ineffective in cancer patients. These people can benefit by eating smaller meals, sipping clear beverages slowly, and eating foods cold rather than hot, since hot foods give off more aromas, which often cause nausea.

The taste alterations that often result from cancer frequently decrease the ability to taste salt and sugar; patients also often complain that meat smells rotten. In these cases, substitutions of milk, eggs, and cheeses provide sources of protein.

Oral feeding is always the method of choice. However, due to persistent anorexia, malnutrition, and the side effects of therapy, tube feeding and parenteral nutrition may have to be used. Until recently, parenteral nutrition was not used extensively for treating cancer. The reason was the fear that this aggressive nutritional support would cause increased growth of the tumor. However, studies show that tube feedings and parenteral nutrition enable a cancer patient to tolerate larger doses of chemotherapy and radiation therapy.[10]

CASE STUDY: CANCER PATIENT

Mr. S is a 50-year-old man who has lung cancer. He has been receiving chemotherapy once a week. Currently, he is hospitalized for the management of anemia, which is often a side effect of chemotherapy.

Physical Findings	Normal Values
Height: 5 ft 10 in.	
Body weight: 141 lb (64 kg)	151–163 lb (medium frame)
Laboratory Findings	
Blood albumin: 2.5 g/dl	3.5–5.0 g/dl
Hemoglobin: 11.5 g/dl	13.5–18.0 g/dl
Hematocrit: 35%	40–54%
Ascorbic acid: 0.1 mg/dl	0.4–2.0 mg/dl
Vitamin A: 10 μg/dl	15–60 μg/dl

Using the above data and the information in this chapter, answer the following questions.

1. The above data indicate that Mr. S may be suffering from the nutritional problem called _____.
   A. neoplasm
   B. carcinoma
   C. cachexia
   D. myeloma

2. Mr. S is probably in a negative nitrogen balance, which is indicated by the low:
   A. ascorbic acid value
   B. blood albumin value
   C. vitamin A value
   D. hemoglobin value

3. Mr. S's condition and body weight indicate that the amount of protein he should be consuming is _____ g.
   A. 35–50
   B. 51–64
   C. 64–80
   D. 128–192

4. Mr. S's diet should contain approximately _____ kcal.
   A. 800–1,200
   B. 1,200–1,500
   C. 1,500–1,800
   D. 2,000–4,000

5. According to the data, Mr. S is anemic; therefore, increased amounts of _____ should be given to alleviate this problem.
   A. vitamins A and C
   B. vitamin B_{12} and folacin
   C. vitamins E and K
   D. vitamins C and K

6. Mr. S is anorexic; to help him increase his intake of kilocalories and protein, the following might be tried:
   A. add milk powder to milk, cereals, soups, gravies, and ground meat
   B. add ground meat and cheese to dishes like soups and sauces
   C. increase the consumption of foods like eggs and peanut butter by adding them to other dishes
   D. increase the consumption of citrus fruits
   E. A, B, C

7. Since Mr. S is undergoing chemotherapy, _____ and _____ might enable him to tolerate larger doses.
   A. weight loss—exercise
   B. enteral feedings—larger doses of vitamins
   C. weight gain—overnutrition
   D. tube feedings—parenteral nutrition

SUMMARY

- Cancer is a neoplasm of body cells and is more common in older rather than younger people.
- Breast cancer is possibly related to a diet high in animal fat, as is colon cancer.
- Dietary recommendations to possibly reduce the risk of cancer: 1) reduce saturated and unsaturated fats to no more than 30% of the daily kcal; 2) consume more fruits and vegetables, especially those high in vitamins A and C; 3) eat whole-grain cereals daily; 4) restrict the intake of salt-cured, salt-pickled, and smoked foods; 5) use alcohol in moderation; and 6) avoid high-dose supplements of individual nutrients.
- Possible reasons for anorexia in cancer patients are altered tastes, a feeling of fullness, altered metabolism, and nausea or vomiting.
- Characteristics of cachexia are extreme weight loss, weakness, and severe wasting of tissues. A major problem is the loss of tissue protein. Complications include increased susceptibility to infections and decreased tolerance of cancer therapies.
- Diet therapy for cancer patients include a high-protein diet, with approximately 1 g protein/kg of ideal body weight for well-nourished patients and 2–3 g/kg of ideal body weight for a malnourished patient; high kcal with 2,000–4,000 kcal/day; increased vitamin intake of A, C, thiamin, vitamin B_{12}, and folacin; smaller meals; and allowing the patient to sip clear beverages, eat cold foods, and substitute milk, eggs, and cheese for meats.

REVIEW QUESTIONS

True (A) or False (B)

1. Cancer is as prevalent in younger people as it is in older ones.
2. Anorexia is the primary nutritional problem in cancer and is a major cause of cachexia.
3. Cachexia is characterized by weight gain and decreased metabolism.
4. The major complications of cachexia are weight loss and edema.
5. Diet therapy for cancer includes low levels of protein in order to reduce stress on the kidneys.
6. The diet for a cancer patient should be high in fat as a source of kilocalories.
7. Foods served cold are tolerated by anorexic and nauseated patients better than they are when served warm.
8. A major advantage of tube feeding and parenteral nutrition is the intake of a large amount nutrients despite anorexia or nausea.

CRITICAL THINKING CHALLENGE

1. The American Cancer Society has identified seven recommendations to prevent cancer. Identify the exchange groups and some specific foods that can be used to achieve recommendations 1–6.
2. You are caring for a client diagnosed with cancer. Prepare a teaching plan to assist the primary caregiver to meet the client's nutritional needs. Include requirements for protein, kilocalories, and vitamins and specific foods to meet the needs.

REVIEW QUESTIONS FOR NCLEX

Situation. Mr. F is hospitalized with lung cancer. His wife asks you to discuss what can be done nutritionally to reduce the risks that she will get cancer and possibly prevent her husband from developing future cancerous growths.

1. In reference to weight you would tell Mrs. F to avoid obesity because women who are 40 percent or more overweight have a _____ greater chance of developing cancer than normal weight individuals.
   A. 33%
   B. 40%
   C. 50%
   D. 55%
2. Increasing intake of high-fiber foods to 20–30 g/day possibly reduces the incidence of _____ cancer.
   A. breast and lung
   B. lung and G.I.
   C. colon and rectum
   D. mouth and esophageal
3. Including foods rich in vitamins _____ and _____ in daily diets, may lower the risk of developing cancer of the larynx, esophagus, and lung.
   A. B12; C
   B. D; C
   C. A; C
   D. B6; D

4. Two common nutritional problems associated with Mr. F's cancer as well as other cancers are _____ and _____.
   A. anorexia; cachexia
   B. increased BEE; diarrhea
   C. edema; constipation
   D. increased appetite; weight gain

5. Diet therapy for Mr. F includes _____.
   A. low protein, low kcal, and increased vitamins B12 and C
   B. high protein, high kcal, and increased vitamins A and C
   C. high kcal, low fat, increased vitamins E and folic acid
   D. low protein, low fat, and increased amounts of iron and potassium

6. Due to persistent anorexia, malnutrition and the side effects of therapy a cancer patient may have to be fed by _____ and _____.
   A. oral route; tube feeding
   B. tube feeding; parenterally
   C. oral route; liquid formulas
   D. liquid diets; lactose free formulas

REFERENCES

1. American Cancer Society. (1988). *Cancer facts and figures.* New York: American Cancer Society.

2. Wolff, G. L. (1987). Body weight and cancer. *American Journal of Clinical Nutrition, 45,* 168.

3. DeCosse, J. J., Miller, H. H., & Lesser, M. L. (1989). Effect of wheat fiber and vitamins C and E on rectal polyps in patients with familial adenamatous polyps. *Journal of National Cancer Institute, 81,* 1290.

4. Carroll, K. K. et al. (1986). Fat and cancer. *Cancer, 58,* 1818.

5. Hennekens, C. H., Mayrent, S. C., & Willett, W. (1986). Vitamin A carotenoids and retinoids. *Cancer, 58,* 1837.

6. Glatthaar, B. E., Hornig, D. H., & Mosser, U. (1986). The role of ascorbic acid in carcinogenesis. *Advances in Experimental Medicine and Biology, 206,* 357.

7. Weisberger, J. H. (1986). Role of fat, fiber, nitrate, and food additives in carcinogenesis: A critical evaluation of recommendations. *Nutrition and Cancer, 8,* 47.

8. Rogers, A. E., & Conner, M. W. (1986). Alcohol and cancer. *Advances in Experimental Medicine and Biology, 206,* 473.

9. Trant, A. S. (1986). Taste and anorexia in cancer patients: A review. *Topics in Clinical Nutrition, 1*(2), 17.

10. American College of Physicians. (1989). Parenteral nutrition in patients receiving cancer chemotherapy. *Annals of Internal Medicine, 110,* 734.

22

PRE- AND POSTOPERATIVE NUTRITION

OBJECTIVES

Upon completion of this chapter, you should be able to:

1. State three ways in which pre-operative nutrition is important.
2. Describe how kilocalories, proteins, vitamins, and minerals are important in the preoperative nutrition of an under-nourished person.
3. Compare the difference in the pre-operative diet 24 hours and 8 hours before surgery.

4. Describe a postoperative diet progression.
5. Give four ways in which a post-operative regular diet is beneficial to a person.
6. Describe the nutritional support for stages 1, 2, and 3 of burn care.

INTRODUCTION

Patients benefit from optimal nutrition preoperatively and postoperatively. A patient who is well nourished before surgery faces less chance of complications during and after surgery. A patient who is well nourished following surgery heals more quickly, fights infection better, loses less muscle tissue, and has a more positive attitude than a poorly nourished one.

PREOPERATIVE NUTRITION

Preoperative nutrition is important to meet the metabolic stress of surgery, improve wound healing, and increase resistance to infection. Two major nutritional problems in the preoperative period are undernutrition and obesity. The nutrients most needed by an undernourished patient are kilocalories, proteins, vitamins, and minerals. The importance of these nutrients for an undernourished patient before surgery are discussed next.

Kilocalories

Surgery is very stressful to the organ systems; an undernourished patient cannot compensate for the stress as effectively as a well-nourished one. There may not always be enough time to provide a high-kilocalorie diet orally before surgery. However, central vein total parenteral nutrition (TPN) is a way of providing a large amount of nutrients in a short period of time.

Protein

During surgery, a patient who is deficient in protein (hypoproteinemia) is more susceptible to shock than one who is not, especially with great loss of blood. The liver is more threatened by anesthesia toxicity, and more edema occurs at the site of incision, all as a result of a low protein level. In contrast, adequate protein intake fortifies the patient for blood losses during surgery and for tissue catabolism.

In addition to these problems during surgery, a low protein level decreases the person's resistance to infection due to decreased synthesis of antibodies.

Vitamins and Minerals

A deficiency of water-soluble vitamins hinders carbohydrate metabolism, which is increased during surgery. A deficiency of potassium may cause malfunction of the heart. Calcium and sodium are important for muscle and nerve activity. Vitamin K is important for blood clotting.

Obesity, the second major preoperative nutritional problem, presents a variety of potential problems:

- Fat tissue decreases the effects of some anesthetic agents.
- Greater strain on the heart is caused by increased fat.
- There is an increased chance of infection due to decreased resistance of fat tissue.

PREOPERATIVE DIET

If there is enough time before surgery, an undernourished patient should be provided with a high-kilocalorie, high-protein, high-carbohydrate diet. Even a week of this type of diet can be valuable to the undernourished patient. Tube feeding and TPN may be required for some people who cannot consume food orally (see Chapter 14 for details on enteral-parenteral nutrition). An obese person should be placed on a weight-loss diet.

Twenty-four hours before surgery, the diet should provide nutrients that cannot be stored by the body. These nutrients include glucose (the body has only about a 24-hour supply in the form of glycogen), B complex vitamins, and vitamin C. A high fluid intake is valuable during this time until fluids are withheld. If the person is iron deficient, iron supplementation is required.

Eight hours before surgery, all fluids and food are withheld. The reason is to help decrease regurgitation and aspiration of food, which can occur during anesthesia. If surgery is to be performed on the gastrointestinal tract, a restricted-residue diet is given for 2 or 3 days before surgery. The purpose of the diet is to reduce the amount of feces, which could interfere with surgery and lead to distention after surgery. A restricted-residue diet limits the amount of milk, fruits, and vegetables and allows only white bread. Many hospitals are now using synthetic low-residue and residue-free diets, since they contain simple carbohydrates, amino acids, essential fatty acids, minerals, and vitamins. They provide the important nutrients but are readily absorbed, with no remaining residue.[1]

POSTOPERATIVE DIET

During surgery there is a loss of fluids and electrolytes; therefore, the immediate concern after surgery is to replace these losses. More fluids may be lost after surgery from vomiting, draining wounds, and diarrhea. Initially, fluids and electrolytes are replaced parenterally or enterally, since the person is usually nauseated and may be vomiting.

Once peristaltic contractions resume, the person can start receiving food orally. Frequently, a physician will order a diet progression from clear liquid to full liquid to a soft diet to a regular diet. See the sample menus for clear liquid and full liquid diets. Whether a progression through all of these diets is necessary, and at what rate, depends on the patient and on the severity and type of surgery. The faster the person can progress to a regular diet, the better. A regular diet, with its level of nutrients, enables the person to achieve a positive nitrogen balance, prevent weight loss, resist infection, and increase healing. Tables 22-1 through 22-4 present the principles of these diets.

Sample Menu for a Clear Liquid Diet

Exchange	
	Breakfast
1 fruit	$\frac{1}{3}$ cup apple juice
	1 cup beef broth
	1 cup coffee
	1 tsp sugar
	Mid-morning Snack
	8 oz (1 cup) gingerale
	Lunch
	1 cup chicken broth
1 fruit	$\frac{1}{2}$ cup strained orange juice
	$\frac{1}{2}$ cup grape-flavored gelatin
	1 cup hot tea plus sugar
	Mid-Afternoon Snack
	8 oz grape juice

Dinner

	1 cup beef broth
1 fruit	4 oz sweetened cranberry juice
	$\frac{1}{2}$ cup lime-flavored gelatin
	1 cup coffee or tea with sugar

Bedtime Snack

$\frac{1}{2}$ cup lime gelatin

Analysis and Comments

- An analysis of this diet shows that it contains 3 fruit exchanges. The miscellaneous foods contain various amounts of nutrients. Milk is not given since it is high in residue.
- Gelatin provides protein and the soups provide both protein and carbohydrate. Gingerale supplies carbohydrates and the fruit juices (orange and apple) supply carbohydrates along with some vitamin C and potassium.
- The amount of fluid given in a feeding is usually restricted to 30–60 ml/hour until the patient's tolerance improves.
- If the diet is given after gastric surgery or myocardial infarction, the coffee and other caffeine beverages should be eliminated, since they stimulate hydrochloric acid secretion and increased heart rate.

Source: Menu adapted from American Dietetic Association, *Handbook of Clinical Dietetics.* New Haven, Conn.: Yale University Press, 1981. Reprinted by permission.

TABLE 22-1 CLEAR (SURGICAL) LIQUID DIET

Purpose:	To minimize the amount of undigested material in the gastrointestinal tract.
Use:	Patients who have experienced surgery, vomiting, diarrhea, infections, and gastrointestinal problems will receive these diets.
Examples of foods:	Clear broth, plain gelatin, water ice, all clear and strained fruit-juices of fruit drinks, tea, decaffeinated coffee, commercial low-residue, high-protein, high-calorie oral supplements; *no milk products are used, since they are high in residue.*
Adequacy:	Inadequate in all nutrients except vitamin C and should not be used for more than 1 or 2 days.

Source: Chicago Dietetic Association, *Manual of Clinical Dietetics*, 4th ed. Philadelphia: W.B. Saunders Company, 1981. Reprinted by permission.

TABLE 22-2 FULL LIQUID DIET

Purpose:	To provide more nourishing fluids as the patient's gastrointestinal functions return to normal.
Use:	Transitional diet between the Clear Liquid Diet and the Soft Diet.
Examples of foods:	Milk and dairy products, fruit juices, strained vegetable juice, cooked or refined cereals, plain gelatin, and smooth pudding; the major difference between Full Liquid and Clear Liquid diets is the inclusion of milk and dairy products.
Adequacy:	May be low in protein, calories, iron, thiamin; vitamin and mineral supplements should be ordered if the diet continues for more than 3 to 4 days.

Source: Chicago Dietetic Association, *Manual of Clinical Dietetics,* 4th ed. Philadelphia, W.B. Saunders Company, 1981. Reprinted by permission.

Depending on the surgery and on whether the person is undernourished, TPN or tube feeding may be required. These diets are high in kilocalories and especially in proteins. In addition, it is important that the diets be high in the B complex vitamins, vitamin C, and vitamin K.[2]

DIET THERAPY FOR BURN PATIENTS

A person who has received extensive burns is in a hypermetabolic state. The body systems are stressed to the point where their energy needs can

TABLE 22-3 SOFT DIET

Purpose:	For patients who are physically or psychologically unable to tolerate a general diet.
Use:	A transitional diet between the Full Liquid Diet and the General Diet.
Examples of foods:	Foods that a patient can tolerate; fried foods, most raw fruits and vegetables, and very coarse breads and cereals may not be tolerated.
Adequacy:	This diet can be planned to provide all the nutrients necessary to be adequate.

Source: Chicago Dietetic Association, *Manual of Clinical Dietetics,* 4th ed. Philadelphia, W.B. Saunders Company, 1981. Reprinted by permission.

TABLE 22-4 MECHANICAL SOFT DIET

Purpose:	To minimize the amount of chewing necessary for ingestion of food.
Use:	Used for people who have chewing difficulties due to poor or missing teeth, stroke, and oral surgery.
Examples of foods:	Allows same foods as the Regular Diet except that meat, poultry, and fish should be modified by chopping, grinding, or pureeing (straining) and served with enough broth or gravy to ease swallowing; fruits and vegetables should be cooked, mashed, or strained.
Adequacy:	This diet is adequate in all nutrients.

Source: Chicago Dietetic Association, *Manual of Clinical Dietetics,* 4th ed. Philadelphia, W.B. Saunders Company, 1981 Reprinted by permission.

Sample Menu for a Full Liquid Diet

Exchange	
	Breakfast
1 fruit	½ cup orange juice
1 bread	½ cup farina (cereal rich in protein and easily digested)
1 milk	1 cup milk
1 fat	1 tbsp light cream
	4 tsp sugar
	Mid-Morning Snack
	½ cup custard
	Lunch
	6 oz strained cream soup
	½ cup gelatin
1 fat	2 tbsp light cream
	8 oz eggnog
	1 cup tea
	2 tsp sugar

	Mid-Afternoon Snack
	½ cup vanilla pudding
	½ cup grape juice

	Dinner
	6 oz beef broth
	½ cup ice cream
1 milk	1 cup skim milk
2 fruit	⅔ cup apple juice
	1 cup coffee
1 fat	2 tbsp light cream
	2 tsp sugar

	Bedtime Snack
	10 oz malted milk shake
	½ cup jello

Analysis and Comments

- An analysis of this menu shows that it contains 2 milk, 0 vegetable, 3 fruit, 1 bread, 0 meat, and 3 fat.
- In addition to the individual milk exchanges, milk is present in the puddings, eggnog, cream soup, and malted milk. Milk is important to provide some protein, since there are no meat exchanges. Additional protein can be gained by incorporating nonfat dry milk into foods such as milk and puddings.
- If the diet is to be given to a lactose-intolerant person, lactose-free supplements are available.
- The one bread exchange is a cereal (farina) that is easily digested and contains primarily carbohydrates.
- Many of the foods on the menu are from the miscellaneous group (e.g., eggnog, malted milk, pudding, ice cream, and custard) and supply primarily carbohydrates. In addition to these foods, oral supplements that are low in residue, high in protein, and high in calories can be given.
- This menu is inadequate in niacin, folacin, and iron. If the abovementioned supplements are given, the diet may be adequate in all nutrients.

Source: Menu adapted from Chicago Dietetic Association, *Manual of Clinical Dietetics,* 4th ed. Philadelphia: W.B. Saunders Company, 1981. Reprinted by permission.

be met only by metabolizing fat and protein stores. As a result of this situation, plus exposure of areas of the body to bacteria, the person will experience tissue catabolism and rapid loss of body mass. Nutritional support is critical for survival and healing for a person who has been burned over 20% or more of the body.

The aggressiveness and importance of nutritional support depend on how seriously the person is burned. A person whose burns cover less than 20% of the **body surface area (BSA)** has what many consider to be **small burns.** This person can usually recover adequately on a regular diet. However, a person who has burns covering more than 20% of the BSA usually needs very aggressive nutritional support. The specifics of the diet depend upon the three stages of burn care.

Body surface area (BSA) An estimate of the total body surface area. This measurement is important in burn situations for determining the level of nutritional care.

small burns Burns that cover less than 20% of the BSA.

metabolic acidosis An acidic state of the blood as a result of the accumulation of ketones.

Nutritional Support for Stage 1 of Burn Care

Loss of fluids is a major concern immediately after a serious burn. The loss of fluids and edema at the burn site result from loss of skin, loss of fluids from exposed blood vessels, and shifting of fluids from tissue spaces. As a result of the fluid loss, the person's blood volume decreases, which may result in shock and decreased urinary output. In addition to incurring a major problem from fluid loss during the first 48 hours after a burn, the person may also develop a potassium excess and a sodium deficit. The potassium excess results from its release from damaged cells. The sodium deficit results from a shift of sodium out of the body in the edematous fluid. **Metabolic acidosis** may occur as a result of a shift of bicarbonate ions out of the blood with sodium. The nutritional support and the reasons for stage 1 of burn care are as follows:

Nutritional Support	Reasons for Stage 1
Replacement of fluids and electrolytes	Primarily important to prevent irreversible shock and renal shutdown. From 3 to 5 liters of fluid generally are needed to replace fluid losses per day.
	Saline lactated Ringer's solution (sodium chloride, potassium chloride, and calcium chloride) is used to replace lost electrolytes.
Replacement of bicarbonate ions	Helps to prevent metabolic acidosis.
Replacement of glucose and amino acids	Counteracts tissue catabolism.

paralytic ileus   Absence of
peristalsis.

Generally, nutritional support for stage 1 is supplied parenterally for 1–3 days or until the risk of shock is over and fluid and electrolyte levels are stabilized. Oral feeding is not normally used, since **paralytic ileus** normally occurs in stage 1.

Antibiotics are usually prescribed to protect against infection, and a tetanus shot is usually given.

Nutritional Support for Stage 2 of Burn Care

After stabilization of the fluid and electrolyte levels, there is a period of increased diuresis. This is an indication that the replacement therapy has been effective. In addition, tissue wasting is reversed and oral feeding can begin, since paralytic ileus usually ceases and normal peristalsis is present.

During stage 2, nutritional support is important for wound care and closure and for prevention and treatment of complications, including infection. In order to achieve these goals, the diet is high in kilocalories, protein, vitamins, minerals and electrolytes. The details of the diet are as follows:

High kilocalories

Adults
25 kcal/kg (preburn body weight) + (40 kcal × % BSA burned)

Example: 58-kg woman with 50% BSA
25 kcal × 58 kg + (40 kcal × 50)
1,450 kcal + 2,000 kcal = 3,450 kcal total daily requirement

  or

60 kcal/kg preburn weight/day
60 kcal × 58 kg = 3,480 kcal/day[3]

High protein

2 to 3 g protein per kilogram of preburn body weight per day. This compares with 0.8 g per kilogram of preburn body weight for an unburned person.

Example:

58 kg × 3 g/kg/day = 175 g protein per day.

This high level of protein is needed to establish a positive nitrogen balance to allow healing of the wounds and synthesis of antibodies to fight infection.

High vitamins

Two standard multivitamin tablets per day plus 1–2 g vitamin C.

The B complex vitamins are important for metabolism of the nutrients. Vitamin C is important for the synthesis of collagen, which is critical for the synthesis of new tissues.

Minerals

Generally, adequate amounts are provided by the high protein and kilocalorie intake. However, sodium and potassium levels especially need to be monitored because of diuresis. High intakes of zinc appear to promote more rapid wound healing, and a high protein intake should provide an adequate amount.

Fluids

Fluid intake should be based on output, which may be significant as a result of increased diuresis. However, it is important to avoid excessive water intake to the point of water intoxication.

In order to achieve these high levels of nutrients, oral feeding usually has to be supplemented with tube feedings and parenteral nutrition. Frequent small feedings are used to increase compliance with the diet, since the patient usually is in pain, depressed, anorexic, and subjected to many dressing changes. Constipation is a common problem and can be reduced by increasing the intake of fluid, fiber, fruit, and vegetables. Anemia is a common problem due to blood losses and reduced bone marrow activity. Transfusion has been found to be more effective than drug and diet therapy in treating anemia.

Infection is almost always a problem with burn treatment; therefore, antibiotics are usually added to the intravenous solutions.

Stage 2 continues until the burned area is covered with new tissue or until skin grafting begins.

Nutritional Support for Stage 3 of Burn Care

Stage 3 is characterized by reconstruction, with grafting and plastic surgery occurring during this time. Optimal nutritional care is important during this time for these procedures to be successful. The diet generally does not have to contain as high a level of nutrients as it does during stage 2, since by this time the metabolism is usually back to normal.

CASE STUDY: SEVERE BURN PATIENT

Mrs. G is a 57-year-old woman who was admitted to the hospital with severe full-thickness (third-degree) and partial-thickness (second-degree) burns over 60% of her body. A physical examination reveals that she is in acute distress.

Physical Findings	Normal Values
Height: 5 ft 4 in.	
Weight: 121 lb	114–127 lbs (medium frame)
Blood pressure: $\dfrac{106 \text{ mm Hg}}{80 \text{ mm Hg}}$	$\dfrac{95\text{–}140 \text{ mm Hg}}{60\text{–}90 \text{ mm Hg}}$
Pulse: 128 beats/min	60–80 beats/min
Laboratory Findings	
Serum sodium: 125 mEq/liter	135–145 mEq/liter
Serum potassium: 5.8 mEq/liter	3.5–5.5 mEq/liter
Serum albumin: 2.6 g/dl	3.5–5.0 g/dl
Hematocrit: 53%	38–47%
Serum bicarbonate: 14 mEq/liter	20–30 mEq/liter

Using the information above and in this chapter, answer the following questions.

1. The potassium excess results from _____ and the sodium deficit from _____.
   A. destruction of kidneys—destruction of cells
   B. decreased urination—edema
   C. release from damaged cells—loss in edematous fluid
   D. hypovolemia—release from damaged cells
2. Nutritional support for stage 1 of burn care consists of
   A. glucose and amino acids
   B. amino acids and electrolytes
   C. minerals
   D. bicarbonate ions and fluids
3. The best feeding method for stage 1 of burn care is _____ because _____ normally is present.
   A. enteral—destruction of blood vessels (eliminating parenteral nutrition)
   B. parenteral—paralytic ileus (absence of peristalsis)
   C. oral—malnutrition
   D. parenteral—destruction of the upper gastrointestinal tract
4. During stage 2 of burn care for Mrs. G, based on physical findings, her protein intake should be _____ and her energy intake should be _____ kcal.
   A. 23–35 g—1,683
   B. 44–55 g—2,400
   C. 110–165 g—3,775
   D. 150–235 g—1,375

5. In order to achieve the levels of nutrients necessary for stage 2 of Mrs. G's recovery, oral feeding usually has to be supplemented with _____ and _____.
   A. increased fluid intake—a high level of vitamin C
   B. increased minerals—increased antibiotics
   C. tube feedings—parenteral nutrition
   D. increased fiber—increased feedings

6. Mrs. G. is experiencing constipation; the following compensatory changes are made in her diet:
   A. increased fiber
   B. high protein
   C. increased vitamins
   D. high fat

SUMMARY

- Preoperative nutrition is important to meet the metabolic stress of surgery, improve wound healing, and increase resistance to infection.
- A sufficient amount of kilocalories is important to resist the stress of surgery; protein is important to reduce shock, as well as the risks of anesthesia toxicity to the liver, edema at the site of incision, and infection. A deficiency of vitamins hinders carbohydrate metabolism; a deficiency of potassium may cause malfunction of the heart; and a deficiency of calcium and sodium may cause abnormal muscle and nerve activity.
- Twenty-four hours before surgery the diet should provide nutrients that cannot be stored, specifically glucose, B complex vitamins, and vitamin C, and a high fluid intake is invaluable; eight hours before surgery all fluids and foods are withheld to reduce risk of regurgitation and aspiration.
- Postoperative diet progression is as follows: clear liquid→full liquid→soft diet→regular diet.
- Nutritional support for stage 1 of burn care includes replacement of fluids and electrolytes, bicarbonate ions, and glucose and amino acids. Nutritional support for stage 2 of burn care includes a high kcal diet, a high protein intake with 2–3 g/kg of preburn body weight, and a high vitamin intake; fluids should be based on output. At stage 3 of burn care, optimal nutritional care is important for grafting and plastic surgery.

REVIEW QUESTIONS

True (A) or False (B)

1. Two major nutritional problems in the preoperative period are undernutrition and obesity. (T)
2. A major problem an undernourished person faces in surgery if he or she is deficient in proteins is shock. (T)
3. Obesity interferes with surgery by hindering muscle and nerve activity. (F)
4. A preoperative diet high in kilocalories, protein, and carbohydrate, is of benefit even if consumed for only a week. (T)
5. Nutrients should be given to a presurgery patient up to the time of surgery for maximum benefit. (F)

6. Following surgery a common diet progression is soft diet → clear liquid → regular → full liquid. (F)
7. Aggressive nutritional support is important for all burn patients, no matter what percent of their body surface area (BSA) is burned. (F)
8. Nutritional support immediately after a burn prevents shock and decreases urinary output.
9. Immediately after a burn the person may develop a potassium excess and a sodium deficit.
10. Replacement of bicarbonate ions in nutritional support for stage 1 of burn care is important to counteract tissue catabolism.
11. Oral feeding is started almost immediately after a burn in order to instill the maximum amount of nutrients into the body.
12. During stage 2 of nutritional support for burn care, the most important factor to correct is increased diuresis.
13. The high-kilocalorie diet for stage 2 is often calculated at the rate of 60 kcal/kg preburn weight/day.
14. The kilocalorie intake given in question 13 can be provided only by oral intake.
15. Vitamin C should be given in amounts of 1–2 g per day for the synthesis of collagen.

REVIEW QUESTIONS FOR NCLEX

Situation. Mr. O is admitted to the hospital with 3rd degree burns over 30% of his body. Mr. O's preburn body weight is 71 kg.

1. In addition to fluid loss during the first 48 hours after a burn, what two mineral or electrolyte problems might possibly develop?
   A. potassium excess and sodium deficit
   B. calcium and iron deficit
   C. magnesium and zinc surpluses
   D. potassium deficit and iron surplus
2. Nutritional support for Mr. O during stage 1 of burn care is _____, _____, and _____.
   A. large increase in kcal, protein, and iron
   B. large increase in water, B-complex vitamins, and kcal
   C. replacement of body fluids, bicarbonate ions, and glucose
   D. replacement of fluids, lost proteins, and B-complex vitamins

3. Nutritional support for Mr. O is supplied _____.
   A. orally from the beginning of his treatment in order for him to get the level of kcal he needs
   B. enterally with low kcal fluids being used, in order to avoid stressing the digestive tract
   C. parenterally for 1–3 days or until the risk of shock is over and fluid electrolyte levels are stabilized
   D. parenterally for as long as possible in order to avoid stressing the gastrointestinal tract
4. During stage 2 of his burn care, which of the following details of his diet are correctly given?
   A. high kcal, high protein, low vitamins, and restrict fluid intake
   B. high kcal, high protein, high vitamins, monitor level of some minerals
   C. low kcal, low protein, high vitamins, and high levels of B-complex vitamins
   D. low kcal, high protein, low vitamins, and high levels of B-complex vitamins
5. Based on Mr. O's preburn body weight and % body surface burned and utilizing the burn formula, what should be his total daily kcal requirements?

A. 2475 kcal
B. 2675 kcal
C. 2975 kcal
D. 3375 kcal

REFERENCES

1. Dempsey, D. T., Mullen, J. L., & Buzby, G. P. (1988). The link between nutritional status and clinical outcome: Can nutritional intervention modify it? *American Journal of Clinical Nutrition*, 47(Suppl. 2), 352.
2. Veterans Administration cooperative trial of perioperative total parenteral nutrition in malnourished surgical patients: Background, rationale and study protocol. (1988) *American Journal of Clinical Nutrition*, 47(Suppl. 2), 351–391.
3. Cunningham, J. J., et al. (1989). Measured and predicted calorie requirements of adults during recovery from severe burn trauma. *American Journal of Clinical Nutrition*, 49, 404.

APPENDIXES

APPENDIX A: EXCHANGE LISTS FOR MEAL PLANNING

LIST 1 STARCH/BREAD EXCHANGES

Each item in this list contains approximately 15 grams of carbohydrate, 3 grams of protein, a trace of fat, and 80 calories. Whole grain products average about 2 grams of fiber per serving. Some foods are higher in fiber. Those foods that contain 3 or more grams of fiber per serving are identified by being set in italic.

You can choose your starch exchanges from any of the items on this list. If you want to eat a starch food that is not on this list, the general rule is that:

> ½ cup of cereal, grain or pasta is one serving
> 1 ounce of a bread product is one serving.

Your dietitian can help you be more exact.

Cereals/Grains/Pasta

Bran cereals, concentrated	*⅓ cup*
Bran cereals, flaked	*½ cup*
(such as Bran Buds,® All Bran®)	
Bulgur (cooked)	½ cup
Cooked cereals	½ cup
Cornmeal (dry)	2½ Tbsp.
Grapenuts	3 Tbsp.
Grits (cooked)	½ cup
Other ready-to-eat unsweetened cereals	¾ cup
Pasta (cooked)	½ cup
Puffed cereal	1½ cup
Rice, white or brown (cooked)	⅓ cup
Shredded wheat	½ cup
Wheat germ	*3 Tbsp.*

Dried Beans/Peas/Lentils

Beans and peas (cooked)	*⅓ cup*
(such as kidney, white, split, blackeye)	
Lentils (cooked)	*⅓ cup*
Baked beans	*¼ cup*

Starchy Vegetables

Corn	*½ cup*
Corn on cob, 6 in. long	*1*
Lima beans	*½ cup*
Peas, green (canned or frozen)	*½ cup*
Plantain	*½ cup*
Potato, baked	1 small (3 oz.)
Potato, mashed	½ cup
Squash, winter (acorn, butternut)	¾ cup
Yam, sweet potato, plain	⅓ cup

(continued)

LIST 1 (*Continued*)

Bread

Bagel	½ (1 oz.)
Bread sticks, crisp, 4 in. long × ½ in.	2 (2/3 oz.)
Croutons, low fat	1 cup
English muffin	½
Frankfurter or hamburger bun	½ (1 oz.)
Pita, 6 in. across	½
Plain roll, small	1 (1 oz.)
Raisin, unfrosted	1 slice (1 oz.)
Rye, pumpernickel	*1 slice (1 oz.)*
Tortilla, 6 in. across	1
White (including French, Italian)	1 slice (1 oz.)
Whole wheat	1 slice (1 oz.)

Crackers/Snacks

Animal crackers	8
Graham crackers, 2½ in. square	3
Matzoth	¾ oz.
Melba toast	5 slices
Oyster crackers	24
Popcorn (popped, no fat added)	3 cups
Pretzels	¾ oz.
Rye crisp, 2 in. × 3½ in.	4
Saltine-type crackers	6
Whole wheat crackers, no fat added (crisp breads, such as Finn®, Kavli®, Wasa®)	2-4 slices (¾ oz.)

Starch Foods Prepared With Fat
(Count as 1 starch/bread serving, plus 1 fat serving.)

Biscuit, 2½ in. across	1
Chow mein noodles	½ cup
Corn bread, 2 in. cube	1 (2 oz.)
Cracker, round butter type	6
French fried potatoes, 2 in. to 3½ in. long	10 (1½ oz.)
Muffin, plain, small	1
Pancake, 4 in. across	2
Stuffing, bread (prepared)	¼ cup
Taco shell, 6 in. across	2
Waffle, 4½ in. square	1
Whole wheat crackers, fat added (such as Triscuits®)	4-6 (1 oz.)

LIST 2 MEAT EXCHANGES

Each serving of meat and substitutes on this list contains about 7 grams of protein. The amount of fat and number of calories varies, depending on what kind of meat or substitute you choose. The list is divided into three parts based on the amount of fat and calories: lean meat, medium-fat meat, and high-fat meat. One ounce (one meat exchange) of each of these includes:

	Carbohydrate (grams)	Protein (grams)	Fat (grams)	Calories
Lean	0	7	3	55
Medium-Fat	0	7	5	75
High-Fat	0	7	8	100

You are encouraged to use more lean and medium-fat meat, poultry, and fish in your meal plan. This will help decrease your fat intake, which may help decrease your risk for heart disease. The items from the high-fat group are high in saturated fat, cholesterol, and calories. You should limit your choices from the high-fat group to three (3) times per week. Meat and substitutes do not contribute any fiber to your meal plan.

TIPS

1. Bake, roast, broil, grill, or boil these foods rather than frying them with added fat.
2. Use a nonstick pan spray or a nonstick pan to brown or fry these foods.
3. Trim off visible fat before and after cooking.
4. Do not add flour, bread crumbs, coating mixes, or fat to these foods when preparing them.
5. Weigh meat after removing bones and fat, and after cooking. Three ounces of cooked meat is about equal to 4 ounces of raw meat. Some examples of meat portions are:

    2 ounces meat (2 meat exchanges) =
    1 small chicken leg or thigh
    ½ cup cottage cheese or tuna

    3 ounces meat (3 meat exchanges) =
    1 medium pork chop
    1 small hamburger
    ½ of a whole chicken breast
    1 unbreaded fish fillet
    cooked meat, about the size of a deck of cards

6. Restaurants usually serve prime cuts of meat, which are high in fat and calories.

(continued)

LIST 2 MEAT EXCHANGES (Continued)

LEAN MEAT AND SUBSTITUTES

(One exchange is equal to any one of the following items.)

Beef:	USDA Good or Choice grades of lean beef, such as round, sirloin, and flank steak; tenderloin; and chipped beef[a]	1 oz.
Pork:	Lean pork, such as fresh ham; canned, cured or boiled ham[a]; Canadian bacon[a], tenderloin.	1 oz.
Veal:	All cuts are lean except for veal cutlets (ground or cubed). Examples of lean veal are chops and roasts.	1 oz.
Poultry:	Chicken, turkey, Cornish hen (without skin)	1 oz.
Fish:	All fresh and frozen fish	1 oz.
	Crab, lobster, scallops, shrimp, clams (fresh or canned in water)[a]	2 oz.
	Oysters	6 medium
	Tuna[a] (canned in water)	¼ cup
	Herring (uncreamed or smoked)	1 oz.
	Sardines (canned)	2 medium
Wild Game:	Venison, rabbit, squirrel	1 oz.
	Pheasant, duck, goose (without skin)	1 oz.
Cheese:	Any cottage cheese	¼ cup
	Grated parmesan	2 Tbsp.
	Diet cheeses[a] (with less than 55 calories per ounce)	1 oz.
Other:	95% fat-free luncheon meat	1 oz.
	Egg whites	3 whites
	Egg substitutes with less than 55 calories per ¼ cup	¼ cup

[a] 400 mg or more of sodium per exchange

(continued)

LIST 2 *(Continued)*

MEDIUM-FAT MEAT AND SUBSTITUTES

(One exchange is equal to any one of the following items.)

Beef:	Most beef products fall into this category. Examples are: all ground beef, roast (rib, chuck, rump), steak (cubed, Porterhouse, T-bone), and meatloaf.	1 oz.
Pork:	Most pork products fall into this category. Examples are: chops, loin roast, Boston butt, cutlets.	1 oz.
Lamb:	Most lamb products fall into this category. Examples are: chops, leg, and roast.	1 oz.
Veal:	Cutlet (ground or cubed, unbreaded)	1 oz.
Poultry:	Chicken (with skin), domestic duck or goose (well-drained of fat), ground turkey	1 oz.
Fish:	Tuna[a] (canned in oil and drained)	¼ cup
	Salmon[a] (canned)	¼ cup
Cheese:	Skim or part-skim milk cheeses, such as:	
	Ricotta	¼ cup
	Mozzarella	1 oz.
	Diet cheeses[a] (with 56–80 calories per ounce)	1 oz.
Other:	86% fat-free luncheon meat[a]	1 oz.
	Egg (high in cholesterol, limit to 3 per week)	1
	Egg substitutes with 56–80 calories per ¼ cup	¼ cup
	Tofu (2½ in. × 2¾ in. × 1 in.)	4 oz.
	Liver, heart, kidney, sweetbreads (high in cholesterol)	1 oz.

[a] 400 mg or more of sodium per exchange

(continued)

LIST 2 *(Continued)*

HIGH-FAT MEAT AND SUBSTITUTES

Remember, these items are high in saturated fat, cholesterol, and calories, and should be used only three (3) times per week.
(One exchange is equal to any one of the following items.)

Beef:	Most USDA Prime cuts of beef, such as ribs, corned beef[a]	1 oz.
Pork:	Spareribs, ground pork, pork sausage[a] (patty or link)	1 oz.
Lamb:	Patties (ground lamb)	1 oz.
Fish:	Any fried fish product	1 oz.
Cheese:	All regular cheeses[a], such as American, Blue, Cheddar, Monterey, Swiss	1 oz.
Other:	Luncheon meat[a], such as bologna, salami, pimento loaf	1 oz.
	Sausage[a], such as Polish, Italian	1 oz.
	Knockwurst, smoked	1 oz.
	Bratwurst[a]	1 oz.
	Frankfurter[a] (turkey or chicken)	1 frank (10/lb.)
	Peanut butter (contains unsaturated fat)	1 Tbsp

Count as one high-fat meat plus one fat exchange:

	Frankfurter[a] (beef, pork, or combination)	1 frank (10/lb.)

[a] 400 mg or more of sodium per exchange

LIST 3 VEGETABLE EXCHANGES

Each vegetable serving on this list contains about 5 grams of carbohydrate, 2 grams of protein, and 25 calories. Vegetables contain 2–3 grams of dietary fiber. Vegetables which contain 400 mg of sodium per serving are identified by being set in italic.

Vegetables are a good source of vitamins and minerals. Fresh and frozen vegetables have more vitamins and less added salt. Rinsing canned vegetables will remove much of the salt.

Unless otherwise noted, the serving size for vegetables (one vegetable exchange) is:

½ cup of cooked vegetables or vegetable juice
1 cup of raw vegetables

Artichoke (½ medium)	Mushrooms, cooked
Asparagus	Okra
Beans (green, wax, Italian)	Onions
Bean sprouts	Pea pods
Beets	Peppers (green)
Broccoli	Rutabaga
Brussels sprouts	*Sauerkraut*
Cabbage, cooked	Spinach, cooked
Carrots	Summer squash (crookneck)
Cauliflower	Tomato (one large)
Eggplant	*Tomato/vegetable juice*
Greens (collard, mustard, turnip)	Turnips
Kohlrabi	Water chestnuts
Leeks	Zucchini, cooked

Starchy vegetables such as corn, peas, and potatoes are found on the Starch/Bread List

LIST 4 FRUIT EXCHANGES

Each item on this list contains about 15 grams of carbohydrate, and 60 calories. Fresh, frozen, and dry fruits have about 2 grams of fiber per serving. Fruits that have 3 or more grams of fiber per serving are identified by being set in italic. Fruit juices contain very little dietary fiber.

The carbohydrate and calorie content for a fruit serving are based on the usual serving of the most commonly eaten fruits. Use fresh fruits or fruits frozen or canned without sugar added. Whole fruit is more filling than fruit juice and may be a better choice for those who are trying to lose weight. Unless otherwise noted, the serving size for one fruit serving is:

½ cup of fresh fruit or fruit juice
¼ cup of dried fruit

Fresh, Frozen, and Unsweetened Canned Fruit

Apple (raw, 2 in. across)	1 apple
Applesauce (unsweetened)	½ cup
Apricots (medium, raw) or	4 apricots
Apricots (canned)	½ cup, or 4 halves
Banana (9 in. long)	½ banana
Blackberries (raw)	*¾ cup*
Blueberries (raw)	*¾ cup*
Cantaloupe (5 in. across)	⅓ melon
(cubes)	1 cup
Cherries (large, raw)	12 cherries
Cherries (canned)	½ cup
Figs (raw, 2 in. across)	2 figs
Fruit cocktail (canned)	½ cup
Grapefruit (medium)	½ grapefruit
Grapefruit (segments)	¾ cup
Grapes (small)	15 grapes
Honeydew melon (medium)	⅛ melon
(cubes)	1 cup
Kiwi (large)	1 kiwi
Mandarin oranges	¾ cup
Mango (small)	½ mango
Nectarine (1½ in. across)	*1 nectarine*
Orange (2½ in. across)	1 orange
Papaya	1 cup
Peach (2¾ in. across)	1 peach, or ¾ cup
Peaches (canned)	½ cup, or 2 halves
Pear	½ large, or 1 small
Pears (canned)	½ cup or 2 halves
Persimmon (medium, native)	2 persimmons
Pineapple (raw)	¾ cup

(continued)

LIST 4 *(Continued)*

Pineapple (canned)	⅓ cup
Plum (raw, 2 in. across)	2 plums
Pomegranate	*½ pomegranate*
Raspberries (raw)	*1 cup*
Strawberries (raw, whole)	*1¼ cup*
Tangerine (2½ in. across)	2 tangerines
Watermelon (cubes)	1¼ cup

Dried Fruit

Apples	*4 rings*
Apricots	*7 halves*
Dates	2½ medium
Figs	*1½*
Prunes	*3 medium*
Raisins	2 Tbsp.

Fruit Juice

Apple juice/cider	½ cup
Cranberry juice cocktail	⅓ cup
Grapefruit juice	½ cup
Grape juice	⅓ cup
Orange juice	½ cup
Pineapple juice	½ cup
Prune juice	⅓ cup

LIST 5 MILK EXCHANGES

Each serving of milk or milk products on this list contains about 12 grams of carbohydrate and 8 grams of protein. The amount of fat in milk is measured in percent (%) of butterfat. The calories vary, depending on what kind of milk you choose. The list is divided into three parts based on the amount of fat and calories: skim/very lowfat milk, lowfat milk, and whole milk. One serving (one milk exchange) of each of these includes:

	Carbohydrate (grams)	Protein (grams)	Fat (grams)	Calories
Skim/Very Lowfat	12	8	trace	90
Lowfat	12	8	5	120
Whole	12	8	8	150

Milk is the body's main source of calcium, the mineral needed for growth and repair of bones. Yogurt is also a good source of calcium. Yogurt and many dry or powdered milk products have different amounts of fat. If you have questions about a particular item, read the label to find out the fat and calorie content.

Milk is good to drink, but it can also be added to cereal, and to other foods. Many tasty dishes such as sugar-free pudding are made with milk (see the Combination Foods list). Add life to plain yogurt by adding one of your fruit servings to it.

Skim and Very Lowfat Milk

skim milk	1 cup
½% milk	1 cup
1% milk	1 cup
lowfat buttermilk	1 cup
evaporated skim milk	½ cup
dry nonfat milk	⅓ cup
plain nonfat yogurt	8 oz.

Lowfat Milk

2% milk	1 cup fluid
plain lowfat yogurt (with added nonfat milk solids)	8 oz.

Whole Milk

The whole milk group has much more fat per serving than the skim and lowfat groups. Whole milk has more than 3¼% butterfat. Try to limit your choices from the whole milk group as much as possible.

whole milk	1 cup
evaporated whole milk	½ cup
whole plain yogurt	8 oz.

LIST 6 FAT EXCHANGES

Each serving on the fat list contains about 5 grams of fat and 45 calories.

The foods on the fat list contain mostly fat, although some items may also contain a small amount of protein. All fats are high in calories and should be carefully measured. Everyone should modify fat intake by eating unsaturated fats instead of saturated fats. The sodium content of these foods varies widely. Check the label for sodium information; 400 mg. or more of sodium per serving are identified by being set in italic.

Unsaturated Fats

Avocado	⅛ medium
Margarine	1 tsp.
*Margarine, diet	1 Tbsp.
Mayonnaise	1 tsp.
*Mayonnaise, reduced-calorie	1 Tbsp.

Nuts and Seeds:

Almonds, dry roasted	6 whole
Cashews, dry roasted	1 Tbsp.
Pecans	2 whole
Peanuts	20 small or 10 large
Walnuts	2 whole
Other nuts	1 Tbsp.
Seeds, pine nuts, sunflower (without shells)	1 Tbsp.
Pumpkin seeds	2 tsp.
Oil (corn, cottonseed, safflower, soybean, sunflower, olive, peanut)	1 tsp.
*Olives	10 small or 5 large
Salad dressing, mayonnaise-type	2 tsp.
Salad dressing, mayonnaise-type, reduced-calorie	1 Tbsp.
*Salad dressing (all varieties)	1 Tbsp.
Salad dressing, reduced-calorie	*2 Tbsp.*

(Two tablespoons of low-calorie salad dressing is a free food.)

Saturated Fats

Butter	1 tsp.
*Bacon	1 slice
Chitterlings	½ ounce
Coconut, shredded	2 Tbsp.
Coffee whitener, liquid	2 Tbsp.
Coffee whitener, powder	4 tsp.
Cream (light, coffee, table)	2 Tbsp.
Cream, sour	2 Tbsp.
Cream (heavy, whipping)	1 Tbsp.
Cream cheese	1 Tbsp.
*Salt pork	¼ ounce

*If more than one or two servings are eaten, these foods have 400 mg. or more of sodium.

(continued)

LIST 6 *(Continued)*

Free Foods

A free food is any food or drink that contains less than 20 calories per serving. You can eat as much as you want of those items that have no serving size specified. You may eat two or three servings per day of those items that have a specific serving size. Be sure to spread them out through the day.

Drinks:

Bouillon or broth without fat
Bouillon, low-sodium
Carbonated drinks, sugar-free
Carbonated water
Club soda
Cocoa powder, unsweetened
   (1 Tbsp.)
Coffee / Tea
Drink mixes, sugar-free
Tonic water, sugar-free

Nonstick pan spray

Fruit:

Cranberries, unsweetened (½ cup)
Rhubarb, unsweetened (½ cup)

Vegetables:
(raw, 1 cup)
Cabbage
Celery
Chinese cabbage[a]
Cucumber
Green onion
Hot peppers
Mushrooms
Radishes
Zucchini[a]

Salad greens:

Endive
Escarole
Lettuce
Romaine
Spinach

Sweet Substitutes:

Candy, hard, sugar-free
Gelatin, sugar-free
Gum, sugar-free
Jam / Jelly, sugar-free (2 tsp.)
Pancake syrup, sugar-free
   (1-2 Tbsp.)
Sugar substitutes (saccharin,
   aspartame)
Whipped topping (2 Tbsp.)

Condiments:

Catsup (1 Tbsp.)
Horseradish
Mustard
Pickles, dill, unsweetened
Salad dressing, low-calorie
   (2 Tbsp.)
Taco sauce (1 Tbsp.)
Vinegar

(continued)

LIST 6 (*Continued*)

Seasonings can be very helpful in making food taste better. Be careful of how much sodium you use. Read the label, and choose those seasonings that do not contain sodium or salt.

Basil (fresh)
Celery seeds
Cinnamon
Chili powder
Chives
Curry
Dill
Flavoring extracts (vanilla, almond, walnut, peppermint, butter, lemon, etc.)
Garlic
Garlic powder
Herbs
Hot pepper sauce
Lemon

Lemon juice
Lemon pepper
Lime
Lime juice
Mint
Onion powder
Oregano
Paprika
Pepper
Pimento
Spices
Soy sauce
Soy sauce, low sodium ("lite")
Wine, used in cooking (¼ cup)
Worcestershire sauce

[a]3 grams or more of fiber per serving

APPENDIX B: CHOLESTEROL VALUE OF SELECTED FOODS

Food	Cholesterol (mg)	Food	Cholesterol (mg)
Milk		**Eggs**	
Whole, 3.5% fat (1 cup)	34	Whole (large size)	252
Nonfat (skim) (1 cup)	5	White of egg	0
Low-fat (1 cup)	22	Yolk of egg	252
Cheese		**Meat, poultry, fish, shellfish, related products**	
Blue or Roquefort type (1 cu in.)	15	Bacon (2 slices)	16
Camembert (1 wedge)	35	Beef (lean only) (2.5 oz)	66
Cheddar (1 cu in.)	17	Hamburger, broiled, lean (3 oz)	77
Cottage cheese, creamed (1 pkg)	65	Rib roast, oven cooked, lean and fat (3 oz)	80
Cottage cheese, uncreamed (1 pkg)	24	Rib roast, oven cooked, lean only (1.8 oz)	46
Cream cheese (1 pkg, 3 oz)	94	Steak, broiled, lean and fat (6 oz)	160
Parmesan (1 tbsp)	5	Steak, broiled, lean only (6 oz)	153
Swiss cheese (1 cu in.)	15	Corned beef (3 oz)	85
Processed cheese (1 cu in.)	16	Chicken, flesh only, broiled (3 oz)	74
American pasteurized process cheese food (1 tbsp)	10	Chicken, breast, fried (with bone), (3 oz)	75
American process cheese spread (1 oz)	18	Chicken, breast, fried (flesh and skin only) (2.7 oz)	68
Cream		Chili con carne, canned, with beans (1 cup)	77
Half-and-half (1 tbsp)	6	Chili con carne, canned, without beans (1 cup)	153
Light, coffee or table (1 tbsp)	10	Lamb chop, broiled with bone (1 chop) (4.8 oz)	74
Sour (1 tbsp)	8	Roast leg of lamb, lean and fat (3 oz)	83
Whipped topping (1 cup), pressurized	51	Roast lam shoulder, lean and fat (3 oz)	83
Milk beverages		Beef liver, fried (2 oz)	250
Cocoa, homemade (1 cup)	35	Roast ham, lean and fat (3 oz)	76
Chocolate-flavored drink (skim milk) (1 cup)	20	Boiled ham, sliced (2 oz)	51
Milk desserts		Canned, spiced or unspiced ham (2 oz)	51
Custard, baked (1 cup)	278	Pork chop, thick with bone (1 chop) (3.5 oz)	59
Ice cream, regular (1 cup)	53		
Ice milk, hardened (1 cup)	26		
Ice milk, soft serve (1 cup)	36		
Yogurt (made from partially skimmed milk) (1 cup)	17		
Yogurt (made from whole milk) (1 cup)	30		
Yogurt (sweetened with fruit added) (1 cup)	15		

APPENDIX B: (*Continued*)

Food	Cholesterol (mg)	Food	Cholesterol (mg)
Pork chop, lean only (1 chop) (1.7 oz)	42	Yellow cake (1 piece)	36
Bologna (2 slices)	26	Brownies with nuts (1 brownie)	17
Braunschweiger (2 slices)	20	Doughnuts, cake type (1)	27
Frankfurter, heated (1 frank)	56	Macaroni and cheese, baked (1 cup)	42
Pork links, cooked (2 links)	26	Muffins (1)	21
Salami, dry type (1 oz)	28	Egg noodles (1 cup)	50
Vienna sausage, canned (1 sausage)	16	Pancakes (1 cake)	20
Veal cutlet (3 oz)	86	Apple pie (1 piece)	0
Veal roast (3 oz)	86	Custard pie (1 piece)	137
Bluefish, baked (3 oz)	60	Lemon meringue pie (1 piece)	112
Clams, raw (3 oz)	43	Mince pie (1 piece)	16
Clams, canned (3 oz)	86	Pecan pie (1 piece)	57
Crabmeat, canned (3 oz)	86	Pumpkin pie (1 piece)	79
Fishsticks, frozen (2 sticks)	46	Spaghetti with meat balls and tomato sauce (1 cup)	75
Haddock, fried (3 oz)	51	Spaghetti with meat balls and tomato sauce, canned (1 cup)	39
Ocean perch, fried (3 oz)	51		
Oysters, raw (1 cup)	120	Waffles (1)	45
Salmon, pink, canned (3 oz)	30	Fats and oils	
Sardines, Atlantic (3 oz)	119	Butter (1 tbsp)	35
Shrimp, canned (3 oz)	128	Butter (1 pat)	13
Tuna, canned in oil (3 oz)	55	Whipped butter (1 tbsp)	22
Grain products		Whipped butter (1 pat)	10
Angel-food cake (whole cake) (1 cake)	0	Lard (1 tbsp)	12
Devil's-food cake with chocolate icing (1 cake)	531	Mayonnaise, regular (1 tbsp)	8
Cupcake (1)	17	Sugars and sweets	
Gingerbread (1 cake)	6	Chocolate candy, milk, plain (1 oz)	21
White layer cake with chocolate icing (1 cake)	23	Miscellaneous items	
Boston cream pie (1 piece)	33	Chocolate pudding (1 cup)	30
Fruitcake, dark (1 slice)	7	Vanilla pudding (1 cup)	35
Pound cake (1 slice)	30	Tapioca cream pudding (1 cup)	159
Sponge cake (1 piece)	162		
Yellow cake without icing (1 piece)	26		

Source: F.J. Stare and M. McWilliams, *Living Nutrition*, 4th ed. New York: John Wiley & Sons, Inc., © 1984. Reprinted by permission.

APPENDIX C: NUTRITIVE VALUES OF THE EDIBLE PART OF FOODS

				Nutrients in Indicated Quantity			
Item No. (A)	Foods, approximate measures, units, and weight (edible part unless footnote indicate otherwise) (B)		g	Water (C) %	Food Energy (D) kcal	Pro- tein (E) g	Fat (F) g

Key to Abbreviations:
% = Percent   g = Grams   IU = International Units
kcal = Kilocalories   mg = Milligrams   TR = Trace

Dairy Products (Cheese, Cream, Imitation Cream, Milk & Related Products)

Butter. See Fats, oils; related products, items 103–108.

Cheese

Natural

Item No.	Food	Measure	g	Water %	Food Energy kcal	Protein g	Fat g
1	Blue	1 oz	28	42	100	6	8
2	Camembert (3 wedges per 4-oz container)	1 wedge	38	52	115	8	9
	Cheddar						
3	Cut pieces	1 oz	28	37	115	7	9
4		1 cu in	17.2	37	70	4	6
5	Shredded	1 cup	113	37	455	28	37
	Cottage (curd not pressed down)						
	Creamed (cottage cheese, 4% fat)						
6	Large curd	1 cup	225	79	235	28	10
7	Small curd	1 cup	210	79	220	26	9
8	Low fat (2%)	1 cup	226	79	205	31	4
9	Low fat (1%)	1 cup	226	82	165	28	2
10	Uncreamed (cottage cheese dry curd, less than ½% fat).	1 cup	145	80	125	25	1
11	Cream	1 oz	28	54	100	2	10
	Mozzarella, made with:						
12	Whole milk	1 oz	28	48	90	6	7
13	Part skim milk	1 oz	28	49	80	8	5
	Parmesan, grated						
14	Cup, not pressed down	1 cup	100	18	455	42	30
15	Tablespoon	1 tbsp	5	18	25	2	2
16	Ounce	1 oz	28	18	130	12	9
17	Provolone	1 oz	28	41	100	7	8
	Ricotta, made with:						
18	Whole milk	1 cup	246	72	430	28	32

Source: C. F. Adams, and M. Richardson, *Nutritive Value of Foods,* Home and Garden Bulletin 72, Agricultural Research Service, U.S. Department of Agriculture, Washington, D.C., revised 1982.

Note: Dashes (—) denote lack of reliable data for a constituent believed to be present in measurable amount.

		Nutrients in Indicated Quantity											

Fatty Acids													
Satu-rated (Total) (G) g	Unsaturated		Carbo-hydrate (J) g	Calcium (K) mg	Phos-phorus (L) mg	Iron (M) mg	Potas-sium (N) mg	Vitamin A Value (O) I.U.	Thiamin (P) mg	Ribo-flavin (Q) mg	Niacin (R) mg	Ascorbic Acid (S) mg
	Oleic (H) g	Lino-leic (I) g										
5.3	1.9	0.2	1	150	110	0.1	73	200	0.01	0.11	0.3	0
5.8	2.2	0.2	TR	147	132	0.1	71	350	0.01	0.19	0.2	0
6.1	2.1	0.2	TR	204	145	0.2	28	300	0.01	0.11	TR	0
3.7	1.3	0.1	TR	124	88	0.1	17	180	TR	0.06	TR	0
24.2	8.5	0.7	1	815	579	0.8	111	1,200	0.03	0.42	0.1	0
6.4	2.4	0.2	6	135	297	0.3	190	370	0.05	0.37	0.3	TR
6.0	2.2	0.2	6	126	277	0.3	177	340	0.04	0.34	0.3	TR
2.8	1.0	0.1	8	155	340	0.4	217	160	0.05	0.42	0.3	TR
1.5	0.5	0.1	6	138	302	0.3	193	80	0.05	0.37	0.3	TR
0.4	0.1	TR	3	46	151	0.3	47	40	0.04	0.21	0.2	0
6.2	2.4	0.2	1	23	30	0.3	34	400	TR	0.06	TR	0
4.4	1.7	0.2	1	163	117	0.1	21	260	TR	0.08	TR	0
3.1	1.2	0.1	1	207	149	0.1	27	180	0.01	0.10	TR	0
19.1	7.7	0.3	4	1,376	807	1.0	107	700	0.05	0.39	0.3	0
1.0	0.4	TR	TR	69	40	TR	5	40	TR	0.02	TR	0
5.4	2.2	0.1	1	390	229	0.3	30	200	0.01	0.11	0.1	0
4.8	1.7	0.1	1	214	141	0.1	39	230	0.01	0.09	TR	0
20.4	7.1	0.7	7	509	389	0.9	257	1,210	0.03	0.48	0.3	0

(Continued)

APPENDIX C: (*Continued*)

					Nutrients in Indicated Quantity		

Item No. (A)	Foods, approximate measures, units, and weight (edible part unless footnote indicate otherwise) (B)			Water (C) %	Food Energy (D) kcal	Pro-tein (E) g	Fat (F) g
			g				
Dairy Products (Cheese, Cream, Imitation Cream, Milk & Related Products)							
	Cheese—Continued						
	Natural—Continued						
	Ricotta, made with:—Continued						
19	Part skim milk	1 cup	246	74	340	28	19
20	Romano	1 oz	28	31	110	9	8
21	Swiss	1 oz	28	37	105	8	8
	Pasteurized process cheese						
22	American	1 oz	28	39	105	6	9
23	Swiss	1 oz	28	42	95	7	7
24	Pasteurized process cheese food, American	1 oz	28	43	95	6	7
25	Pasteurized process cheese spread, American	1 oz	28	48	80	5	6
	Cream, sweet						
26	Half-and-half (cream and milk)	1 cup	242	81	315	7	28
27		1 tbsp	15	81	20	TR	2
28	Light, coffee, or table	1 cup	240	74	470	6	46
29		1 tbsp	15	74	30	TR	3
30	Light	1 cup	239	64	700	5	74
31		1 tbsp	15	64	45	TR	5
32	Heavy	1 cup	238	58	820	5	88
33		1 tbsp	15	58	80	TR	6
34	Whipped topping (pressurized)	1 cup	60	61	155	2	13
35		1 tbsp	3	61	10	TR	1
36	Cream, sour	1 cup	230	71	495	7	48
37		1 tbsp	12	71	25	TR	3
	Cream products, imitation (made with vegetable fat)						
	Sweet						
	Creamers						
38	Liquid (frozen)	1 cup	245	77	335	2	24
39		1 tbsp	15	77	20	TR	1
40	Powdered	1 cup	94	2	515	5	33
41		1 tsp	2	2	10	TR	1
	Whipped topping						
42	Frozen	1 cup	75	50	240	1	19
43		1 tbsp	4	50	15	TR	1

[1]Vitamin A value is largely from beta-carotene used for coloring. Riboflavin value for items 40–41 apply to product with added riboflavin.

					Nutrients in Indicated Quantity							
Fatty Acids												
	Unsaturated											
Satu-rated (Total) (G) g	Oleic (H) g	Lino-leic (I) g	Carbo-hydrate (J) g	Calcium (K) mg	Phos-phorus (L) mg	Iron (M) mg	Potas-sium (N) mg	Vitamin A Value (O) I.U.	Thiamin (P) mg	Ribo-flavin (Q) mg	Niacin (R) mg	Ascorbic Acid (S) mg
12.1	4.7	0.5	13	669	449	1.1	308	1,060	0.05	0.46	0.2	0
—	—	—	1	302	215	—	—	160	—	0.11	TR	0
5.0	1.7	0.2	1	272	171	TR	31	240	0.01	0.10	TR	0
5.6	2.1	0.2	TR	174	211	0.1	46	340	0.01	0.10	TR	0
4.5	1.7	0.1	1	219	216	0.2	61	230	TR	0.08	TR	0
4.4	1.7	0.1	2	163	130	0.2	79	260	0.01	0.13	TR	0
3.8	1.5	0.1	2	159	202	0.1	69	220	0.01	0.12	TR	0
17.3	7.0	0.6	10	254	230	0.2	314	260	0.08	0.36	0.2	2
1.1	0.4	TR	1	16	14	TR	19	20	0.01	0.02	TR	TR
28.8	11.7	1.0	9	231	192	0.1	292	1,730	0.08	0.36	0.1	2
1.8	0.7	0.1	1	14	12	TR	18	110	TR	0.02	TR	TR
46.2	18.3	1.5	7	166	146	0.1	231	2,690	0.06	0.30	0.1	1
2.9	1.1	0.1	TR	10	9	TR	15	170	TR	0.02	TR	TR
54.8	22.2	2.0	TR	154	149	TR	179	3,500	0.05	0.26	0.1	1
3.5	1.4	0.1	TR	10	9	TR	11	220	TR	0.02	TR	TR
8.3	3.4	0.3	7	61	54	TR	88	550	0.02	0.04	TR	0
0.4	0.2	TR	TR	3	3	TR	4	30	TR	TR	TR	0
30.0	12.1	1.1	10	268	195	0.1	331	1,820	0.08	0.34	0.2	2
1.6	0.6	0.1	1	14	10	TR	17	90	TR	0.02	TR	TR
22.8	0.3	TR	28	23	157	0.1	467	[1]220	0	0	0	0
1.4	TR	0	2	1	10	TR	29	[1]10	0	0	0	0
30.6	0.9	TR	52	21	397	0.1	763	[1]190	0	0.16	0	0
0.7	TR	0	1	TR	8	TR	16	[1]TR	0	[1]TR	0	0
16.3	1.0	0.2	17	5	6	0.1	14	[1]650	0	0	0	0
0.9	0.1	TR	1	TR	TR	TR	1	[1]30	0	0	0	0

(Continued)

APPENDIX C: (*Continued*)

				Nutrients in Indicated Quantity			

Item No. (A)	Foods, approximate measures, units, and weight (edible part unless footnote indicate otherwise) (B)		g	Water (C) %	Food Energy (D) kcal	Pro-tein (E) g	Fat (F) g
Dairy Products (Cheese, Cream, Imitation Cream, Milk & Related Products)							
	Cream products, imitation (made with vegetable fat—Continued)						
	Sweet—Continued						
	Whipped topping—Continued						
44	Powdered, made with whole milk	1 cup	80	67	150	3	10
45		1 tbsp	4	67	10	TR	TR
46	Pressurized	1 cup	70	60	185	1	16
47		1 tbsp	4	60	10	TR	1
48	Sour dressing (imitation sour cream) made with nonfat dry milk	1 cup	235	75	415	8	39
49		1 tbsp	12	75	20	TR	2
	Ice cream. See Milk desserts, frozen (items 75–80)						
	Ice milk. See Milk desserts, frozen (items 81–83)						
	Milk						
	Fluid						
50	Whole (3.3% fat)	1 cup	244	88	150	8	8
	Lowfat (2%)						
51	No milk solids added	1 cup	244	89	120	8	5
	Milk solids added						
52	Label claims less than 10 g of protein per cup	1 cup	245	89	125	9	5
53	Label claim 10 or more grams of protein per cup (protein fortified)	1 cup	246	88	135	10	5
	Lowfat (1%)						
54	No milk solids added	1 cup	244	90	100	8	3
	Milk solids added						
55	Label claim less than 10 g of protein per cup	1 cup	245	90	105	9	2
56	Label claim 10 or more grams of protein per cup (protein fortified)	1 cup	246	89	120	10	3
57	Nonfat (skim)						
	No milk solids added	1 cup	245	91	85	8	TR
	Milk solids added						
58	Label claim less than 10 g of protein per cup	1 cup	245	90	90	9	1
59	Label claim 10 or more grams of protein per cup (protein fortified)	1 cup	246	89	100	10	1

[2]Applies to product without added vitamin A. With added vitamin A, value is 500 International Units (IU).

								Nutrients in Indicated Quantity					
Fatty Acids													
	Unsaturated												
Satu-rated (Total) (G) g	Oleic (H) g	Lino-leic (I) g	Carbo-hydrate (J) g	Calcium (K) mg	Phos-phorus (L) mg	Iron (M) mg	Potas-sium (N) mg	Vitamin A Value (O) I.U.	Thiamin (P) mg	Ribo-flavin (Q) mg	Niacin (R) mg	Ascorbic Acid (S) mg
8.5	0.6	0.1	13	72	69	TR	121	[1]290	0.02	0.09	TR	1
0.4	TR	TR	1	4	3	TR	6	[1]10	TR	TR	TR	TR
13.2	1.4	0.2	11	4	13	TR	13	[1]330	0	0	0	0
0.8	0.1	TR	1	TR	1	TR	1	[1]20	0	0	0	0
31.2	4.4	1.1	11	286	205	0.1	380	[1]20	0.09	0.38	0.2	2
1.6	0.2	0.1	1	14	10	TR	19	[1]TR	0.01	0.02	TR	TR
5.1	2.1	0.2	11	291	228	0.1	370	[2]310	0.09	0.40	0.2	2
2.9	1.2	0.1	12	297	232	0.1	377	500	0.10	0.40	0.2	2
2.9	1.2	0.1	12	313	245	0.1	397	500	0.10	0.42	0.2	2
3.0	1.2	0.1	14	352	276	0.1	447	500	0.11	0.48	0.2	2
1.6	0.7	0.1	12	300	235	0.1	381	500	0.10	0.41	0.2	2
1.5	0.6	0.1	12	313	245	0.1	397	500	0.10	0.42	0.2	2
1.8	0.7	0.1	14	349	273	0.1	444	500	0.11	0.47	0.2	2
0.3	0.1	TR	12	302	247	0.1	406	500	0.09	0.37	0.2	2
0.4	0.1	TR	12	316	255	0.1	418	500	0.10	0.43	0.2	2
0.4	0.1	TR	14	352	275	0.1	446	500	0.11	0.48	0.2	3

(Continued)

APPENDIX C: (*Continued*)

Nutrients in Indicated Quantity

Item No. (A)	Foods, approximate measures, units, and weight (edible part unless footnotes indicate otherwise) (B)		g	Water (C) %	Food Energy (D) kcal	Pro-tein (E) g	Fat (F) g
Dairy Products (Cheese, Cream, Imitation Cream, Milk & Related Products)—Con.							
	Milk—Continued						
	Fluid—Continued						
60	Buttermilk	1 cup	245	90	100	8	2
	Canned						
	Evaporated, unsweetened						
61	Whole milk	1 cup	252	74	340	17	19
62	Skim milk	1 cup	255	79	200	19	1
63	Sweetened, condensed	1 cup	306	27	980	24	27
	Dried						
64	Buttermilk	1 cup	120	3	465	41	7
	Nonfat instant						
65	Envelope, net wt., 3.2 oz[5]	1 envelope	91	4	325	32	1
66	Cup[7]	1 cup	68	4	245	24	TR
	Milk beverages						
	Chocolate milk (commercial)						
67	Regular	1 cup	250	82	210	8	8
68	Lowfat (2%)	1 cup	250	84	180	8	5
69	Lowfat (1%)	1 cup	250	85	160	8	3
70	Eggnog (commercial)	1 cup	254	74	340	10	19
	Malted milk, home prepared with 1 cup of whole milk and 2 to 3 heaping tsp of malted milk powder (about ¾ oz)						
71	Chocolate + ¾ oz of powder	1 cup of milk	265	81	235	9	9
72	Natural + ¾ oz of powder	1 cup of milk	265	81	235	11	10
	Shakes, thick[8]						
73	Chocolate, container, net wt., 10.6 oz	1 container	300	72	355	9	8
74	Vanilla, container, net wt., 11 oz	1 container	313	74	350	12	9

[3]Applies to product without vitamin A added.
[4]Applies to product with added vitamin A. Without added vitamin A, value is 20 IU.
[5]Yields 1 qt of fluid milk when reconstituted according to package directions.
[6]Applies to product with added vitamin A.
[7]Weight applies to product with label claim of 1⅓ cups equal to 3.2 oz.
[8]Applies to products made from thick shake mixes and that do not contain added ice cream. Products made from milk shake mixes are higher in fat and usually contain added ice cream.

					Nutrients in Indicated Quantity							
Fatty Acids												
	Unsaturated											
Satu-rated (Total) (G) g	*Oleic (H)* g	*Lino-leic (I)* g	*Carbo-hydrate (J)* g	*Calcium (K)* mg	*Phos-phorus (L)* mg	*Iron (M)* mg	*Potas-sium (N)* mg	*Vitamin A Value (O)* I.U.	*Thiamin (P)* mg	*Ribo-flavin (Q)* mg	*Niacin (R)* mg	*Ascorbic Acid (S)* mg
1.3	0.5	TR	12	285	219	0.1	371	[3]80	0.08	0.38	0.1	2
11.6	5.3	0.4	25	657	510	0.5	764	[3]610	0.12	0.80	0.5	5
0.3	0.1	TR	29	738	497	0.7	845	[4]1,000	0.11	0.79	0.4	3
16.8	6.7	0.7	166	868	775	0.6	1,136	[3]1,000	0.28	1.27	0.6	8
4.3	1.7	0.2	59	1,421	1,119	0.4	1,910	[3]260	0.47	1.90	1.1	7
0.4	0.1	TR	47	1,120	896	0.3	1,552	[6]2,160	0.38	1.59	0.8	5
0.3	0.1	TR	35	837	670	0.2	1,160	[6]1,610	0.28	1.19	0.6	4
5.3	2.2	0.2	26	280	251	0.6	417	[3]300	0.09	0.41	0.3	2
3.1	1.3	0.1	26	284	254	0.6	422	500	0.10	0.42	0.3	2
1.5	0.7	0.1	26	287	257	0.6	426	500	0.10	0.40	0.2	2
11.3	5.0	0.6	34	330	278	0.5	420	890	0.09	0.48	0.3	4
5.5	—	—	29	304	265	0.5	500	330	0.14	0.43	0.7	2
6.0	—	—	27	347	307	0.3	529	380	0.20	0.54	1.3	2
5.0	2.0	0.2	63	396	378	0.9	672	260	0.14	0.67	0.4	0
5.9	2.4	0.2	56	457	361	0.3	572	360	0.09	0.61	0.5	0

(Continued)

APPENDIX C: *(Continued)*

Item No. (A)	Foods, approximate measures, units, and weight (edible part unless footnote indicate otherwise) (B)		g	Water (C) %	Food Energy (D) kcal	Pro- tein (E) g	Fat (F) g
Dairy Products (Cheese, Cream, Imitation Cream, Milk & Related Products)—Con.							
	Milk desserts, frozen						
	Ice cream						
	Regular (about 11% fat)						
75	Hardened	½ gal	1,064	61	2,155	38	115
76		1 cup	133	61	270	5	14
77		3-fl oz	50	61	100	2	5
78	Soft serve (frozen custard)	1 cup	173	60	375	7	23
79	Rich (about 16% fat), hardened	½ gal	1,188	59	2,805	33	190
80		1 cup	148	59	350	4	24
	Ice milk						
81	Hardened (about 4.3% fat)	½ gal	1,048	69	1,470	41	45
82		1 cup	131	69	185	5	6
83	Soft serve (about 2.6% fat)	1 cup	175	70	225	8	5
84	Sherbet (about 2% fat)	½ gal	1,542	66	2,160	17	31
85		1 cup	193	66	270	2	4
	Milk desserts, other						
86	Custard, baked	1 cup	265	77	305	14	15
	Puddings						
	From home recipe						
	Starch base						
87	Chocolate	1 cup	260	66	385	8	12
88	Vanilla (blancmange)	1 cup	255	76	285	9	10
89	Tapioca cream	1 cup	165	72	220	8	8
	From mix (chocolate) and milk						
90	Regular (cooked)	1 cup	260	70	320	9	8
91	Instant	1 cup	260	69	325	8	7
	Yogurt						
	With added milk solids						
	Made with lowfat milk						
92	Fruit-flavored[9]	1 8-oz container	227	75	230	10	3
93	Plain	1 container	227	85	145	12	4
94	Made with nonfat milk	1 8-oz container	227	85	125	13	TR
	Without added milk solds						
95	Made with whole milk	1 8-oz container	227	88	140	8	7

[9]Content of fat, vitamin A, and carbohydrate varies. Consult the label when precise values are needed for special diets.
[10]Applies to product made with milk containing no added vitamin A.

						Nutrients in Indicated Quantity							
Fatty Acids													
	Unsaturated												
Satu-rated (Total) (G) g	Oleic (H) g	Lino-leic (I) g	Carbo-hydrate (J) g	Calcium (K) mg	Phos-phorus (L) mg	Iron (M) mg	Potas-sium (N) mg	Vitamin A Value (O) I.U.	Thiamin (P) mg	Ribo-flavin (Q) mg	Niacin (R) mg	Ascorbic Acid (S) mg
71.3	28.8	2.6	254	1,406	1,075	1.0	2,052	4,340	0.42	2.63	1.1	6
8.9	3.6	0.3	32	176	134	0.1	257	540	0.05	0.33	0.1	1
3.4	1.4	0.1	12	66	51	TR	96	200	0.02	0.12	0.1	TR
13.5	5.9	0.6	38	236	199	0.4	338	790	0.08	0.45	0.2	1
118.3	47.8	4.3	256	1,213	927	0.8	1,771	7,200	0.36	2.27	0.9	5
14.7	6.0	0.5	32	151	115	0.1	221	900	0.04	0.28	0.1	1
28.1	11.3	1.0	232	1,409	1,035	1.5	2,117	1,710	0.61	2.78	0.9	6
3.5	1.4	0.1	29	176	129	0.1	265	210	0.08	0.35	0.1	1
2.9	1.2	0.1	38	274	202	0.3	412	180	0.12	0.54	0.2	1
19.0	7.7	0.7	469	827	594	2.5	1,585	1,480	0.26	0.71	1.0	31
2.4	1.0	0.1	59	103	74	0.3	198	190	0.03	0.09	0.1	4
6.8	5.4	0.7	29	297	310	1.1	387	930	0.11	0.50	0.3	1
7.6	3.3	0.3	67	250	255	1.3	445	390	0.05	0.36	0.3	1
6.2	2.5	0.2	41	298	232	TR	352	410	0.08	0.41	0.3	2
4.1	2.5	0.5	28	173	180	0.7	223	480	0.07	0.30	0.2	2
4.3	2.6	0.2	59	265	247	0.8	354	340	0.05	0.39	0.3	2
3.6	2.2	0.3	63	374	237	1.3	335	340	0.08	0.39	0.3	2
1.8	0.6	0.1	42	343	269	0.2	439	[10]120	0.08	0.40	0.2	1
2.3	0.8	0.1	16	415	326	0.2	531	[10]150	0.10	0.49	0.3	2
0.3	0.1	TR	17	452	355	0.2	579	[10]20	0.11	0.53	0.3	2
4.8	1.7	0.1	11	274	215	0.1	351	280	0.07	0.32	0.2	1

(Continued)

APPENDIX C: *(Continued)*

Nutrients in Indicated Quantity

Item No. (A)	Foods, approximate measures, units, and weight (edible part unless footnote indicate otherwise) (B)		g	Water (C) %	Food Energy (D) kcal	Pro-tein (E) g	Fat (F) g
Eggs							
	Eggs, large (24 oz per dozen)						
	Raw						
96	Whole, without shell	1 egg	50	75	80	6	6
97	White	1 white	33	88	15	3	TR
98	Yolk	1 yolk	17	49	65	3	6
	Cooked						
99	Fried in butter	1 egg	46	72	85	5	6
100	Hard-cooked, shell removed	1 egg	50	75	80	6	6
101	Poached	1 egg	50	74	80	6	6
102	Scrambled (milk added) in butter. Also omelet	1 egg	64	76	95	6	7
Fats, Oils, Related Products							
	Butter						
	Regular (1 brick or 4 sticks per lb)						
103	Stick (½ cup)	1 stick	113	16	815	1	92
104	Tablespoon (about ⅛ stick)	1 tbsp	14	16	100	TR	12
105	Pat (1 in square, ⅓ in high; 90 per lb)	1 pat	5	16	35	TR	4
	Whipped (6 sticks or two 8-oz containers per lb)						
106	Stick (½ cup)	1 stick	76	16	540	1	61
107	Tablespoon (about ⅛ stick)	1 tbsp	9	16	65	TR	8
108	Pat (1¼ in square, ⅓ in high; 120 per lb)	1 pat	4	16	25	TR	3
109	Fats, cooking (vegetable shortenings)	1 cup	200	0	1,770	0	200
110		1 tbsp	13	0	110	0	13
111	Lard	1 cup	205	0	1,850	0	205
112		1 tbsp	13	0	115	0	13
	Margarine						
	Regular (1 brick or 4 sticks per lb)						
113	Stick (½ cup)	1 stick	113	16	815	1	92
114	Tablespoon (about ⅛ stick)	1 tbsp	14	16	100	TR	12
115	Pat (1 in square, ⅓ in. high; 90 per lb)	1 pat	5	16	35	TR	4
116	Soft, two 8-oz containers per lb	1 container	227	16	1,635	1	184
117		1 tbsp	14	16	100	TR	12
	Whipped (6 sticks per lb)						
118	Stick (½ cup)	1 stick	76	16	545	TR	61

[11]Based on year-round average.

[12]Based on average vitamin A content of fortified margarine. Federal specifications for fortified margarine require a minimum of 15,000 International Units (IU) of vitamin A per pound.

| | Fatty Acids | | | | | | | | | | | |
| | | Unsaturated | | | | | | | | | | |
Saturated (Total) (G) g	Oleic (H) g	Linoleic (I) g	Carbohydrate (J) g	Calcium (K) mg	Phosphorus (L) mg	Iron (M) mg	Potassium (N) mg	Vitamin A Value (O) I.U.	Thiamin (P) mg	Riboflavin (Q) mg	Niacin (R) mg	Ascorbic Acid (S) mg
1.7	2.0	0.6	1	28	90	1.0	65	260	0.04	0.15	TR	0
0	0	0	TR	4	4	TR	45	0	TR	0.09	TR	0
1.7	2.1	0.6	TR	26	86	0.9	15	310	0.04	0.07	TR	0
2.4	2.2	0.6	1	26	80	0.9	58	290	0.03	0.13	TR	0
1.7	2.0	0.6	1	28	90	1.0	65	260	0.04	0.14	TR	0
1.7	2.0	0.6	1	28	90	1.0	65	260	0.04	0.13	TR	0
2.8	2.3	0.6	1	47	97	0.9	85	310	0.04	0.16	TR	0
57.3	23.1	2.1	TR	27	26	0.2	29	[11]3,470	0.01	0.04	TR	0
7.2	2.9	0.3	TR	3	3	TR	4	[11]430	TR	TR	TR	0
2.5	1.0	0.1	TR	1	1	TR	1	[11]150	TR	TR	TR	0
38.2	15.4	1.4	TR	18	17	0.1	20	[11]2,310	TR	0.03	TR	0
4.7	1.9	0.2	TR	2	2	TR	2	[11]290	TR	TR	TR	0
1.9	0.8	0.1	TR	1	1	TR	1	[11]120	0	TR	TR	0
48.8	88.2	48.4	0	0	0	0	0	—	0	0	0	0
3.2	5.7	3.1	0	0	0	0	0	—	0	0	0	0
81.0	83.8	20.5	0	0	0	0	0	0	0	0	0	0
5.1	5.3	1.3	0	0	0	0	0	0	0	0	0	0
16.7	42.9	24.9	TR	27	26	0.2	29	[12]3,750	0.01	0.04	TR	0
2.1	5.3	3.1	TR	3	3	TR	4	[12]470	TR	TR	TR	0
0.7	1.9	1.1	TR	1	1	TR	1	[12]170	TR	TR	TR	0
32.5	71.5	65.4	TR	53	52	0.4	59	[12]7,500	0.01	0.08	0.1	0
2.0	4.5	4.1	TR	3	3	TR	4	[12]470	TR	TR	TR	0
11.2	28.7	16.7	TR	18	17	0.1	20	[12]2,500	TR	0.03	TR	0

(Continued)

APPENDIX C: (*Continued*)

Item No. (A)	Foods, approximate measures, units, and weight (edible part unless footnote indicate otherwise) (B)		g	Water (C) %	Food Energy (D) kcal	Pro-tein (E) g	Fat (F) g
	Nutrients in Indicated Quantity						

Fats, Oils, Related Products—Con.

Margarine—Continued

Whipped (6 sticks per lb)—Continued

Item No. (A)	Foods (B)		g	Water (C) %	Food Energy (D) kcal	Protein (E) g	Fat (F) g
119	Tablespoon (about ⅛ stick)	1 tbsp	9	16	70	TR	8
	Oils, salad or cooking						
120	Corn	1 cup	218	0	1,925	0	218
121		1 tbsp	14	0	120	0	14
122	Olive	1 cup	216	0	1,910	0	216
123		1 tbsp	14	0	120	0	14
124	Peanut	1 cup	216	0	1,910	0	216
125		1 tbsp	14	0	120	0	14
126	Safflower	1 cup	218	0	1,925	0	218
127		1 tbsp	14	0	120	0	14
128	Soybean oil, hydrogenated (partially hardened)	1 cup	218	0	1,925	0	218
129		1 tbsp	14	0	120	0	14
130	Soybean-cottonseed oil blend, hydrogenated	1 cup	218	0	1,925	0	218
131		1 tbsp	14	0	120	0	14
	Salad dressings						
	Commercial						
	Blue cheese						
132	Regular	1 tbsp	15	32	75	1	8
133	Low calorie (5 cal/tsp)	1 tbsp	16	84	10	TR	1
	French						
134	Regular	1 tbsp	16	39	65	TR	6
135	Low calorie (5 cal/tsp)	1 tbsp	16	77	15	TR	1
	Italian						
136	Regular	1 tbsp	15	28	85	TR	9
137	Low calorie (2 cal/tsp)	1 tbsp	15	90	10	TR	1
138	Mayonnaise	1 tbsp	14	15	100	TR	11
	Mayonnaise type						
139	Regular	1 tbsp	15	41	65	TR	6
140	Low calorie (8 cal/tsp)	1 tbsp	16	81	20	TR	2
141	Tartar sauce, regular	1 tbsp	14	34	75	TR	8
	Thousand Island						
142	Regular	1 tbsp	16	32	80	TR	8
143	Low calorie (10 cal/tsp)	1 tbsp	15	68	25	TR	2

								Nutrients in Indicated Quantity				
Fatty Acids												
	Unsaturated											
Satu- rated (Total) (G) g	Oleic (H) g	Lino- leic (I) g	Carbo- hydrate (J) g	Calcium (K) mg	Phos- phorus (L) mg	Iron (M) mg	Potas- sium (N) mg	Vitamin A Value (O) I.U.	Thiamin (P) mg	Ribo- flavin (Q) mg	Niacin (R) mg	Ascorbic Acid (S) mg
1.4	3.6	2.1	TR	2	2	TR	2	[12]310	TR	TR	TR	0
27.7	53.6	125.1	0	0	0	0	0	—	0	0	0	0
1.7	3.3	7.8	0	0	0	0	0	—	0	0	0	0
30.7	154.4	17.7	0	0	0	0	0	—	0	0	0	0
1.9	9.7	1.1	0	0	0	0	0	—	0	0	0	0
37.4	98.5	67.0	0	0	0	0	0	—	0	0	0	0
2.3	6.2	4.2	0	0	0	0	0	—	0	0	0	0
20.5	25.9	159.8	0	0	0	0	0	—	0	0	0	0
1.3	1.6	10.0	0	0	0	0	0	—	0	0	0	0
31.8	93.1	75.6	0	0	0	0	0	—	0	0	0	0
2.0	5.8	4.7	0	0	0	0	0	—	0	0	0	0
38.2	63.0	99.6	0	0	0	0	0	—	0	0	0	0
2.4	3.9	6.2	0	0	0	0	0	—	0	0	0	0
1.6	1.7	3.8	1	12	11	TR	6	30	TR	0.02	TR	TR
0.5	0.3	TR	1	10	8	TR	5	30	TR	0.01	TR	TR
1.1	1.3	3.2	3	2	2	0.1	13	—	—	—	—	—
0.1	0.1	0.4	2	2	2	0.1	13	—	—	—	—	—
1.6	1.9	4.7	1	2	1	TR	2	TR	TR	TR	TR	—
0.1	0.1	0.4	TR	TR	1	TR	2	TR	TR	TR	TR	—
2.0	2.4	5.6	TR	3	4	0.1	5	40	TR	0.01	TR	—
1.1	1.4	3.2	2	2	4	TR	1	30	TR	TR	TR	—
0.4	0.4	1.0	2	3	4	TR	1	40	TR	TR	TR	—
1.5	1.8	4.1	1	3	4	0.1	11	30	TR	TR	TR	TR
1.4	1.7	4.0	2	2	3	0.1	18	50	TR	TR	TR	TR
0.4	0.4	1.0	2	2	3	0.1	17	50	TR	TR	TR	TR

(Continued)

APPENDIX C: (*Continued*)

				Nutrients in Indicated Quantity			
Item No. (A)	Foods, approximate measures, units, and weight (edible part unless footnote indicate otherwise) (B)			Water (C)	Food Energy (D)	Pro- tein (E)	Fat (F)
		g		%	kcal	g	g

Fats, Oils, Related Products—Con.
Salad dressings—Continued

From home recipe

| 144 | Cooked type[13] | 1 tbsp | 16 | 68 | 25 | 1 | 2 |

Fish, Shellfish, Meat, Poultry; Related Products
Fish and Shellfish

145	Bluefish, baked with butter or margarine	3 oz	85	68	135	22	4
	Clams						
146	Raw, meat only	3 oz	85	82	65	11	1
147	Canned, solids and liquid	3 oz	85	86	45	7	1
148	Crabmeat (white or king), canned, not pressed down	1 cup	135	77	135	24	3
149	Fish sticks, breaded, cooked, frozen (stick, 4 by 1 by ½ in)	1 fish stick	28	66	50	5	3
150	Haddock, breaded, fried[14]	3 oz	85	66	140	17	5
151	Ocean perch, breaded, fried[14]	1 fillet	85	59	195	16	11
152	Oysters, raw, meat only (13–19 medium Selects)	1 cup	240	85	160	20	4
153	Salmon, pink, canned, solids and liquid	3 oz	85	71	120	17	5
154	Sardines, Atlantic, canned in oil, drained solids	3 oz	85	62	175	20	9
155	Scallops, frozen, breaded, fried, reheated	6 scallops	90	60	175	16	8
156	Shad, baked with butter or margarine, bacon	3 oz	85	64	170	20	10
	Shrimp						
157	Canned meat	3 oz	85	70	100	21	1
158	French fried[16]	3 oz	85	57	190	17	9
159	Tuna, canned in oil, drained solids	3 oz	85	61	170	24	7
160	Tuna salad[17]	1 cup	205	70	350	30	22
	Meat and meat products						
161	Bacon, (20 slices per lb, raw), broiled or fried, crisp	2 slices	15	8	85	4	8
	Beef,[18] cooked						
	Cuts braised, simmered or pot roasted						
162	Lean and fat (piece, 2½ by 2½ by ¾ in)	3 oz	85	53	245	23	16

[13]Fatty acid values apply to product made with regular-type margarine.
[14]Dipped in egg, milk or water, and breadcrumbs; fried in vegetable shortening.
[15]If bones are discarded, value for calcium will be greatly reduced.
[16]Dipped in egg, breadcrumbs, and flour or batter.
[17]Prepared with tuna, celery, salad dressing (mayonnaise type), pickle, onion, and egg.
[18]Outer layer of fat on the cut was removed to within approximately ½ in. of the lean. Deposits of fat within the cut were not removed.

	Nutrients in Indicated Quantity											
Fatty Acids												
	Unsaturated											
Satu-rated (Total) (G) g	Oleic (H) g	Lino-leic (I) g	Carbo-hydrate (J) g	Calcium (K) mg	Phos-phorus (L) mg	Iron (M) mg	Potas-sium (N) mg	Vitamin A Value (O) I.U.	Thiamin (P) mg	Ribo-flavin (Q) mg	Niacin (R) mg	Ascorbic Acid (S) mg
0.5	0.6	0.3	2	14	15	0.1	19	80	0.01	0.03	TR	TR
—	—	—	0	25	244	0.6	—	40	0.09	0.08	1.6	—
—	—	—	2	59	138	5.2	154	90	0.08	0.15	1.1	8
0.2	TR	TR	2	47	116	3.5	119	—	0.01	0.09	0.9	—
0.6	0.4	0.1	1	61	246	1.1	149	—	0.11	0.11	2.6	—
—	—	—	2	3	47	0.1	—	0	0.01	0.02	0.5	—
1.4	2.2	1.2	5	34	210	1.0	296	—	0.03	0.06	2.7	2
2.7	4.4	2.3	6	28	192	1.1	242	—	0.10	0.10	1.6	—
1.3	0.2	0.1	8	226	343	13.2	290	740	0.34	0.43	6.0	—
0.9	0.8	0.1	0	[15]167	243	0.7	307	60	0.03	0.16	6.8	—
3.0	2.5	0.5	0	372	424	2.5	502	190	0.02	0.17	4.6	—
—	—	—	9	—	—	—	—	—	—	—	—	—
—	—	—	0	20	266	0.5	320	30	0.11	0.22	7.3	—
0.1	0.1	TR	1	98	224	2.6	104	50	0.01	0.03	1.5	—
2.3	3.7	2.0	9	61	162	1.7	195	—	0.03	0.07	2.3	—
1.7	1.7	0.7	0	7	199	1.6	—	70	0.04	0.10	10.1	—
4.3	6.3	6.7	7	41	291	2.7	—	590	0.08	0.23	10.3	2
2.5	3.7	0.7	TR	2	34	0.5	35	0	0.08	0.05	0.8	—
6.8	6.5	0.4	0	10	114	2.9	184	30	0.04	0.18	3.6	—

(Continued)

APPENDIX C: (*Continued*)

				Nutrients in Indicated Quantity			
Item No. (A)	Foods, approximate measures, units, and weight (edible part unless footnotes indicate otherwise) (B)		g	Water (C) %	Food Energy (D) kcal	Pro-tein (E) g	Fat (F) g

Fish, Shellfish, Meat, Poultry; Related Products—Con.

Meat and meat products—Continued

Beef,[18] cooked—Continued

Cuts braised, simmered or pot roasted—Continued

163	Lean only from item 162	2.5 oz	72	62	140	22	5
	Ground beef, broiled:						
164	Lean with 10% fat	3-oz patty	85	60	185	23	10
165	Lean with 21% fat	2.9-oz patty	82	54	235	20	17
	Roast, oven cooked, no liquid added						
	Relatively fat, such as rib						
166	Lean and fat (2 pieces, 4⅛ by 2¼ by ¼ in)	3 oz	85	40	375	17	33
167	Lean only from item 166	1.8 oz	51	57	125	14	7
	Relatively lean, such as heel of round						
168	Lean and fat (2 pieces, 4⅛ by 2¼ by ¼ in)	3 oz	85	62	165	25	7
169	Lean only from item 168	2.8 oz	78	65	125	24	3
	Steak						
	Relatively fat-sirloin, broiled						
170	Lean and fat (piece, 2½ by 2½ by ¾ in.)	3 oz	85	44	330	20	27
171	Lean only from item 170	2.0 oz	56	59	115	18	4
	Relatively lean-round, braised						
172	Lean and fat (piece, 4⅛ by 2¼ by ½ in.)	3 oz	85	55	220	24	13
173	Lean only from item 172	2.4 oz	68	61	130	21	4
	Beef, canned						
174	Corned beef	3 oz	85	59	185	22	10
175	Corned beef hash	1 cup	220	67	400	19	25
176	Beef, dried, chipped	2½-oz jar	71	48	145	24	4
177	Beef and vegetable stew	1 cup	245	82	220	16	11
178	Beef potpie ((home recipe), baked[19] (piece, ⅓ of 9-in. diam. pie)	1 piece	210	55	515	21	30
179	Chili con carne with beans, canned	1 cup	255	72	340	19	16
180	Chop suey with beef and pork (home recipe)	1 cup	250	75	300	26	17
181	Heart, beef, lean, braised	3 oz	85	61	160	27	5
	Lamb, cooked						
	Chop, rib (cut 3 per lb with bone), broiled						
182	Lean and fat	3.1 oz	89	43	360	18	32

[18]Outer layer of fat on the cut was removed to within approximately ½ in of the lean. Deposits of fat within the cut were not removed.
[19]Crust made with vegetable shortening and enriched flour.

								Nutrients in Indicated Quantity					
Fatty Acids													
	Unsaturated												
Satu-rated (Total) (G) g	Oleic (H) g	Lino-leic (I) g	Carbo-hydrate (J) g	Calcium (K) mg	Phos-phorus (L) mg	Iron (M) mg	Potas-sium (N) mg	Vitamin A Value (O) I.U.	Thiamin (P) mg	Ribo-flavin (Q) mg	Niacin (R) mg	Ascorbic Acid (S) mg
2.1	1.8	0.2	0	10	108	2.7	176	10	0.04	0.17	3.3	—
4.0	3.9	0.3	0	10	196	3.0	261	20	0.08	0.20	5.1	—
7.0	6.7	0.4	0	9	159	2.6	221	30	0.07	0.17	4.4	—
14.0	13.6	0.8	0	8	158	2.2	189	70	0.05	0.13	3.1	—
3.0	2.5	0.3	0	6	131	1.8	161	10	0.04	0.11	2.6	—
2.8	2.7	0.2	0	11	208	3.2	279	10	0.06	0.19	4.5	—
1.2	1.0	0.1	0	10	199	3.0	268	TR	0.06	0.18	4.3	—
11.3	11.1	0.6	0	9	162	2.5	220	50	0.05	0.15	4.0	—
1.8	1.6	0.2	0	7	146	2.2	202	10	0.05	0.14	3.6	—
5.5	5.2	0.4	0	10	213	3.0	272	20	0.07	0.19	4.8	—
1.7	1.5	0.2	0	9	182	2.5	238	10	0.05	0.16	4.1	—
4.9	4.5	0.2	0	17	90	3.7	—	—	0.01	0.20	2.9	—
11.9	10.9	0.5	24	29	147	4.4	440	—	0.02	0.20	4.6	—
2.1	2.0	0.1	0	14	287	3.6	142	—	0.05	0.23	2.7	0
4.9	4.5	0.2	15	29	184	2.9	613	2,400	0.15	0.17	4.7	17
7.9	12.8	6.7	39	29	149	3.8	334	1,720	0.30	0.30	5.5	6
7.5	6.8	0.3	31	82	321	4.3	594	150	0.08	0.18	3.3	—
8.5	6.2	0.7	13	60	248	4.8	425	600	0.28	0.38	5.0	33
1.5	1.1	0.6	1	5	154	5.0	197	20	0.21	1.04	6.5	1
14.8	12.1	1.2	0	8	139	1.0	200	—	0.11	0.19	4.1	—

(Continued)

APPENDIX C: (*Continued*)

Item No. (A)	Foods, approximate measures, units, and weight (edible part unless footnote indicate otherwise) (B)		g	Water (C) %	Food Energy (D) kcal	Pro-tein (E) g	Fat (F) g
					Nutrients in Indicated Quantity		

Fish, Shellfish, Meat, Poultry; Related Products—Con.
    Meat and meat products—Continued
      Lamb, cooked—Continued
        Chop, rib (cut 3 per lb with bone), broiled—Continued

Item No.	Foods	Measure	g	Water %	Food Energy kcal	Protein g	Fat g
183	Lean only from item 182	2 oz	57	60	120	16	6
	Leg, roasted						
184	Lean and fat (2 pieces, 4⅛ by 2¼ by ¼ in.)	3 oz	85	54	235	22	16
185	Lean only from item 184	2.5 oz	71	62	130	20	5
	Shoulder, roasted						
186	Lean and fat (3 pieces, 2½ by 2½ by ¼ in.)	3 oz	85	50	285	18	23
187	Lean only from item 186	2.3 oz	64	61	130	17	6
188	Liver, beef, fried[20] (slice, 6½ by 2⅜ by ⅜ in.)	3 oz	85	56	195	22	9
	Pork, cured, cooked						
189	Ham, light cure, lean and fat, roasted (2 pieces, 4⅛ by 2¼ by ¼ in.)[22]	3 oz	85	54	245	18	19
	Luncheon meat						
190	Boiled ham, slice (8 per 8-oz pkg.)	1 oz	28	59	65	5	5
	Canned, spiced or unspiced						
191	Slice, approx. 3 by 2 by ½ in.	1 slice	60	55	175	9	15
	Pork, fresh,[18] cooked						
	Chop, loin (cut 3 per lb with bone), broiled						
192	Lean and fat	2.7 oz	78	42	305	19	25
193	Lean only from item 192	2 oz	56	53	150	17	9
	Roast, oven cooked, no liquid added						
194	Lean and fat (piece, 2½ by 2½ by ¾ in.)	3 oz	85	46	310	21	24
195	Lean only from item 194	2.4 oz	68	55	175	20	10
	Shoulder cut, simmered						
196	Lean and fat (3 pieces, 2½ by 2½ by ¼ in.)	3 oz	85	46	320	20	26
197	Lean only from item 196	2.2 oz	63	60	135	18	6
	Sausages (see also Luncheon meat (items 190–191))						
198	Bologna, slice (8 per 8-oz pkg.)	1 slice	28	56	85	3	8
199	Braunschweiger, slice (6 per 6-oz pkg.)	1 slice	28	53	90	4	8
200	Brown and serve (10–11 per 8-oz pkg.), browned	1 link	17	40	70	3	6

[20]Regular-type margarine used.
[21]Value varies widely.
[22]About one-fourth of the outer layer of fat on the cut was removed. Deposits of fat within the cut were not removed.

								Nutrients in Indicated Quantity				
Fatty Acids												
Satu- rated (Total) (G) g	Unsaturated		Carbo- hydrate (J) g	Calcium (K) mg	Phos- phorus (L) mg	Iron (M) mg	Potas- sium (N) mg	Vitamin A Value (O) I.U.	Thiamin (P) mg	Ribo- flavin (Q) mg	Niacin (R) mg	Ascorbic Acid (S) mg
	Oleic (H) g	Lino- leic (I) g										
2.5	2.1	0.2	0	6	121	1.1	174	—	0.09	0.15	3.4	—
7.3	6.0	0.6	0	9	177	1.4	241	—	0.13	0.23	4.7	—
2.1	1.8	0.2	0	9	169	1.4	227	—	0.12	0.21	4.4	—
10.8	8.8	0.9	0	9	146	1.0	206	—	0.11	0.20	4.0	—
3.6	2.3	0.2	0	8	140	1.0	193	—	0.10	0.18	3.7	—
2.5	3.5	0.9	5	9	405	7.5	323	[21]45,390	0.22	3.56	14.0	23
6.8	7.9	1.7	0	8	146	2.2	199	0	0.40	0.15	3.1	—
1.7	2.0	0.4	0	3	47	0.8	—	0	0.12	0.04	0.7	—
5.4	6.7	1.0	1	5	65	1.3	133	0	0.19	0.13	1.8	—
8.9	10.4	2.2	0	9	209	2.7	216	0	0.75	0.22	4.5	—
3.1	3.6	0.8	0	7	181	2.2	192	0	0.63	0.18	3.8	—
8.7	10.2	2.2	0	9	218	2.7	233	0	0.78	0.22	4.8	—
3.5	4.1	0.8	0	9	211	2.6	224	0	0.73	0.21	4.4	—
9.3	10.9	2.3	0	9	118	2.6	158	0	0.46	0.21	4.1	—
2.2	2.6	0.6	0	8	111	2.3	146	0	0.42	0.19	3.7	—
3.0	3.4	0.5		2	36	0.5	65	—	0.05	0.06	0.7	—
2.6	3.4	0.8	1	3	69	1.7	—	1,850	0.05	0.41	2.3	—
2.3	2.8	0.7	—	—	—	—	—	—	—	—	—	—

(Continued)

APPENDIX C: (*Continued*)

					Nutrients in Indicated Quantity			
Item No. (A)	Foods, approximate measures, units, and weight (edible part unless footnotes indicate otherwise) (B)			Water (C) %	Food Energy (D) kcal	Pro-tein (E) g	Fat (F) g
			g				

Fish, Shellfish, Meat, Poultry; Related Products—Con.

Meat and meat products—Continued

Sausages (see also Luncheon meat (items 190–191))—Continued

201	Deviled ham, canned	1 tbsp	13	51	45	2	4
202	Frankfurter (8 per 1-lb pkg.), cooked (reheated)	1 frankfurter	56	57	170	7	15
203	Meat, potted (beef, chicken, turkey), canned	1 tbsp	13	61	30	2	2
204	Pork link (16 per 1-lb pkg.), cooked	1 link	13	35	60	2	6
	Salami						
205	Dry type, slice (12 per 4-oz pkg.)	1 slice	10	30	45	2	4
206	Cooked type, slice (8 per 8-oz pkg.)	1 slice	28	51	90	5	7
207	Vienna sausage (7 per 4-oz can)	1 sausage	16	63	40	2	3
	Veal, medium fat, cooked, bone removed						
208	Cutlet (4⅛ by 2¼ by ½ in.), braised or broiled	3 oz	85	60	185	23	9
209	Rib (2 pieces, 4⅛ by 2¼ by ¼ in.), roasted	3 oz	85	55	230	23	14
	Poultry and poultry products						
	Chicken, cooked						
210	Breast, fried,[23] bones removed, ½ breast (3.3 oz with bones)	2.8 oz	79	58	160	26	5
211	Drumstick, fried,[23] bones removed (2 oz with bones)	1.3 oz	38	55	90	12	4
212	Half broiler, broiled, bones removed (10.4 oz with bones)	6.2 oz	176	71	240	42	7
213	Chicken, canned, boneless	3 oz	85	65	170	18	10
214	Chicken a la king, cooked (home recipe)	1 cup	245	68	470	27	34
215	Chicken and noodles, cooked (home recipe)	1 cup	240	71	365	22	18
	Chicken chow mein						
216	Canned	1 cup	250	89	95	7	TR
217	From home recipe	1 cup	250	78	255	31	10
218	Chicken potpie (home recipe), baked,[19] piece (⅓ or 9-in. diam. pie)	1 piece	232	57	545	23	31
	Turkey, roasted, flesh without skin						
219	Dark meat, piece, 2½ by 1⅝ by ¼ in.	4 pieces	85	61	175	26	7
220	Light meat, piece, 4 by 2 by ¼ in.	2 pieces	85	62	150	28	3
	Light and dark meat						
221	Chopped or diced	1 cup	140	61	265	44	9
222	Pieces (1 slice white meat, 4 by 2 by ¼ in with 2 slices dark meat, 2½ by 1⅝ by ¼ in)	3 pieces	85	61	160	27	5

[23]Vegetable shortening used.

						Nutrients in Indicated Quantity						
Fatty Acids												
	Unsaturated											
Satu-rated (Total) (G) g	Oleic (H) g	Lino-leic (I) g	Carbo-hydrate (J) g	Calcium (K) mg	Phos-phorus (L) mg	Iron (M) mg	Potas-sium (N) mg	Vitamin A Value (O) I.U.	Thiamin (P) mg	Ribo-flavin (Q) mg	Niacin (R) mg	Ascorbic Acid (S) mg
1.5	1.8	0.4	0	1	12	0.3	—	0	0.02	0.01	0.2	—
5.6	6.5	1.2	1	3	57	0.8	—	—	0.08	0.11	1.4	—
—	—	—	0	—	—	—	—	—		0.03	0.2	—
2.1	2.4	0.5		1	21	0.3	35	0	0.10	0.04	0.5	—
1.6	1.6	0.1		1	28	0.4	—	—	0.04	0.03	0.5	—
3.1	3.0	0.2		3	57	0.7	—	—	0.07	0.07	1.2	—
1.2	1.4	0.2		1	24	0.3	—	—	0.01	0.02	0.4	—
4.0	3.4	0.4	0	9	196	2.7	258	—	0.06	0.21	4.6	—
6.1	5.1	0.6	0	10	211	2.9	259	—	0.11	0.26	6.6	—
1.4	1.8	1.1	1	9	218	1.3	—	70	0.04	0.17	11.6	—
1.1	1.3	0.9		6	89	0.9	—	50	0.03	0.15	2.7	—
2.2	2.5	1.3	0	16	355	3.0	483	160	0.09	0.34	15.5	—
3.2	3.8	2.0	0	18	210	1.3	117	200	0.03	0.11	3.7	3
2.7	14.3	3.3	12	127	358	2.5	404	1,130	0.10	0.42	5.4	12
5.9	7.1	3.5	26	26	247	2.2	149	430	0.05	0.17	4.3	
—	—	—	18	45	35	1.3	418	150	0.05	0.10	1.0	13
2.4	3.4	3.1	10	58	293	2.5	473	280	0.08	0.23	4.3	10
11.3	10.9	5.6	42	70	232	3.0	343	3,090	0.34	0.31	5.5	5
2.1	1.5	1.5	0	—	—	2.0	338	—	0.03	0.20	3.6	—
0.9	0.6	0.7	0	—	—	1.0	349	—	0.04	0.12	9.4	—
2.5	1.7	1.8	0	11	351	2.5	514	—	0.07	0.25	10.8	—
1.5	1.0	1.1	0	7	213	1.5	312	—	0.04	0.15	6.5	—

(Continued)

APPENDIX C: (*Continued*)

							Nutrients in Indicated Quantity

Item No. (A)	Foods, approximate measures, units, and weight (edible part unless footnote indicate otherwise) (B)		g	Water (C) %	Food Energy (D) kcal	Pro- tein (E) g	Fat (F) g
Fruits and Fruit Products							
	Apples, raw, unpeeled, without cores:						
223	2¾-in diam. (about 3 per lb with cores)	1 apple	138	84	80	TR	1
224	3¼-in diam. (about 2 per lb with cores)	1 apple	212	84	125	TR	1
225	Applejuice, bottled or canned[24]	1 cup	248	88	120	TR	TR
	Applesauce, canned						
226	Sweetened	1 cup	255	76	230	1	TR
227	Unsweetened	1 cup	244	89	100	TR	TR
	Apricots						
228	Raw, without pits (about 12 per lb with pits)	3 apricots	107	85	55	1	TR
229	Canned in heavy sirup (halves and sirup)	1 cup	258	77	220	2	TR
	Dried						
230	Uncooked (28 large or 37 medium halves per cup)	1 cup	130	25	340	7	1
231	Cooked, unsweetened, fruit and liquid	1 cup	250	76	215	4	1
232	Apricot nectar, canned	1 cup	251	85	145	1	TR
	Avocados, raw, whole, without skins and seeds						
233	California, mid- and late-winter (with skin and seed, 3⅛-in diam.; wt., 10 oz)	1 avocado	216	74	370	5	37
234	Florida, late summer and fall (with skin and seed, 3⅝-in. diam.; wt., 1 lb)	1 avocado	304	78	390	4	33
235	Banana without peel (about 2.6 per lb with peel)	1 banana	119	76	100	1	TR
236	Banana flakes	1 tbsp	6	3	20	TR	TR
237	Blackberries, raw	1 cup	144	85	85	2	1
238	Blueberries, raw	1 cup	145	83	90	1	1
	Cantaloupe. See Muskmelons (item 271)						
	Cherries						
239	Sour (tart), red, pitted, canned, water pack	1 cup	244	88	105	2	TR
240	Sweet, raw, without pits and stems	10 cherries	68	80	45	1	TR
241	Cranberry juice cocktail, bottled, sweetened	1 cup	253	83	165	TR	TR
242	Cranberry sauce, sweetened, canned, strained.	1 cup	277	62	405	TR	1
	Dates						
243	Whole, without pits	10 dates	80	23	220	2	TR
244	Chopped	1 cup	178	23	490	4	1

[24]Also applies to pasteurized apple cider.
[25]Applies to product without added ascorbic acid. For value of product with added ascorbic acid, refer to label.
[26]Based on product with label claim of 45% of U.S. RDA in 6 fl oz.
[27]Based on product with label claim of 100% of U.S. RDA in 6 fl oz.

								**Nutrients in Indicated Quantity**				
Fatty Acids												
	Unsaturated											
Satu-rated (Total) (G) g	**Oleic (H) g**	**Lino-leic (I) g**	**Carbo-hydrate (J) g**	**Calcium (K) mg**	**Phos-phorus (L) mg**	**Iron (M) mg**	**Potas-sium (N) mg**	**Vitamin A Value (O) I.U.**	**Thiamin (P) mg**	**Ribo-flavin (Q) mg**	**Niacin (R) mg**	**Ascorbic Acid (S) mg**
—	—	—	20	10	14	0.4	152	120	0.04	0.03	0.1	6
—	—	—	31	15	21	0.6	233	190	0.06	0.04	0.2	8
—	—	—	30	15	22	1.5	250	—	0.02	0.05	0.2	[25]2
—	—	—	61	10	13	1.3	166	100	0.05	0.03	0.1	[25]3
—	—	—	26	10	12	1.2	190	100	0.05	0.02	0.1	[25]2
—	—	—	14	18	25	0.5	301	2,890	0.03	0.04	0.6	11
—	—	—	57	28	39	0.8	604	4,490	0.05	0.05	1.0	10
—	—	—	86	87	140	7.2	1,273	14,170	0.01	0.21	4.3	16
—.	—	—	54	55	88	4.5	795	7,500	0.01	0.13	2.5	8
—	—	—	37	23	30	0.5	379	2,380	0.03	0.03	0.5	[26]36
5.5	22.0	3.7	13	22	91	1.3	1,303	630	0.24	0.43	3.5	30
6.7	15.7	5.3	27	30	128	1.8	1,836	880	0.33	0.61	4.9	43
—	—	—	26	10	31	0.8	440	230	0.06	0.07	0.8	12
—	—	—	5	2	6	0.2	92	50	0.01	0.01	0.2	
—	—	—	19	46	27	1.3	245	290	0.04	0.06	0.6	30
—	—	—	22	22	19	1.5	117	150	0.04	0.09	0.7	20
—	—	—	26	37	32	0.7	317	1,660	0.07	0.05	0.5	12
—	—	—	12	15	13	0.3	129	70	0.03	0.04	0.3	7
—	—	—	42	13	8	0.8	25	TR	0.03	0.03	0.1	[27]81
—	—	—	104	17	11	0.6	83	60	0.03	0.03	0.1	6
—	—	—	58	47	50	2.4	518	40	0.07	0.08	1.8	0
—	—	—	130	105	112	5.3	1,153	90	0.16	0.18	3.9	0

(Continued)

APPENDIX C: *(Continued)*

Nutrients in Indicated Quantity

Item No. (A)	Foods, approximate measures, units, and weight (edible part unless footnote indicate otherwise) (B)		g	Water (C) %	Food Energy (D) kcal	Pro-tein (E) g	Fat (F) g
Fruits and Fruit Products—Con.							
245	Fruit cocktail, canned, in heavy sirup	1 cup	255	80	195	1	TR
	Grapefruit						
	Raw, medium, 3¾-in diam. (about 1 lb 1 oz)						
246	Pink or red	½ grapefruit[28]	241	89	50	1	TR
247	White	½ grapefruit[28]	241	89	45	1	TR
248	Canned, sections with sirup	1 cup	254	81	180	2	TR
	Grapefruit juice						
249	Raw, pink, red, or white	1 cup	246	90	95	1	TR
	Canned, white						
250	Unsweetened	1 cup	247	89	100	1	TR
251	Sweetened	1 cup	250	86	135	1	TR
	Frozen, concentrate, unsweetened						
252	Undiluted, 6-fl oz can	1 can	207	62	300	4	1
253	Diluted with 3 parts water by volume	1 cup	247	89	100	1	TR
254	Dehydrated crystals, prepared with water (1 lb yields about 1 gal)	1 cup	247	90	100	1	TR
	Grapes, European type (adherent skin), raw						
255	Thompson Seedless	10 grapes	50	81	35	TR	TR
256	Tokay and Emperor, seeded types	10 grapes[30]	60	81	40	TR	TR
	Grape juice						
257	Canned or bottled	1 cup	253	83	165	1	TR
	Frozen concentrate, sweetened						
258	Undiluted, 6-fl oz can	1 can	216	53	395	1	TR
259	Diluted with 3 parts water by volume	1 cup	250	86	135	1	TR
260	Grape drink, canned	1 cup	250	86	135	TR	TR
261	Lemon, raw, size 165, without peel and seeds (about 4 per lb with peels and seeds)	1 lemon	74	90	20	1	TR
	Lemon juice						
262	Raw	1 cup	244	91	60	1	TR

[28]Weight includes peel and membranes between sections. Without these parts, the weight of the edible portion is 123 g for item 246 and 118 g for item 247.

[29]For white-fleshed varieties, value is about 20 International Units (I.U.) per cup; for red-fleshed varieties, 1,080 I.U.

[30]Weight includes seeds. Without seeds, weight of the edible portion is 57 g.

[31]Applies to product without added ascorbic acid. With added ascorbic acid, based on claim that 6 fl oz of reconstituted juice contain 45% or 50% of the U.S. RDA, value in milligrams is 108 or 120 for a 6-fl oz can (item 258), 36 or 40 for 1 cup of diluted juice (item 259).

[32]For products with added thiamin and riboflavin but without added ascorbic acid, values in milligrams would be 0.60 for thiamin, 0.80 for riboflavin, and trace for ascorbic acid. For products with only ascorbic acid added, value varies with the brand. Consult the label.

						Nutrients in Indicated Quantity						
Fatty Acids												
	Unsaturated											
Satu-rated (Total) (G) g	*Oleic (H) g*	*Lino-leic (I) g*	*Carbo-hydrate (J) g*	*Calcium (K) mg*	*Phos-phorus (L) mg*	*Iron (M) mg*	*Potas-sium (N) mg*	*Vitamin A Value (O) I.U.*	*Thiamin (P) mg*	*Ribo-flavin (Q) mg*	*Niacin (R) mg*	*Ascorbic Acid (S) mg*
—	—	—	50	23	31	1.0	411	360	0.05	0.03	1.0	5
—	—	—	13	20	20	0.5	166	540	0.05	0.02	0.2	44
—	—	—	12	19	19	0.5	159	10	0.05	0.02	0.2	44
—	—	—	45	33	36	0.8	343	30	0.08	0.05	0.5	76
—	—	—	23	22	37	0.5	399	([29])	0.10	0.05	0.5	93
—	—	—	24	20	35	1.0	400	20	0.07	0.05	0.5	84
—	—	—	32	20	35	1.0	405	30	0.08	0.05	0.5	78
—	—	—	72	70	124	0.8	1,250	60	0.29	0.12	1.4	286
—	—	—	24	25	42	0.2	420	20	0.10	0.04	0.5	96
—	—	—	24	22	40	0.2	412	20	0.10	0.05	0.5	91
—	—	—	9	6	10	0.2	87	50	0.03	0.02	0.2	2
—	—	—	10	7	11	0.2	99	60	0.03	0.02	0.2	2
—	—	—	42	28	30	0.8	293	—	0.10	0.05	0.5	[25]TR
—	—	—	100	22	32	0.9	255	40	0.13	0.22	1.5	[31]32
—	—	—	33	8	10	0.3	85	10	0.05	0.08	0.5	[31]10
—	—	—	35	8	10	0.3	88	—	[32]0.03	[32]0.03	0.3	([32])
—	—	—	6	19	12	0.4	102	10	0.03	0.01	0.1	39
—	—	—	20	17	24	0.5	344	50	0.07	0.02	0.2	112

(Continued)

APPENDIX C: (*Continued*)

					Food	Pro-	
							Nutrients in Indicated Quantity

Item No. (A)	Foods, approximate measures, units, and weight (edible part unless footnotes indicate otherwise) (B)		g	Water (C) %	Food Energy (D) kcal	Pro- tein (E) g	Fat (F) g
	Fruits and Fruit Products—Con.						
	Lemon juice—Continued						
263	Canned, or bottled, unsweetened	1 cup	244	92	55	1	TR
264	Frozen, single strength, unsweetened, 6-fl oz can	1 can	183	92	40	1	TR
	Lemonade concentrate, frozen						
265	Undiluted, 6-fl oz can	1 can	219	49	425	TR	TR
266	Diluted with 4⅓ parts water by volume	1 cup	248	89	105	TR	TR
	Limeade concentrate, frozen						
267	Undiluted, 6-fl oz can	1 can	218	50	410	TR	TR
268	Diluted with 4⅓ parts water by volume	1 cup	247	89	100	TR	TR
	Limejuice						
269	Raw	1 cup	246	90	65	1	TR
270	Canned, unsweetened	1 cup	246	90	65	1	TR
	Muskmelons, raw, with rind, without seed cavity						
271	Cantaloupe, orange-fleshed (with rind and seed cavity, 5-in. diam., 2⅓ lb)	½ melon with rind[33]	477	91	80	2	TR
272	Honeydew (with rind and seed cavity, 6½-in. diam., 5¼ lb)	1/10 melon with rind[33]	226	91	50	1	TR
	Oranges, all commercial varieties, raw						
273	Whole, 2⅝-in diam., without peel and seeds (about 2½ per lb with peel and seeds)	1 orange	131	86	65	1	TR
274	Sections without membrane	1 cup	180	86	90	2	TR
	Orange juice						
275	Raw, all varieties	1 cup	248	88	110	2	TR
276	Canned, unsweetened	1 cup	249	87	120	2	TR
	Frozen concentrate						
277	Undiluted, 6-fl oz can	1 can	213	55	360	5	TR
278	Diluted with 3 parts water by volume	1 cup	249	87	120	2	TR
279	Dehydrated crystals, prepared with water (1 lb yields about 1 gal)	1 cup	248	88	115	1	TR
	Orange and grapefruit juice						
	Frozen concentrate						
280	Undiluted, 6-fl oz can	1 can	210	59	330	4	1
281	Diluted with 3 parts water by volume	1 cup	248	88	110	1	TR
282	Papayas, raw, ½-in cubes	1 cup	140	89	55	1	TR

[33]Weight includes rind. Without rind, the weight of the edible portion is 272 g for item 271 and 149 g for item 272.

								Nutrients in Indicated Quantity				
Fatty Acids												
	Unsaturated											
Satu-rated (Total) (G) g	*Oleic (H) g*	*Lino-leic (I) g*	*Carbo-hydrate (J) g*	*Calcium (K) mg*	*Phos-phorus (L) mg*	*Iron (M) mg*	*Potas-sium (N) mg*	*Vitamin A Value (O) I.U.*	*Thiamin (P) mg*	*Ribo-flavin (Q) mg*	*Niacin (R) mg*	*Ascorbic Acid (S) mg*
—	—	—	19	17	24	0.5	344	50	0.07	0.02	0.2	102
—	—	—	13	13	16	0.5	258	40	0.05	0.02	0.2	81
—	—	—	112	9	13	0.4	153	40	0.05	0.06	0.7	66
—	—	—	28	2	3	0.1	40	10	0.01	0.02	0.2	17
—	—	—	108	11	13	0.2	129	TR	0.02	0.02	0.2	26
—	—	—	27	3	3	TR	32	TR	TR	TR	TR	6
—	—	—	22	22	27	0.5	256	20	0.05	0.02	0.2	79
—	—	—	22	22	27	0.5	256	20	0.05	0.02	0.2	52
—	—	—	20	38	44	1.1	682	9,240	0.11	0.08	1.6	90
—	—	—	11	21	24	0.6	374	60	0.06	0.04	0.9	34
—	—	—	16	54	26	0.5	263	260	0.13	0.05	0.5	66
—	—	—	22	74	36	0.7	360	360	0.18	0.07	0.7	90
—	—	—	26	27	42	0.5	496	500	0.22	0.07	1.0	124
—	—	—	28	25	45	1.0	496	500	0.17	0.05	0.7	100
—	—	—	87	75	126	0.9	1,500	1,620	0.68	0.11	2.8	360
—	—	—	29	25	42	0.2	503	540	0.23	0.03	0.9	120
—	—	—	27	25	40	0.5	518	500	0.20	0.07	1.0	109
—	—	—	78	61	99	0.8	1,308	800	0.48	0.06	2.3	302
—	—	—	26	20	32	0.2	439	270	0.15	0.02	0.7	102
—	—	—	14	28	22	0.4	328	2,450	0.06	0.06	0.4	78

(Continued)

APPENDIX C: (*Continued*)

Item No. (A)	Foods, approximate measures, units, and weight (edible part unless footnote indicate otherwise) (B)		g	Water (C) %	Food Energy (D) kcal	Pro-tein (E) g	Fat (F) g
	Fruits and Fruit Products—Con.						
	Peaches						
	Raw						
283	Whole, 2½-in diam., peeled, pitted (about 4 per lb with peels and pits)	1 peach	100	89	40	1	TR
284	Sliced	1 cup	170	89	65	1	TR
	Canned, yellow-fleshed, solids and liquid (halves or slices)						
285	Sirup pack	1 cup	256	79	200	1	TR
286	Water pack	1 cup	244	91	75	1	TR
	Dried						
287	Uncooked	1 cup	160	25	420	5	1
288	Cooked, unsweetened, halves and juice	1 cup	250	77	205	3	1
	Frozen, sliced, sweetened						
289	10-oz container	1 container	284	77	250	1	TR
290	Cup	1 cup	250	77	220	1	TR
	Pears						
	Raw, with skin, cored						
291	Bartlett, 2½-in diam. (about 2½ per lb with cores and stems)	1 pear	164	83	100	1	1
292	Bosc, 2½-in diam. (about 3 per lb with cores and stems)	1 pear	141	83	85	1	1
293	D'Anjou, 3-in diam. (about 2 per lb with cores and stems)	1 pear	200	83	120	1	1
294	Canned, solids and liquid, syrup pack, heavy (halves or slices)	1 cup	255	80	195	1	1
	Pineapple						
295	Raw, diced	1 cup	155	85	80	1	TR
	Canned, heavy sirup pack, solids and liquid						
296	Crushed, chunks, tidbits	1 cup	255	80	190	1	TR
	Slices and liquid						
297	Large	1 slice; 2¼ tbsp of liquid	105	80	80	TR	TR
298	Medium	1 slice; 1¼ tbsp of liquid	58	80	45	TR	TR
299	Pineapple juice, unsweetened, canned	1 cup	250	86	140	1	TR

[34]Represents yellow-fleshed varieties. For white-fleshed varieties, value is 50 International Units (I.U.) for 1 peach, 90 I.U. for 1 cup of slices.

[35]Value represents products with added ascorbic acid. For products without added ascorbic acid, value in milligrams is 116 for a 10-oz container, 103 for 1 cup.

							Nutrients in Indicated Quantity					
Fatty Acids												
	Unsaturated											
Satu-rated (Total) (G) g	Oleic (H) g	Lino-leic (I) g	Carbo-hydrate (J) g	Calcium (K) mg	Phos-phorus (L) mg	Iron (M) mg	Potas-sium (N) mg	Vitamin A Value (O) I.U.	Thiamin (P) mg	Ribo-flavin (Q) mg	Niacin (R) mg	Ascorbic Acid (S) mg
—	—	—	10	9	19	0.5	202	[34]1,330	0.02	0.05	1.0	7
—	—	—	16	15	32	0.9	343	[34]2,260	0.03	0.09	1.7	12
—	—	—	51	10	31	0.8	333	1,100	0.03	0.05	1.5	8
—	—	—	20	10	32	0.7	334	1,100	0.02	0.07	1.5	7
—	—	—	109	77	187	9.6	1,520	6,240	0.02	0.30	8.5	29
—	—	—	54	38	93	4.8	743	3,050	0.01	0.15	3.8	5
—	—	—	64	11	37	1.4	352	1,850	0.03	0.11	2.0	[35]116
—	—	—	57	10	33	1.3	310	1,630	0.03	0.10	1.8	[35]103
—	—	—	25	13	18	0.5	213	30	0.03	0.07	0.2	7
—	—	—	22	11	16	0.4	83	30	0.03	0.06	0.1	6
—	—	—	31	16	22	0.6	260	40	0.04	0.08	0.2	8
—	—	—	50	13	18	0.5	214	10	0.03	0.05	0.3	3
—	—	—	21	26	12	0.8	226	110	0.14	0.05	0.3	26
—	—	—	49	28	13	0.8	245	130	0.20	0.05	0.5	18
—	—	—	20	12	5	0.3	101	50	0.08	0.02	0.2	7
—	—	—	11	6	3	0.2	56	30	0.05	0.01	0.1	4
—	—	—	34	38	23	0.8	373	130	0.13	0.05	0.5	[27]80

(Continued)

APPENDIX C: *(Continued)*

Nutrients in Indicated Quantity

Item No. (A)	Foods, approximate measures, units, and weight (edible part unless footnotes indicate otherwise) (B)		g	Water (C) %	Food Energy (D) kcal	Pro-tein (E) g	Fat (F) g
Fruits and Fruit Products—Con.							
	Plums						
	Raw, without pits						
300	Japanese and hybrid (2⅛-in diam., about 6½ per lb with pits)	1 plum	66	87	30	TR	TR
301	Prune-type (1½-in diam., about 15 per lb with pits)	1 plum	28	79	20	TR	TR
	Canned, heavy sirup pack (Italian prunes), with pits and liquid						
302	Cup	1 cup[36]	272	77	215	1	TR
303	Portion	3 plums; 2¾ tbsp of liquid[36]	140	77	110	1	TR
	Prunes, dried, "softenized," with pits						
304	Uncooked	4 extra large or 5 large prunes[36]	49	28	110	1	TR
305	Cooked, unsweetened, all sizes, fruit and liquid	1 cup[36]	250	66	255	2	1
306	Prune juice, canned or bottled	1 cup	256	80	195	1	TR
	Raisins, seedless						
307	Cup, not pressed down	1 cup	145	18	420	4	TR
308	Packet, ½ oz (1½ tbsp)	1 packet	14	18	40	TR	TR
	Raspberries, red						
309	Raw, capped, whole	1 cup	123	84	70	1	1
310	Frozen, sweetened, 10-oz container	1 container	284	74	280	2	1
	Rhubarb, cooked, added sugar						
311	From raw	1 cup	270	63	380	1	TR
312	From frozen, sweetened	1 cup	270	63	385	1	1
	Strawberries						
313	Raw, whole berries, capped	1 cup	149	90	55	1	1
	Frozen, sweetened						
314	Sliced, 10-oz container	1 container	284	71	310	1	1
315	Whole, 1-lb container (about 1¾ cups)	1 container	454	76	415	2	1
316	Tangerine, raw, 2⅜-in diam., size 176, without peel (about 4 per lb with peels and seeds)	1 tangerine	86	87	40	1	TR
317	Tangerine juice, canned, sweetened	1 cup	249	87	125	1	TR
318	Watermelon, raw, 4 by 8 in wedge with rind and seeds (1/16 of 32⅔-lb melon, 10 by 16 in.)	1 wedge[37]	926	93	110	2	1

[36]Weight includes pits. After removal of the pits, the weight of the edible portion is 258 g for item 302, 133 g for item 303, 43 g for item 304, and 213 g for item 305.
[37]Weight includes rind and seeds. Without rind and seeds, weight of the edible portion is 426 g.

							Nutrients in Indicated Quantity					
Fatty Acids												
	Unsaturated											
Satu-rated (Total) (G) g	Oleic (H) g	Lino-leic (I) g	Carbo-hydrate (J) g	Calcium (K) mg	Phos-phorus (L) mg	Iron (M) mg	Potas-sium (N) mg	Vitamin A Value (O) I.U.	Thiamin (P) mg	Ribo-flavin (Q) mg	Niacin (R) mg	Ascorbic Acid (S) mg
—	—	—	8	8	12	0.3	112	160	0.02	0.02	0.3	4
—	—	—	6	3	5	0.1	48	80	0.01	0.01	0.1	1
—	—	—	56	23	26	2.3	367	3,130	0.05	0.05	1.0	5
—	—	—	29	12	13	1.2	189	1,610	0.03	0.03	0.5	3
—	—	—	29	22	34	1.7	298	690	0.04	0.07	0.7	1
—	—	—	67	51	79	3.8	695	1,590	0.07	0.15	1.5	2
—	—	—	49	36	51	1.8	602	—	0.03	0.03	1.0	5
—	—	—	112	90	146	5.1	1,106	30	0.16	0.12	0.7	1
—	—	—	11	9	14	0.5	107	TR	0.02	0.01	0.1	TR
—	—	—	17	27	27	1.1	207	160	0.04	0.11	1.1	31
—	—	—	70	37	48	1.7	284	200	0.06	0.17	1.7	60
—	—	—	97	211	41	1.6	548	220	0.05	0.14	0.8	16
—	—	—	98	211	32	1.9	475	190	0.05	0.11	0.5	16
—	—	—	13	31	31	1.5	244	90	0.04	0.10	0.9	88
—	—	—	79	40	48	2.0	318	90	0.06	0.17	1.4	151
—	—	—	107	59	73	2.7	472	140	0.09	0.27	2.3	249
—	—	—	10	34	15	0.3	108	360	0.05	0.02	0.1	27
—	—	—	30	44	35	0.5	440	1,040	0.15	0.05	0.2	54
—	—	—	27	30	43	2.1	426	2,510	0.13	0.13	0.9	30

(Continued)

APPENDIX C: (Continued)

Item No. (A)	Foods, approximate measures, units, and weight (edible part unless footnote indicate otherwise) (B)		g	Water (C) %	Food Energy (D) kcal	Pro-tein (E) g	Fat (F) g
					Nutrients in Indicated Quantity		
Grain Products							
	Bagel, 3-in diam.						
319	Egg	1 bagel	55	32	165	6	2
320	Water	1 bagel	55	29	165	6	1
321	Barley, pearled, light, uncooked	1 cup	200	11	700	16	2
	Biscuits, baking powder, 2-in diam. (enriched flour, vegetable shortening)						
322	From home recipe	1 biscuit	28	27	105	2	5
323	From mix	1 biscuit	28	29	90	2	3
	Breadcrumbs (enriched)[38]						
324	Dry, grated	1 cup	100	7	390	13	5
	Soft. See White bread (items 349–350)						
	Breads						
325	Boston brown bread, canned, slice, 3¼ by ½ in.[38]	1 slice	45	45	95	2	1
	Cracked-wheat bread (¾ enriched wheat flour, ¼ cracked wheat):[38]						
326	Loaf, 1 lb	1 loaf	454	35	1,195	39	10
327	Slice (18 per loaf)	1 slice	25	35	65	2	1
	French or Vienna bread, enriched:[38]						
328	Loaf, 1 lb	1 loaf	454	31	1,315	41	14
	Slice						
329	French (5 by 2½ by 1 in)	1 slice	35	31	100	3	1
330	Vienna (4¾ by 4 by ½ in)	1 slice	25	31	75	2	1
	Italian bread, enriched:						
331	Loaf, 1 lb	1 loaf	454	32	1,250	41	4
332	Slice, 4½ by 3¼ by ¾ in.	1 slice	30	32	85	3	TR
	Raisin bread, enriched:[38]						
333	Loaf, 1 lb	1 loaf	454	35	1,190	30	13
334	Slice (18 per loaf)	1 slice	25	35	65	2	1
	Rye bread						
	American, light (⅔ enriched wheat flour, ⅓ rye flour)						
335	Loaf, 1 lb	1 loaf	454	36	1,100	41	5
336	Slice (4¾ by 3¾ by 7/16 in)	1 slice	25	36	60	2	TR

[38]Made with vegetable shortening.
[39]Applies to product made with white cornmeal. With yellow cornmeal, value is 30 International Units (I.U.).

							Nutrients in Indicated Quantity					
Fatty Acids												
	Unsaturated											
Satu-rated (Total) (G) g	Oleic (H) g	Lino-leic (I) g	Carbo-hydrate (J) g	Calcium (K) mg	Phos-phorus (L) mg	Iron (M) mg	Potas-sium (N) mg	Vitamin A Value (O) I.U.	Thiamin (P) mg	Ribo-flavin (Q) mg	Niacin (R) mg	Ascorbic Acid (S) mg
0.5	0.9	0.8	28	9	43	1.2	41	30	0.14	0.10	1.2	0
0.2	0.4	0.6	30	8	41	1.2	42	0	0.15	0.11	1.4	0
0.3	0.2	0.8	158	32	378	4.0	320	0	0.24	0.10	6.2	0
1.2	2.0	1.2	13	34	49	0.4	33	TR	0.08	0.08	0.7	TR
0.6	1.1	0.7	15	19	65	0.6	32	TR	0.09	0.08	0.8	TR
1.0	1.6	1.4	73	122	141	3.6	152	TR	0.35	0.35	4.8	TR
0.1	0.2	0.2	21	41	72	0.9	131	[39]0	0.06	0.04	0.7	0
2.2	3.0	3.9	236	399	581	9.5	608	TR	1.52	1.13	14.4	TR
0.1	0.2	0.2	13	22	32	0.5	34	TR	0.08	0.06	0.8	TR
3.2	4.7	4.6	251	195	386	10.0	408	TR	1.80	1.10	15.0	TR
0.2	0.4	0.4	19	15	30	0.8	32	TR	0.14	0.08	1.2	TR
0.2	0.3	0.3	14	11	21	0.6	23	TR	0.10	0.06	0.8	TR
0.6	0.3	1.5	256	77	349	10.0	336	0	1.80	1.10	15.0	0
TR	TR	0.1	17	5	23	0.7	22	0	0.12	0.07	1.0	0
3.0	4.7	3.9	243	322	395	10.0	1,057	TR	1.70	1.07	10.7	TR
0.2	0.3	0.2	13	18	22	0.6	58	TR	0.09	0.06	0.6	TR
0.7	0.5	2.2	236	340	667	9.1	658	0	1.35	0.98	12.9	0
TR	TR	0.1	13	19	37	0.5	36	0	0.07	0.05	0.7	0

(Continued)

APPENDIX C: (Continued)

Item No. (A)	Foods, approximate measures, units, and weight (edible part unless footnote indicate otherwise) (B)		g	Water (C) %	Food Energy (D) kcal	Pro-tein (E) g	Fat (F) g
Grain Products—Con.							
	Rye bread—Continued						
	Pumpernickel ($\frac{2}{3}$ rye flour, $\frac{1}{3}$ enriched wheat flour)						
337	Loaf, 1 lb	1 loaf	454	34	1,115	41	5
338	Slice (5 by 4 by $\frac{3}{8}$ in)	1 slice	32	34	80	3	TR
	White bread, enriched[38]						
	Soft-crumb type						
339	Loaf, 1 lb	1 loaf	454	36	1,225	39	15
340	Slice (18 per loaf)	1 slice	25	36	70	2	1
341	Slice, toasted	1 slice	22	25	70	2	1
342	Slice (22 per loaf)	1 slice	20	36	55	2	1
343	Slice, toasted	1 slice	17	25	55	2	1
344	Loaf, 1$\frac{1}{2}$ lb	1 loaf	680	36	1,835	59	22
345	Slice (24 per loaf)	1 slice	28	36	75	2	1
346	Slice, toasted	1 slice	24	25	75	2	1
347	Slice (28 per loaf)	1 slice	24	36	65	2	1
348	Slice, toasted	1 slice	21	25	65	2	1
349	Cubes	1 cup	30	36	80	3	1
350	Crumbs	1 cup	45	36	120	4	1
	Firm-crumb type						
351	Loaf, 1 lb	1 loaf	454	35	1,245	41	17
352	Slice (20 per loaf)	1 slice	23	35	65	2	1
353	Slice, toasted	1 slice	20	24	65	2	1
354	Loaf, 2 lb	1 loaf	907	35	2,495	82	34
355	Slice (34 per loaf)	1 slice	27	35	75	2	1
356	Slice, toasted	1 slice	23	24	75	2	1
	Whole-wheat bread						
	Soft-crumb type[38]						
357	Loaf, 1 lb	1 loaf	454	36	1,095	41	12
358	Slice (16 per loaf)	1 slice	28	36	65	3	1
359	Slice, toasted	1 slice	24	24	65	3	1
	Firm-crumb type[38]						
360	Loaf, 1 lb	1 loaf	454	36	1,100	48	14
361	Slice (18 per loaf)	1 slice	25	36	60	3	1
362	Slice, toasted	1 slice	21	24	60	3	1

Nutrients in Indicated Quantity

						Nutrients in Indicated Quantity							
Fatty Acids													
	Unsaturated												
Satu-rated (Total) (G) g	*Oleic (H) g*	*Lino-leic (I) g*	*Carbo-hydrate (J) g*	*Calcium (K) mg*	*Phos-phorus (L) mg*	*Iron (M) mg*	*Potas-sium (N) mg*	*Vitamin A Value (O) I.U.*	*Thiamin (P) mg*	*Ribo-flavin (Q) mg*	*Niacin (R) mg*	*Ascorbic Acid (S) mg*
0.7	0.5	2.4	241	381	1,039	11.8	2,059	0	1.30	0.93	8.5	0
0.1	TR	0.2	17	27	73	0.8	145	0	0.09	0.07	0.6	0
3.4	5.3	4.6	229	381	440	11.3	476	TR	1.80	1.10	15.0	TR
0.2	0.3	0.3	13	21	24	0.6	26	TR	0.10	0.06	0.8	TR
0.2	0.3	0.3	13	21	24	0.6	26	TR	0.08	0.06	0.8	TR
0.2	0.2	0.2	10	17	19	0.5	21	TR	0.08	0.05	0.7	TR
0.2	0.2	0.2	10	17	19	0.5	21	TR	0.06	0.05	0.7	TR
5.2	7.9	6.9	343	571	660	17.0	714	TR	2.70	1.65	22.5	TR
0.2	0.3	0.3	14	24	27	0.7	29	TR	0.11	0.07	0.9	TR
0.2	0.3	0.3	14	24	27	0.7	29	TR	0.09	0.07	0.9	TR
0.2	0.3	0.2	12	20	23	0.6	25	TR	0.10	0.06	0.8	TR
0.2	0.3	0.2	12	20	23	0.6	25	TR	0.08	0.06	0.8	TR
0.2	0.3	0.3	15	25	29	0.8	32	TR	0.12	0.07	1.0	TR
0.3	0.5	0.5	23	38	44	1.1	47	TR	0.18	0.11	1.5	TR
3.9	5.9	5.2	228	435	463	11.3	549	TR	1.80	1.10	15.0	TR
0.2	0.3	0.3	12	22	23	0.6	28	TR	0.09	0.06	0.8	TR
0.2	0.3	0.3	12	22	23	0.6	28	TR	0.07	0.06	0.8	TR
7.7	11.8	10.4	455	871	925	22.7	1,097	TR	3.60	2.20	30.0	TR
0.2	0.3	0.3	14	26	28	0.7	33	TR	0.11	0.06	0.9	TR
0.2	0.3	0.3	14	26	28	0.7	33	TR	0.09	0.06	0.9	TR
2.2	2.9	4.2	224	381	1,152	13.6	1,161	TR	1.37	0.45	12.7	TR
0.1	0.2	0.2	14	24	71	0.8	72	TR	0.09	0.03	0.8	TR
0.1	0.2	0.2	14	24	71	0.8	72	TR	0.07	0.03	0.8	TR
2.5	3.3	4.9	216	449	1,034	13.6	1,238	TR	1.17	0.54	12.7	TR
0.1	0.2	0.3	12	25	57	0.8	68	TR	0.06	0.03	0.7	TR
0.1	0.2	0.3	12	25	57	0.8	68	TR	0.05	0.03	0.7	TR

(Continued)

APPENDIX C: (*Continued*)

				Nutrients in Indicated Quantity		

Item No. (A)	Foods, approximate measures, units, and weight (edible part unless footnotes indicate otherwise) (B)		g	Water (C) %	Food Energy (D) kcal	Pro- tein (E) g	Fat (F) g
Grain Products—Con.							
	Breakfast cereals						
	Hot type, cooked						
	Corn (hominy) grits, degermed						
363	Enriched	1 cup	245	87	125	3	TR
364	Unenriched	1 cup	245	87	125	3	TR
365	Farina, quick-cooking, enriched	1 cup	245	89	105	3	TR
366	Oatmeal or rolled oats	1 cup	240	87	130	5	2
367	Wheat, rolled	1 cup	240	80	180	5	1
368	Wheat, whole-meal	1 cup	245	88	110	4	1
	Ready-to-eat:						
369	Bran flakes (40% bran), added sugar, salt, iron, vitamins	1 cup	35	3	105	4	1
370	Bran flakes with raisins, added sugar, salt, iron, vitamins	1 cup	50	7	145	4	1
	Corn flakes						
371	Plain, added sugar, salt, iron, vitamins.	1 cup	25	4	95	2	TR
372	Sugar-coated, added salt, iron, vitamins	1 cup	40	2	155	2	TR
373	Corn, oat flour, puffed, added sugar, salt, iron, vitamins	1 cup	20	4	80	2	1
374	Corn, shredded, added sugar, salt, iron, thiamin, niacin	1 cup	25	3	95	2	TR
375	Oats, puffed, added sugar, salt, minerals, vitamins	1 cup	25	3	100	3	1
	Rice, puffed						
376	Plain, added iron, thiamin, niacin	1 cup	15	4	60	1	TR
377	Presweetened, added salt, iron, vitamins	1 cup	28	3	115	1	0
378	Wheat flakes, added sugar, salt, iron, vitamins	1 cup	30	4	105	3	TR
	Wheat, puffed						
379	Plain, added iron, thiamin, niacin	1 cup	15	3	55	2	TR
380	Presweetened, added salt, iron, vitamins	1 cup	38	3	140	3	TR

[40] Applies to white varieties. For yellow varieties, value is 150 International Units (I.U.).
[41] Applies to products that do not contain di-sodium phosphate. If di-sodium phosphate is an ingredient, value is 162 mg.
[42] Value may range from less than 1 mg to about 8 mg depending on the brand. Consult the label.
[43] Applies to product with added nutrient. Without added nutrient, value is trace.
[44] Value varies with the brand. Consult the label.
[45] Applies to product with added nutrient. Without added nutrient, value is trace.

								Nutrients in Indicated Quantity					
Fatty Acids													
	Unsaturated												
Satu-rated (Total) (G) g	Oleic (H) g	Lino-leic (I) g	Carbo-hydrate (J) g	Calcium (K) mg	Phos-phorus (L) mg	Iron (M) mg	Potas-sium (N) mg	Vitamin A Value (O) I.U.	Thiamin (P) mg	Ribo-flavin (Q) mg	Niacin (R) mg	Ascorbic Acid (S) mg
TR	TR	0.1	27	2	25	0.7	27	[40]TR	0.10	0.07	1.0	0
TR	TR	0.1	27	2	25	0.2	27	[40]TR	0.05	0.02	0.5	0
TR	TR	0.1	22	147	[41]113	([42])	25	0	0.12	0.07	1.0	0
0.4	0.8	0.9	23	22	137	1.4	146	0	0.19	0.05	0.2	0
—	—	—	41	19	182	1.7	202	0	0.17	0.07	2.2	0
—	—	—	23	17	127	1.2	118	0	0.15	0.05	1.5	0
—	—	—	28	19	125	5.6	137	1,540	0.46	0.52	6.2	0
—	—	—	40	28	146	7.9	154	[43]2,200	([44])	([44])	([44])	0
—	—	—	21	([44])	9	([44])	30	([44])	([44])	([44])	([44])	[45]13
—	—	—	37	1	10	([44])	27	1,760	0.53	0.60	7.1	[45]21
—	—	—	16	4	18	5.7	—	880	0.26	0.30	3.5	11
—	—	—	22	1	10	0.6	—	0	0.33	0.05	4.4	13
—	—	—	19	44	102	4.0	—	1,100	0.33	0.38	4.4	13
—	—	—	13	3	14	0.3	15	0	0.07	0.01	0.7	0
—	—	—	26	3	14	([44])	43	[45]1,240	([44])	([44])	([44])	[45]15
—	—	—	24	12	83	4.8	81	1,320	0.40	0.45	5.3	16
—	—	—	12	4	48	0.6	51	0	0.08	0.03	1.2	0
—	—	—	33	7	52	([44])	63	1,680	0.50	0.57	6.7	[45]20

(Continued)

APPENDIX C: (Continued)

Item No. (A)	Foods, approximate measures, units, and weight (edible part unless footnote indicate otherwise) (B)		g	Water (C) %	Food Energy (D) kcal	Pro- tein (E) g	Fat (F) g
					Nutrients in Indicated Quantity		
Grain Products—Con.							
	Breakfast cereals—Continued						
	Ready-to-eat—Continued						
381	Wheat, shredded, plain	1 oblong biscuit or ½ cup spoon-size biscuits	25	7	90	2	1
382	Wheat germ, without salt and sugar, toasted	1 tbsp	6	4	25	2	1
383	Buckwheat flour, light, sifted	1 cup	98	12	340	6	1
384	Bulgur, canned, seasoned	1 cup	135	56	245	8	4
	Cake icings. See Sugars and Sweets (items 532–536)						
	Cakes made from cake mixes with enriched flour[46]						
	Angelfood						
385	Whole cake (9¾-in diam. tube cake)	1 cake	635	34	1,645	36	1
386	Piece, 1⁄12 of cake	1 piece	53	34	135	3	TR
	Coffee cake						
387	Whole cake (7¾ by 5⅝ by 1¼ in)	1 cake	430	30	1,385	27	41
388	Piece, ⅙ of cake	1 piece	72	30	230	5	7
	Cupcakes, made with egg, milk, 2½-in diam.						
389	Without icing	1 cupcake	25	26	90	1	3
390	With chocolate icing	1 cupcake	36	22	130	2	5
	Devil's food with chocolate icing						
391	Whole, 2 layer cake (8- or 9-in diam.)	1 cake	1,107	24	3,755	49	136
392	Piece, 1⁄16 of cake	1 piece	69	24	235	3	8
393	Cupcake, 2½-in diam.	1 cupcake	35	24	120	2	4
	Gingerbread						
394	Whole cake (8-in square)	1 cake	570	37	1,575	18	39
395	Piece, ⅑ of cake	1 piece	63	37	175	2	4
	White, 2 layer with chocolate icing						
396	Whole cake (8- or 9-in. diam.)	1 cake	1,140	21	4,000	44	122
397	Piece 1⁄16 of cake	1 piece	71	21	250	3	8
	Yellow, 2 layer with chocolate icing						
398	Whole cake (8- or 9-in. diam.)	1 cake	1,108	26	3,735	45	125
399	Piece, 1⁄16 of cake	1 piece	69	26	235	3	8

[46]Excepting angelfood cake, cakes were made from mixes containing vegetable shortening; icings, with butter.

								Nutrients in Indicated Quantity					
Fatty Acids													
	Unsaturated												
Satu-rated (Total) (G) g	Oleic (H) g	Lino-leic (I) g	Carbo-hydrate (J) g	Calcium (K) mg	Phos-phorus (L) mg	Iron (M) mg	Potas-sium (N) mg	Vitamin A Value (O) I.U.	Thiamin (P) mg	Ribo-flavin (Q) mg	Niacin (R) mg	Ascorbic Acid (S) mg
---	---	---	---	---	---	---	---	---	---	---	---	---
—	—	—	20	11	97	0.9	87	0	0.06	0.03	1.1	0
—	—	—	3	3	70	0.5	57	10	0.11	0.05	0.3	1
0.2	0.4	0.4	78	11	86	1.0	314	0	0.08	0.04	0.4	0
—	—	—	44	27	263	1.9	151	0	0.08	0.05	4.1	0
—	—	—	377	603	756	2.5	381	0	0.37	0.95	3.6	0
—	—	—	32	50	63	0.2	32	0	0.03	0.08	0.3	0
11.7	16.3	8.8	225	262	748	6.9	469	690	0.82	0.91	7.7	1
2.0	2.7	1.5	38	44	125	1.2	78	120	0.14	0.15	1.3	TR
0.8	1.2	0.7	14	40	59	0.3	21	40	0.05	0.05	0.4	TR
2.0	1.6	0.6	21	47	71	0.4	42	60	0.05	0.06	0.4	TR
50.0	44.9	17.0	645	653	1,162	16.6	1,439	1,660	1.06	1.65	10.1	1
3.1	2.8	1.1	40	41	72	1.0	90	100	0.07	0.10	0.6	TR
1.6	1.4	0.5	20	21	37	0.5	46	50	0.03	0.05	0.3	TR
9.7	16.6	10.0	291	513	570	8.6	1,562	TR	0.84	1.00	7.4	TR
1.1	1.8	1.1	32	57	63	0.9	173	TR	0.09	0.11	0.8	TR
48.2	46.4	20.0	716	1,129	2,041	11.4	1,322	680	1.50	1.77	12.5	2
3.0	2.9	1.2	45	70	127	0.7	82	40	0.09	0.11	0.8	TR
47.8	47.8	20.3	638	1,008	2,017	12.2	1,208	1,550	1.24	1.67	10.6	2
3.0	3.0	1.3	40	63	126	0.8	75	100	0.08	0.10	0.7	TR

(Continued)

APPENDIX C: (*Continued*)

Item No. (A)	Foods, approximate measures, units, and weight (edible part unless footnote indicate otherwise) (B)		g	Water (C) %	Food Energy (D) kcal	Pro- tein (E) g	Fat (F) g
Grain Products—Con.							
	Cakes made from home recipes using enriched flour[47]						
	Boston cream pie with custard filling						
400	Whole cake (8-in. diam.)	1 cake	825	35	2,490	41	78
401	Piece, $\frac{1}{12}$ of cake	1 piece	69	35	210	3	6
	Fruitcake, dark						
402	Loaf, 1-lb ($7\frac{1}{2}$ by 2 by $1\frac{1}{2}$ in.)	1 loaf	454	18	1,720	22	69
403	Slice, $\frac{1}{30}$ of loaf	1 slice	15	18	55	1	2
	Plain, sheet cake						
	Without icing						
404	Whole cake (9-in. square)	1 cake	777	25	2,830	35	108
405	Piece, $\frac{1}{9}$ of cake	1 piece	86	25	315	4	12
	With uncooked white icing						
406	Whole cake (9-in. square)	1 cake	1,096	21	4,020	37	129
407	Piece, $\frac{1}{9}$ of cake	1 piece	121	21	445	4	14
	Pound[49]						
408	Loaf, $8\frac{1}{2}$ by $3\frac{1}{2}$ by $3\frac{1}{4}$ in.	1 loaf	565	16	2,725	31	170
409	Slice, $\frac{1}{17}$ of loaf	1 slice	33	16	160	2	10
	Spongecake:						
410	Whole cake ($9\frac{3}{4}$-in diam. tube cake)	1 cake	790	32	2,345	60	45
411	Piece, $\frac{1}{12}$ of cake	1 piece	66	32	195	5	4
	Cookies made with enriched flour[50,51]						
	Brownies with nuts						
	Home-prepared, $1\frac{3}{4}$ by $1\frac{3}{4}$ by $\frac{7}{8}$ in.						
412	From home recipe	1 brownie	20	10	95	1	6
413	From commercial recipe	1 brownie	20	11	85	1	4
414	Frozen, with chocolate icing,[52] 1½ by 1¾ by ⅞ in.	1 brownie	25	13	105	1	5

[47]Excepting spongecake, vegetable shortening used for cake portion; butter, for icing. If butter or margarine used for cake portion, vitamin A values would be higher.

[48]Applies to product made with a sodium aluminum-sulfate type baking powder. With a low-sodium type baking powder containing potassium, value would be about twice the amount shown.

[49]Equal weights of flour, sugar, eggs, and vegetable shortening.

[50]Products are commercial unless otherwise specified.

[51]Made with enriched flour and vegetable shortening except for macaroons which do not contain flour or shortening.

[52]Icing made with butter.

	Nutrients in Indicated Quantity												
Fatty Acids													
Satu-rated (Total) (G) g	Unsaturated		Carbo-hydrate (J) g	Calcium (K) mg	Phos-phorus (L) mg	Iron (M) mg	Potas-sium (N) mg	Vitamin A Value (O) I.U.	Thiamin (P) mg	Ribo-flavin (Q) mg	Niacin (R) mg	Ascorbic Acid (S) mg
	Oleic (H) g	Lino-leic (I) g										
23.0	30.1	15.2	412	553	833	8.2	[48]734	1,730	1.04	1.27	9.6	2
1.9	2.5	1.3	34	46	70	0.7	[48]61	140	0.09	0.11	0.8	TR
14.4	33.5	14.8	271	327	513	11.8	2,250	540	0.72	0.73	4.9	2
0.5	1.1	0.5	9	11	17	0.4	74	20	0.02	0.02	0.2	TR
29.5	44.4	23.9	434	497	793	8.5	[48]614	1,320	1.21	1.40	10.2	2
3.3	4.9	2.6	48	55	88	0.9	[48]68	150	0.13	0.15	1.1	TR
42.2	49.5	24.4	694	548	822	8.2	[48]669	2,190	1.22	1.47	10.2	2
4.7	5.5	2.7	77	61	91	0.8	[48]74	240	0.14	0.16	1.1	TR
42.9	73.1	39.6	273	107	418	7.9	345	1,410	0.90	0.99	7.3	0
2.5	4.3	2.3	16	6	24	0.5	20	80	0.05	0.06	0.4	0
13.1	15.8	5.7	427	237	885	13.4	687	3,560	1.10	1.64	7.4	TR
1.1	1.3	0.5	36	20	74	1.1	57	300	0.09	0.14	0.6	TR
1.5	3.0	1.2	10	8	30	0.4	38	40	0.04	0.03	0.2	TR
0.9	1.4	1.3	13	9	27	0.4	34	20	0.03	0.02	0.2	TR
2.0	2.2	0.7	15	10	31	0.4	44	50	0.03	0.03	0.2	TR

(Continued)

APPENDIX C: (Continued)

Item No. (A)	Foods, approximate measures, units, and weight (edible part unless footnotes indicate otherwise) (B)		g	Water (C) %	Nutrients in Indicated Quantity Food Energy (D) kcal	Pro- tein (E) g	Fat (F) g
Grain Products—Con.							
	Cookies made with enriched flour[50,51]—Continued						
	Chocolate chip						
415	Commercial, 2¼-in. diam., ⅜ in. thick	4 cookies	42	3	200	2	9
416	From home recipe, 2⅓-in. diam.	4 cookies	40	3	205	2	12
417	Fig bars, square (1⅝ by 1⅝ by ⅜ in.) or rectangular (1½ by 1¾ by ½ in.)	4 cookies	56	14	200	2	3
418	Gingersnaps, 2-in diam., ¼ in thick	4 cookies	28	3	90	2	2
419	Macaroons, 2¾-in diam., ¼ in thick	2 cookies	38	4	180	2	9
420	Oatmeal with raisins, 2⅝-in diam., ¼ in thick	4 cookies	52	3	235	3	8
421	Plain, prepared from commercial chilled dough, 2½-in diam., ¼ in thick	4 cookies	48	5	240	2	12
422	Sandwich type (chocolate or vanilla), 1¾-in diam., ⅜ in thick	4 cookies	40	2	200	2	9
423	Vanilla wafers, 1¾-in diam., ¼ in. thick	10 cookies	40	3	185	2	6
	Cornmeal						
424	Whole-ground, unbolted, dry form	1 cup	122	12	435	11	5
425	Bolted (nearly whole-grain), dry form	1 cup	122	12	440	11	4
	Degermed, enriched						
426	Dry form	1 cup	138	12	500	11	2
427	Cooked	1 cup	240	88	120	3	TR
	Degermed, unenriched						
428	Dry form	1 cup	138	12	500	11	2
429	Cooked	1 cup	240	88	120	3	TR
	Crackers[38]						
430	Graham, plain, 2½-in square	2 crackers	14	6	55	1	1
431	Rye wafers, whole-grain, 1⅞ by 3½ in.	2 wafers	13	6	45	2	TR
432	Saltines, made with enriched flour	4 crackers	11	4	50	1	1
	Danish pastry (enriched flour), plain without fruit or nuts:[54]						
433	Packaged ring, 12 oz	1 ring	340	22	1,435	25	80
434	Round piece, about 4¼-in diam. by 1 in.	1 pastry	65	22	275	5	15
435	Ounce	1 oz	28	22	120	2	7
	Doughnuts, made with enriched flour:[38]						
436	Cake type, plain, 2½-in diam., 1 in high	1 doughnut	25	24	100	1	5
437	Yeast-leavened, glazed, 3¾-in diam., 1¼ in high	1 doughnut	50	26	205	3	11

[53]Applies to yellow varieties; white varieties contain only a trace.
[54]Contains vegetable shortening and butter.

						Nutrients in Indicated Quantity						
Fatty Acids												
Satu-rated (Total) (G) g	*Unsaturated*		Carbo-hydrate (J) g	Calcium (K) mg	Phos-phorus (L) mg	Iron (M) mg	Potas-sium (N) mg	Vitamin A Value (O) I.U.	Thiamin (P) mg	Ribo-flavin (Q) mg	Niacin (R) mg	Ascorbic Acid (S) mg
	Oleic (H) g	Lino-leic (I) g										
2.8	2.9	2.2	29	16	48	1.0	56	50	0.10	0.17	0.9	TR
3.5	4.5	2.9	24	14	40	0.8	47	40	0.06	0.06	0.5	TR
0.8	1.2	0.7	42	44	34	1.0	111	60	0.04	0.14	0.9	TR
0.7	1.0	0.6	22	20	13	0.7	129	20	0.08	0.06	0.7	0
—	—	—	25	10	32	0.3	176	0	0.02	0.06	0.2	0
2.0	3.3	2.0	38	11	53	1.4	192	30	0.15	0.10	1.0	TR
3.0	5.2	2.9	31	17	35	0.6	23	30	0.10	0.08	0.9	0
2.2	3.9	2.2	28	10	96	0.7	15	0	0.06	0.10	0.7	0
—	—	—	30	16	25	0.6	29	50	0.10	0.09	0.8	0
0.5	1.0	2.5	90	24	312	2.9	246	[53]620	0.46	0.13	2.4	0
0.5	0.9	2.1	91	21	272	2.2	303	[53]590	0.37	0.10	2.3	0
0.2	0.4	0.9	108	8	137	4.0	166	[53]610	0.61	0.36	4.8	0
TR	0.1	0.2	26	2	34	1.0	38	[53]140	0.14	0.10	1.2	0
0.2	0.4	0.9	108	8	137	1.5	166	[53]610	0.19	0.07	1.4	0
TR	0.1	0.2	26	2	34	0.5	38	[53]140	0.05	0.02	0.2	0
0.3	0.5	0.3	10	6	21	0.5	55	0	0.02	0.08	0.5	0
—	—	—	10	7	50	0.5	78	0	0.04	0.03	0.2	0
0.3	0.5	0.4	8	2	10	0.5	13	0	0.05	0.05	0.4	0
24.3	31.7	16.5	155	170	371	6.1	381	1,050	0.97	1.01	8.6	TR
4.7	6.1	3.2	30	33	71	1.2	73	200	0.18	0.19	1.7	TR
2.0	2.7	1.4	13	14	31	0.5	32	90	0.08	0.08	0.7	TR
1.2	2.0	1.1	13	10	48	0.4	23	20	0.05	0.05	0.4	TR
3.3	5.8	3.3	22	16	33	0.6	34	25	0.10	0.10	0.8	0

(Continued)

APPENDIX C: (*Continued*)

				Nutrients in Indicated Quantity			
Item No. (A)	Foods, approximate measures, units, and weight (edible part unless footnote indicate otherwise) (B)		g	Water (C) %	Food Energy (D) kcal	Pro-tein (E) g	Fat (F) g

Grain Products—Con.							
	Macaroni, enriched, cooked (cut lengths, elbows, shells)						
438	Firm stage (hot)	1 cup	130	64	190	7	1
	Tender stage						
439	Cold macaroni	1 cup	105	73	115	4	TR
440	Hot macaroni	1 cup	140	73	155	5	1
	Macaroni (enriched) and cheese:						
441	Canned[55]	1 cup	240	80	230	9	10
442	From home recipe (served hot)[56]	1 cup	200	58	430	17	22
	Muffins made with enriched flour:[38]						
	From home recipe						
443	Blueberry, $2\frac{3}{8}$-in diam., $1\frac{1}{2}$ in high	1 muffin	40	39	110	3	4
444	Bran	1 muffin	40	35	105	3	4
445	Corn (enriched degermed cornmeal and flour), $2\frac{3}{8}$-in. diam., $1\frac{1}{2}$ in high	1 muffin	40	33	125	3	4
446	Plain, 3-in diam., $1\frac{1}{2}$ in high	1 muffin	40	38	120	3	4
	From mix, egg, milk						
447	Corn, $2\frac{3}{8}$-in diam., $1\frac{1}{2}$ in high[58]	1 muffin	40	30	130	3	4
448	Noodles (egg noodles), enriched, cooked	1 cup	160	71	200	7	2
449	Noodles, chow mein, canned	1 cup	45	1	220	6	11
	Pancakes, (4-in diam.)[38]						
450	Buckwheat, made from mix (with buckwheat and enriched flours), egg and milk added	1 cake	27	58	55	2	2
	Plain						
451	Made from home recipe using enriched flour	1 cake	27	50	60	2	2
452	Made from mix with enriched flour, egg and milk added	1 cake	27	51	60	2	2
	Pies, piecrust made with enriched flour, vegetable shortening (9-in diam.)						
	Apple						
453	Whole	1 pie	945	48	2,420	21	105
454	Sector, $\frac{1}{7}$ of pie	1 sector	135	48	345	3	15

[55]Made with corn oil.
[56]Made with regular margarine.
[57]Applies to product made with yellow cornmeal.
[58]Made with enriched degermed cornmeal and enriched flour.

						Nutrients in Indicated Quantity						
Fatty Acids												
	Unsaturated											
Satu-rated (Total) (G) g	Oleic (H) g	Lino-leic (I) g	Carbo-hydrate (J) g	Calcium (K) mg	Phos-phorus (L) mg	Iron (M) mg	Potas-sium (N) mg	Vitamin A Value (O) I.U.	Thiamin (P) mg	Ribo-flavin (Q) mg	Niacin (R) mg	Ascorbic Acid (S) mg
—	—	—	39	14	85	1.4	103	0	0.23	0.13	1.8	0
—	—	—	24	8	53	0.9	64	0	0.15	0.08	1.2	0
—	—	—	32	11	70	1.3	85	0	0.20	0.11	1.5	0
4.2	3.1	1.4	26	199	182	1.0	139	260	0.12	0.24	1.0	TR
8.9	8.8	2.9	40	362	322	1.8	240	860	0.20	0.40	1.8	TR
1.1	1.4	0.7	17	34	53	0.6	46	90	0.09	0.10	0.7	TR
1.2	1.4	0.8	17	57	162	1.5	172	90	0.07	0.10	1.7	TR
1.2	1.6	0.9	19	42	68	0.7	54	[57]120	0.10	0.10	0.7	TR
1.0	1.7	1.0	17	42	60	0.6	50	40	0.09	0.12	0.9	TR
1.2	1.7	0.9	20	96	152	0.6	44	[57]100	0.08	0.09	0.7	TR
—	—	—	37	16	94	1.4	70	110	0.22	0.13	1.9	0
—	—	—	26	—	—	—	—	—	—	—	—	—
0.8	0.9	0.4	6	59	91	0.4	66	60	0.04	0.05	0.2	TR
0.5	0.8	0.5	9	27	38	0.4	33	30	0.06	0.07	0.5	TR
0.7	0.7	0.3	9	58	70	0.3	42	70	0.04	0.06	0.2	TR
27.0	44.5	25.2	360	76	208	6.6	756	280	1.06	0.79	9.3	9
3.9	6.4	3.6	51	11	30	0.9	108	40	0.15	0.11	1.3	2

(Continued)

APPENDIX C: (*Continued*)

				Nutrients in Indicated Quantity			

Item No. (A)	Foods, approximate measures, units, and weight (edible part unless footnote indicate otherwise) (B)		g	Water (C) %	Food Energy (D) kcal	Pro- tein (E) g	Fat (F) g
Grain Products—Con.							
	Pies, piecrust made with enriched flour, vegetable shortening (9-in diam.)—Continued						
	Banana cream						
455	Whole	1 pie	910	54	2,010	41	85
456	Sector, ⅓ of pie	1 sector	130	54	285	6	12
	Blueberry						
457	Whole	1 pie	945	51	2,285	23	102
458	Sector, ⅓ of pie	1 sector	135	51	325	3	15
	Cherry						
459	Whole	1 pie	945	47	2,465	25	107
460	Sector, ⅓ of pie	1 sector	135	47	350	4	15
	Custard						
461	Whole	1 pie	910	58	1,985	56	101
462	Sector, ⅓ of pie	1 sector	130	58	285	8	14
	Lemon meringue						
463	Whole	1 pie	840	47	2,140	31	86
464	Sector, ⅓ of pie	1 sector	120	47	305	4	12
	Mince						
465	Whole	1 pie	945	43	2,560	24	109
466	Sector, ⅓ of pie	1 sector	135	43	365	3	16
	Peach						
467	Whole	1 pie	945	48	2,410	24	101
468	Sector, ⅓ of pie	1 sector	135	48	345	3	14
	Pecan						
469	Whole	1 pie	825	20	3,450	42	189
470	Sector, ⅓ of pie	1 sector	118	20	495	6	27
	Pumpkin						
471	Whole	1 pie	910	59	1,920	36	102
472	Sector, ⅓ of pie	1 sector	130	59	275	5	15
473	Piecrust (home recipe) made with enriched flour and vegetable shortening, baked	1 pie shell, 9 in diam.	180	15	900	11	60
474	Piecrust mix with enriched flour and vegetable shortening, 10-oz pkg. prepared and baked	Piecrust for 2 crust pie 9-in diam.	320	19	1,485	20	93
475	Pizza (cheese) baked, 4¾-in sector; ⅛ of 12-in diam. pie.[19]	1 sector	60	45	145	6	4
	Popcorn, popped						
476	Plain, large kernel	1 cup	6	4	25	1	TR

							Nutrients in Indicated Quantity					
Fatty Acids												
	Unsaturated											
Satu-rated (Total) (G) g	Oleic (H) g	Lino-leic (I) g	Carbo-hydrate (J) g	Calcium (K) mg	Phos-phorus (L) mg	Iron (M) mg	Potas-sium (N) mg	Vitamin A Value (O) I.U.	Thiamin (P) mg	Ribo-flavin (Q) mg	Niacin (R) mg	Ascorbic Acid (S) mg
26.7	33.2	16.2	279	601	746	7.3	1,847	2,280	0.77	1.51	7.0	9
3.8	4.7	2.3	40	86	107	1.0	264	330	0.11	0.22	1.0	1
24.8	43.7	25.1	330	104	217	9.5	614	280	1.03	0.80	10.0	28
3.5	6.2	3.6	47	15	31	1.4	88	40	0.15	0.11	1.4	4
28.2	45.0	25.3	363	132	236	6.6	992	4,160	1.09	0.84	9.8	TR
4.0	6.4	3.6	52	19	34	0.9	142	590	0.16	0.12	1.4	TR
33.9	38.5	17.5	213	874	1,028	8.2	1,247	2,090	0.79	1.92	5.6	0
4.8	5.5	2.5	30	125	147	1.2	178	300	0.11	0.27	0.8	0
26.1	33.8	16.4	317	118	412	6.7	420	1,430	0.61	0.84	5.2	25
3.7	4.8	2.3	45	17	59	1.0	60	200	0.09	0.12	0.7	4
28.0	45.9	25.2	389	265	359	13.3	1,682	20	0.96	0.86	9.8	9
4.0	6.6	3.6	56	38	51	1.9	240	TR	0.14	0.12	1.4	1
24.8	43.7	25.1	361	95	274	8.5	1,408	6,900	1.04	0.97	14.0	28
3.5	6.2	3.6	52	14	39	1.2	201	990	0.15	0.14	2.0	4
27.8	101.0	44.2	423	388	850	25.6	1,015	1,320	1.80	0.95	6.9	TR
4.0	14.4	6.3	61	55	122	3.7	145	190	0.26	0.14	1.0	TR
37.4	37.5	16.6	223	464	628	7.3	1,456	22,480	0.78	1.27	7.0	TR
5.4	5.4	2.4	32	66	90	1.0	208	3,210	0.11	0.18	1.0	TR
14.8	26.1	14.9	79	25	90	3.1	89	0	0.47	0.40	5.0	0
22.7	39.7	23.4	141	131	272	6.1	179	0	1.07	0.79	9.9	0
1.7	1.5	0.6	22	86	89	1.1	67	230	0.16	0.18	1.6	4
TR	0.1	0.2	5	1	17	0.2	—	—	—	0.01	0.1	0

(Continued)

APPENDIX C: *(Continued)*

Item No. (A)	Foods, approximate measures, units, and weight (edible part unless footnotes indicate otherwise) (B)		g	Water (C) %	Food Energy (D) kcal	Pro- tein (E) g	Fat (F) g
Grain Products—Con.							
	Popcorn, popped—Continued						
477	With oil (coconut) and salt added, large kernel	1 cup	9	3	40	1	2
478	Sugar coated	1 cup	35	4	135	2	1
	Pretzels, made with enriched flour						
479	Dutch, twisted, 2¾ by 2⅝ in.	1 pretzel	16	5	60	2	1
480	Thin, twisted, 3¼ by 2¼ by ¼ in.	10 pretzels	60	5	235	6	3
481	Stick, 2¼ in long	10 pretzels	3	5	10	TR	TR
	Rice, white, enriched						
482	Instant, ready-to-serve, hot	1 cup	165	73	180	4	TR
	Long grain						
483	Raw	1 cup	185	12	670	12	1
484	Cooked, served hot	1 cup	205	73	225	4	TR
	Parboiled						
485	Raw	1 cup	185	10	685	14	1
486	Cooked, served hot	1 cup	175	73	185	4	TR
	Rolls, enriched:[38]						
	Commercial						
487	Brown-and-serve (12 per 12-oz pkg.), browned	1 roll	26	27	85	2	2
488	Cloverleaf or pan, 2½-in diam., 2 in. high	1 roll	28	31	85	2	2
489	Frankfurter and hamburger (8 per 11½-oz pkg.)	1 roll	40	31	120	3	2
490	Hard, 3¾-in diam., 2 in high	1 roll	50	25	155	5	2
491	Hoagie or submarine, 11½ by 3 by 2½ in.	1 roll	135	31	390	12	4
	From home recipe						
492	Cloverleaf, 2½-in diam., 2 in high	1 roll	35	26	120	3	3
	Spaghetti, enriched, cooked:						
493	Firm stage, "al dente," served hot	1 cup	130	64	190	7	1
494	Tender stage, served hot	1 cup	140	73	155	5	1
	Spaghetti (enriched) in tomato sauce with cheese						
495	From home recipe	1 cup	250	77	260	9	9
496	Canned	1 cup	250	80	190	6	2
	Spaghetti (enriched) with meat balls and tomato sauce						
497	From home recipe	1 cup	248	70	330	19	12

[59]Product may or may not be enriched with riboflavin. Consult the label.

						Nutrients in Indicated Quantity							
Fatty Acids													
	Unsaturated												
Satu-rated (Total) (G) g	Oleic (H) g	Lino-leic (I) g	Carbo-hydrate (J) g	Calcium (K) mg	Phos-phorus (L) mg	Iron (M) mg	Potas-sium (N) mg	Vitamin A Value (O) I.U.	Thiamin (P) mg	Ribo-flavin (Q) mg	Niacin (R) mg	Ascorbic Acid (S) mg
1.5	0.2	0.2	5	1	19	0.2	—	—	—	0.01	0.2	0
0.5	0.2	0.4	30	2	47	0.5	—	—	—	0.02	0.4	0
—	—	—	12	4	21	0.2	21	0	0.05	0.04	0.7	0
—	—	—	46	13	79	0.9	78	0	0.20	0.15	2.5	0
—	—	—	2	1	4	TR	4	0	0.01	0.01	0.1	0
TR	TR	TR	40	5	31	1.3	—	0	0.21	([59])	1.7	0
0.2	0.2	0.2	149	44	174	5.4	170	0	0.81	0.06	6.5	0
0.1	0.1	0.1	50	21	57	1.8	57	0	0.23	0.02	2.1	0
0.2	0.1	0.2	150	111	370	5.4	278	0	0.81	0.07	6.5	0
0.1	0.1	0.1	41	33	100	1.4	75	0	0.19	0.02	2.1	0
0.4	0.7	0.5	14	20	23	0.5	25	TR	0.10	0.06	0.9	TR
0.4	0.6	0.4	15	21	24	0.5	27	TR	0.11	0.07	0.9	TR
0.5	0.8	0.6	21	30	34	0.8	38	TR	0.16	0.10	1.3	TR
0.4	0.6	0.5	30	24	46	1.2	49	TR	0.20	0.12	1.7	TR
0.9	1.4	1.4	75	58	115	3.0	122	TR	0.54	0.32	4.5	TR
0.8	1.1	0.7	20	16	36	0.7	41	30	0.12	0.12	1.2	
—	—	—	39	14	85	1.4	103	0	0.23	0.13	1.8	0
—	—	—	32	11	70	1.3	85	0	0.20	0.11	1.5	0
2.0	5.4	0.7	37	80	135	2.3	408	1,080	0.25	0.18	2.3	13
0.5	0.3	0.4	39	40	88	2.8	303	930	0.35	0.28	4.5	10
3.3	6.3	0.9	39	124	236	3.7	665	1,590	0.25	0.30	4.0	22

(Continued)

APPENDIX C: *(Continued)*

							Nutrients in Indicated Quantity

Item No. (A)	Foods, approximate measures, units, and weight (edible part unless footnote indicate otherwise) (B)		g	Water (C) %	Food Energy (D) kcal	Pro-tein (E) g	Fat (F) g
Grain Products—Con.							
	Spaghetti (enriched) with meatballs and tomato sauce—Continued						
498	Canned	1 cup	250	78	260	12	10
499	Toaster pastries	1 pastry	50	12	200	3	6
	Waffles, made with enriched flour, 7-in diam.[38]						
500	From home recipe	1 waffle	75	41	210	7	7
501	From mix, egg and milk added	1 waffle	75	42	205	7	8
	Wheat flours						
	All-purpose or family flour, enriched						
502	Sifted, spooned	1 cup	115	12	420	12	1
503	Unsifted, spooned	1 cup	125	12	455	13	1
504	Cake or pastry flour, enriched, sifted, spooned	1 cup	96	12	350	7	1
505	Self-rising, enriched, unsifted, spooned	1 cup	125	12	440	12	1
506	Whole-wheat, from hard wheats, stirred	1 cup	120	12	400	16	2
Legumes (Dry), Nuts, Seeds; Related Products							
	Almonds, shelled						
507	Chopped (about 130 almonds)	1 cup	130	5	775	24	70
508	Slivered, not pressed down (about 115 almonds).	1 cup	115	5	690	21	62
	Beans, dry						
	Common varieties as Great Northern, navy, and others						
	Cooked, drained						
509	Great Northern	1 cup	180	69	210	14	1
510	Pea (navy)	1 cup	190	69	225	15	1
	Canned, solids and liquid						
	White with:						
511	Frankfurters (sliced)	1 cup	255	71	365	19	18
512	Pork and tomato sauce	1 cup	255	71	310	16	7
513	Pork and sweet sauce	1 cup	255	66	385	16	12
514	Red kidney	1 cup	255	76	230	15	1
515	Lima, cooked, drained	1 cup	190	64	260	16	1
516	Blackeye peas, dry, cooked (with residual cooking liquid)	1 cup	250	80	190	13	1
517	Brazil nuts, shelled (6–8 large kernels)	1 oz	28	5	185	4	19
518	Cashew nuts, roasted in oil	1 cup	140	5	785	24	64

[60]Value varies with the brand. Consult the label.

							Nutrients in Indicated Quantity					
Fatty Acids												
Satu-rated (Total) (G) g	Unsaturated		Carbo-hydrate (J) g	Calcium (K) mg	Phos-phorus (L) mg	Iron (M) mg	Potas-sium (N) mg	Vitamin A Value (O) I.U.	Thiamin (P) mg	Ribo-flavin (Q) mg	Niacin (R) mg	Ascorbic Acid (S) mg
	Oleic (H) g	Lino-leic (I) g										
2.2	3.3	3.9	29	53	113	3.3	245	1,000	0.15	0.18	2.3	5
—	—	—	36	[60]54	[60]67	1.9	[60]74	500	0.16	0.17	2.1	([60])
2.3	2.8	1.4	28	85	130	1.3	109	250	0.17	0.23	1.4	TR
2.8	2.9	1.2	27	179	257	1.0	146	170	0.14	0.22	0.9	TR
0.2	0.1	0.5	88	18	100	3.3	109	0	0.74	0.46	6.1	0
0.2	0.1	0.5	95	20	109	3.6	119	0	0.80	0.50	6.6	0
0.1	0.1	0.3	76	16	70	2.8	91	0	0.61	0.38	5.1	0
0.2	0.1	0.5	93	331	583	3.6	—	0	0.80	0.50	6.6	0
0.4	0.2	1.0	85	49	446	4.0	444	0	0.66	0.14	5.2	0
5.6	47.7	12.8	25	304	655	6.1	1,005	0	0.31	1.20	4.6	TR
5.0	42.2	11.3	22	269	580	5.4	889	0	0.28	1.06	4.0	TR
—	—	—	38	90	266	4.9	749	0	0.25	0.13	1.3	0
—	—	—	40	95	281	5.1	790	0	0.27	0.13	1.3	0
—	—	—	32	94	303	4.8	668	330	0.18	0.15	3.3	TR
2.4	2.8	0.6	48	138	235	4.6	536	330	0.20	0.08	1.5	5
4.3	5.0	1.1	54	161	291	5.9	—	—	0.15	0.10	1.3	—
—	—	—	42	74	278	4.6	673	10	0.13	0.10	1.5	—
—	—	—	49	55	293	5.9	1,163	—	0.25	0.11	1.3	—
—	—	—	35	43	238	3.3	573	30	0.40	0.10	1.0	—
4.8	6.2	7.1	3	53	196	1.0	203	TR	0.27	0.03	0.5	—
12.9	36.8	10.2	41	53	522	5.3	650	140	0.60	0.35	2.5	—

(Continued)

APPENDIX C: (Continued)

				Nutrients in Indicated Quantity			

Item No. (A)	Foods, approximate measures, units, and weight (edible part unless footnotes indicate otherwise) (B)		g	Water (C) %	Food Energy (D) kcal	Pro- tein (E) g	Fat (F) g
Legumes (Dry), Nuts, Seeds; Related Products							
	Coconut meat, fresh						
519	Piece, about 2 by 2 by ½ in.	1 piece	45	51	155	2	16
520	Shredded or grated, not pressed down	1 cup	80	51	275	3	28
521	Filberts (hazelnuts), chopped (about 80 kernels)	1 cup	115	6	730	14	72
522	Lentils, whole, cooked	1 cup	200	72	210	16	TR
523	Peanuts, roasted in oil, salted (whole, halves, chopped)	1 cup	144	2	840	37	72
524	Peanut butter	1 tbsp	16	2	95	4	8
525	Peas, split, dry, cooked	1 cup	200	70	230	16	1
526	Pecans, chopped or pieces (about 120 large halves)	1 cup	118	3	810	11	84
527	Pumpkin and squash kernels, dry, hulled	1 cup	140	4	775	41	65
528	Sunflower seeds, dry, hulled	1 cup	145	5	810	35	69
	Walnuts						
	Black:						
529	Chopped or broken kernels	1 cup	125	3	785	26	74
530	Ground (finely)	1 cup	80	3	500	16	47
531	Persian or English, chopped (about 60 halves)	1 cup	120	4	780	18	77
Sugars and Sweets							
	Cake icings						
	Boiled, white						
532	Plain	1 cup	94	18	295	1	0
533	With coconut	1 cup	166	15	605	3	13
	Uncooked						
534	Chocolate made with milk and butter	1 cup	275	14	1,035	9	38
535	Creamy fudge from mix and water	1 cup	245	15	830	7	16
536	White	1 cup	319	11	1,200	2	21
	Candy						
537	Caramels, plain or chocolate	1 oz	28	8	115	1	3
	Chocolate						
538	Milk, plain	1 oz	28	1	145	2	9
539	Semisweet, small pieces (60 per oz)	1 cup or 6-oz pkg	170	1	860	7	61
540	Chocolate-coated peanuts	1 oz	28	1	160	5	12
541	Fondant, uncoated (mints, candy corn, other)	1 oz	28	8	105	TR	1
542	Fudge, chocolate, plain	1 oz	28	8	115	1	3
543	Gum drops	1 oz	28	12	100	TR	TR

							Nutrients in Indicated Quantity					
Fatty Acids												
	Unsaturated											
Satu-rated (Total) (G) g	Oleic (H) g	Lino-leic (I) g	Carbo-hydrate (J) g	Calcium (K) mg	Phos-phorus (L) mg	Iron (M) mg	Potas-sium (N) mg	Vitamin A Value (O) I.U.	Thiamin (P) mg	Ribo-flavin (Q) mg	Niacin (R) mg	Ascorbic Acid (S) mg
14.0	0.9	0.3	4	6	43	0.8	115	0	0.02	0.01	0.2	1
24.8	1.6	0.5	8	10	76	1.4	205	0	0.04	0.02	0.4	2
5.1	55.2	7.3	19	240	388	3.9	810	—	0.53	—	1.0	TR
—	—	—	39	50	238	4.2	498	40	0.14	0.12	1.2	0
13.7	33.0	20.7	27	107	577	3.0	971	—	0.46	0.19	24.8	0
1.5	3.7	2.3	3	9	61	0.3	100	—	0.02	0.02	2.4	0
—	—	—	42	22	178	3.4	592	80	0.30	0.18	1.8	—
7.2	50.5	20.0	17	86	341	2.8	712	150	1.01	0.15	1.1	2
11.8	23.5	27.5	21	71	1,602	15.7	1,386	100	0.34	0.27	3.4	—
8.2	13.7	43.2	29	174	1,214	10.3	1,334	70	2.84	0.33	7.8	—
6.3	13.3	45.7	19	TR	713	7.5	575	380	0.28	0.14	0.9	—
4.0	8.5	29.2	12	TR	456	4.8	368	240	0.18	0.09	0.6	—
8.4	11.8	42.2	19	119	456	3.7	540	40	0.40	0.16	1.1	2
0	0	0	75	2	2	TR	17	0	TR	0.03	TR	0
11.0	0.9	TR	124	10	50	0.8	277	0	0.02	0.07	0.3	0
23.4	11.7	1.0	185	165	305	3.3	536	580	0.06	0.28	0.6	1
5.1	6.7	3.1	183	96	218	2.7	238	TR	0.05	0.20	0.7	TR
12.7	5.1	0.5	260	48	38	TR	57	860	TR	0.06	TR	TR
1.6	1.1	0.1	22	42	35	0.4	54	TR	0.01	0.05	0.1	TR
5.5	3.0	0.3	16	65	65	0.3	109	80	0.02	0.10	0.1	TR
36.2	19.8	1.7	97	51	255	4.4	553	30	0.02	0.14	0.9	0
4.0	4.7	2.1	11	33	84	0.4	143	TR	0.10	0.05	2.1	TR
0.1	0.3	0.1	25	4	2	0.3	1	0	TR	TR	TR	0
1.3	1.4	0.6	21	22	24	0.3	42	TR	0.01	0.03	0.1	TR
—	—	—	25	2	TR	0.1	1	0	0	TR	TR	0

(Continued)

APPENDIX C: (Continued)

					Nutrients in Indicated Quantity	

Item No. (A)	Foods, approximate measures, units, and weight (edible part unless footnote indicate otherwise) (B)		g	Water (C) %	Food Energy (D) kcal	Pro- tein (E) g	Fat (F) g

Sugars and Sweets

Candy—Continued

544	Hard	1 oz	28	1	110	0	TR
545	Marshmallows	1 oz	28	17	90	1	TR
	Chocolate-flavored beverage powders (about 4 heaping tsp per oz)						
546	With nonfat dry milk	1 oz	28	2	100	5	1
547	Without milk	1 oz	28	1	100	1	1
548	Honey, strained or extracted	1 tbsp	21	17	65	TR	0
549	Jams and preserves	1 tbsp	20	29	55	TR	TR
550		1 packet	14	29	40	TR	TR
551	Jellies	1 tbsp	18	29	50	TR	TR
552		1 packet	14	29	40	TR	TR
	Sirups						
	Chocolate-flavored sirup or topping						
553	Thin type	1 fl oz or 2 tbsp	38	32	90	1	1
554	Fudge type	1 fl oz or 2 tbsp	38	25	125	2	5
	Molasses, cane						
555	Light (first extraction)	1 tbsp	20	24	50	—	—
556	Blackstrap (third extraction)	1 tbsp	20	24	45	—	—
557	Sorghum	1 tbsp	21	23	55	—	—
558	Table blends, chiefly corn, light and dark	1 tbsp	21	24	60	0	0
	Sugars						
559	Brown, pressed down	1 cup	220	2	820	0	0
	White						
560	Granulated	1 cup	200	1	770	0	0
561		1 tbsp	12	1	45	0	0
562		1 packet	6	1	23	0	0
563	Powdered, sifted, spooned into cup.	1 cup	100	1	385	0	0

Vegetable and Vegetable Products

Asparagus, green:

Cooked, drained

Cuts and tips, 1½- to 2-in lengths

564	From raw	1 cup	145	94	30	3	TR
565	From frozen	1 cup	180	93	40	6	TR
	Spears, ½-in diam. at base:						
566	From raw	4 spears	60	94	10	1	TR

								Nutrients in Indicated Quantity					
Fatty Acids													
	Unsaturated												
Satu-rated (Total) (G) g	Oleic (H) g	Lino-leic (I) g	Carbo-hydrate (J) g	Calcium (K) mg	Phos-phorus (L) mg	Iron (M) mg	Potas-sium (N) mg	Vitamin A Value (O) I.U.	Thiamin (P) mg	Ribo-flavin (Q) mg	Niacin (R) mg	Ascorbic Acid (S) mg
—	—	—	28	6	2	0.5	1	0	0	0	0	0
—	—	—	23	5	2	0.5	2	0	0	TR	TR	0
0.5	0.3	TR	20	167	155	0.5	227	10	0.04	0.21	0.2	1
0.4	0.2	TR	25	9	48	0.6	142	—	0.01	0.03	0.1	0
0	0	0	17	1	1	0.1	11	0	TR	0.01	0.1	TR
—	—	—	14	4	2	0.2	18	TR	TR	0.01	TR	TR
—	—	—	10	3	1	0.1	12	TR	TR	TR	TR	TR
—	—	—	13	4	1	0.3	14	TR	TR	0.01	TR	1
—	—	—	10	3	1	0.2	11	TR	TR	TR	TR	1
0.5	0.3	TR	24	6	35	0.6	106	TR	0.01	0.03	0.2	0
3.1	1.6	0.1	20	48	60	0.5	107	60	0.02	0.08	0.2	TR
—	—	—	13	33	9	0.9	183	—	0.01	0.01	TR	—
—	—	—	11	137	17	3.2	585	—	0.02	0.04	0.4	—
—	—	—	14	35	5	2.6	—	—	—	0.02	TR	—
0	0	0	15	9	3	0.8	1	0	0	0	0	0
0	0	0	212	187	42	7.5	757	0	0.02	0.07	0.4	0
0	0	0	199	0	0	0.2	6	0	0	0	0	0
0	0	0	12	0	0	TR	TR	0	0	0	0	0
0	0	0	6	0	0	TR	TR	0	0	0	0	0
0	0	0	100	0	0	0.1	3	0	0	0	0	0
—	—	—	5	30	73	0.9	265	1,310	0.23	0.26	2.0	38
—	—	—	6	40	115	2.2	396	1,530	0.25	0.23	1.8	41
—	—	—	2	13	30	0.4	110	540	0.10	0.11	0.8	16

(Continued)

APPENDIX C: (*Continued*)

				Nutrients in Indicated Quantity		

Item No. (A)	Foods, approximate measures, units, and weight (edible part unless footnote indicate otherwise) (B)		g	Water (C) %	Food Energy (D) kcal	Pro-tein (E) g	Fat (F) g
Vegetable and Vegetable Products—Con.							
	Asparagus, green:—Continued						
567	From frozen	4 spears	60	92	15	2	TR
568	Canned, spears, ½-in diam. at base	4 spears	80	93	15	2	TR
	Beans						
	Lima, immature seeds, frozen, cooked, drained						
569	Thick-seeded types (Fordhooks)	1 cup	170	74	170	10	TR
570	Thin-seeded types (baby limas)	1 cup	180	69	210	13	TR
	Snap						
	Green						
	Cooked, drained						
571	From raw (cuts and French style)	1 cup	125	92	30	2	TR
	From frozen						
572	Cuts	1 cup	135	92	35	2	TR
573	French style	1 cup	130	92	35	2	TR
574	Canned, drained solids (cuts)	1 cup	135	92	30	2	TR
	Yellow or wax						
	Cooked, drained						
575	From raw (cuts and French style)	1 cup	125	93	30	2	TR
576	From frozen (cuts)	1 cup	135	92	35	2	TR
577	Canned, drained solids (cuts)	1 cup	135	92	30	2	TR
	Beans, mature. See Beans, dry (items 509–515) and Blackeye peas, dry (item 516).						
	Bean sprouts (mung)						
578	Raw	1 cup	105	89	35	4	TR
579	Cooked, drained	1 cup	125	91	35	4	TR
	Beets						
	Cooked, drained, peeled						
580	Whole beets, 2-in diam.	2 beets	100	91	30	1	TR
581	Diced or sliced	1 cup	170	91	55	2	TR
	Canned, drained solids						
582	Whole beets, small	1 cup	160	89	60	2	TR
583	Diced or sliced	1 cup	170	89	65	2	TR
584	Beet greens, leaves and stems, cooked, drained	1 cup	145	94	25	2	TR

				Nutrients in Indicated Quantity								

Fatty Acids												
	Unsaturated											
Satu-rated (Total) (G) g	Oleic (H) g	Lino-leic (I) g	Carbo-hydrate (J) g	Calcium (K) mg	Phos-phorus (L) mg	Iron (M) mg	Potas-sium (N) mg	Vitamin A Value (O) I.U.	Thiamin (P) mg	Ribo-flavin (Q) mg	Niacin (R) mg	Ascorbic Acid (S) mg
—	—	—	2	13	40	0.7	143	470	0.10	0.08	0.7	16
—	—	—	3	15	42	1.5	133	640	0.05	0.08	0.6	12
—	—	—	32	34	153	2.9	724	390	0.12	0.09	1.7	29
—	—	—	40	63	227	4.7	709	400	0.16	0.09	2.2	22
—	—	—	7	63	46	0.8	189	680	0.09	0.11	0.6	15
—	—	—	8	54	43	0.9	205	780	0.09	0.12	0.5	7
—	—	—	8	49	39	1.2	177	690	0.08	0.10	0.4	9
—	—	—	7	61	34	2.0	128	630	0.04	0.07	0.4	5
—	—	—	6	63	46	0.8	189	290	0.09	0.11	0.6	16
—	—	—	8	47	42	0.9	221	140	0.09	0.11	0.5	8
—	—	—	7	61	34	2.0	128	140	0.04	0.07	0.4	7
—	—	—	7	20	67	1.4	234	20	0.14	0.14	0.8	20
—	—	—	7	21	60	1.1	195	30	0.11	0.13	0.9	8
—	—	—	7	14	23	0.5	208	20	0.03	0.04	0.3	6
—	—	—	12	24	39	0.9	354	30	0.05	0.07	0.5	10
—	—	—	14	30	29	1.1	267	30	0.02	0.05	0.2	5
—	—	—	15	32	31	1.2	284	30	0.02	0.05	0.2	5
—	—	—	5	144	36	2.8	481	7,400	0.10	0.22	0.4	22

(Continued)

APPENDIX C: (*Continued*)

Item No. (A)	Foods, approximate measures, units, and weight (edible part unless footnotes indicate otherwise) (B)		g	Water (C) %	Food Energy (D) kcal	Pro-tein (E) g	Fat (F) g
Vegetable and Vegetable Products—Con.							
	Blackeye peas, immature seeds, cooked and drained						
585	From raw	1 cup	165	72	180	13	1
586	From frozen	1 cup	170	66	220	15	1
	Broccoli, cooked, drained						
	From raw						
587	Stalk, medium size	1 stalk	180	91	45	6	1
588	Stalks cut into ½-in. pieces	1 cup	155	91	40	5	TR
	From frozen:						
589	Stalk, 4½ to 5 in. long	1 stalk	30	91	10	1	TR
590	Chopped	1 cup	185	92	50	5	1
	Brussels sprouts, cooked, drained:						
591	From raw, 7–8 sprouts (1¼- to 1½-in. diam.)	1 cup	155	88	55	7	1
592	From frozen	1 cup	155	89	50	5	TR
	Cabbage						
	Common varieties						
	Raw						
593	Coarsely shredded or sliced	1 cup	70	92	15	1	TR
594	Finely shredded or chopped	1 cup	90	92	20	1	TR
595	Cooked, drained	1 cup	145	94	30	2	TR
596	Red, raw, coarsely shredded or sliced	1 cup	70	90	20	1	TR
597	Savoy, raw, coarsely shredded or sliced	1 cup	70	92	15	2	TR
598	Cabbage, celery (also called *pe-tsai* or *wongbok*), raw, 1-in pieces	1 cup	75	95	10	1	TR
599	Cabbage, white mustard (also called *bokchoy* or *pakchoy*), cooked, drained	1 cup	170	95	25	2	TR
	Carrots						
	Raw, without crowns and tips, scraped						
600	Whole, 7½ by 1⅛ in, or strips, 2½ to 3 in long	1 carrot or 18 strips	72	88	30	1	TR
601	Grated	1 cup	110	88	45	1	TR
602	Cooked (crosswise cuts), drained	1 cup	155	91	50	1	TR
	Canned						
603	Sliced, drained solids	1 cup	155	91	45	1	TR
604	Strained or junior (baby food)	1 oz (1⅞ to 2 tbsp)	28	92	10	TR	TR
	Cauliflower						
605	Raw, chopped	1 cup	115	91	31	3	TR

	Fatty Acids											

Nutrients in Indicated Quantity

Saturated (Total) (G) g	Oleic (H) g	Linoleic (I) g	Carbohydrate (J) g	Calcium (K) mg	Phosphorus (L) mg	Iron (M) mg	Potassium (N) mg	Vitamin A Value (O) I.U.	Thiamin (P) mg	Riboflavin (Q) mg	Niacin (R) mg	Ascorbic Acid (S) mg
—	—	—	30	40	241	3.5	625	580	0.50	0.18	2.3	28
—	—	—	40	43	286	4.8	573	290	0.68	0.19	2.4	15
—	—	—	8	158	112	1.4	481	4,500	0.16	0.36	1.4	162
—	—	—	7	136	96	1.2	414	3,880	0.14	0.31	1.2	140
—	—	—	1	12	17	0.2	66	570	0.02	0.03	0.2	22
—	—	—	9	100	104	1.3	392	4,810	0.11	0.22	0.9	105
—	—	—	10	50	112	1.7	423	810	0.12	0.22	1.2	135
—	—	—	10	33	95	1.2	457	880	0.12	0.16	0.9	126
—	—	—	4	34	20	0.3	163	90	0.04	0.04	0.2	33
—	—	—	5	44	26	0.4	210	120	0.05	0.05	0.3	42
—	—	—	6	64	29	0.4	236	190	0.06	0.06	0.4	48
—	—	—	5	29	25	0.6	188	30	0.06	0.04	0.3	43
—	—	—	3	47	38	0.6	188	140	0.04	0.06	0.2	39
—	—	—	2	32	30	0.5	190	110	0.04	0.03	0.5	19
—	—	—	4	252	56	1.0	364	5,270	0.07	0.14	1.2	26
—	—	—	7	27	26	0.5	246	7,930	0.04	0.04	0.4	6
—	—	—	11	41	40	0.8	375	12,100	0.07	0.06	0.7	9
—	—	—	11	51	48	0.9	344	16,280	0.08	0.08	0.8	9
—	—	—	10	47	34	1.1	186	23,250	0.03	0.05	0.6	3
—	—	—	2	7	6	0.1	51	3,690	0.01	0.01	0.1	1
—	—	—	6	29	64	1.3	339	70	0.13	0.12	0.8	90

(Continued)

APPENDIX C: (*Continued*)

Item No. (A)	Foods, approximate measures, units, and weight (edible part unless footnote indicate otherwise) (B)		g	Water (C) %	Food Energy (D) kcal	Pro- tein (E) g	Fat (F) g
					Nutrients in Indicated Quantity		

Vegetable and Vegetable Products—Con.

Item No. (A)	Foods, approximate measures, units, and weight (B)		g	Water (C) %	Food Energy (D) kcal	Pro- tein (E) g	Fat (F) g
	Cauliflower—Continued						
	Cooked, drained						
606	From raw (flower buds)	1 cup	125	93	30	3	TR
607	From frozen (flowerets)	1 cup	180	94	30	3	TR
	Celery, Pascal type, raw						
608	Stalk, large outer, 8 by 1½ in, at root end	1 stalk	40	94	5	TR	TR
609	Pieces, diced	1 cup	120	94	20	1	TR
	Collards, cooked, drained						
610	From raw (leaves without stems)	1 cup	190	90	65	7	1
611	From frozen (chopped)	1 cup	170	90	50	5	1
	Corn, sweet						
	Cooked, drained						
612	From raw, ear 5 by 1¾ in	1 ear[61]	140	74	70	2	1
	From frozen						
613	Ear, 5 in long	1 ear[61]	229	73	120	4	1
614	Kernels	1 cup	165	77	130	5	1
	Canned:						
615	Cream style	1 cup	256	76	210	5	2
	Whole kernel						
616	Vacuum pack	1 cup	210	76	175	5	1
617	Wet pack, drained solids	1 cup	165	76	140	4	1
	Cowpeas. See Blackeye peas (Items 585–586)						
	Cucumber slices, ⅛ in thick (large, 2¼-in diam.; small, 1¾-in diam.)						
618	With peel	6 large or 8 small slices		95	5	TR	TR
619	Without peel	6½ large or 9 small pieces	28	96	5	TR	TR
620	Dandelion greens, cooked, drained	1 cup	105	90	35	2	1
621	Endive, curly (including escarole), raw, small pieces	1 cup	50	93	10	1	TR
	Kale, cooked, drained						
622	From raw (leaves without stems and midribs)	1 cup	110	88	45	5	1
623	From frozen (leaf style)	1 cup	130	91	40	4	1

[61]Weight includes cob. Without cob, weight is 77 g for item 612, 126 g for item 613.
[62]Based on yellow varieties. For white varieties, value is trace.

| | Fatty Acids | | | | | | | | | | | |
| | | Unsaturated | | | | | | | | | | |
Satu-rated (Total) (G) g	Oleic (H) g	Lino-leic (I) g	Carbo-hydrate (J) g	Calcium (K) mg	Phos-phorus (L) mg	Iron (M) mg	Potas-sium (N) mg	Vitamin A Value (O) I.U.	Thiamin (P) mg	Ribo-flavin (Q) mg	Niacin (R) mg	Ascorbic Acid (S) mg
—	—	—	5	26	53	0.9	258	80	0.11	0.10	0.8	69
—	—	—	6	31	68	0.9	373	50	0.07	0.09	0.7	74
—	—	—	2	16	11	0.1	136	110	0.01	0.01	0.1	4
—	—	—	5	47	34	0.4	409	320	0.04	0.04	0.4	11
—	—	—	10	357	99	1.5	498	14,820	0.21	0.38	2.3	144
—	—	—	10	299	87	1.7	401	11,560	0.10	0.24	1.0	56
—	—	—	16	2	69	0.5	151	[62]310	0.09	0.08	1.1	7
—	—	—	27	4	121	1.0	291	[62]440	0.18	0.10	2.1	9
—	—	—	31	5	120	1.3	304	[62]580	0.15	0.10	2.5	8
—	—	—	51	8	143	1.5	248	[62]840	0.08	0.13	2.6	13
—	—	—	43	6	153	1.1	204	[62]740	0.06	0.13	2.3	11
—	—	—	33	8	81	0.8	160	[62]580	0.05	0.08	1.5	7
—	—	—	1	7	8	0.3	45	70	0.01	0.01	0.1	3
—	—	—	1	5	5	0.1	45	TR	0.01	0.01	0.1	3
—	—	—	7	147	44	1.9	244	12,290	0.14	0.17	—	19
—	—	—	2	41	27	0.9	147	1,650	0.04	0.07	0.3	5
—	—	—	7	206	64	1.8	243	9,130	0.11	0.20	1.8	102
—	—	—	7	157	62	1.3	251	10,660	0.08	0.20	0.9	49

(Continued)

APPENDIX C: (Continued)

				Nutrients in Indicated Quantity		

Item No. (A)	Foods, approximate measures, units, and weight (edible part unless footnote indicate otherwise) (B)		Water (C) %	Food Energy (D) kcal	Pro-tein (E) g	Fat (F) g
		g				
Vegetable and Vegetable Products—Con.						
	Lettuce, raw					
	Butterhead, as Boston types					
624	Head, 5-in diam.	1 head[63]	220	95	25	2	TR
625	Leaves	1 outer or 2 inner or 3 heart leaves	15	95	TR	TR	TR
	Crisphead, as Iceberg					
626	Head, 6-in diam.	1 head[64]	567	96	70	5	1
627	Wedge, ¼ of head	1 wedge	135	96	20	1	TR
628	Pieces, chopped or shredded	1 cup	55	96	5	TR	TR
629	Looseleaf (bunching varieties including romaine or cos), chopped or shredded pieces	1 cup	55	94	10	1	TR
630	Mushrooms, raw, sliced or chopped	1 cup	70	90	20	2	TR
631	Mustard greens, without stems and midribs, cooked, drained	1 cup	140	93	30	3	1
632	Okra pods, 3 by ⅝ in, cooked	10 pods	106	91	30	2	TR
	Onions					
	Mature					
	Raw					
633	Chopped	1 cup	170	89	65	3	TR
634	Sliced	1 cup	115	89	45	2	TR
635	Cooked (whole or sliced), drained	1 cup	210	92	60	3	TR
636	Young green, bulb (⅜ in diam.) and white portion of top	6 onions	30	88	15	TR	TR
637	Parsley, raw, chopped	1 tbsp	4	85	TR	TR	TR
638	Parsnips, cooked (diced or 2-in. lengths)	1 cup	155	82	100	2	1
	Peas, green					
	Canned					
639	Whole, drained solids	1 cup	170	77	150	8	1
640	Strained (baby food)	1 oz (1¾ to 2 tbsp)	28	86	15	1	TR
641	Frozen, cooked, drained	1 cup	160	82	110	8	TR
642	Peppers, hot, red, without seeds, dried (ground chili powder, added seasonings)	1 tsp	2	9	5	TR	TR

[63]Weight includes refuse of outer leaves and core. Without these parts, weight is 163 g.
[64]Weight includes core. Without core, weight is 539 g.
[65]Value based on white-fleshed varieties. For yellow-fleshed varieties, value is International Units (I.U.) is 70 for item 633, 50 for item 634, and 80 for item 635.

| Fatty Acids | | | | | | | | | | | | |
| Satu-rated (Total) (G) g | Unsaturated | | Carbo-hydrate (J) g | Calcium (K) mg | Phos-phorus (L) mg | Iron (M) mg | Potas-sium (N) mg | Vitamin A Value (O) I.U. | Thiamin (P) mg | Ribo-flavin (Q) mg | Niacin (R) mg | Ascorbic Acid (S) mg |
	Oleic (H) g	Lino-leic (I) g										
—	—	—	4	57	42	3.3	430	1,580	0.10	0.10	0.5	13
—	—	—	TR	5	4	0.3	40	150	0.01	0.01	TR	1
—	—	—	16	108	118	2.7	943	1,780	0.32	0.32	1.6	32
—	—	—	4	27	30	0.7	236	450	0.08	0.08	0.4	8
—	—	—	2	11	12	0.3	96	180	0.03	0.03	0.2	3
—	—	—	2	37	14	0.8	145	1,050	0.03	0.04	0.2	10
—	—	—	3	4	81	0.6	290	TR	0.07	0.32	2.9	2
—	—	—	6	193	45	2.5	308	8,120	0.11	0.20	0.8	67
—	—	—	6	98	43	0.5	184	520	0.14	0.19	1.0	21
—	—	—	15	46	61	0.9	267	[65]TR	0.05	0.07	0.3	17
—	—	—	10	31	41	0.6	181	[65]TR	0.03	0.05	0.2	12
—	—	—	14	50	61	0.8	231	[65]TR	0.06	0.06	0.4	15
—	—	—	3	12	12	0.2	69	TR	0.02	0.01	0.1	8
—	—	—	TR	7	2	0.2	25	300	TR	0.01	TR	6
—	—	—	23	70	96	0.9	587	50	0.11	0.12	0.2	16
—	—	—	29	44	129	3.2	163	1,170	0.15	0.10	1.4	14
—	—	—	3	3	18	0.3	28	140	0.02	0.03	0.3	3
—	—	—	19	30	138	3.0	216	960	0.43	0.14	2.7	21
—	—	—	1	5	4	0.3	20	1,300	TR	0.02	0.2	TR

Nutrients in Indicated Quantity

(Continued)

APPENDIX C: (*Continued*)

Item No. (A)	Foods, approximate measures, units, and weight (edible part unless footnotes indicate otherwise) (B)		g	Water (C) %	Food Energy (D) kcal	Pro-tein (E) g	Fat (F) g
					Nutrients in Indicated Quantity		
Vegetable and Vegetable Products—Con.							
	Peppers, sweet (about 5 per lb, whole), stem and seeds removed						
643	Raw	1 pod	74	93	15	1	TR
644	Cooked, boiled, drained	1 pod	73	95	15	1	TR
	Potatoes, cooked						
645	Baked, peeled after baking (about 2 per lb, raw)	1 potato	156	75	145	4	TR
	Boiled (about 3 per lb, raw):						
646	Peeled after boiling	1 potato	137	80	105	3	TR
647	Peeled before boiling	1 potato	135	83	90	3	TR
	French-fried, strip, 2 to 3½ in long						
648	Prepared from raw	10 strips	50	45	135	2	7
649	Frozen, oven heated	10 strips	50	53	110	2	4
650	Hashed brown, prepared from frozen	1 cup	155	56	345	3	18
	Mashed, prepared from—						
	Raw						
651	Milk added	1 cup	210	83	135	4	2
652	Milk and butter added	1 cup	210	80	195	4	9
653	Dehydrated flakes (without milk), water, milk, butter, and salt added.	1 cup	210	79	195	4	7
654	Potato chips, 1¾ by 2½ in oval cross section	10 chips	20	2	115	1	8
655	Potato salad, made with cooked salad dressing	1 cup	250	76	250	7	7
656	Pumpkin, canned	1 cup	245	90	80	2	1
657	Radishes, raw (prepackaged) stem ends, rootless cut off	4 radishes	18	95	5	TR	TR
658	Sauerkraut, canned, solids and liquid	1 cup	235	93	40	2	TR
	Southern peas. See Blackeye peas (items 585–586)						
	Spinach						
659	Raw, chopped	1 cup	55	91	15	2	TR
	Cooked, drained						
660	From raw	1 cup	180	92	40	5	1
	From frozen						
661	Chopped	1 cup	205	92	45	6	1
662	Leaf	1 cup	190	92	45	6	1
663	Canned, drained solids	1 cup	205	91	50	6	1

								Nutrients in Indicated Quantity				
Fatty Acids												
	Unsaturated											
Satu-rated (Total) (G) g	Oleic (H) g	Lino-leic (I) g	Carbo-hydrate (J) g	Calcium (K) mg	Phos-phorus (L) mg	Iron (M) mg	Potas-sium (N) mg	Vitamin A Value (O) I.U.	Thiamin (P) mg	Ribo-flavin (Q) mg	Niacin (R) mg	Ascorbic Acid (S) mg
—	—	—	4	7	16	0.5	157	310	0.06	0.06	0.4	94
—	—	—	3	7	12	0.4	109	310	0.05	0.05	0.4	70
—	—	—	33	14	101	1.1	782	TR	0.15	0.07	2.7	31
—	—	—	23	10	72	0.8	556	TR	0.12	0.05	2.0	22
—	—	—	20	8	57	0.7	385	TR	0.12	0.05	1.6	22
1.7	1.2	3.3	18	8	56	0.7	427	TR	0.07	0.04	1.6	11
1.1	0.8	2.1	17	5	43	0.9	326	TR	0.07	0.01	1.3	11
4.6	3.2	9.0	45	28	78	1.9	439	TR	0.11	0.03	1.6	12
0.7	0.4	TR	27	50	103	0.8	548	40	0.17	0.11	2.1	21
5.6	2.3	0.2	26	50	101	0.8	525	360	0.17	0.11	2.1	19
3.6	2.1	0.2	30	65	99	0.6	601	270	0.08	0.08	1.9	11
2.1	1.4	4.0	10	8	28	0.4	226	TR	0.04	0.01	1.0	3
2.0	2.7	1.3	41	80	160	1.5	798	350	0.20	0.18	2.8	28
—	—	—	19	61	64	1.0	588	15,680	0.07	0.12	1.5	12
—	—	—	1	5	6	0.2	58	TR	0.01	0.01	0.1	5
—	—	—	9	85	42	1.2	329	120	0.07	0.09	0.5	33
—	—	—	2	51	28	1.7	259	4,460	0.06	0.11	0.3	28
—	—	—	6	167	68	4.0	583	14,580	0.13	0.25	0.9	50
—	—	—	8	232	90	4.3	683	16,200	0.14	0.31	0.8	39
—	—	—	7	200	84	4.8	688	15,390	0.15	0.27	1.0	53
—	—	—	7	242	53	5.3	513	16,400	0.04	0.25	0.6	29

(Continued)

APPENDIX C: (Continued)

Item No. (A)	Foods, approximate measures, units, and weight (edible part unless footnote indicate otherwise) (B)		Nutrients in Indicated Quantity			
		g	Water (C) %	Food Energy (D) kcal	Pro- tein (E) g	Fat (F) g
Vegetable and Vegetable Products—Con.						
	Squash, cooked					
664	Summer (all varieties), diced, drained	1 cup	210	96	30	2	TR
665	Winter (all varieties), baked, mashed	1 cup	205	81	130	4	1
	Sweet potatoes					
	Cooked (raw, 5 by 2 in.; about 2½ per lb)					
666	Baked in skin, peeled	1 potato	114	64	160	2	1
667	Boiled in skin, peeled	1 potato	151	71	170	3	1
668	Candied, 2½ by 2-in piece	1 piece	105	60	175	1	3
	Canned					
669	Solid pack (mashed)	1 cup	255	72	275	5	1
670	Vacuum pack, piece 2¾ by 1 in.	1 piece	40	72	45	1	TR
	Tomatoes					
671	Raw, 2⅜-in diam. (3 per 12 oz pkg.)	1 tomato[66]	135	94	25	1	TR
672	Canned, solids and liquid	1 cup	241	94	50	2	TR
673	Tomato catsup	1 cup	273	69	290	5	1
674		1 tbsp	15	69	15	TR	TR
	Tomato juice, canned					
675	Cup	1 cup	243	94	45	2	TR
676	Glass (6 fl oz)	1 glass	182	94	35	2	TR
677	Turnips, cooked, diced	1 cup	155	94	35	1	TR
	Turnip greens, cooked, drained					
678	From raw (leaves and stems)	1 cup	145	94	30	3	TR
679	From frozen (chopped)	1 cup	165	93	40	4	TR
680	Vegetables, mixed, frozen, cooked	1 cup	182	83	115	6	1
Miscellaneous Items						
	Baking powders for home use					
	Sodium aluminum sulfate					
681	With monocalcium phosphate monohydrate	1 tsp	3.0	2	5	TR	TR

[66]Weight includes cores and stem ends. Without these parts, weight is 123 g.

[67]Based on year-round average. For tomatoes marketed from November through May, value is about 12 mg; from June through October, 32 mg.

[68]Applies to product without calcium salts added. Value for products with calcium salts added may be as much as 63 mg for whole tomatoes, 241 mg for cut forms.

								Nutrients in Indicated Quantity				
Fatty Acids												
Saturated (Total) (G) g	Unsaturated		Carbohydrate (J) g	Calcium (K) mg	Phosphorus (L) mg	Iron (M) mg	Potassium (N) mg	Vitamin A Value (O) I.U.	Thiamin (P) mg	Riboflavin (Q) mg	Niacin (R) mg	Ascorbic Acid (S) mg
	Oleic (H) g	Linoleic (I) g										
—	—	—	7	53	53	0.8	296	820	0.11	0.17	1.7	21
—	—	—	32	57	98	1.6	945	8,610	0.10	0.27	1.4	27
—	—	—	37	46	66	1.0	342	9,230	0.10	0.08	0.8	25
—	—	—	40	48	71	1.1	367	11,940	0.14	0.09	0.9	26
2.0	0.8	0.1	36	39	45	0.9	200	6,620	0.06	0.04	0.4	11
—	—	—	63	64	105	2.0	510	19,890	0.13	0.10	1.5	36
—	—	—	10	10	16	0.3	80	3,120	0.02	0.02	0.2	6
—	—	—	6	16	33	0.6	300	1,110	0.07	0.05	0.9	[67]28
—	—	—	10	[68]14	46	1.2	523	2,170	0.12	0.07	1.7	41
—	—	—	69	60	137	2.2	991	3,820	0.25	0.19	4.4	41
—	—	—	4	3	8	0.1	54	210	0.01	0.01	0.2	2
—	—	—	10	17	44	2.2	552	1,940	0.12	0.07	1.9	39
—	—	—	8	13	33	1.6	413	1,460	0.09	0.05	1.5	29
—	—	—	8	54	37	0.6	291	TR	0.06	0.08	0.5	34
—	—	—	5	252	49	1.5	—	8,270	0.15	0.33	0.7	68
—	—	—	6	195	64	2.6	246	11,390	0.08	0.15	0.7	31
—	—	—	24	46	115	2.4	348	9,010	0.22	0.13	2.0	15
0	0	0	1	58	87	—	5	0	0	0	0	0

(Continued)

APPENDIX C: (Continued)

Item No. (A)	Foods, approximate measures, units, and weight (edible part unless footnote indicate otherwise) (B)		g	Water (C) %	Food Energy (D) kcal	Pro-tein (E) g	Fat (F) g
Miscellaneous Items—Con.							
	Baking powders for home use—Continued						
	Sodium aluminum sulfate—Continued						
682	With monocalcium phosphate monohydrate, calcium sulfate	1 tsp	2.9	1	5	TR	TR
683	Straight phosphate	1 tsp	3.8	2	5	TR	TR
684	Low sodium	1 tsp	4.3	2	5	TR	TR
685	Barbecue sauce	1 cup	250	81	230	4	17
	Beverages, alcoholic						
686	Beer	12 fl oz	360	92	150	1	0
	Gin, rum, vodka, whisky:						
687	80-proof	1½-fl oz jigger	42	67	95	—	—
688	86-proof	1½-fl oz jigger	42	64	105	—	—
689	90-proof	1½-fl oz jigger	42	62	110	—	—
	Wines						
690	Dessert	3½-fl oz glass	103	77	140	TR	0
691	Table	3½-fl oz glass	102	86	85	TR	0
	Beverages, carbonated, sweetened, nonalcoholic						
692	Carbonated water	12 fl oz	366	92	115	0	0
693	Cola type	12 fl oz	369	90	145	0	0
694	Fruit-flavored sodas and Tom Collins mixer	12 fl oz	372	88	170	0	0
695	Ginger ale	12 fl oz	366	92	115	0	0
696	Root beer	12 fl oz	370	90	150	0	0
	Chili powder. See Peppers, hot, red (item 642)						
	Chocolate						
697	Bitter or baking	1 oz	28	2	145	3	15
	Semisweet, see Candy, chocolate (item 539)						
698	Gelatin, dry	1, 7-g envelope	7	13	25	6	TR
699	Gelatin dessert prepared with gelatin dessert powder and water	1 cup	240	84	140	4	0
700	Mustard, prepared, yellow	1 tsp or individual serving pouch or cup.	5	80	5	TR	TR
	Olives, pickled, canned:						
701	Green	4 medium or 3 extra large or 2 giant.[69]	16	78	15	TR	2
702	Ripe, Mission	3 small or 2 large[69]	10	73	15	TR	2

Nutrients in Indicated Quantity

[69]Weight includes pits. Without pits, weight is 13 g for item 701, 9 g for item 702.

									Nutrients in Indicated Quantity				
Fatty Acids													
	Unsaturated												
Satu-rated (Total) (G) g	Oleic (H) g	Lino-leic (I) g	Carbo-hydrate (J) g	Calcium (K) mg	Phos-phorus (L) mg	Iron (M) mg	Potas-sium (N) mg	Vitamin A Value (O) I.U.	Thiamin (P) mg	Ribo-flavin (Q) mg	Niacin (R) mg	Ascorbic Acid (S) mg
0	0	0	1	183	45	—	—	0	0	0	0	0
0	0	0	1	239	359	—	6	0	0	0	0	0
0	0	0	2	207	314	—	471	0	0	0	0	0
2.2	4.3	10.0	20	53	50	2.0	435	900	0.03	0.03	0.8	13
0	0	0	14	18	108	TR	90	—	0.01	0.11	2.2	—
0	0	0	TR	—	—	—	1	—	—	—	—	—
0	0	0	TR	—	—	—	1	—	—	—	—	—
0	0	0	TR	—	—	—	1	—	—	—	—	—
0	0	0	8	8	—	—	77	—	0.01	0.02	0.2	—
0	0	0	4	9	10	0.4	94	—	TR	0.01	0.1	—
0	0	0	29	—	—	—	—	0	0	0	0	0
0	0	0	37	—	—	—	—	0	0	0	0	0
0	0	0	45	—	—	—	—	0	0	0	0	0
0	0	0	29	—	—	—	0	0	0	0	0	0
0	0	0	39	—	—	—	0	0	0	0	0	0
8.9	4.9	0.4	8	22	109	1.9	235	20	0.01	0.07	0.4	0
0	0	0	0	—	—	—	—	—	—	—	—	—
0	0	0	34	—	—	—	—	—	—	—	—	—
—	—	—	TR	4	4	0.1	7	—	—	—	—	—
0.2	1.2	0.1	TR	8	2	0.2	7	40	—	—	—	—
0.2	1.2	0.1	TR	9	1	0.1	2	10	TR	TR	—	—

(Continued)

APPENDIX C: (Continued)

Nutrients in Indicated Quantity

Item No. (A)	Foods, approximate measures, units, and weight (edible part unless footnotes indicate otherwise) (B)		g	Water (C) %	Food Energy (D) kcal	Pro- tein (E) g	Fat (F) g
Miscellaneous Items—Con.							
	Pickles, cucumber						
703	Dill, medium, whole, 3¾ in long, 1¼-in diam.	1 pickle	65	93	5	TR	TR
704	Fresh-pack, slices 1½-in diam., ¼ in thick	2 slices	15	79	10	TR	TR
705	Sweet, gherkin, small, whole, about 2½ in long, ¾-in diam.	1 pickle	15	61	20	TR	TR
706	Relish, finely chopped, sweet	1 tbsp	15	63	20	TR	TR
	Popcorn. See items 476–478						
707	Popsicle, 3-fl oz size	1 popsicle	95	80	70	0	0
	Soups						
	Canned, condensed						
	Prepared with equal volume of milk						
708	Cream of chicken	1 cup	245	85	180	7	10
709	Cream of mushroom	1 cup	245	83	215	7	14
710	Tomato	1 cup	250	84	175	7	7
	Prepared with equal volume of water						
711	Bean with pork	1 cup	250	84	170	8	6
712	Beef broth, bouillon, consomme	1 cup	240	96	30	5	0
713	Beef noodle	1 cup	240	93	65	4	3
714	Clam chowder, Manhattan type (with tomatoes, without milk)	1 cup	245	92	80	2	3
715	Cream of chicken	1 cup	240	92	95	3	6
716	Cream of mushroom	1 cup	240	90	135	2	10
717	Minestrone	1 cup	245	90	105	5	3
718	Split pea	1 cuᵢ	245	85	145	9	3
719	Tomato	1 cup	245	91	90	2	3
720	Vegetable beef	1 cup	245	92	80	5	2
721	Vegetarian	1 cup	245	92	80	2	2
	Dehydrated						
722	Bouillon cube, ½ in.	1 cube	4	4	5	1	TR
	Mixes:						
	Unprepared						
723	Onion	1½-oz pkg.	43	3	150	6	5
	Prepared with water						
724	Chicken noodle	1 cup	240	95	55	2	1
725	Onion	1 cup	240	96	35	1	1
726	Tomato vegetable with noodles	1 cup	240	93	65	1	1

Nutrients in Indicated Quantity

| Fatty Acids | | | | | | | | | | | | |
| Saturated (Total) (G) g | Unsaturated | | Carbo-hydrate (J) g | Calcium (K) mg | Phos-phorus (L) mg | Iron (M) mg | Potas-sium (N) mg | Vitamin A Value (O) I.U. | Thiamin (P) mg | Ribo-flavin (Q) mg | Niacin (R) mg | Ascorbic Acid (S) mg |
	Oleic (H) g	Lino-leic (I) g										
—	—	—	1	17	14	0.7	130	70	TR	0.01	TR	4
—	—	—	3	5	4	0.3	—	20	TR	TR	TR	1
—	—	—	5	2	2	0.2	—	10	TR	TR	TR	1
—	—	—	5	3	2	0.1	—	—	—	—	—	—
0	0	0	18	0	—	TR	—	0	0	0	0	0
4.2	3.6	1.3	15	172	152	0.5	260	610	0.05	0.27	0.7	2
5.4	2.9	4.6	16	191	169	0.5	279	250	0.05	0.34	0.7	1
3.4	1.7	1.0	23	168	155	0.8	418	1,200	0.10	0.25	1.3	15
1.2	1.8	2.4	22	63	128	2.3	395	650	0.13	0.08	1.0	3
0	0	0	3	TR	31	0.5	130	TR	TR	0.02	1.2	—
0.6	0.7	0.8	7	7	48	1.0	77	50	0.05	0.07	1.0	TR
0.5	0.4	1.3	12	34	47	1.0	184	880	0.02	0.02	1.0	—
1.6	2.3	1.1	8	24	34	0.5	79	410	0.02	0.05	0.5	TR
2.6	1.7	4.5	10	41	50	0.5	98	70	0.02	0.12	0.7	TR
0.7	0.9	1.3	14	37	59	1.0	314	2,350	0.07	0.05	1.0	—
1.1	1.2	0.4	21	29	149	1.5	270	440	0.25	0.15	1.5	1
0.5	0.5	1.0	16	15	34	0.7	230	1,000	0.05	0.05	1.2	12
—	—	—	10	12	49	0.7	162	2,700	0.05	0.05	1.0	—
—	—	—	13	20	39	1.0	172	2,940	0.05	0.05	1.0	—
—	—	—	TR	—	—	—	4	—	—	—	—	—
1.1	2.3	1.0	23	42	49	0.6	238	30	0.05	0.03	0.3	6
—	—	—	8	7	19	0.2	19	50	0.07	0.05	0.5	TR
—	—	—	6	10	12	0.2	58	TR	TR	TR	TR	2
—	—	—	12	7	19	0.2	29	480	0.05	0.02	0.5	5

(Continued)

APPENDIX C: (*Continued*)

Nutrients in Indicated Quantity

Item No. (A)	Foods, approximate measures, units, and weight (edible part unless footnote indicate otherwise) (B)		Water (C) %	Food Energy (D) kcal	Pro- tein (E) g	Fat (F) g
		g				
Miscellaneous Items—Con.						
727	Vinegar, cider	1 tbsp	15	94	TR	TR	0
728	White sauce, medium, with enriched flour	1 cup	250	73	405	10	31
	Yeast						
729	Baker's, dry, active	1 pkg	7	5	20	3	TR
730	Brewer's, dry	1 tbsp	8	5	25	3	TR

[70]Value may vary from 6 to 60 mg.

							Nutrients in Indicated Quantity						
Fatty Acids													
	Unsaturated												
Satu-rated (Total) (G) g	Oleic (H) g	Lino-leic (I) g	Carbo-hydrate (J) g	Calcium (K) mg	Phos-phorus (L) mg	Iron (M) mg	Potas-sium (N) mg	Vitamin A Value (O) I.U.	Thiamin (P) mg	Ribo-flavin (Q) mg	Niacin (R) mg	Ascorbic Acid (S) mg
0	0	0	1	1	1	0.1	15	—	—	—	—	—
19.3	7.8	0.8	22	288	233	0.5	348	1,150	0.12	0.43	0.7	2
—	—	—	3	3	90	1.1	140	TR	0.16	0.38	2.6	TR
—	—	—	3	[70]17	140	1.4	152	TR	1.25	0.34	3.0	TR

APPENDIX D: RELATIVE RATIOS OF POLYUNSATURATED FAT AND SATURATED FAT (P:S RATIO) IN REPRESENTATIVE FOODS

P:S Ratio	Foods
High >2.5:1	Almonds Corn oil Cottonseed oil Mayonnaise (made with oils in this group) Safflower oil Sesame oil Soft margarines Soybean oil Sunflower oil Walnuts
Medium high 2:1	Chicken Fish Peanut oil Semisolid margarines
Medium 1:1	Beef heart and liver Hydrogenated or hardened vegetable oils (shortenings, special products) Pecans Peanuts, peanut butter Solid margarines
Low 0.1–0.5:1	Chicken liver Lamb Lard Olive oil Palm oil Pork Veal
Very low <0.1:1	Beef Butter, cream Coconut oil Egg yolk Whole milk and milk products

APPENDIX E: SODIUM AND POTASSIUM CONTENT OF FOODS

Food	Approximate Amount	Weight (gm)	Sodium (mEq)	Potassium (mEq)
Meat Group				
Meat (cooked)				
Beef	1 oz	30	0.8	2.8
Ham	1 oz	30	14.3	2.6
Lamb	1 oz	30	0.9	2.2
Pork	1 oz	30	0.9	3.0
Veal	1 oz	30	1.0	3.8
Liver	1 oz	30	2.4	3.2
Sausage, pork	2 links	40	16.5	2.8
Beef, dried	2 slices	20	37.0	1.0
Cold cuts	1 slice	45	25.0	2.7
Frankfurters	1	50	24.0	3.0
Fowl				
Chicken	1 oz	30	1.0	3.0
Goose	1 oz	30	1.6	4.6
Duck	1 oz	30	1.0	2.2
Turkey	1 oz	30	1.2	2.8
Egg	1	50	2.7	1.8
Fish	1 oz	30	1.0	2.6
Salmon				
Fresh	$\frac{1}{4}$ cup	30	0.6	2.3
Canned	$\frac{1}{4}$ cup	30	4.6	2.6
Tuna				
Fresh	$\frac{1}{4}$ cup	30	0.5	2.2
Canned	$\frac{1}{4}$ cup	30	10.4	2.3
Sardines	3 medium	35	12.5	4.5
Shellfish				
Clams	5 small	50	2.6	2.3
Lobster	1 small tail	40	3.7	1.8
Oysters	5 small	70	2.1	1.5
Scallops	1 large	50	5.7	6.0
Shrimp	5 small	30	1.8	1.7
Cheese				
Cheese, American or Cheddar type	1 slice	30	9.1	0.6
Cheese foods	1 slice	30	15.0	0.8
Cheese spreads	2 tbsp	30	15.0	0.8
Cottage cheese	$\frac{1}{4}$ cup	50	5.0	1.1
Peanut butter	2 tbsp	30	7.8	5.0
Peanuts, unsalted	25	25	—	4.5

(Continued)

APPENDIX E: (Continued)

Food	Approximate Amount	Weight (gm)	Sodium (mEq)	Potassium (mEq)
Fat Group				
Avocado	$\frac{1}{8}$	30	—	4.6
Bacon	1 slice	5	2.2	0.6
Butter or margarine	1 tsp	5	2.2	—
Cooking fat	1 tsp	5	—	—
Cream				
Half and half	2 tbsp	30	0.6	1.0
Sour	2 tbsp	30	0.4	—
Whipped	2 tbsp	15	0.3	1.0
Cream cheese	1 tbsp	15	1.7	—
Mayonnaise	1 tsp	5	1.3	—
Nuts				
Almonds, slivered	5 (2 tsp)	6	—	0.8
Pecans	4 halves	5	—	0.8
Walnuts	5 halves	10	—	1.0
Oil, salad	1 tsp	5	—	—
Olives, green	3 medium	30	31.3	0.4
Bread Group				
Bread	1 slice	25	5.5	0.7
Biscuit	1 (2-in. diameter)	35	9.6	0.7
Muffin	1 (2-in. diameter)	35	7.3	1.2
Cornbread	1 ($1\frac{1}{2}$-in. cube)	35	11.3	1.7
Roll	1 (2-in. diameter)	25	5.5	0.6
Bun	1	30	6.6	0.7
Pancake	1 (4-in. diameter)	45	8.8	1.1
Waffle	$\frac{1}{2}$ square	35	8.5	1.0
Cereals				
Cooked	$\frac{2}{3}$ cup	140	8.7	2.0
Dry, flake	$\frac{2}{3}$ cup	20	8.7	0.6
Dry, puffed	$1\frac{1}{2}$ cups	20	—	1.5
Shredded wheat	1 biscuit	20	—	2.2
Crackers				
Graham	3	20	5.8	2.0
Melba toast	4	20	5.5	0.7
Oyster	20	20	9.6	0.6
Ritz	6	20	9.5	0.5
Rye-Krisp	3	30	11.5	3.0
Saltines	6	20	9.6	0.6
Soda	3	20	9.6	0.6
Dessert				
Commercial gelatin	$\frac{1}{2}$ cup	100	2.2	—
Ice cream	$\frac{1}{2}$ cup	75	2.0	3.0

APPENDIX E: (*Continued*)

Food	Approximate Amount	Weight (gm)	Sodium (mEq)	Potassium (mEq)
Sherbet	$\frac{1}{3}$ cup	50	—	—
Angel food cake	$1\frac{1}{2} \times 1\frac{1}{2}$ i.	25	3.0	0.6
Sponge cake	$1\frac{1}{2} \times 1\frac{1}{2}$ in.	25	1.8	0.6
Vanilla wafers	5	15	1.7	—
Floor products				
Cornstarch	2 tbsp	15	—	—
Macaroni	$\frac{1}{4}$ cup	50	—	0.8
Noodles	$\frac{1}{4}$ cup	50	—	0.6
Rice	$\frac{1}{4}$ cup	50	—	0.9
Spaghetti	$\frac{1}{4}$ cup	50	—	0.8
Tapioca	2 tbsp	15	—	—
Vegetable Group[a]				
Artichokes	1 large bud	100	1.3	7.7
Asparagus				
Cooked	$\frac{1}{2}$ cup	100	—	4.7
Canned[b]	$\frac{1}{2}$ cup	100	10.0	3.6
Frozen	$\frac{1}{2}$ cup	100	—	5.5
Beans, dried (cooked)	$\frac{1}{2}$ cup	90	—	10.0
Beans, lima	$\frac{1}{2}$ cup	90	—	9.5
Bean sprouts	$\frac{1}{2}$ cup	100	—	4.0
Beans, green or wax				
Fresh or frozen	$\frac{1}{2}$ cup	100	—	4.0
Canned[b]	$\frac{1}{2}$ cup	100	10.0	2.5
Beet greens	$\frac{1}{2}$ cup	100	3.0	8.5
Beets	$\frac{1}{2}$ cup	100	1.8	5.0
Broccoli	$\frac{1}{2}$ cup	100	—	7.0
Brussels sprouts	$\frac{2}{3}$ cup	100	—	7.6
Cabbage, cooked	$\frac{1}{2}$ cup	100	0.6	4.2
Raw	1 cup	100	0.9	6.0
Carrots, cooked	$\frac{1}{2}$ cup	100	1.4	5.7
Raw	1 large	100	2.0	8.8
Cauliflower, cooked	1 cup	100	0.4	5.2
Celery, raw	1 cup	100	5.4	9.0
Chard, Swiss	$\frac{3}{5}$ cup	100	3.7	8.0
Collards	$\frac{1}{2}$ cup	100	0.8	6.0
Corn				
Canned[b]	$\frac{1}{3}$ cup	80	8.0	2.0
Fresh	$\frac{1}{2}$ ear	100	—	2.0
Frozen	$\frac{1}{3}$ cup	80	—	3.7
Cress, garden (cooked)	$\frac{1}{2}$ cup	100	0.5	7.2
Cucumber	1 medium	100	0.3	4.0

(*Continued*)

APPENDIX E: (Continued)

Food	Approximate Amount	Weight (gm)	Sodium (mEq)	Potassium (mEq)
Vegetable Group[a] (Continued)				
Dandelion greens	½ cup	100	2.0	6.0
Eggplant	½ cup	100	—	3.8
Hominy (dry)	¼ cup	36	4.1	—
Kale, cooked	¾ cup	100	2.0	5.6
Frozen	½ cup	100	1.0	5.0
Kohlrabi	⅔ cup	100	—	6.6
Leeks, raw	3–4	100	—	9.0
Lettuce	varies	100	0.4	4.5
Mushrooms, raw	4 large	100	0.7	10.6
Mustard greens	½ cup	100	0.8	4.4
Okra	½ cup	100	—	4.4
Onions, cooked	½ cup	100	—	2.8
Parsnips	⅔ cup	100	0.3	9.7
Peas				
Canned[b]	½ cup	100	10.0	1.2
Dried	½ cup	90	1.5	6.8
Fresh	½ cup	100	—	2.5
Frozen	½ cup	100	2.5	1.7
Pepper, green or red				
Cooked	½ cup	100	—	5.5
Raw	1	100	0.5	4.0
Popcorn	1 cup	15	—	—
Potato				
Potato chips	1 oz	30	13.0	3.7
White, baked	½ cup	100	—	13.0
White, boiled	½ cup	100	—	7.3
Sweet, baked	¼ cup	50	0.4	4.0
Pumpkin	½ cup	100	—	6.3
Radishes	10	100	0.8	8.0
Rutabagas	½ cup	100	—	4.4
Sauerkraut	⅔ cup	100	32.0	3.5
Spinach	½ cup	100	2.2	8.5
Squash	½ cup	100	—	3.5
Squash, winter				
Baked	½ cup	100	—	12.0
Boiled	½ cup	100	—	6.5
Tomatoes	½ cup	100	—	6.5
Tomato juice	½ cup	100	0.7	3.8
Turnip greens	½ cup	100	0.7	3.8
Turnips	½ cup	100	1.5	4.8

APPENDIX E: (*Continued*)

Food	Approximate Amount	Weight (gm)	Sodium (mEq)	Potassium (mEq)
Milk Group				
Whole milk	1 cup	240	5.2	8.8
Evaporated whole milk	½ cup	120	6.0	9.2
Powdered whole milk	¼ cup	30	5.2	10.0
Buttermilk	1 cup	240	13.6	8.5
Skim milk	1 cup	240	5.2	8.8
Powdered skim milk	¼ cup	30	6.9	13.5
Fruit Group				
Figs				
Canned	½ cup	120	—	4.6
Dried	1 small	15	—	2.5
Fresh	1 large	60	—	5.0
Fruit cocktail	½ cup	120	—	5.0
Grapes				
Canned	⅓ cup	80	—	2.2
Fresh	15	80	—	3.2
Juice				
Bottled	¼ cup	60	—	2.8
Frozen	⅓ cup	80	—	2.4
Grapefruit				
Fresh	½ medium	120	—	3.6
Juice	½ cup	120	—	4.1
Sections	¾ cup	150	—	5.1
Mandarin orange	¾ cup	200	—	6.5
Mango	½ small	70	—	3.4
Melon				
Cantaloupe	½ small	200	—	13.0
Honeydew	¼ medium	200	—	13.0
Watermelon	½ slice	200	—	5.0
Nectarine	1 medium	80	—	6.0
Orange				
Fresh	1 medium	100	—	5.1
Juice	½ cup	120	—	5.7
Sections	½ cup	100	—	5.1
Papaya	½ cup	120	—	7.0
Peach				
Canned	½ cup	120	—	4.0
Dried	2 halves	20	—	5.0
Fresh	1 medium	120	—	6.2
Nectar	½ cup	120	—	2.4

(*Continued*)

APPENDIX E: *(Continued)*

Food	Approximate Amount	Weight (gm)	Sodium (mEq)	Potassium (mEq)
Fruit Group (Continued)				
Pear				
Canned	½ cup	120	—	2.5
Dried	2 halves	20	—	3.0
Fresh	1 small	80	—	2.6
Nectar	⅓ cup	80	—	0.9
Pineapple				
Canned	½ cup	120	—	3.0
Fresh	½ cup	80	—	3.0
Juice	⅓ cup	80	—	3.0
Plums				
Canned	½ cup	120	—	4.5
Fresh	2 medium	80	—	4.1
Prunes	2 medium	15	—	2.6
Juice	¼ cup	60	—	3.6
Raisins	1 tbsp	15	—	2.9
Rhubarb	½ cup	100	—	6.5
Tangerines				
Fresh	2 small	100	—	3.2
Juice	½ cup	120	—	5.5
Sections	½ cup	100	—	3.2

Source: Reproduced with permission from *Mayo Clinic Diet Manual,* 4th ed. Philadelphia: W.B. Saunders Company, 1971.

[a]Value for products without added salt.

[b]Estimated average based on addition of salt, approximately 0.6% of the finished product.

Note: To convert mEq to mg multiply mEq by 23 (sodium) or 39 (potassium) mEq × 23 = mg of sodium mEq × 39 = mg of potassium.

GLOSSARY

Abscess Localized collection of pus in cavities formed by the disintegration of tissues.

Acetylcholine A neurotransmitter that transmits nerve impulses between certain types of neurons.

Acid ash diet A diet that includes foods that will form an acid urine.

Acidic An acid-forming substance. Some foods cause an acidic pH in the urine.

Acidosis A condition in which the pH of blood is below 7.35; can result in the denaturation of proteins.

Acid-base balance A balance of the amount of acid and base ions so that blood pH is within the normal range, 7.35–7.45.

Acid-resistant Something that is resistant to acid but susceptible to bases. An example is the enteric coating on some drugs.

Active transport Movement of molecules from a low concentration to a high concentration. Energy is required and involves carrier molecules.

Acute fulminating A condition that occurs suddenly with great intensity.

Acute glomerulonephritis A form of kidney disease that involves inflammation of the glomeruli.

Acute renal disease Sudden onset of kidney disease.

Acute renal failure Sudden onset of renal failure.

Acute respiratory failure (ARF) Inadequacy of the respiratory function in maintaining the body's need for an oxygen supply and for carbon dioxide removal while at rest.

Addison's disease A disease caused by insufficient secretion of adrenal hormones.

Adipose tissue Fat tissue.

Adolescence The period of life from 12 to about 20 years of age.

Adrenal gland A gland located on top of the kidneys that secretes several different hormones.

Adrenocorticotrophic hormone (ACTH) A hormone that is secreted by the anterior pituitary gland.

Adult respiratory distress syndrome (ARDS) A variety of acute lung lesions that cause deficient oxygenation of the blood.

Adult-onset obesity Obesity beginning in adulthood.

Aerobic respiration A process in cell respiration in which ATP molecules are synthesized and oxygen is required.

Air embolism Air bubbles in the blood as a result of air leaks through a catheter.

Albumin A blood protein that regulates the osmotic pressure of the blood.

Albuminuria Albumin in the urine.

Aldosterone A hormone secreted from the adrenal gland that regulates the levels of sodium and potassium.

Alimentary canal A muscular tube that extends from the mouth to the anus.

Alkalosis A condition in which the pH of blood is above 7.45; can result in the denaturation of proteins.

Alveolar surfactant A protein compound that is important in inflating the lungs.

Alzheimer's disease A condition that results from a depletion of acetylcholine and causes losses of neurons in the brain.

Amino acid The fundamental building block of proteins.

Amino acid content The number of essential amino acids present in a particular food.

Amino acid pool A region in which large numbers of amino acids are maintained, such as in the liver.

From the liver, the amino acids are distributed to the tissues.

Anabolic steroid Male hormone that is naturally secreted in large quantities during sexual maturity.

Anabolism A metabolic process whereby large molecules are synthesized from small ones.

Anaerobic (glycolysis) respiration A process in cell respiration in which ATP molecules are synthesized and oxygen is not required.

Anemia A condition in which the total quantity of red blood cells and hemoglobin is less than normal.

Angina pectoris Acute pain in the chest resulting from ischemia of the heart muscle.

Anhydrous Lacking water molecules; an example is anhydrous dextrose, which is found in food.

Anion Mineral that is negatively charged.

Anorexia A loss of appetite.

Anorexia nervosa A self-starvation disease that is characterized by severe disruption of the person's eating behavior.

Anthropometric measurement Measurement of the size, weight, and proportions of the human body.

Antiarrhythmic Agent that prevents variations of the normal heart rhythm.

Antibiotic Chemical substance produced by bacteria, yeasts, and molds that is damaging to other cells such as disease-producing bacteria.

Antibody Protein formed by the body to combat antigens.

Anticholinergic drug Drug that blocks the passage of impulses through the parasympathetic nerves.

Anticonvulsant Agent that suppresses convulsions; the drug Dilantin is an example of an anticonvulsant.

Antifungal An agent that destroys or checks the growth of fungi.

Antigen Foreign substance (usually a protein) that invades the body; can cause infections and allergic reactions.

Antihistamine Drug that counteracts inflammation or allergies.

Antihypertensive agent Agent that reduces high blood pressure.

Antineoplastic agent Cancer-fighting drug.

Antioxidant A compound that prevents oxidation.

Antipsychotic drugs Drugs that control the symptoms of mental disorders but not the causes.

Anti-inflammatory agent An agent that counteracts inflammation.

Anuria Less than 50 ml of urine per day excreted from the body.

Appetite A learned psychological response to food that is initiated for reasons other than the need for food.

Arachidonic A fatty acid that is derived from linoleic acid.

Ascending colon The portion of the large intestine that ascends upward on the right side of the body from the cecum to the liver.

Ascites The accumulation of fluids in the abdominal cavity.

Aseptic Free from infection or infectious material.

Aspiration pneumonia Regurgitation of the stomach contents and inhalation into the lungs.

Asthma A respiratory condition, characterized by recurrent attacks of wheezing, that may be due to bronchitis.

ATP Adenosine triphosphate. A high-energy compound that supplies energy for body processes.

Ataxia Uncoordinated gait.

Atelectasis A collapsed state of the lungs, which may involve all or part of the lungs.

Atheroma An abnormal mass of fatty or lipid material with a fibrous covering often found in the inner lining of arteries.

Atherosclerosis Accumulation of fatty plaques within medium-sized and large arteries.

Atrial arrhythmia Abnormal rhythm in the contractions of the atria in the heart.

Atrophy A decrease in the size of a normally developed organ.

Attention deficit disorder (ADD) Disorder such as hyperkinesia that can be seen in children.

Autodigestion Self-digestion.

Autoimmunity A condition in which the body forms antibodies against its own tissues.

Autosomal dominant trait A dominant gene that is present on one of the 22 pairs of genes known as *autosomes*.

Azotemia Presence of excess nitrogen in the blood.

Bacterial pneumonia A type of pneumonia in which the alveoli become filled with exudate that interferes with the exchange of gases.

Barrel chest An appearance of the chest often seen in people who suffer from chronic asthma attacks.

Basal energy expenditure (BEE) The amount of energy expended by a person at rest.

Basal metabolic rate The rate at which the body uses energy for maintenance of homeostasis at rest.

Basal region A region located at the base of the brain.

Basic A base-forming substance. Some foods cause a basic pH in the urine.

Behavior modification An approach to the correction of undesirable eating habits. This procedure involves the manipulation of environmental and behavioral variables.

Beta cell Cell in the pancreas that secretes insulin. These cells are often damaged in IDDM, causing an insulin deficiency.

Bile A fluid secreted by the liver that emulsifies fat molecules in the small intestine.

Bile salt Clear yellow or orange fluid secreted by the liver.

Biliary atresia Congenital destruction or closure of one or more bile ducts in the liver.

Bilirubin A pigment produced by the breakdown of heme and secreted into bile.

Binder compound Substance that inhibits absorption of calcium.

Binge eating Consumption of large amounts of food in a short period of time.

Biological value (BV) Measures the absorbed nitrogen that is retained for growth or maintenance and not excreted through the feces, urine, or skin.

Blackhead A plug of sebum within a hair follicle.

Bland diet A diet that restricts the use of many spicy foods.

Blood acidosis A condition in which blood pH is below 7.35. This condition can result from an excess amount of ketones.

Blood capillary Microscopic blood vessels through which nutrients and wastes are exchanged.

Blood lipid profile A measurement of the amounts of different classes of lipoproteins.

Blood urea nitrogen (BUN) Nitrogenous waste product formed in the liver when amino acids are deaminized.

Body composition The percentage of total body weight that is composed of fat, muscle, and water.

Body frame size The size of a person's body frame, with small, medium, and large being the three possibilities.

Body size Height and weight.

Body surface area (BSA) An estimate of the total body surface area. This measurement is important in burn situations for determining the level of nutritional care.

Bolus A round mass of food.

Bolus feeding Intermittent feeding of a formula as meals.

Bonding The formation of an emotional link between the mother and infant.

Bowman's capsule A proximal portion of a renal tubule that encloses the glomerulus of a nephron.

Bronchial pneumonia Inflammation of the bronchi in the lungs.

Bronchiogenic cancer A malignant tumor of the lung that originates in the epithelial lining of the bronchi.

Bronchitis Inflammation of the bronchi, the passageways to the lungs.

Buffer Compound in the blood that resists changes in pH with the addition of acids and bases.

Bulimarexia Purging of food.

Bulimia An enormous appetite that is satisfied by eating binges.

Cachexia A problem characterized by extreme weight loss, weakness, and severe wasting of tissues.

Calcidiol The inactive form of vitamin D that is stored in the liver.

Calcification The hardening of soft tissues due to an accumulation of calcium.

Calcitriol The active form of vitamin D.

Calcium antagonist Antiarrhythmic drug that is effective in managing some types of arrhythmias.

Calipers   An instrument with two bent or curved legs. It is frequently used for measuring skinfold thickness.

Calorie (cal)   The amount of heat required to raise the temperature of 1 g of water 1°C.

Carbohydrate   Organic compound composed of carbon, hydrogen, and oxygen, with a 2:1 ratio of hydrogen to oxygen atoms.

Carcinogenic   A cancer-causing substance.

Cardiotonic glycoside   Drug that increases the strength of heart contractions.

Cardiovascular disease   Disease of the blood vessels and the heart.

Carotene   A precursor of vitamin A.

Caseous necrosis   Necrosis of the tubules in which the dead tissue assumes a cheesy appearance.

Catabolic steroid   Steroid hormone that promotes catabolism.

Catabolism   A breakdown phase that involves oxidation (the loss of hydrogen atoms and energy) of glucose.

Catabolized   Broken down.

Cathartic   Laxative drugs.

Catheter   A slender, flexible tube of rubber or plastic that is inserted into a channel such as a vein.

Cation   Mineral that is positively charged.

Cecum   The first portion of the large intestine to which the small intestine attaches and from which the appendix extends.

Celiac crisis   An attack of watery diarrhea and vomiting.

Celiac disease   A disease characterized by the degeneration and atrophy of the intestinal villi, induced by the ingestion of foods containing gluten.

Cellulose   Fiber.

Celsius (C)   A unit of temperature measurement on the Celsius scale.

Central vein   A vein located in the center or midline of the body; an example is the superior vena cava.

Central vein total parenteral nutrition   Infusion of nutrients through a catheter into the subclavian vein and their guidance into the superior vena cava.

Cephalin   A phospholipid found in the body.

Cerebrovascular accident   A rupture or blockage of a blood vessel in the brain.

Cheilosis   Cracks at the corner of the mouth due to a deficiency of vitamin B_2.

Chemically defined (elemental) diet   Formula that is composed of purified or synthetic nutrients.

Chlorophyll   The green pigment found in most plant cells that is important for photosynthesis.

Cholecalciferol   Chemical name for vitamin D.

Cholecystectomy   Surgical removal of the gallbladder.

Cholecystitis   An inflammation of the gallbladder that results from bacterial infection or gallstones.

Cholecystokinin   A hormone that stimulates the gallbladder to contract and release bile.

Cholelithiasis   The formation of stones in the gallbladder.

Cholesterol   A lipid that is produced by the body and used in the synthesis of steroid hormones and excreted in bile.

Choline   A compound that is synthesized in the body from serine and methionine amino acids.

Chromosome   Rod-like structure that appears in the nucleus of the cell during mitosis. The chromosomes contain genes.

Chronic continuous   A condition that persists for a long time and shows either little change or an extremely slow progression over a long period.

Chronic intermittent (recurrent) colitis   A type of ulcerative colitis that is characterized by mild diarrhea and intermittent, slight bleeding.

Chronic obstructive pulmonary disease (COPD)   A chronic, persistent obstruction of the air flow into the bronchi of the lung. Asthma, bronchitis, and emphysema are the main causes of this condition.

Chronic persistent hepatitis.   An inflammation of the liver that may last for 4–8 months.

Chronic renal disease   Gradual onset of kidney disease.

Chronic renal failure   Gradual onset of renal failure.

Chylomicron   Lipoprotein synthesized in the intestines that transports triglycerides through the lymph and blood to the liver.

Chyme   Semifluid mass of food that is formed in the stomach and released into the duodenum.

Cirrhosis   Inflammation and scarring of interstitial

(between parts) tissue; commonly occurs in liver tissue.

Citric acid cycle (Krebs Cycle) A series of aerobic respiration reactions that result in the release of hydrogen atoms and CO_2 molecules and the synthesis of one ATP molecule.

Clear liquid diet A diet limited to liquids such as broths, gelatin, and strained fruit juices.

Clinical care process A series of activities (assessment, planning, implementation, and evaluation) used by health professionals to identify and meet patients' needs.

Coenzyme A small nonprotein molecule that combines with an inactive protein to make it an active enzyme.

Colic A spasm in an organ accompanied by pain.

Collagen A protein that is important in the structure of skin, teeth, bones, and muscle.

Collateral channel Vein that is used as detour routes from the liver connecting to veins from the lower esophagus.

Collecting duct A duct that carries urine from the distal convoluted tubule of the nephron to the pelvic region.

Colonic diverticulosis A condition characterized by small, saclike herniations of the colon mucosa called diverticula.

Complementary protein supplementation A strategy that involves eating two or more foods that are complementary to each other in amino acids.

Complete protein Protein that contains all of the essential amino acids in amounts needed by the body.

Cone Receptor cell in the retina of the eye that is sensitive to bright light and colors.

Confabulation Recitation of imaginary experiences to fill gaps in memory.

Congenital lactase deficiency A rare inherited intolerance of lactase throughout life.

Congenital metabolic disorder An inherited metabolic disorder that a child is born with, such as phenylketonuria (PKU).

Congestive heart failure A failure of the heart to pump the blood adequately to the tissues. It results in an accumulation of blood and fluids in the tissues and therefore causes congestion.

Convulsion Involuntary spasm or contraction of groups of muscles.

Cor pulmonale Hypertrophy of the right side of the heart.

Cornea The outer covering of the eye.

Coronary artery Artery that supplies blood to the myocardium (heart tissue).

Cortisone A hormone secreted from the cortex region of the adrenal glands. It increases the blood glucose level.

Creatinine A nitrogenous waste that is formed from protein, muscle, and purine metabolism.

Creatinine clearance The rate at which the nitrogen compound creatinine is filtered out of the blood by the kidneys.

Creatinine height index A laboratory test that measures the amount of creatinine excreted in the urine. Creatinine results from muscle metabolism; therefore, it is indicative of the skeletal muscle mass.

Cretinism A condition caused by an iodine deficiency in an infant.

Crohn's disease An inflammatory disease that is located primarily in the ileum region of the small intestine and may extend into the large intestine.

Crude fiber The residue left after laboratory treatment of food with acid and alkali.

Culture The concept, skills, and broad-based characteristics of a given population.

Cushing's disease A condition caused by an excessive secretion of hormones from the cortex region of the adrenal glands.

Cyanotic Bluish color of the skin due to reduced level of oxygen.

Cystic duct A duct that drains bile from the gallbladder to the common bile duct.

Cystic fibrosis A hereditary disease characterized by secretion and accumulation of excessively thick mucus that blocks the secretion of pancreatic enzymes.

Cytochrome A molecule in the electron transport system.

DDT (dichloro diphenyl trichloroethane) An insecticide that is toxic to insects and humans. It has been found in human breast milk.

Deamination The removal of an amine group (NH_2) from each amino acid.

Decompensation The inability of the heart to maintain adequate circulation. It is characterized by edema, cyanosis, and dyspnea.

Decubiti Bed sores or skin ulcers that result from interference with blood circulation to the skin.

Dehydration An excess loss of fluids from tissues.

Deltoid muscle Triangular-shaped muscle at the cap of the shoulder. It is frequently used as a site of injections.

Dementia A severe mental disorder involving impairment of mental ability.

Demographic The study of human populations in terms of size, growth, density, and other vital statistics.

Denaturation A change in the chemical structure of a molecule; often occurs with protein molecules when certain conditions exist.

Densitometry A method of determining the body composition and body fatness of a person. The method involves measuring the body's specific gravity by immersing the individual in water.

Dental caries Decay or cavities of the teeth.

Deoxyribonucleic acid (DNA) A nucleic acid found in the cell nucleus. It contains genetic information for the synthesis of specific proteins.

Dermatitis Inflammation of the skin, evidenced by itching and redness.

Descending colon The portion of the large intestine that extends downward along the left side of the abdomen.

Developmental lactase deficiency A condition that results from a gradual decrease in lactase during childhood and adolescence.

Dextrin Product of starch digestion in the mouth.

Diabetes insipidus A type of diabetes that is caused by inadequate secretion of the antidiuretic hormone (ADH).

Diabetes mellitus Disease of the pancreas that causes inadequate secretion of insulin, thereby resulting in an inability to regulate blood glucose level normally.

Diabetic ketoacidosis (DKA) A buildup of ketones in the blood that results from uncontrolled IDDM.

Diabetic nephropathy Kidney disease caused by damage to blood vessels that results from diabetes.

Diabetic retinopathy Damage to the retinal blood capillaries as a result of diabetes.

Dialysate A fluid that bathes semipermeable dialysis membranes.

Dialysis The separation of small molecules from large ones by passage through a semipermeable membrane.

Diastolic The pressure created by the relaxation of the heart ventricles.

Diet therapy The use of modified diets to help a person overcome or cope with an illness or inter-related illnesses.

Dietary fiber Fiber resistant to the human digestive enzymes.

Diffusion Movement of molecules from high concentration to low concentration.

Digestibility Pertains to the ease of digestion.

Dipeptides Molecules composed of two amino acids.

Diplopia Double vision.

Disaccharide Double sugar.

Distal convoluted tubule The portion of the renal tubule that is farthest from Bowman's tubule. Some water reabsorption and secretion occur here.

Diuresis Increased urine flow.

Diuretics Agents that promote urine excretion and are used to alleviate edema.

Diverticulitis Inflammatory condition of diverticula caused by bacterial growth and action arising from food residues and fecal matter.

Diverticulosis Presence of diverticula (outpouching of the colon wall).

Dorsal plexus A network of veins located near the dorsal surface of the foot.

Dorsum The back or posterior surface of a body or part.

Drug Chemical substance that is intended to have a therapeutic effect on a patient.

Dumping syndrome A number of physical problems (nausea, vomiting, sweating, and palpitations) that develop from a gastrectomy. The problems develop when the stomach contents enter the duodenum too rapidly and large amounts of fluid shift out of the blood into the duodenum.

Duodenal ulcer A deterioration of the mucosal lining of the duodenum.

Duodenum First region of the small intestine.

Dysphagia Difficulty in swallowing.

Dyspnea Labored breathing.

Eclampsia High blood pressure accompanied by convulsions and coma.

Eczema Redness and small blisters on the skin.

Edema Accumulation of water in tissues.

Edematous Refers to a condition of edema.

Elderly People who are 65 years of age or older.

Electrolyte depletion A reduction in the amount of electrolytes below the normal level.

Electron transport system Composed of cytochrome molecules by which the pairs of hydrogen electrons released from glycolysis and citric acid cycles are carried.

Elemental formula Liquid formula that contains simple sugars and amino acids.

Emphysema A disease characterized by the gradual destruction of alveoli, enlargement of distal air spaces, and trapping of air.

Emulsifying agent Substance that increases the surface area of fats for ease of absorption.

Endotracheal tube An airway catheter inserted into the trachea that removes secretions and maintains an adequate air passageway.

End-stage renal disease (ESRD) The stage of chronic renal failure in which 90% of the kidney tissue is damaged.

Energy The capacity to do work.

Energy balance The amount of energy remaining in the body when energy output is subtracted from energy input.

Energy intake Energy supplied by the three energy nutrients: carbohydrates, fats, and proteins.

Enteral nutrition The movement of nutrients through the intestine into the blood.

Enteric Pertains to the small intestine. An enteric coat prevents the release and absorption of the drug until it reaches the small intestine.

Epigastric distress (pain) Pain and discomfort in the epigastrium region, which is the upper central region of the abdomen.

Epinephrine A hormone secreted by the adrenal gland in times of stress.

Epithelial Cells that form the outer layer of the skin.

Erythrocyte Red blood cell.

Erythropoiesis The synthesis of red blood cells.

Erythropoietin A hormone, secreted by the kidneys, that stimulates erythropoiesis.

Esophageal reflux Backward and upward flow of food through the esophagus.

Esophageal varices Dilation of esophageal veins.

Esophagotomy Introduction of a tube through the skin into the esophagus.

Essential amino acids Amino acids that must be present in the diet since they cannot be synthesized by the body.

Essential fatty acid A fatty acid (e.g., linoleic acid) that cannot be manufactured by the body in adequate quantities and, therefore, must be obtained from the diet.

Essential hypertension A type of hypertension for which there is no known cause.

Essential nutrient Compound that the body cannot synthesize.

Estrogen The female sex hormone secreted by the ovaries. It stimulates the development of the female secondary sex characteristics.

Etiology Cause.

Exacerbation Increased severity and complications.

Exogenous Outside of the body.

Extracellular Fluid outside cells, such as plasma and interstitial fluid.

Extrinsic factor A compound that refers to vitamin B_{12} and is formed outside the body.

Exudate Fluid with a high content of protein and cellular debris.

Fasting blood glucose/sugar (FBG or FBS) A blood glucose test performed on a person's blood after an overnight fast.

Fasting hypoglycemia A type of hypoglycemia that occurs either long after a meal, in the middle of the night, or before breakfast.

Fat cell hypothesis The theory that the body has the potential to accumulate an excess number of fat cells during three periods of life: the last 3 months of fetal development, the first 3 years of life, and adolescence.

Fat soluble Able to be dissolved in fats.

Fatty acid Chain of carbon and hydrogen atoms that functions as a building block of fat molecules.

Ferric Chemical form of iron, Fe^{3+}; a less absorbable form than ferrous iron.

Ferritin A form of iron that is stored in the liver, spleen, and bone marrow.

Ferrous Chemical form of iron, Fe^{2+}; more absorbable form than ferric iron.

Ferrous sulfate An oral iron supplement that is often given to correct iron deficiency anemia.

Fetal alcohol syndrome (FAS) Characterized by growth retardation, physical deformities, behavioral defects, and mental retardation in a baby born to an alcoholic mother.

Fever Elevation of body temperature above normal.

Fibrinogen A blood protein that contributes to blood clotting.

Filtrate A fluid present in Bowman's capsule. It is formed by filtration of blood in the glomeruli.

Fistula Abnormal tube-like passage within the body tissue, usually between two internal organs.

Flavin adenine dinucleotide (FAD) An electron transfer compound that transfers electrons and hydrogen atoms from the Krebs cycle through the cytochrome system to oxygen.

Flavin A chemical that is fluorescent.

Food diary A record of what a person eats, the mood he or she is in while eating, and the circumstances in which eating occurs.

Food fallacy False, deceptive idea about food and its effects in the body.

Food frequency record A method that is used to determine how many times per day, week, month, or year a person consumes certain foods from the Food Pyramid.

Fortified The addition of nutrients to a food to make it richer than the unprocessed food.

Fructose Fruit sugar.

Functional hypoglycemia A type of hypoglycemia that occurs 3–4 hours after eating or in response to a meal.

Galactosemia A genetic disease in which galactose is not properly metabolized due to the lack of an enzyme.

Gallstone Stonelike mass that forms in the gallbladder.

Gangrene Death of body tissue due to a loss of the vascular supply, followed by bacterial invasion and putrefaction.

Gastrectomy Surgical removal of the stomach.

Gastric ulcer A deterioration of the gastric mucosa generally located along the lesser curvature of the stomach.

Gastritis Inflammation of the stomach lining.

Gastrostomy Feeding directly into the stomach through a specially created opening.

Generic Chemical name of a drug.

Gene The portion of DNA molecules that contains information necessary to synthesize an enzyme.

Genetic Congenital or inherited.

Giordano-Giovannetti (G-G) diet A diet used to treat chronic renal failure.

Globule Small mass of material. Fat globules are small masses of fat that result from the interaction of large fat masses with bile.

Glomerular filtration rate (GFR) The amount of filtrate formed.

Glomerulus A capillary tuft within the Bowman's capsule of a nephron.

Glossitis Smooth, purplish appearance of the tongue due to a deficiency of vitamin B_2.

Glucagon A hormone secreted by the pancreas.

Glucose tolerance factor A compound that helps to bind insulin to cell membranes.

Glucostatic theory The theory that when the blood glucose level is high, a person will feel full, and when it is low, the person will feel hungry.

Gluten A water-soluble protein found in wheat, rye, barley, and oats.

Gluten intolerance (gluten-induced enteropathy) A disorder in which gluten (protein) causes the destruction of intestinal villi, thereby preventing the absorption of fats and other nutrients.

Glyceride A fat, such as monoglyceride, diglyceride, and triglyceride.

Glycogen Branched chain polysaccharide composed of glucose molecules.

Glycogenesis Synthesis of glycogen.

Glycogenolysis The catabolism of glycogen.

Glycolysated hemoglobin (HbA$_{1c}$) A test that measures the amount of hemoglobin to which glucose is attached.

Goal A statement of the desired outcome in a patient.

Goiter Abnormal enlargement of the thyroid gland due to an inbalance in the amount of the mineral iodine.

Goitrogen Substance that blocks the absorption or use of iodine.

Gout A metabolic disease characterized by an inability to metabolize purines and an elevated uric acid level in the blood.

Granuloma A tumor-like mass of granulation tissue.

Gravity-drip method A method by which liquid formulas flow slowly by gravity through a nasogastric tube.

Gum A water-soluble, nonstructural polysaccharide.

Hematocrit A percentage of RBCs in a sample of whole blood.

Hematuria Blood in the urine.

Hemicellulose A polysaccharide that is similar to cellulose.

Hemochromatosis An inherited disease in which a person absorbs and deposits excessive amounts of iron in the liver.

Hemodialysis Circulation of arterial blood from the body into a machine called a dialyzer. Through diffusion and osmosis, nitrogenous wastes, excess fluid, and electrolytes are exchanged from the blood into the dialysate. The cleansed blood is then returned to the body.

Hemoglobin A protein molecule composed of four amino acid chains with one iron atom in each.

Hemolytic anemia A condition that results in the destruction of red blood cells (RBCs) at a faster than normal rate.

Hemolyzed Broken down.

Hemorrhage An escape of blood from a ruptured or damaged vessel.

Hemosiderin An insoluble form of iron that is stored in the liver.

Hemothorax Presence of blood in the chest.

Heparin An anticoagulant or substance that prevents blood clotting.

Hepatic cirrhosis The degeneration of liver cells with the formation of fibrous scar tissue.

Hepatic coma A coma that results from the buildup of ammonia, which increases as a result of the liver's inability to convert ammonia to urea.

Hepatic encephalopathy A condition caused by increased levels of ammonia in the blood, which leads to a malfunction of brain tissue.

Hepatic vein Vein that drains the blood from the liver into the inferior vena cava.

Hepatitis A viral infection that results in inflammation of the liver tissue.

Hiatal hernia A condition in which the stomach protrudes through an opening in the diaphragm through which the esophagus passes.

High-fiber diet A diet that contains large amounts of fiber (greater than 40 g) such as fresh fruits, vegetables, and bran cereals.

High-potassium diet A diet that contains foods that are rich in potassium such as bacon, bran, instant coffee, and oatmeal.

Hives Itching and burning swellings of the skin.

Human lymphocyte antigens (HLA) A lymphocyte (a type of white blood cell) that has an antigen attached to its surface.

Hunger An inborn instinct that causes a physiological response to the body's need for food.

Hydrochloric acid Acid secreted by cells in the stomach that changes pepsinogen to pepsin.

Hydrogen transport molecule Molecule in cell respiration that transports hydrogen atoms from glucose to cytochrome molecules.

Hydrogenation A process by which an unsaturated fat is changed to a solid saturated fat by forcing hydrogens into the substance.

Hydrolysate Solution with amino acids.

Hydrometry A method of determining the body composition and body fatness of a person. It involves injection of deuterium oxide (heavy water) into the body.

Hydrothorax Fluid in the chest.

Hyperactivity Abnormally increased activity that is often referred to as hyperkinesia in children.

Hyperaldosteronism An increased level of the hormone aldosterone.

Hyperalimentation Injection of hyperosmolar fluids directly into the superior vena cava vein.

Hyperammonemia Excess ammonia in the blood.

Hypercalcemia A condition in which the blood calcium level is elevated.

Hypercholesterolemia High level of cholesterol in the blood.

Hyperglycemia A condition characterized by an excess amount of glucose in the blood.

Hyperkalemia Elevated blood potassium levels.

Hyperlipidemia Elevated level of lipids in the blood.

Hyperlipoproteinemia Elevated blood lipoprotein level.

Hypermetabolic A high metabolic rate following problems like major trauma or burns.

Hyperosmolar hyperglycemic nonketotic coma (HHNK) A complication of type II or noninsulin-dependent diabetes mellitus. Hyperglycemia causes a loss of fluids and electrolytes that can result in coma and death.

Hyperparathyroidism An excessive secretion of the parathyroid hormone from the gland.

Hyperphosphatemia An excess of phosphate in the blood.

Hyperplasia A dramatic increase in the number of fat cells.

Hypertension Sustained high arterial blood pressure, either diastolic, systolic, or both.

Hyperthyroidism Excessive activity of the thyroid gland, which results in increased secretion of thyroxine.

Hypertonic A food or solution that has an osmolality of at least 340 mOsm or higher.

Hypertrophy An increase in the size of fat cells.

Hypervitaminosis A An excess amount of vitamin A that results in a toxicity condition.

Hypoalbuminemia A low level of albumin in the blood.

Hypochromic Pale in color.

Hypochromic microcytic anemia Anemic condition characterized by RBCs that are smaller in size and pale in color.

Hypoglycemia Abnormally low level of blood glucose.

Hypoglycemic agent A drug that decreases blood glucose levels.

Hypokalemia Decreased blood potassium levels.

Hyponatremia Deficiency of sodium in the blood.

Hypophosphatemia A deficiency of phosphates in the blood.

Hypothalamus An area at the base of the brain that contains centers of hunger and satiety and secretes the antidiuretic hormone.

Hypothyroidism Decreased activity of the thyroid gland which results in an underproduction of thyroxine.

Hypotonic A food or solution that has an osmolality of 240 mOsm or lower.

Hypovolemic shock Shock caused by low blood volume.

Hypoxia A decreased amount of oxygen available to the tissues.

Iatrogenic malnutrition Physician-induced malnutrition.

Ileocecal valve A valve that is located between the ileum and the cecum.

Ileostomy An opening into the ileum for drainage of fecal matter.

Ileum The terminal portion of the small intestine that is connected to the large intestine.

Inborn error of metabolism An inherited metabolic disorder.

Incomplete protein Protein lacking one or more of the essential amino acids.

Infancy The period from time of birth through the first year.

Inferior vena cava The vein that drains the blood from the lower part of the body to the right atrium of the heart.

Inorganic nutrient Substance that does not contain carbon atoms.

Insensible water loss Fluid lost through the skin, vomiting, diarrhea, and fever.

Insulin A hormone secreted by the pancreas that aids in both the diffusion of glucose into the liver and muscle cells and the synthesis of glycogen.

Insulin resistance The deactivation of insulin.

Insulin shock (insulin reaction) A condition caused by a blood glucose level below 50 mg/dl.

Insulinoma A small noncancerous pancreatic tumor that causes secretion of an excessive amount of insulin.

Insulin-dependent diabetes mellitus (IDDM) A type of diabetes in which the person does not secrete enough insulin to control the blood glucose level.

Intermittent positive-pressure breathing The use of a ventilator for treatment of patients with inadequate breathing.

Interstitial Between parts. Interstitial fluid, which is located between cells, is an example.

Intestinal flora Bacteria in the large intestine.

Intestinal villi Small mucous projections lining the small intestine.

Intracellular Fluid within cells.

Intralipid A fat emulsion solution that is administered intravenously to supply essential fatty acids and kilocalories.

Intramuscular injections Injections of substances into muscles.

Intramuscularly Within a muscle.

Intrauterine devices (IUDS) Objects inserted into the uterus for contraceptive purposes.

Intrinsic Functional substances in blood or urine.

Intrinsic factor A protein that is secreted by the gastric mucosa and combines with vitamin B_{12}, thereby making its absorption possible.

Involution The contraction of the enlarged uterus after birth.

Iodine number Number of grams of iodine absorbed by 100 g of fat.

Ionize Chemical process by which substances break apart into ions.

Ion Atom or molecule that has either a positive or a negative charge.

Iron deficiency anemia A reduced number of RBCs that are smaller than normal.

Ischemia The lack of blood flow and oxygen to a body part that is often due to an obstruction of an artery, as in atherosclerosis.

Islet cell antibodies Antibodies formed in response to islet of Langerhans cell fragments.

Islets of Langerhans Irregular microscopic structures scattered throughout the pancreas. They are composed of alpha cells that secrete glucagon and beta cells that secrete insulin.

Isotonic A food or solution that has the approximate osmolality of body fluids: 300 mOsm.

Jaundice Yellow discoloration of the whites of the eyes and the skin due to buildup of bile in blood.

Jejunostomy Feeding directly into the jejunum region of the small intestine through a specially created opening.

Jejunum The region of the small intestine that extends from the duodenum to the ileum.

Juvenile-onset obesity Obesity beginning during the last 3 months of fetal life, the first 3 years of life, and adolescence.

Keratin A protein substance in hair and nails.

Keratinized To become hard or horny.

Ketoacidosis High blood level of ketones (acids).

Ketone Product of incomplete metabolism of fats (acetone is an example of a ketone).

Kidney stones The stones formed in the kidneys as a result of certain dietary and chemical changes.

Kilocalorie (kcal) A unit of energy measurement that is calculated and expressed in relation to nutrition. A *calorie* is often called a *small calorie*, since 1,000 small calories equal 1 kilocalorie.

Kwashiorkor A type of protein-calorie malnutrition that results from a decreased protein intake.

Lactation Production of milk by the mammary glands.

Lacteal Lymph vessel.

Lactose Milk sugar.

Lacto-ovo vegetarian A vegan diet that includes milk, eggs, and other dairy products.

Laennec's cirrhosis Cirrhosis caused by chronic alcoholism.

Large-vessel disease The development of atherosclerosis in various arteries.

Lecithin A phospholipid found in the body.

Left subclavian vein Vein that receives the majority of lymph and chylomicrons.

Legume Seed of plants such as kidney beans, soybeans, garden peas, and lima beans.

Lethargic Sluggishness, slowness, and sleepiness that often result from drugs.

Liberal diet A diet that allows a variety of foods.

Lignin A noncarbohydrate substance that functions as a structured bonding agent in plants.

Linoleic A PUFA that is obtained from food and serves as a precursor of arachidonic and linolenic acids.

Linolenic A fatty acid that is derived from linoleic acid.

Lipid A biological substance that has an oily or greasy touch and is insoluble in water. Lipids are soluble in organic solvents such as ether and alcohol.

Lipoatrophy Loss of fat at an injection site, resulting in indentation.

Lipoprotein Lipid with a protein coat around it.

Lipostatic theory The theory that the tissues, especially the fat tissues, signal the brain when the level of fat is increased above or decreased below a certain level.

Lipotropic factor Compound that contributes to the formation of lipoproteins that transports fats out of the liver.

Liquefaction Conversion into a liquid form.

Long chain fatty acid Fatty acid that is 18 to 20 carbon atoms in length.

Low birth weight (LBW) baby A baby that weighs less than 5.5 lb (2500 g).

Low-residue diet A diet low in residue and fiber; it is also called a low-fiber diet.

Low-sodium diet A diet that allows no salt in cooking or at the table; all cured and canned meats are also eliminated.

Lumen Inner open space in a tube such as blood vessel or the intestine.

Luminal effect Change that occurs in the lumen of the small intestine.

Lymph Fluid in lymphatic vessels that originates in tissue spaces.

Lymphocytopenia A low level of lymphocytes that help provide immunity.

Macrocytic anemia A type of anemia in which red blood cells are larger than normal.

Major mineral Mineral that is present in the body in quantities greater than 5 g and is required at levels of 100 mg/day.

Maltose Malt sugar.

Mammary gland Specialized gland in the breast that secretes milk during pregnancy.

Marasmus A type of protein-calorie malnutrition that results from a deficiency of proteins and calories.

Massive (morbid) obesity Body weight that is more than 100% above the ideal weight.

Maturity-onset diabetes of youth (MODY) NIDDM that occurs in people under 40.

Mechanical soft diet Same as a soft diet.

Medium chain fatty acid Fatty acid that contains 14 to 16 carbon atoms.

Megaloblastic anemia Anemia characterized by large, immature, nucleated red blood cells called megaloblasts.

Menopause A permanent cessation of menstruation when ovaries, fallopian tubes, uterus, vagina, and breasts atrophy.

Metabolic acidosis An acidic state of the blood as a result of the accumulation of ketones.

Metabolic factor (internal) An internal factor that can lead to obesity.

Metabolism All chemical reactions that absorbed molecules undergo inside cells.

Metastasis The transfer of a cancerous tumor.

Microcytic An RBC that is smaller in size than normal.

Midarm muscle circumference (MAMC) A measurement of the circumference of the arm. Usually done approximately midway between the shoulder and elbow. Using the formula, it is a good indicator of lean body or muscle mass.

Milk anemia Anemia that results from feeding older infants only milk that is low in iron.

Milliosmole (mOsm) Equals 1/1,000th of an osmole.

Mineral Small, inorganic element that yields no energy.

Miscarriage (spontaneous abortion) Interrupted pregnancy before the seventh month.

Modified (therapeutic) A normal diet that has modifications of nutritional components.

Monoglyceride Glyceride that contains one fatty acid chain.

Monohydrous Containing one water molecule; an example is monohydrous dextrose, which contains one water molecule connected to a dextrose molecule.

Monosaccharide Simple sugar.

Monounsaturated fatty acid A fatty acid that contains one double bond.

Morning sickness Nausea and vomiting experienced by pregnant women.

Motility Spontaneous movement. The contractions of the gastrointestinal tract are an example.

Mucosal effect Change that occurs in the mucosal lining of the gastrointestinal tract or inactivation of enzyme systems.

Mucous membrane Membrane that lines the cavities that open to the outside of the body.

Myelin sheath A sheath, composed of fatty material, that surrounds and insulates some nerve fibers.

Myocardial infarction A condition in which a portion of the heart tissue becomes necrotic. Commonly referred to as a heart attack.

Myoglobin (heme iron) A protein molecule composed of four amino acid chains, with one iron atom in each that is found in muscle tissue.

Nasogastric Referring to a tube of soft rubber or plastic that is inserted through a nostril into the stomach. It is used to instill liquid foods or withdraw gastric contents.

Naturally occurring sugar Sugar found naturally in foods, such as glucose and fructose, as opposed to artificial sugar, such as sorbital and xylitol.

Necrosis Death of tissue.

Negative energy balance A situation in which energy expenditure is greater than energy input.

Negative nitrogen balance A state that occurs when more nitrogen is excreted than ingested.

Neoplasm Tumor.

Nephron The structural and functional unit of the kidney.

Nephrosis Kidney disease that is characterized by a large loss of proteins in the urine and edema.

Nephrotic syndrome A stage of kidney disease that is characterized by large losses of protein in the urine, severe edema, low serum protein levels, elevated levels of cholesterol and other serum lipids, and anemia.

Night blindness The inability to see well in dim light.

Nitrogen equilibrium Conditions in which the amount of nitrogen consumed is equal to the amount excreted.

Nitrogen-fixing bacteria Bacteria that can take in nitrogen from the air and soil and convert it into proteins.

Noncaloric Non-energy-yielding.

Nonessential amino acid Amino acid that can be synthesized by the adult body from carbohydrates, lipids, and other amino acids.

Nonessential fatty acid A fatty acid that is synthesized by the body if a person consumes adequate quantities of food containing carbon, hydrogen, and oxygen atoms.

Nontropical sprue An alternative term for adult celiac disease (malabsorption disorder).

Noninsulin-dependent diabetes mellitus (NIDDM) A type of diabetes mellitus that is not caused by an insulin deficiency but rather by the ineffectiveness of insulin in moving glucose into the cells.

Norepinephrine A neurotransmitter secreted by the sympathetic nerves and as a hormone secreted from the adrenal gland.

Normal diet A diet that consists of any and all foods and provides the RDAs and adequacy by means of the Food Pyramid.

Nutrition The combination of processes by which the body receives and utilizes the materials necessary to maintain homeostasis.

Nystagmus Rapid movement of the eyeballs.

Obesity Body weight that is 15–25% above ideal weight.

Objective A statement of a short-term specific step to be used to help achieve a goal.

Oliguria Diminished urine output.

Omenta A serous membrane attached to the visceral organs.

Opsin A protein pigment that combines with retinene in the rods to form rhodopsin.

Oral glucose tolerance test (OGTT) A blood glucose test in which a person fasts overnight and is then given a measured amount of glucose in an oral glucose drink.

Organic compound Substance that contains carbon atoms.

Orthomolecular approach An approach that consists of giving large doses of vitamins, especially niacin (vitamin B_3, nicotinic acid) and vitamin C (ascorbic acid) to schizophrenic patients.

Osmolality The number of osmoles per kilogram of solvent.

Osmole The standard unit of measure of osmotic pressure.

Osmosis The movement of water from a low-solute concentration to a high-solute concentration through a membrane permeable to water only.

Osmotic overload A condition that results in the movement of large amounts of water into the intestines from the blood.

Osmotic pressure Pressure on the cell membrane due to the inability of solutes to pass through it.

Osteomalacia The softening of the bones due to the loss of calcium or demineralization.

Osteoporosis A progressive demineralization of bones that results in the reduction of bone tissue.

Overfat Disproportionately high percentage of fat tissue.

Overt Open and observable.

Overweight Body weight that is more than 10% above ideal weight.

Oxalic acid An acid found in some foods such as cocoa, rhubarb, and spinach. It inhibits the absorption of calcium, iron, and magnesium.

Oxidized A chemical reaction in which an atom or molecule either loses hydrogen atoms and electrons or accepts oxygen.

Oxytocin A pituitary hormone that stimulates uterine contractions.

Palmar erythema Bright red palms.

Pancreatic amylase An enzyme secreted by the pancreas that breaks down dextrins into maltose.

Pancreatic enzyme deficiency A deficiency in the amount of enzymes secreted by the pancreas. This deficiency is especially a problem with pancreatic lipase, which breaks down triglycerides.

Pancreatitis Inflammation of the pancreas.

Paralytic ileus Absence of peristalsis.

Parenteral feeding Feeding that bypasses the intestine and is infused directly into the veins.

Parenteral nutrition The movement of nutrients that bypass the intestine and are infused directly into the veins.

Partial gastrectomy An operation in which a portion of the stomach is removed. The remaining section is joined to the duodenum.

Pectin A water-soluble, nonstructural polysaccharide.

Pellagra A condition that is caused by a niacin deficiency.

Pelvic girdle A ring of bones in the pelvic region composed of two hip bones joined to the sacrum.

Pepsin A gastric enzyme that breaks down proteins into short chain polypeptides, proteoses, and peptides.

Peptic ulcer A deterioration or lesion in the mucosal lining of the stomach or duodenum.

Peptidase enzyme An enzyme that catalyzes the degradation of a harmful peptide.

Peptide bond Chemical bond that connects amino acids.

Peptone Intermediate-sized protein segment.

Perforation An opening through the gastric or duodenal wall.

Peripheral edema Excess accumulation of interstitial fluids within the extremities.

Peripheral neuritis Degenerative changes in the peripheral nerves.

Peripheral resistance Resistance to the passage of blood through small blood vessels, especially the arterioles.

Peripheral vein A vein near the skin surface in the arm and forearm.

Peristalsis Wavelike, muscular contractions that propel food and wastes through the gastrointestinal tract.

Peristaltic contraction Rhythmic wave of smooth muscle contraction.

Peritoneal dialysis Infusion of dialysate fluid through a tube into the abdominal cavity. Nitrogenous wastes, excess fluids, and electrolytes are exchanged from the blood through the peritoneum into the dialysate fluid. The fluid is then drained out.

Peritoneum membrane A membrane that covers most of the abdominal pelvic organs and through which exchange of nutrients and wastes occurs in peritoneal dialysis.

Permeability A state of being permeable, or allowing the passage of materials.

Pernicious anemia Anemia that results from a deficiency of vitamin B_{12} because of a lack of the intrinsic factor.

Phagocytic cell Cell that carries on phagocytosis, such as some white blood cells.

Pharmacologic dose Dose of a nutrient that exceeds the normal requirements to the point where drug-like effects are observed.

Pharmacologic effect A drug-like effect.

Phenothiazine tranquilizer Tranquilizers used in the treatment of severe mental illnesses.

Phenylalanine An essential amino acid.

Phenylalanine hydroxylase An enzyme that synthesizes tyrosine from phenylalanine.

Phenylketonuria (PKU) A disorder in an infant caused by the absence of the enzyme phenylalanine hydroxylase, which oxidizes phenylalanine to tyrosine.

Phlebitis Inflammation of a vein.

Phospholipid A lipid subclass. Each phospholipid is composed of two fatty acid molecules connected to a glycerol molecule.

Photophobia Sensitivity of the eyes to light and strain.

Physical activity The amount of energy expended by the body to contract the skeletal muscles in voluntary activities.

Physiological solution Solution in which the osmotic pressure exerted by the solutions is equal to that of body fluids.

Phytic acid A binder compound that forms an insoluble calcium complex.

Pimple Small, elevated area of pus containing lesions of the skin. It is often called a blackhead.

Placenta A structure present within the uterus of a pregnant woman that is connected to the developing fetus and exchanges wastes and nutrients.

Placental lactogen A hormone secreted by the placenta that enhances lactation and inhibits insulin activity in the mother.

Plaque Mound of lipid material, smooth muscle cells, and calcium.

Plateau Period during weight reduction in which the person is not losing weight.

Pleurisy Inflammation of the pleura membrane that lines and covers the lungs in the thoracic cavity.

Pneumonia An acute infection of the lung tissue.

Pneumothorax Air or gas in the chest.

Polychlorinated biphenyl (PCB) Chemical used in the manufacture of plastics. It is not biodegradable and has been found in breast milk.

Polycythemia A condition characterized by an excessive number of red blood cells.

Polydipsia Increased thirst.

Polyphagia Increased hunger.

Polysaccharide Complex sugar.

Polyunsaturated fatty acid A fatty acid that contains two or more double bonds.

Polyuria Increased urination.

Porosity The state of being porous.

Portal hypertension Abnormally increased pressure in the portal circulation.

Portal vein Vein that brings blood rich in nutrients into the liver. Blood from the intestines, stomach, and spleen drain into the portal vein.

Positive energy balance A situation in which energy input is greater than energy expenditure.

Positive nitrogen balance A state that occurs when more nitrogen is ingested than excreted.

Potassium-40 A radioactive isotope that is naturally present in the body, but in low quantities in fat tissue.

Preeclampsia Sudden high blood pressure or an increase of 20–30 mmHg in systolic pressure and 10–15 mmHg in diastolic pressure.

Pregnancy-induced hypertension (PIH) Formerly called toxemia of pregnancy and characterized by proteinuria, hypertension, and edema.

Premature (preterm) baby Birth of a baby prior to the 38th week of pregnancy.

Preschooler Child from 3 to 6 years of age.

Presenile dementia   Mental disorder occurring in people under the age of 65.

Primary aldosteronism   An excessive secretion of the hormone aldosterone from the adrenal gland. It is characterized by hypertension, hypokalemia, muscular weakness, and polydipsia.

Primary level   Health care that is aimed at averting the occurrence of disease and protecting the health of the general public.

Primary malnutrition   Malnutrition that results from diet alone. Alcoholics often suffer from primary malnutrition as a result of an inadequate diet.

Problem-oriented medical record (POMR)   A communication tool that focuses on a patient's health problems and the structuring of cooperative health care plans to cope with the identified problems.

Progesterone   A female hormone that is important in the menstrual cycle and in pregnancy.

Protein   The most fundamental constituent of living matter. Proteins are essential for the growth and repair of animal tissue.

Protein efficiency ratio (PER)   Measures the growth of rats in relation to the amounts of protein eaten.

Proteinuria   The loss of protein in the urine.

Protein-calorie malnutrition (PCM)   Malnutrition that is caused by deficits of calories, proteins, or both.

Protein-sparing solution   A solution that supplies the needed kilocalories so that proteins can be spared as a source of kilocalories.

Proteoses   Intermediate-sized protein segment.

Prothrombin   A blood protein that contributes to blood clotting.

Proximal tubule   The portion of the renal tubule attached to Bowman's capsule. Most reabsorption of nutrients occurs here.

Pruritis vulvae   Itching of the external genitalia of the female.

Psychotherapeutic   Drug used in the treatment of manic-depressive illness.

Psychotherapy   Any of a number of related techniques for treating mental illness by psychological methods. It is often used in the second stage of treating anorexia nervosa.

PUFA   Polyunsaturated fatty acids.

Pulmonary therapy   Treatment of lung diseases.

Pyloric obstruction   A condition in which the pyloric sphincter becomes scarred and stenosed (the opening is narrowed).

Pyloric sphincter valve   A circular muscle that controls the movement of food from the pyloric region of the stomach into the duodenum.

Pyrosis   Heartburn.

Pyruvic acid   An end product of anaerobic respiration.

Quinone   Chemical compound that includes vitamin K.

Quinidine intoxication   A poisoned state due to a buildup of the drug quinidine.

Reactant   A substance that interacts with other substances to produce products.

Reagent   A substance that is used to produce a chemical reaction.

Rebound scurvy   A condition that occurs when a pregnant woman takes megadoses of vitamin C, causing the fetus to adapt to the massive doses. After birth, without continued ingestion of vitamin C, the infant shows signs of scurvy.

Recombinant DNA   DNA in bacteria that has genes spliced into the normal molecule. Frequently, human genes that produce insulin are spliced, thereby forming recombinant DNA insulin; it is also called artificial human insulin.

Recommended Dietary Allowances (RDAs)   Recommended allowances of certain nutrients that are established by the Food and Nutrition Board of the National Academy of Sciences–National Research Council (NAS–NRC).

Reflectance photometer   A special device that measures the intensity of light reflected through urine and thereby the amount of glucose that is present.

Reflux   Regurgitation.

Regulatory factor (external)   An external factor that can lead to obesity.

Regurgitation   Backup of stomach contents through the esophagus.

Renal failure   A condition in which kidney damage is severe enough that the kidneys no longer excrete the nitrogenous wastes or maintain the electrolytes in the blood.

Renal osteodystrophy   A complication of end-stage

renal disease that is characterized by the loss of calcium from the bones and bone mass.

Renin   A hormone that causes the formation of the compound angiotensin.

Repletion   Restoration of body composition.

Respiratory failure   A condition that develops when the blood pH becomes too acidic, the pCO_2 increases, and the PO_2 decreases.

Respiratory insufficiency   A condition that results when the exchange of oxygen and carbon dioxide is insufficient for the body's needs during normal activities.

Retina   The innermost layer of the eye that contains the visual receptors, rods, and cones.

Retinene   A pigment that is derived from vitamin A and results from the breakdown of rhodopsin.

Retinol   A form of vitamin A that is found in food.

Rheumatoid disease   A disease that results in inflammation and degeneration of the connective tissues around joints.

Rhodopsin   The compound secreted by the rods in the retina.

Rickets   A condition caused by a deficiency of vitamin D that leads to decreased absorption of calcium by the bones.

Rod   Receptor cell in the retina of the eye that is sensitive to dim light.

R-group   The rest of the amino acid that is attached to the amine and acid portions of the molecule.

Saccharide   Sugar unit.

Salicylate-like   Analgesic or pain-relieving compounds.

Salivary amylase   An enzyme secreted in the mouth that splits starch into smaller fragments.

Satiety   A sensation of fullness that follows a meal.

Saturated fatty acid   A fatty acid whose carbon atoms are linked by single bonds, and are bonded to as many hydrogen atoms as possible.

Schizophrenia   A mental illness characterized by withdrawal from reality and disturbances in thought and behavior.

School-age child   Child from 6 to 12 years of age.

Sclerosis   Hardening of a vein.

Scurvy   A disease that is characterized by weakness, skin degeneration, ulcerated gums, loss of teeth, and hemorrhages in the skin.

Sebaceous gland   Gland in the skin that secretes the oily substance sebum.

Sebum   An oily secretion of the sebaceous glands. It lubricates and waterproofs the skin and hair.

Secondary lactase deficiency   A condition that may develop as a secondary problem in a person who has a disease of the small intestine such as celiac disease, Crohn's disease, or protein-calorie malnutrition.

Secondary level   Health care that is utilized for early diagnosis of disease and prevention of further complications.

Secondary malnutrition   Malnutrition that results from impaired use of nutrients. It is often seen in alcoholics and results from the toxic effects of alcohol on the liver and the gastrointestinal tract.

Senile dementia   Dementia that occurs in people over the age of 65.

Sepsis   Presence of pathogenic bacteria in the blood.

Septic abortion   An abortion in which a uterine infection is spread to the general circulation.

Serosa   The outer layer of the intestine.

Serous   A fluid that lubricates body walls and organs that are coated with the fluid.

Serum albumin   A protein in the blood that is important for the regulation of osmotic pressure.

Serum transferrin test   A test that measures the amount of globulin protein that transports iron; a sensitive indicator of PCM.

Set point theory   The theory that the body is programmed to maintain a certain amount of fat.

Severe obesity   Body weight that is 30–100% above the ideal weight.

Serum glutamic oxaloacetic transaminase (SGOT)   An enzyme found especially in the heart and liver. An elevated level in the blood is indicative of liver damage.

Serum glutamic pyruvic transaminase (SGPT)   An enzyme found in several tissues including the liver. An elevated level in the blood is indicative of liver disease.

Short bowel   Surgical shortening of the length of the small intestine. Normally done as a therapeutic procedure to aid person in losing weight.

Short chain fatty acid   Fatty acid that contains 8 to 12 carbon atoms.

Sickle cell disease A disease characterized by abnormal hemoglobin that results in sickle-shaped red blood cells.

Sigmoid colon The S-shaped portion of the large intestine between the descending colon and the rectum.

Small burns Burns that cover less than 20% of the body surface area.

Small-vessel disease (microangiopathies) A thickening of small vessels such as arterioles, venules, and capillaries.

SOAP: Subjective, objective, assessment, and planning. This is a format in which progress notes are written.

Sodium-potassium pump Protein carriers in cell membranes that transport sodium and potassium ions back to their original positions.

Soft diet A diet modified in consistency that includes high-protein liquid foods and solid foods low in fiber.

Solute A substance that dissolves in a solvent.

Solvent A fluid that causes a solute to dissolve and form a solution.

Specific dynamic effect The expenditure of energy when food is consumed.

Specific heat The amount of heat required to raise the temperature of 1 g of liquid 1°C (Celsius).

Spermatogenesis The production of sperm cells in the testes.

Spider angioma Spider-shaped blood vessels.

Spleen A large glandular organ composed of lymphatic tissue.

Sputum Mucous secretion from the lungs, bronchi, and trachea.

Steatorrhea Abnormally large amounts of fats in the feces.

Steroid hormone Hormone secreted by the adrenal cortex and other endocrine glands that has a typical steroid shape.

Sterol A subclass of lipids. Molecule is composed of four fused rings (cholesterol is an example of a sterol).

Stillborn infant A baby dead at birth.

Stimuli Changes in an environmental condition that cause a response.

Stroke A rupture or blockage of a blood vessel in the brain, resulting in loss of consciousness, paralysis, or other symptoms; it is also called a cerebrovascular accident.

Subclavian vein A vein in the shoulder region that is often used for insertion of a TPN catheter.

Subcutaneous Under the skin.

Subjective Conditions or changes perceived by the patient rather than by a health examiner.

Sucrose Table sugar.

Superior vena cava A vein that carries blood from the upper part of the body into the heart. A TPN catheter is guided into this vein from the subclavian vein.

Superior vena cava thrombosis A blood clot in the superior vena cava.

Synapse The junction between two neurons where an impulse is transmitted.

Synergistic The combined effect is greater than the sum of the parts.

Synovial A fluid that lubricates bones articulating in joints.

Systemic flushing Redness throughout the body as a whole.

Systolic Pressure created by the contraction of the heart ventricles as blood is pumped into the arteries.

Tachycardia Rapid and irregular heartbeat.

Tardive dyskinesia A condition that occurs in patients with mental disorders as a side effect of long-term treatment with antipsychotic drugs.

Target organ Organ that is stimulated by hormones.

Tertiary level Health care that is designed to educate a patient for the maximum use of his or her remaining capacities.

Testicular degeneration Degeneration of the testes.

Testosterone The male sex hormone secreted by the testes. It stimulates the development of male secondary sex characteristics.

Tetany Continuous, forceful muscle contraction.

Tetracycline An antibiotic that is effective against

microorganisms such as gram-positive and gram-negative bacteria.

Therapeutic nutrition Nutritional care that is used to help a person cope with an illness.

Thoracic cavity Chest cavity.

Threshold level The amount of nutrients that will be reabsorbed into the blood of the nephrons. When this level is reached, no more reabsorption of the nutrients will occur.

Thrombosis Blood clot formation.

Thyroid gland An endocrine gland located below the larynx and in front of the trachea. Secretes thyroxine and triiodothyronine hormones.

Thyroxine (T_4) A thyroid hormone that regulates the body's metabolism. Each thyroxin molecule contains four iodine atoms; therefore, it is designated as T_4.

Toddler Child from 1 to 3 years of age.

Tooth mottling Brown discoloration of the teeth.

Total colectomy Removal of the colon.

Total iron-binding capacity A measurement of the percentage of saturation of transferrin. It evaluates the amount of extra iron that can be carried.

Total parenteral nutrition (TPN) Infusion of solutions composed of dextrose for energy, amino acids for tissue synthesis, fats for energy, and essential fatty acids plus vitamins and minerals.

Toxicity The quality of being poisonous; a condition that can result from consumption of excess amounts of some vitamins.

Trace mineral Mineral that is present in the body in quantities of less than 5 g.

Transferrin (nonheme iron) A combination of iron and a globulin protein; important as the transport form of iron.

Transverse colon The portion of the large intestine that extends across the abdomen from the right to the left.

Triceps A muscle located on the back of the upper arm.

Triceps skinfold thickness Measurement of skin thickness over the triceps brachii muscle; a good indicator of overall fatness.

Tricyclic antidepressant Drug used in the treatment of depression. The drug is thought to work by increasing the amount of norepineprhine and serotonin.

Triglyceride A lipid compound composed of three fatty acids attached to a glycerol molecule.

Triiodothyronine (T_3) A thyroid hormone that regulates the body's metabolism. Each triiodothyronine molecule contains three iodine atoms; therefore, it is designated as T_3.

Trimester A period of 3 months.

Tripeptide Molecule composed of three amino acid molecules.

Tryptophan An amino acid.

Tubercle A small, rounded nodule produced by the bacterium *Mycobacterium tuberculosis*.

Tuberculosis A bacterial infectious disease caused by the bacterium *Mycobacterium tuberculosis*.

24-hour recall A recounting of the kinds and amounts of food consumed during the 24 hours preceding the interview.

Tyrosine A nonessential amino acid.

U100 insulin 100 units per milliter of insulin.

Ulcerative colitis A disease of the large intestine that is characterized by inflammation of the intestinal mucosa and ulcers.

Underweight Body weight that is more than 10% below the ideal weight.

Unproductive No expulsion of sputum.

Unsaturated fatty acid A fatty acid whose carbon atoms are linked by double or triple bonds, and therefore are not bonded to as many hydrogen atoms as possible.

Urea A nitrogen waste product that results from the metabolism or deamination of amino acids and is excreted in the urine.

Uremic syndrome A complex of symptoms that result from an extremely high level of nitrogenous wastes in the blood.

U.S. RDAs Nutrient recommendations established by the U.S. Food and Drug Administration (FDA) that are used as a standard for nutritional labeling.

Usual body weight (UBW) The normal or usual weight of a person.

Usual intake pattern A recounting of the foods that a person first eats or drinks during the day.

Vagus nerve The tenth cranial nerve. It stimulates gastric glands in the stomach to secrete hydrochloric acid and pepsin enzyme.

Vasodilation Increased diameter or size of blood vessels.

Vegan Pure vegetarian diet that uses no animal or dairy products.

Ventilation The ability to move air into and out of the lungs.

Ventricular arrhythmia Abnormal rhythm in the contraction of the ventricles in the heart.

Viscosity The tendency for a fluid to resist flowing.

Vitamin Organic substance that is essential for normal metabolism, growth, and development of the body. It does not generate energy.

Water soluble Refers to substances that dissolve in water. Fats become water soluble when a protein coat is secreted around them.

Wernicke-Korsakoff disease A mental disorder caused by a thiamin deficiency.

Wernicke's syndrome A condition that results from a thiamin deficiency.

Xerophthalmia A condition in which the cornea becomes thickened and opaque.

INDEX

ANSWERS TO REVIEW QUESTIONS

Chapter 1

1. B	6. A	11. B
2. A	7. A	12. A
3. B	8. D	13. B
4. B	9. B	14. D
5. B	10. D	15. B

Review Questions for NCLEX

1. A
2. A
3. A
4. C
5. A

Chapter 2

1. B	11. B	20. A
2. A	12. A	21. C
3. B	13. B	22. B
4. B	14. B	23. C
5. A	15. B	24. A
6. A	16. A	25. D
7. B	17. A	26. B
8. B	18. D	27. A
9. B	19. E	28. B
10. A		

Review Questions for NCLEX

1. D
2. A
3. C
4. A

Chapter 3

1. B	13. B	25. A
2. B	14. B	26. A
3. A	15. A	27. C
4. A	16. B	28. E
5. A	17. B	29. D
6. B	18. B	30. C
7. B	19. A	31. C
8. B	20. A	32. B
9. A	21. A	33. A
10. B	22. B	34. B
11. A	23. B	35. C
12. A	24. B	36. C

Review Questions for NCLEX

1. B	4. A	7. B
2. A	5. C	8. D
3. C	6. B	9. A

Chapter 4

1. A	11. A	21. B
2. A	12. A	22. E
3. B	13. B	23. B
4. B	14. B	24. D
5. B	15. A	25. A
6. B	16. A	26. C
7. A	17. D	27. B
8. A	18. C	28. A
9. A	19. B	29. B
10. B	20. E	

Review Questions for NCLEX

1. B	5. D
2. A	6. C
3. D	7. A
4. A	

Chapter 5

1. B	16. B	31. C
2. A	17. B	32. D
3. B	18. A	33. A
4. A	19. A	34. A
5. B	20. A	35. B
6. B	21. B	36. B
7. B	22. C	37. A
8. B	23. E	38. B
9. A	24. B	39. B
10. A	25. B	40. A
11. A	26. D	41. B
12. B	27. A	42. C
13. A	28. B	43. A
14. B	29. E	44. A
15. A	30. A	45. A

Review Questions for NCLEX

1. D	5. C
2. A	6. B
3. D	7. C
4. D	

Chapter 6

1. B	10. B	19. B
2. B	11. A	20. A
3. A	12. A	21. A
4. B	13. B	22. A
5. A	14. B	23. B
6. B	15. B	24. A
7. A	16. A	25. B
8. B	17. A	26. B
9. B	18. B	27. C

28. E	35. E	41. A
29. C	36. A	42. D
30. A	37. B	43. B
31. E	38. B	44. E
32. E	39. D	45. C
33. E	40. C	46. A
34. B		

Review Questions for NCLEX

1. C	4. A
2. A	5. A
3. D	6. C

Chapter 7

1. A	22. C	43. A
2. A	23. D	44. B
3. A	24. B	45. A
4. B	25. B	46. B
5. A	26. B	47. B
6. B	27. D	48. A
7. B	28. C	49. B
8. B	29. B	50. E
9. A	30. A	51. B
10. A	31. C	52. B
11. A	32. C	53. D
12. B	33. C	54. C
13. A	34. C	55. A
14. B	35. A	56. C
15. B	36. B	57. E
16. B	37. B	58. B
17. A	38. B	59. D
18. A	39. A	60. C
19. B	40. A	61. E
20. A	41. B	62. B
21. A	42. B	63. A

Review Questions for NCLEX

1. D	5. D
2. B	6. D
3. B	7. A
4. D	

Chapter 8

1. B	9. B	17. E
2. B	10. A	18. E
3. A	11. B	19. B
4. A	12. A	20. A
5. B	13. E	21. C
6. A	14. C	22. B
7. A	15. E	23. C
8. A	16. B	24. B

Review Questions for NCLEX

1. B
2. C
3. D
4. C

Chapter 9

1. A	13. B	24. E
2. B	14. A	25. D
3. A	15. A	26. B
4. A	16. B	27. C
5. B	17. A	28. D
6. B	18. B	29. E
7. B	19. B	30. D
8. B	20. B	31. E
9. A	21. A	32. C
10. A	22. A	33. A
11. B	23. A	34. B
12. B		

Review Questions for NCLEX

1. C
2. A
3. D
4. D
5. D

Chapter 10

1. B	3. A	5. B
2. A	4. B	6. B

7. A	13. A	18. A
8. A	14. B	19. A
9. A	15. A	20. D
10. B	16. C	21. C
11. A	17. D	22. B
12. A		

Review Questions for NCLEX

1. B	4. C
2. D	5. A
3. A	6. A

Chapter 11

1. A	10. B	18. B
2. A	11. B	19. B
3. B	12. B	20. A
4. A	13. B	21. B
5. B	14. A	22. E
6. B	15. A	23. E
7. B	16. B	24. B
8. A	17. A	25. C
9. A		

Review Questions for NCLEX

1. C	4. B
2. B	5. B
3. A	6. A

Chapter 12

1. A	5. B	9. B
2. B	6. A	10. C
3. B	7. C	11. A
4. A	8. A	

Review Questions for NCLEX

1. B
2. A
3. C
4. A
5. B

Chapter 13

1. A	12. B	22. A
2. B	13. B	23. D
3. B	14. A	24. E
4. A	15. A	25. E
5. A	16. B	26. E
6. B	17. A	27. E
7. B	18. B	28. C
8. B	19. C	29. D
9. A	20. A	30. A
10. A	21. B	31. B
11. B		

Review Questions for NCLEX

1. C
2. A
3. B
4. C

Chapter 14

1. A	10. A	18. E
2. B	11. A	19. A
3. A	12. B	20. B
4. B	13. B	21. D
5. B	14. B	22. D
6. A	15. A	23. B
7. B	16. C	24. A
8. B	17. E	25. E
9. B		

Review Questions for NCLEX

1. D	5. D
2. A	6. C
3. B	7. A
4. D	

Chapter 15

1. B	16. B	31. A
2. B	17. A	32. B
3. B	18. A	33. A
4. A	19. B	34. A
5. A	20. B	35. C
6. B	21. A	36. D
7. A	22. A	37. C
8. A	23. B	38. B
9. B	24. A	39. A
10. A	25. B	40. B
11. B	26. B	41. B
12. A	27. A	42. A
13. A	28. A	43. B
14. A	29. A	44. C
15. B	30. B	45. A

Review Questions for NCLEX

1. D	6. D
2. B	7. A
3. B	8. D
4. A	9. D
5. B	

Chapter 16

1. A	15. B	28. E
2. A	16. B	29. E
3. B	17. B	30. D
4. B	18. A	31. B
5. B	19. B	32. C
6. A	20. A	33. A
7. B	21. A	34. C
8. A	22. B	35. B
9. A	23. B	36. D
10. B	24. A	37. C
11. B	25. A	38. C
12. A	26. A	39. C
13. A	27. B	40. E
14. A		

Review Questions for NCLEX

1. A
2. D
3. B
4. A
5. C

Chapter 17

1. A	12. A	22. B
2. B	13. B	23. C
3. A	14. B	24. A
4. B	15. A	25. B
5. A	16. A	26. A
6. B	17. B	27. B
7. B	18. B	28. E
8. A	19. B	29. C
9. A	20. A	30. B
10. B	21. A	31. B
11. A		

Review Questions for NCLEX

1. D
2. B
3. C
4. D

Chapter 18

1. B	13. B	24. E
2. A	14. B	25. C
3. A	15. A	26. E
4. B	16. A	27. A
5. A	17. B	28. C
6. A	18. A	29. B
7. B	19. A	30. B
8. B	20. B	31. A
9. A	21. B	32. C
10. A	22. A	33. B
11. B	23. A	34. B
12. B		

Review Questions for NCLEX

1. A
2. C
3. D
4. A
5. D

Chapter 19

1. B	9. B	16. C
2. B	10. B	17. C
3. A	11. A	18. E
4. A	12. B	19. A
5. B	13. A	20. D
6. B	14. B	21. B
7. A	15. A	22. D
8. B		

Review Questions for NCLEX

1. D
2. C
3. A
4. D
5. D

Chapter 20

1. B	10. A	18. B
2. A	11. B	19. A
3. A	12. A	20. D
4. A	13. B	21. E
5. B	14. A	22. D
6. B	15. A	23. A
7. A	16. B	24. B
8. A	17. B	25. C
9. A		

Review Questions for NCLEX

1. B
2. D
3. A
4. D
5. C

Chapter 21

1. B	5. B
2. A	6. A
3. B	7. A
4. B	8. A

Review Questions for NCLEX

1. D
2. C
3. C
4. A
5. B

Chapter 22

1. A	6. B	11. B
2. A	7. B	12. B
3. B	8. A	13. A
4. A	9. A	14. B
5. B	10. B	15. A

Review Questions for NCLEX

1. A
2. C
3. C
4. B
5. C